Designed for the maintenance of good nutrition of practically

all healthy people in the United States

Water-Soluble Vitamins							Minerals							
Vita-min C (mg)	Thia-min (mg)	Ribo-flavin (mg)	Niacin (mg NE)[f]	Vita-min B$_6$ (mg)	Fo-late (µg)	Vita-min B$_{12}$ (µg)	Cal-cium (mg)	Phos-phorus (mg)	Mag-nesium (mg)	Iron (mg)	Zinc (mg)	Iodine (µg)	Sele-nium (µg)
30	0.3	0.4	5	0.3	25	0.3	400	300	40	6	5	40	10
35	0.4	0.5	6	0.6	35	0.5	600	500	60	10	5	50	15
40	0.7	0.8	9	1.0	50	0.7	800	800	80	10	10	70	20
45	0.9	1.1	12	1.1	75	1.0	800	800	120	10	10	90	20
45	1.0	1.2	13	1.4	100	1.4	800	800	170	10	10	120	30
50	1.3	1.5	17	1.7	150	2.0	1,200	1,200	270	12	15	150	40
60	1.5	1.8	20	2.0	200	2.0	1,200	1,200	400	12	15	150	50
60	1.5	1.7	19	2.0	200	2.0	1,200	1,200	350	10	15	150	70
60	1.5	1.7	19	2.0	200	2.0	800	800	350	10	15	150	70
60	1.2	1.4	15	2.0	200	2.0	800	800	350	10	15	150	70
50	1.1	1.3	15	1.4	150	2.0	1,200	1,200	280	15	12	150	45
60	1.1	1.3	15	1.5	180	2.0	1,200	1,200	300	15	12	150	50
60	1.1	1.3	15	1.6	180	2.0	1,200	1,200	280	15	12	150	55
60	1.1	1.3	15	1.6	180	2.0	800	800	280	15	12	150	55
60	1.0	1.2	13	1.6	180	2.0	800	800	280	10	12	150	55
70	1.5	1.6	17	2.2	400	2.2	1,200	1,200	320	30	15	175	65
95	1.6	1.8	20	2.1	280	2.6	1,200	1,200	355	15	19	200	75
90	1.6	1.7	20	2.1	260	2.6	1,200	1,200	340	15	16	200	75

[c] Retinol equivalents. 1 retinol equivalent = 1 µg retinol or 6 µg ß-carotene.

[d] As cholecalciferol. 10 µg cholecalciferol = 400 IU of vitamin D.

[e] α-Tocopherol equivalents. 1 mg d-α tocopherol = 1 α-TE.

[f] 1 NE (niacin equivalent) is equal to 1 mg of niacin or 60 mg of dietary tryptophan.

Estimated Safe and Adequate Daily Dietary Intakes of Selected Vitamins and Minerals[a]

		Vitamins	
Category	Age (years)	Biotin (µg)	Pantothenic Acid (mg)
Infants	0–0.5	10	2
	0.5–1	15	3
Children and adolescents	1–3	20	3
	4–6	25	3–1
	7–10	30	4–5
	11 +	30–100	4–7
Adults		30–100	4–7

		Trace Elements[b]				
Category	Age (years)	Copper (mg)	Man-ganese (mg)	Fluoride (mg)	Chromium (µg)	Molybdenum (µg)
Infants	0–0.5	0.4–0.6	0.3–0.6	0.1–0.5	10–40	15–30
	0.5–1	0.6–0.7	0.6–1.0	0.2–1.0	20–60	20–40
Children and adolescents	1–3	0.7–1.0	1.0–1.5	0.5–1.5	20–80	25–50
	4–6	1.0–1.5	1.5–2.0	1.0–2.5	30–120	30–75
	7–10	1.0–2.0	2.0–3.0	1.5–2.5	50–200	50–150
	11 +	1.5–2.5	2.0–5.0	1.5–2.5	50–200	75–250
Adults		1.5–3.0	2.0–5.0	1.5–4.0	50–200	75–250

[a] Because there is less information on which to base allowances, these figures are not given in the main table of RDA and are provided here in the form of ranges of recommended intakes.

[b] Since the toxic levels for many trace elements may be only several times usual intakes, the upper levels for the trace elements given in this table should not be habitually exceeded.

Times Mirror/Mosby
Series In Nutrition

Guthrie
Introductory Nutrition
7th edition

Owen/Frankle
Nutrition in the Community
2nd edition

Pipes
Nutrition in Infancy and Childhood
4th edition

Schlenker
Nutrition in Aging
1st edition

Wardlaw/Insel
Perspectives in Nutrition
1st edition

Williams
**Essentials of Nutrition
and Diet Therapy**
5th edition

Williams
**Mowry's Basic Nutrition
and Diet Therapy**
8th edition

Williams
Nutrition and Diet Therapy
6th edition

Williams
**Self-Study Guide for Essentials of Nutrition
and Diet Therapy**
5th edition

Williams/Worthington-Roberts, et al.
Nutrition Throughout the Life Cycle
1st edition

Worthington-Roberts/Williams, et al.
Nutrition in Pregnancy and Lactation
4th edition

Essentials of Nutrition and Diet Therapy

Sue Rodwell Williams, Ph.D., M.P.H., R.D.

President, SRW Productions, Inc. and
Director, The Berkeley Nutrition Group, Berkeley, California;
Metabolic Nutritionist, Kaiser-Permanente Northern California
Regional Newborn Screening and Metabolic Program,
Kaiser-Permanente Medical Center, Oakland;
Field Faculty, M.P.H.-Dietetic Internship Program and
Coordinated Undergraduate Program in Dietetics,
University of California, Berkeley, California

Fifth edition

with 80 illustrations

Times Mirror/Mosby College Publishing

ST. LOUIS • TORONTO • BOSTON • LOS ALTOS   1990

Editor: Pat Coryell
Editorial Assistant: Loren M. Stevenson
Project Manager: Peggy Fagen
Manuscript Editor: Barbara Terrell
Design: Liz Fett
Production: Kathy Teal

Photo credits: p. 2 NASA; pp. 29, 192, 252, 275, 302, and 340 H. Armstrong Roberts; pp. 51, 69, 100, 116, 396, 416, 503, and 531 Dan Sindelar; pp. 87, 151, 225, 319, 434, 473, and 562 G. Robert Bishop; p. 364 Stephen Marks/Stockphotos; p. 588 Mallinckrodt Institute of Radiology; and p. 610 R. Tully/Medichrome.

Cover photograph and part opener illustrations of nicotine acid amide (niacin) by Roland Birke, copyright © Peter Arnold, Inc.

Fifth edition

Library of Congress Cataloging-in-Publication Data

Williams, Sue Rodwell.
    Essentials of nutrition and diet therapy / Sue Rodwell Williams.—
5th ed.
        p.   cm.
    An abridgement of: Nutrition and diet therapy. 6th ed.
    Includes bibliographical references.
    ISBN 0-8016-5260-X
    1. Diet therapy.   2. Nutrition.   I. Williams, Sue Rodwell.
Nutrition and diet therapy.   II. Title
    [DNLM: 1. Diet Therapy.   2. Nutrition.   QU 145 W727e]
RM216.W683   1990
613.2—dc20
DNLM/DLC
for Library of Congress   89-13512
                                                              CIP
C/VH/VH 9 8 7 6 5 4 3

To **My Students**
whose "whys" and "hows" and "so whats"
keep my feet to the fire of knowledge
and make the learning process exciting
and ever new to me

Preface

Through four previous editions, this compact "little" book has served the needs of students and teachers in the health sciences in many community colleges, as well as providing a sound but simple reference for busy practitioners. In truth, in all its editions, as its title indicates, it has captured and distilled the essence of my larger, more comprehensive college and university textbook, *Nutrition and Diet Therapy*, to lay a faithful foundation for further study and practice.

In this new fifth edition I have adhered to these same fundamental goals. But as in the previous, completely reformatted edition, here I have rewritten much of the material to reflect advancing knowledge as well as to continue the revised format. Thus its expanded current material and its organization continue to meet the more comprehensive needs of beginning students in the allied health professions today. All the while, it retains its sound, simple, substantive content, thoroughly updated and realistically applied to meet human health needs in our rapidly changing modern world.

Major Changes in This Edition

As indicated, this book is in essence an abridgement of my larger text. It follows a similar format and style to facilitate learning and lay a beginning foundation for sound clinical practice. To achieve these goals in this current edition, I have made a number of changes:

New Chapters

Several new chapters apply the expanding science of nutrition to changing health care needs and provide in our developing technology tools for its clinical practice and management. These new chapters include Chapter 16, "Nutrition and Stress Management," and Chapter 25, "Nutritional Support in Disabling Disease."

New Illustrations

A number of new illustrations enhance the overall design and provide learning support. These added graphs, charts, and photographs portray concepts introduced and help students grasp the clinical problems encountered in patient care.

Enhanced Readability and Student Interest

A large amount of the text has been rewritten to incorporate new material in a writing style designed to capture student interest and present comprehensive subject matter in a sound and simple manner. Many issues of student interest and public-professional controversy are discussed. The many examples used open up meaning and understanding. Topics of current relevance clarify questions and concerns.

Additional Changes New to This Edition

In addition to these major changes, I have made substantive changes in the development and organization of material in this new edition:

Chapter 1 has been rewritten to include an immediate introduction of all types of current nutritional guides used in the United States for health promotion: (1) Nutrient standards: the U.S. Recommended Dietary Allowances (RDA); (2) Food guides: the Basic Four Food Groups and the Exchange Lists Food Guide; and (3) Health promotion guidelines: the general guide, *Nutrition and Your Health: Dietary Guidelines for Americans;* and the specific health guides, *The Prudent Diet* of the American Heart Association, and the report *Diet, Nutrition, and Cancer* of the National Cancer Institute and the American Cancer Society. Here in one place the student or practitioner will have ready access to these frequently used guides, with a description of the development and use of each one. These guides expand the continuing focus in this introductory chapter on changing health care needs in our rapidly changing world. They illustrate especially the vital role of nutrition in our major U.S. health problems in relation to those of the world, and focus on our increasing concern with a preventive team approach to health promotion, both in our health care system and in our public food marketplace.

Part I, "Introduction to Human Nutrition," adds updated and new material based on current research in the nutritional sciences and its application in community and clinical practice. For example, there is new content on the omega-3 fatty acids and additions in apolipoproteins, dietary fiber, vitamins, and trace minerals to help students distinguish faddish claims from sound ideas and practice in their study and patient care.

Part II, "Community Nutrition: The Life Cycle," continues its focus on family and individual nutritional needs through the life cycle with emphasis on *health maintenance.* This emphasis is strengthened by the timely new Chapter 16, "Nutrition and Stress Management," which discusses stress as a significant modern health risk, its far-reaching physiologic effect on the body, sources of stress in our lives, and approaches to high-risk stress management. This new chapter on stress joins updated chapters on physical fitness and weight management to round out the discussion of basic risk factors associated with our modern life-style and environment that contribute to health problems.

Part III, "Introduction to Diet Therapy," presents updated material reflecting current research and practice. This is particularly evident in Chapter 20, "Coronary Heart Disease and Hypertension." This key chapter has been revised to incorporate current knowledge and practice that has moved from controversy to consensus about the relation of nutrition to the underlying disease process atherosclerosis, focusing on the key role of cholesterol and other lipids and launching the National Cholesterol Education Program through National Institutes of Health (NIH). Basic assessment guides and the step-wise diet program being used in this national cholesterol evaluation and education effort are included. This updating carries through in all clinical nutrition chapters. For example, the chapter on diabetes mellitus moves from previous trends into their current application in practice in all phases of therapy, including diet, insulins, self-monitoring of blood glucose, and tighter control to prevent complications. Finally, the new Chapter 25, "Nutrition Support in Disabling Disease," presents a general nutrition support base to meet rehabilitative needs, and a special focus on three particularly debilitating conditions, often having devastating results, that demand specific nutritional therapy: rheumatoid arthritis, chronic obstructive pulmonary disease (COPD), and acquired immune deficiency syndrome (AIDS).

Learning Aids Within the Text

Throughout the text, many learning aids continue to be developed to help unify and teach the comprehensive material:

Chapter openers focus immediate attention on the key chapter topic, giving a brief overview statement, chapter objectives, and a theme photograph.

Chapter headings and subheadings of special type and color help to organize the content, relate key concepts, and make for easy reading.

Marginal material highlights definitions, data, comments, line drawings, and photographs to expand understanding of text discussion.

Boxed material expands or illustrates text discussions with "To Probe Further" and "Clinical Application" nuggets to stimulate thought.

Definitions of terms are clarified in the running text, side margins, and a summary glossary at the end of the book complete with pronunciation guide. This three-level approach to vocabulary development greatly improves overall study and use of the text.

Illustration and color emphasis integrate page design and content with clarifying artwork.

Chapter summaries review chapter highlights and help students place details in the "big picture."

Review questions help test comprehension of chapter material and lead students to analyze and apply key concepts.

Further readings provide brief annotated guides to expanded background sources relevant to chapter topics.

Issues and Answers present short articles, a number of them new to this edition, on current issues and controversies related to chapter material to stimulate thinking, practical application, and questions.

Diet guides in clinical chapters provide sample food lists for patient care and education.

Appendixes include reference tables and tools for use in study projects and practice. Food value tables include nutrient and energy references for a variety of basic foods. Current American Diabetes Association food exchange lists are given for diet calculations, meal planning, and patient education.

The index extends the basic text cross-referencing and provides a quick reference to the book's content topics.

Supplementary Materials

Several available supplements enhance the teaching/learning process. Information on these helpful packages may be obtained from the publisher.

Instructor's Manual

Prepared by Betty J. Elliott of Truckee Meadows Community College, this valuable tool features suggested course syllabuses; chapter reviews; behavioral objectives; key terms; chapter outlines with teaching notes on controversial topics; "Nutrition in the News"; additional resources, including slides, films, and filmstrips; transparency masters; and an extensive test-item band of approximately 1300 questions.

Computerized Test Bank (Diploma)

This tool provides test items from the instructor's manual on floppy disk, compatible with IBM-PC and Apple II and IIe computers. It is free to adopters of the text.

Overhead Transparency Acetates

Illustrations of important, hard-to-understand concepts are available as acetate transparencies. These useful tools facilitate learning of key concepts discussed in the text and are free to adopters of the text.

Self-Study Guide

This concise little companion continues to serve as a general learning aid during initial courses, as well as a tool for review of the text for professional examinations or for practitioners needing to update knowledge. It includes may items to support learning of each chapter's content: chapter focus; summary-review quiz; discussion questions to stimulate thinking; true-false and multiple choice test items to test comprehension; numerous guides for individual and group projects that involve experiments, case studies, and situational problems; and inquiry questions that relate an "Issues and Answers" article to current health care problems.

Personal Approach

My person-centered approach in past editions remains in this new text. It is enhanced by (1) a personal writing style that reflects my own convictions and commitments about student learning and patient care; (2) extensive use of ever-expanding personal files and materials gathered from my own clinical practice, teaching, and biochemical-metabolic work; and (3) practical applications of scientific knowledge in realistic *human* terms to find personal solutions to individual problems.

Acknowledgments

Many persons have helped me in this book project and I am grateful for their contributions. To these persons I give my thanks: to my publisher and editorial staff, especially Pat Coryell and Loren Stevenson for their constant skill and support; to the reviewers for their valuable time and suggestions:

Kathryn Daughton, Asheville Buncombe Technical Community College;
Marsha Ray, Shasta College;

Susan W. Crawford, Minneapolis Community College; and
Cheryl Wrasper, Casper College.

I also thank my own staff for all their personal skills and support, especially to Jim Williams and Tony Rinella, whose computer savvy and personal support kept me and my system going; my many students, interns, colleagues, clients, and patients, all of whom have taught me much; and my family, who never cease to support all my efforts and who always share in whatever I am able to achieve.

Sue Rodwell Williams
Berkeley, California

Contents

Part II   Community Nutrition: The Life Cycle

9   The Food Environment and Food Habits, 192

10   Family Nutrition Counseling: Food Needs and Costs, 225

11   Nutrition During Pregnancy and Lactation, 252

Part III Introduction to Diet Therapy

Appendixes

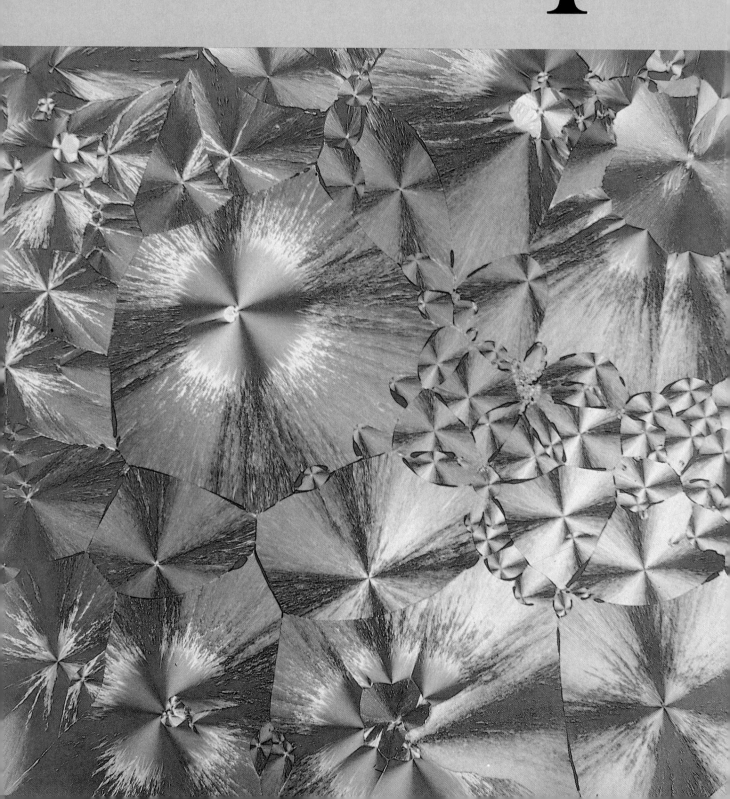

Introduction to Human Nutrition

1 Nutrition and Health

Chapter Objectives

After studying this chapter the student should be able to:

1. Identify today's main world health problems and describe their root causes in terms of food supply.
2. Define the major U.S. health problems and relate them to social and nutritional factors.
3. Distinguish the functions of food and of nutrients and describe levels of nutritional status.
4. Identify four major social influences on our changing concepts of health and disease.
5. Identify four basic changes in the current U.S. health care system and their effects on our health care practices, especially team care.
6. Describe the expanding role of nutrition in health care and define human nutrition in terms of health needs and personal social needs.

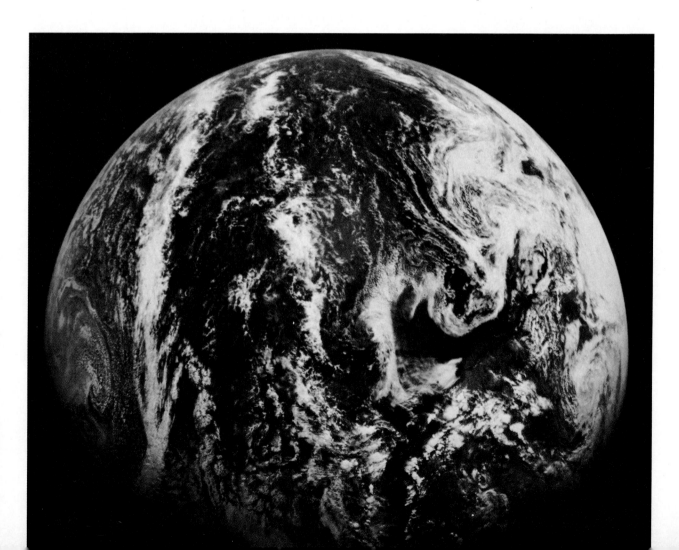

PREVIEW

▪

Why should persons working in health care be concerned about nutrition? What is health? How is nutrition related? What is nutrition? What does it *do*?

To answer such basic questions and meet realistic and practical needs in today's world, the study of nutrition and health must focus first on *change*. Our physical bodies and personalities, our scientific knowledge and society are all constantly changing. These constant life changes must be in some kind of *positive balance* to produce healthy living. Thus in our study the learning concepts of *change* and *balance* will provide a fundamental framework. Although we may view and define health and disease in different ways, a primary basis for promoting health and preventing disease must always be a wholesome food supply for all persons and the sound nutrition it provides.

In this first chapter, then, we introduce three increasingly interdependent issues: a broad world nutrition view, an understanding of our own major U.S. health problems, and a person-centered health team approach for meeting these problems, promoting health, and preventing disease. We will consider the far-reaching effects of change in today's world on nutrition and health, the ways persons define health and disease, and the role of nutrition in health care.

Main World Health Problems

Food Security

Perhaps in no other area do we realize the necessity of mutual interaction and interdependence among the countries of our world more than in the issue of food security and, hence, survival. Today food security is of great concern in international discussions. The Food and Agriculture Organization (FAO) of the United Nations focuses on food security in terms of the three basic issues on which it depends: food production, stability of food supplies, and economic access to food. We have learned, often through sad experience, that in the small world of our planet Earth events in one place cause disrupting effects in other parts as well. We know now that in a very real sense we are all bound together for survival.

Population Expansion and Food Supply

With our expanding world population, the ultimate objective of world food security is to ensure that all people are able to buy or grow the basic food they need. But this is not a simple problem with simple solutions. The world has made some progress in coping with its food problems, but the tasks that still lie ahead are monumental. The surplus food stocks of exporting countries do not fill the bellies of hungry people in a major part of the world. A major determinant of food security in the world is the agricultural production possible in developing countries of south and east Asia, since these countries contain about half of the world's population. But food security in these populous regions is still fragile. Some of the most devasted area is the

Nutrition and World Health

Approximately 15 to 20 million people in the world, principally in the poorer countries, die each year of hunger-related causes. It is estimated that some 450 million persons throughout the world suffer from severe malnutrition, consuming less than 1.2 times the kilocalories required to maintain even the basal metabolic rate.

African sub-Sahara region where countries face staggering problems of appalling famine. Although malnutrition has many roots, several interrelated problems lie at its heart: (1) poverty, (2) population growth, (3) soil deterioration as a result of poor farming methods, (4) political turmoil and war, and (5) maldistribution of the world's food supply.

Malnutrition Diseases

By far the greatest world health problem is **protein-energy malnutrition** with its attendent infectious diseases, followed by *nutritional anemias* principally caused by iron deficiency, and *vitamin A deficiency,* which causes widespread blindness. Other continuing problems include classic nutritional deficiency diseases such as endemic goiter, pellagra, beriberi, scurvy, and rickets. The FAO has begun a long-term program to help raise nutritional standards in the poorest countries by applying nutritional guidelines to all its development projects and assisting in community education and training. FAO also conducts regional workshops to improve national skills in nutrition assessment and planning.

Major U.S. Health Problems

In the past, our killer diseases were infections such as smallpox, diphtheria, pneumonia, and tuberculosis. For these we found "magic bullets" in specific vaccines and antibodies and drugs. Today, however, our problems are more complex and there are no simple solutions. Our major health problems center on the so-called diseases of civilization—heart disease and cancer. Additional problems include those stemming from complications of diabetes mellitus that relate to heart disease and renal disease.

Heart Disease

The major cause of death in the United States and other Western societies for the past half century has been and continues to be diseases of the heart and blood vessels. The magnitude of this health care problem is enormous. In addition to the human toll, heart disease extracts a severe social and economic cost from the families affected. Major nutrition-related problems center on (1) fat and cholesterol in relation to blood vessel health and (2) sodium in relation to hypertension, a major risk factor for heart disease. Look for a detailed discussion of this major U.S. health problem in Chapter 20.

Cancer

In its many forms, cancer has become one of our major public health problems. It accounts for about 20% of the total deaths in the United States, close on the heels of our number one killer, heart disease, which accounts for about 50% of the total. Important relationships between nutrition and cancer seem to exist in (1) prevention by improving the environment and strengthening the body's defense system and (2) nutritional support for medical treatment and rehabilitation. Look for more detail about these nutritional relationships in Chapter 24.

Diabetes Mellitus Complications

In the United States diabetes has become the fifth ranking cause of death from disease. Among older persons with diabetes the cause of death from

---

Protein-energy malnutrition
Malnutrition caused by a deficiency of both protein and kilocalories as compared with protein deficiency in the presence of adequate kilocalories.

Every day about 3400 Americans, more than two each minute, suffer a heart attack. In addition, every day approximately 1600 people suffer strokes. Coronary heart disease alone is responsible for some 650,000 deaths per year, with more than 150,000 of these occurring in people less than 65 years old.

About 440,000 Americans die each year of cancer. A majority of these persons, about 25%, die of lung cancer.

diabetic complications is mainly myocardial infarction, or heart attack. The underlying pathology of coronary heart disease is **atherosclerosis,** which is two to three times more common in persons with diabetes than in the general population. Among younger persons with diabetes the major complicating cause of death is renal failure resulting from **glomerulosclerosis.** Kidney disease is a leading cause of lost work time and income and is the fourth leading health problem in America today. Good dietary control supported by insulin and exercise, monitored by self-testing of blood glucose levels, often helps prevent these diabetic complications. These related problems are discussed in Chapters 21 and 22.

Atherosclerosis
Condition in which yellowish plaques (atheromas) are deposited within the medium-sized and large arteries.

Glomerulosclerosis
Scarring and aging of renal glomeruli.

General Malnutrition and Poverty

Encroaching problems of malnutrition occur in low income American families caught in the grip of unemployment and poverty. General economic problems of regional and racial poverty have caused more and more middle income families to slip below the identified national poverty income level. For the families involved, these problems have enormous repercussions in their standard of living and food intake. Look for details about this food economics problem in Chapter 10.

Food and Nutrients
Basic Definitions

Nutrition and Human Health

To answer our initial questions about what nutrition is or does in relation to health, some basic definitions are first in order. The word *nutrition* comes from a Latin root *nutr-*, meaning to *nurture* or *nourish*. Nourishment is that which sustains life. The science and art of human nutrition both focus on nourishing human life. They do this in many ways. Persons breathe, work, rest, play, sleep, and generally live their lives, all of which require energy. They must replenish that energy with food and its nutrients to sustain physical life. Nutrition thus concerns the food people eat and how their bodies use it. Nutritional science comprises the body of scientific knowledge governing the nutritional requirements of persons for maintenance, growth, activity, and reproduction. In health care, *dietetics* is the health profession having primary responsibility for the practical application of nutritional science to persons and groups of persons in various conditions of health and disease. The *registered dietitian (RD)*, especially the *clinical nutrition specialist*, is the nutrition authority on the health care team and carries the major responsibility for nutritional care of patients and clients, working with other health team members.[1] The *public health nutritionist* is responsible for nutritional care of groups of people in the community, especially those high-risk groups who require assessment of need and community programs planned to meet these needs.

Functions of Food and Nutrients

The respective functions of *food* and *nutrients* in human nutrition also need to be distinguished. First of all, dispense with the myth that any particular food or food combination is required by the body for health. Consider that the human race has subsisted for centuries upon centuries with wide varieties of foods, depending on what was available to eat and what the culture designated as human food. Various foods serve as important vehicles for taking nutrients into the body and bringing human pleasure and comfort. But it is the specific chemical compounds or elements—the *nutrients*—in a wide variety of foods that the body requires. About 40 of these essential nutrients are known, and probably still others are yet to be discovered. The known ones include the *macronutrients*—carbohydrates, fats, and proteins—whose constituent substances supply energy and build tissue, and the *micronutrients*—vitamins and minerals that the body uses in much smaller amounts to regulate and control body processes. And of course there is water, the vital nutrient sustaining all our life processes. The term *metabolism* refers to the sum of all these chemical processes in the body that work on the nutrients in a warm watery internal environment to sustain life and health. The chapters that follow in this first part of the text will cover your study of these vital nutrients.

Levels of Nutritional Status

An individual's nutritional status will vary according to living situation, available food supply, and health condition. You will be concerned with these varying levels in your nutrition study as you assess your own status and that of others.

Sound Nutrition

Evidence of sound positive nutrition includes a well-developed body, ideal weight-for-height and body composition (ratio of muscle mass to fat), and good muscle development and tone. The skin is smooth and clear, the hair glossy, and the eyes clear and bright. Posture is good, and the facial expression is alert. Appetite, digestion, and elimination are normal. Table 1-1 compares characteristics of good and poor states of nutrition. Begin to think about these signs as you get into your nutrition study, and look for them as you become a more skilled observer. Well-nourished persons are much more likely to be alert, both mentally and physically, and to have a positive outlook on life. They are not only meeting their day-to-day needs, but also maintaining essential reserves for resisting infections and generally extending their years of normal functioning.

Borderline Nutrition

As the descriptive label indicates, persons with only a borderline nutritional status may manage from day to day to meet their minimum needs. However, they lack nutritional reserves to meet any added physiologic or metabolic demand from injury or illness or to sustain additional fetal development during pregnancy or proper growth in childhood. This state may exist in persons with poor eating habits or those who are living in stressed environments on low incomes. Dietary surveys have shown that approximately one third of the U.S. population is living on diets below the optimal level. This does not necessarily mean that these Americans are undernourished, because some persons can maintain general health on somewhat less than the optimal amounts of various nutrients. On the average, however, a person receiving less than the desired amounts, especially over extended periods of time, has a greater risk of physical illness than a person in an optimal state of nutrition. The human body has much capacity for adapting to such lowered nu-

Features	Good	Poor
		Table 1-1 Clinical Signs of Nutritional Status
General appearance	Alert, responsive	Listless, apathetic; cachexia
Hair	Shiny, lustrous, healthy scalp	Stringy, dull, brittle, dry, depigmented
Neck glands	No enlargement	Thyroid enlarged
Skin, face and neck	Smooth, slightly moist; good color, reddish pink mucous membranes	Greasy, discolored, scaly
Eyes	Bright, clear; no fatigue circles	Dryness, signs of infection, increased vascularity, glassiness, thickened conjunctivae
Lips	Good color, moist	Dry, scaly, swollen, angular lesions (stomatitis)
Tongue	Good pink color; surface papillae present; no lesions	Papillary atrophy, smooth appearance; swollen, red, beefy (glossitis)
Gums	Good pink color; no swelling or bleeding; firm	Marginal redness or swelling; receding, spongy
Teeth	Straight, no crowding; well-shaped jaw; clean, no discoloration	Unfilled cavities, absent teeth, worn surfaces; mottled, malpositioned
Skin, general	Smooth, slightly moist; good color	Rough, dry, scaly, pale, pigmented, irritated; petechiae, bruises
Abdomen	Flat	Swollen
Legs, feet	No tenderness, weakness, swelling; good color	Edema, tender calf; tingling, weakness
Skeleton	No malformations	Bowlegs, knock-knees, chest deformity at diaphragm, beaded ribs, prominent scapulae
Weight	Normal for height, age, body build	Overweight or underweight
Posture	Erect, arms and legs straight, abdomen in, chest out	Sagging shoulders, sunken chest, humped back

Continued.

Table 1-1
Clinical Signs of
Nutritional Status—
cont'd

Features	Good	Poor
Muscles	Well developed, firm	Flaccid, poor tone; undeveloped, tender
Nervous control	Good attention span for age; does not cry easily; not irritable or restless	Inattentive, irritable
Gastrointestinal function	Good appetite and digestion; normal, regular elimination	Anorexia, indigestion, constipation or diarrhea
General vitality	Endurance; energetic; sleeps well at night; vigorous	Easily fatigued, no energy, falls asleep in school, looks tired, apathetic

tritional states, but it can sustain only a certain amount of physiologic stress before signs of frank malnutrition appear.

Malnutrition

Signs of malnutrition appear when nutritional reserves are depleted and nutrient and energy intake is not sufficient to meet day-to-day needs or added metabolic stress. A large number of malnourished people live in high-risk conditions of poverty. These conditions influence the health of all persons involved, but especially the most vulnerable ones—pregnant women, infants, children, and elderly adults.[2,3] In the United States, one of the wealthiest countries on Earth, many studies document widespread hunger and malnutrition among the poor and homeless. The 1985 Physician Task Force on Hunger in America found that at least 20 million Americans suffer hunger some days each month.[4] Worldwide, about 40,000 to 50,000 people die *each day* from malnutrition, while an estimated 450 million to 1.3 billion people do not have enough to eat.[5]

   We also find frank malnutrition in our hospitals. For example, extended illness, especially among older persons with chronic disease, places added stress on the body, and the person's daily nutrient and energy intake is insufficient to meet needs. If you are working with such patients, observe carefully for signs of malnutrition, using the general guidelines provided in Table 1-1 and results of assessment procedures such as those described in Chapter 17.

Changing Concepts of Health and Disease

Current nutritional care, as well as that of nursing and other health professions, is a fundamental part of rapidly developing changes in our society and our health values and goals. These changing values are having profound effects on our professional practices and on persons' self-care of health or use of professional services. We are all affected, providers and consumers alike.

Reasons for Changes in Health Views
Views of Health and Disease

In the past, health has usually been defined simply as the absence of disease. Thus the basic approach to care was curative. Education and training of hospital and community workers centered primarily on learning certain skills for treatment of illness or for crisis intervention. In contrast, more primitive societies associated disease with evil spirits or mysterious supernatural powers to be driven out of the body. Thus treatment of disease required a religious leader, the shaman, to act as both priest and physician. In underdeveloped countries this approach still exists and is being blended with more modern medical knowledge. Gradually, however, as scientific knowledge has increased, the biologic basis for disease has become well established. In developed countries public and personal hygiene has improved, treatment for specific diseases has become more scientific and skilled, and many of the most lethal childhood diseases have been eliminated.

Human Values and Health Goals

Faced now with the so-called gift of longer life, we view health increasingly in quality-of-life terms. Health concepts have moved from the wholly negative view of absence of disease—*curative* approach—to a more positive view of optimal human fulfillment and productivity—the *preventive* approach of health promotion. During the 1980s, U.S. health officials developed national health and nutrition goals, have projected goals for the 1990s, and are well underway shaping objectives for the year 2000.[6] But health is a relative concept in any culture. Health competes with other values and is relative to a culture's way of life. These differences in needs extend to include moral, philosophical, ethical, and religious dimensions. Perhaps, then, a realistic overall goal for health efforts in any part of the world would be a level of physical and mental health that would make for social well-being within the social system in which the individual must live. Such a goal must provide opportunity for personal productivity and self-fulfillment. To achieve it, today's education for students in the health care fields requires an integrated study of the whole person, the community, and personal health needs.

Social Influences

A number of factors in our rapidly developing society have contributed to changes in health values and practices:

1. **Expansion of scientific knowledge.** The rate of expansion in our scientific knowledge is almost incomprehensible. Knowledge of nutritional science, the body's fascinating and intricate chemistry, and its interaction with our changing environment is constantly increasing. Computers and nutritional analysis software have become regular tools in assessing nutritional status, planning care, and keeping up with scientific literature. And in modern hospitals and medical centers a network of computers now stores, transmits, monitors, and evaluates vital data necessary for valid patient care services. Also, rapidly advancing medical technology challenges and taxes health care facilities. A wide variety of treatment techniques, surgical procedures, drugs, and electronic instruments have become a regular part of medical care. Although life-saving and life-extending in many ways, such rapidly expanding medical science has created problems. Increased specialization

To Probe Further

Our Increasing Health Care Bills

The increasing costs of America's health care system are straining both personal and governmental resources. According to a recent report to the National Committee for Quality Assurance, a number of current trends contribute to this strain: an aging population requiring more specialized services, increased consumer awareness and demands for health screening, increased needs for alcohol- and drug-abuse treatment programs, the AIDS epidemic, the high rate of teenage pregnancies, and the increased use of advanced medical technology, as in neonatal care and organ transplants.

This economic impact is growing daily. Studies indicate that in 1987 Americans spent about $2100 on medical care for every man, woman, and child, and the government's doctor bill was almost $500 billion. This amounts to 11% of the gross national product and nearly twice the national defense cost. In 1988 health insurance bills rose 20% to 40%, and the number of uninsured grew to an estimated 37 million. At least 700 hospitals, including much-needed inner-city and rural facilities, will probably have to close by the year 1995. Advanced life-prolonging medical technology is adding to costs. Spectacular CT scanners and magnetic resonance imaging machines can cost millions. Heart transplants come at about $125,000 apiece; liver transplants, $160,000; bone marrow transplants, $100,000 to $150,000. These situations bring not only economic burden but also moral and ethical questions.

No doubt the U.S. health care system in the year 2000 will have had to find more answers to its increasing cost problems. Treatment advances will divert a large number of patients from the hospital setting, shrinking the hospitalized population to about half its current size. The hospital will become a critical-care hub for a dispersed network of smaller clinical facilities connected by air and ground transport and integrated by clinical information and patient monitoring systems. The increasing supply of physicians will increase competition, make services more available in rural areas, increase time spent with patients, and increase group practice and integrated financing systems such as prepaid health plans and health maintenance organizations (HMOs). With wider gaps between federal and state programs for the poor and the private insurance system, quality health care for the poor is likely to be further compromised.

What are the answers? They are not easy. Increasingly, the hard fact is that the health care system will have to deal with the difficult problem of containing costs without sacrificing human need. The key word in planning health care will have to be "accountability," and cost-benefit studies will have to be part of all services, including nutritional care.

REFERENCES

Goldsmith JC: The US health care system in the year 2000, JAMA 256:3371, Dec 26, 1986.
Russell S: A sick health system, San Francisco Chronicle, May 17, 1988, editorial.

brings fragmented care and a system in which persons often feel lost. Also, with this increasing complexity of care have come increasing costs and ethical questions about the use of our costly new medical technology. (See the box on the facing page.)

2. **Population increase.** The population is increasing in many nations of the world, especially in those that can least afford to feed such growing numbers. According to its 1980 census, the U.S. population had grown to 232.6 million, a total that our next 1990 decade count will no doubt exceed.[7] The "baby-boom" generation of the 1940s continues to create a demographic bulge affecting everything from the housing market to social security payments. This generation is not conforming to historical patterns of American life: they are marrying later, divorcing more frequently, having children later, and setting up smaller households, many with single parents. Immigration has increased, especially Asian and Hispanic, with the influx of thousands of refugees. Resulting health care needs have grown.

In general, the recent American population increase is reflected not only in total numbers but also in percentage shifts in age and location. The percentage of older people is increasing, and overall mobility is greater. Urban-suburban trends have created changes in individual psychologic patterns, in family patterns, and in community and national social patterns. All these changes affect health needs and social values.

3. **Social changes.** Radical changes continue to develop in family and community patterns in our highly industrialized society. Crowded, low-income housing in cities contrasts with sprawling, affluent suburbs. Economic affluence, higher costs of living, and more emphasis on post-secondary education—all in the face of increasing poverty in urban and rural areas—have changed human goals, health values, and medical care programs.

4. **Development of the social sciences.** The behavioral sciences—psychology, sociology, and anthropology—are contributing insights concerning human behavior in response to illness and other life stresses, as well as food habits. There is a renewed effort within the health professions to understand and help the patient or client as a whole person and the family as a primary supportive social unit. More time is given to analyzing the impact of psychosocial, economic, and cultural factors on personal concepts of health.

Effects of Change on Health Care Practices

These scientific and socioeconomic developments, together with changing attitudes toward health and disease, have produced far-reaching effects on the American health care system. These changes reflect changing roles of health care providers and patients-clients, as well as escalating costs of medical care that have priced many persons out of the health care market.

Focus of Care

The change in focus of care includes attention to the social issues that lie at the roots of disease and increase health risks. This goal values and emphasizes preventive health maintenance and promotion, rather than focusing on the exclusive traditional approach of crisis intervention and curative practice only. Health workers at all levels are more involved in person-centered care. They also work in the areas of community and legislative action, family and

1980 census indicates a percentage increase of Asian immigration during the past decade of 127.6%. Most of these people have settled in the West, helping to give California the largest population (23.7 million) among the states and making it the most urban of the states.

At any given point in time, about 20% of our total population is moving to a different place.

Functional illness is recognized as a very real phenomenon. An individual's life situation and reaction to stress must be considered if total health needs are to be met.

community health, and primary family care that includes a focus on nutrition and health education.

Systems of Providing Care

Changes in our health care delivery systems are based on the work of *health care teams* providing primary care in a *variety of settings*. Primary care practitioners in each of the basic health care professions, assisted by support personnel, work in a number of various satellite clinics or health centers, as well as in central-core medical centers. There are extended-care facilities based on degree of care needed; community health centers and special clinics such as those for nutrition, home-management counseling, and maternity and child care; and outreach clinics in more remote rural areas.

Role of Patients and Clients

Patients and clients are taking an increasingly active role in their own care, rather than the traditionally passive role of patients in medical care. Patients need to be involved in planning care and decision making. They must have opportunity for better education in nutrition and general health to help them toward more positive health behavior, wiser use of health care facilities, and good self-care based on knowledge and support rather than blame for their health problems. (See Issues and Answers.)

Payment for Services

The traditional fee-for-service practice of American medicine and the rapidly rising costs of medical care often place such care beyond the reach of many persons who need it most. Changes in payment mechanisms focus on some form of health insurance. These various plans include prepaid group medical practice in health maintenance organizations (HMOs), preferred provider organizations (PPOs) established by corporations contracting with selected local physicians under controlled costs for designated services, and various forms of individual and group health insurance.

Since Medicare legislation of the early 1960s, the U.S. government has provided limited assistance, especially for older adults. More recently, attempts to curtail rising hospital costs for Medicare patients came with the 1983 passage of the Prospective Payment System (Title VI of Public Law 98-21), which has affected the cost, quality, and access of care.[8,9] The basis for payment in this system is the *diagnosis related groupings (DRGs)*. This system classifies patients according to the International Classification of Diseases into 23 major diagnostic categories based on organ systems. Cost-benefit analysis of nutrition services relates their importance to a number of these categories.[10,11]

Changing Health Care Values and Attitudes
The Science and Art of Clinical Care

Science is a body of systematic knowledge, facts, and principles born of controlled research that shows the operation of natural law. Rapid scientific advances have provided all clinicians with a stronger base on which to build professional practice. *Art* is the exceptional ability to conduct any human activity. All practitioners must base their practice on sound scientific knowledge *and* they must know and care about people and their needs. Especially

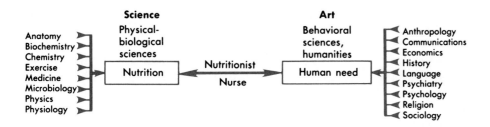

Figure 1-1
The science and art of nutrition applied to human need.

in the field of human nutrition and health, scientific knowledge has little significance apart from application to human needs, both physical and emotional. In many aspects of nutritional care, nutritionists and nurses work together, functioning as catalysts that bring scientific knowledge and skill to bear on human needs at particular points in persons' lives. The diagram in Figure 1-1 illustrates this significant role.

Unique Team Position of Nutritionist and Nurse

Whether functioning in the hospital, the clinic, or the community, the clinical dietitian, or clinical nutrition specialist, and the nurse hold positions on the health team that are uniquely related to the patient. Their roles are changing as their team responsibilities expand. The clinical dietitian (RD), holding both professional certification and graduate degrees in nutritional science, determines nutritional care needs in relation to medical diagnosis and care, as well as individual patient needs, and provides primary nutritional care and counseling.[1] The nurse assists the dietitian with this nutritional care, making consultation and referral skills essential in applying the dietitian's nutritional care plan to general nursing care. In many respects, these two health professionals are closest to the patient and the family and have the opportunity to determine many of the patient's needs. They must coordinate services and help the patient understand and participate in personal care. Such sensitive practitioners realize that their most therapeutic contribution is their genuine involvement and concern.

RD—Registered Dietitian.

In personalized patient care, remember that often your most therapeutic tool is *yourself*.

Changing Concepts of Nutrition

In the midst of such significant changes in society and approaches to health care, nutrition can no longer be viewed in the narrow, isolated sense that may have been common in the past. It is intimately involved in these broader changes in total health care. Several interrelated areas of social and scientific change are reflected in changing nutritional needs, problems, and priorities.

Nutrition in Health Care

Rapidly Changing Food Environment

No longer do we always have "regular food" and home meals as in past generations. The number of "fast-food" outlets has been increasing rapidly. Also, the growing food industry is producing many new processed food products. These include a wide variety of combination, "convenience," synthetic, and textured foods. In general, two basic problem areas result: (1) primary single foods of known nutrient composition tend to be used less often,

From 1970 to 1980 fast-food sales rose 300%, from $6.5 billion to $23 billion per year. About 90% of all Americans eat periodically in a fast-food restaurant; 10% eat fast foods more than five times a week.

so careful label reading is necessary to help determine values and (2) the need for nutrition education in schools, homes, clinics, hospitals, and the marketplace has increased. Confusing claims and counterclaims and misleading advertising, especially in television commercials, increase the difficulty of buying wisely. These concerns are discussed in Chapters 9 and 10.

Increased Consumer Awareness and Action

The development of mass media such as television and the national attention given to nutritional problems of the poor and the aged, as well as the questionable use of pesticides and food additives, have increased public awareness of the role of nutrition in health. Questions are being raised and consumers are seeking answers and sound nutrition information.

Changing Socioeconomic and Population Trends

Shifts in population patterns and an increased number of older persons have focused attention on nutrition problems in two basic areas:

1. **Malnutrition in poverty areas.** An increasing number of persons in large cities, especially among minority groups, migrant working populations, and those in rural areas, face the pressure of unemployment and reduced income.
2. **Malnutrition and chronic health problems in elderly persons.** Attitudes of our youth-and-action-oriented society toward the aged, compounded by problems of health and economic security, often isolate and bring despair to elderly persons. Realistic programs are needed to provide food assistance and nutrition education related to chronic conditions such as heart disease and diabetes.

Definition of Human Nutrition
Human Health Needs

At its fundamental level, then, distinctly *human nutrition* may be distinguished from general nutritional science. It may be defined as the process of meeting human health needs in the context of basic human personal needs by nutritional means. Four basic frames of reference help us identify these human health needs in our patients and clients:

1. **Age group needs.** Human beings progress through normal growth and development from the prenatal period, birth, infancy, and childhood through adulthood in the continuing aging process leading eventually to death. In each of these stages specific physical growth patterns and psychosocial development occur. Each age group has its special needs and nutritional requirements, as outlined in Chapters 11 through 13 on the life cycle. Food habits specifically relate to this growth and development process within an individual's own culture.

2. **Stress factors.** Stresses in individual life situations bring physical, mental, and emotional problems. Depending on personal strength, reserves, and resources available, the stress may be handled well or not. The effect of stress on the body and the degree of adjustment or method of coping has to be considered in determining needs. These stress factors are discussed in Chapter 16.

3. **Health status.** A person's degree of health or disease, not only the actual situation but the situation as each person perceives it, influences nutritional

or food modification needs. These clinical needs are the basis of all the final chapters in Part Three.

4. **Basic human needs.** Certain basic general needs are common to all human beings. These needs form an ordered hierarchy. For example, such physiologic survival needs as food and water and safety and comfort, respectively, must be met before the higher human needs for love, self-esteem, and creative growth can be met. Basic nutrition and health needs relate to each of these general human needs in achieving the overall goal of personal integrity. This basic thread of person-centered care based on identified individual needs is a key structure running throughout this book.

Relation of Nutrition to Health

It is evident, then, that nutrition is specifically related to both physical and emotional health.

1. **Physical health.** Life in its most fundamental sense—survival—depends on air, water, and food. These basic life-support materials supply the body with certain essential chemicals that enable it to do its work. Oxygen from the air combines with chemical substances—nutrients—in food and water to make it possible for the body to carry on all its physiologic functions. We must have energy for metabolic work and physical activities, and we must build and maintain body cells and tissues. The necessary nutrients supply the fuel and building blocks for carrying on these activities. In a biologic sense, we are indeed what we eat.

2. **Human personal health.** Although air, water, and food are essential for physical survival, we do not breathe, drink, and eat to sustain our physical body alone. Food especially has many meanings and helps us meet a number of personal, social, and cultural needs. In fact, unmet personal needs may contribute to actual physical illness. Nutrition and food, then, are essential to both physical and psychosocial health.

Nutritional Guides for Health Promotion

Since the early 1900s, a number of food and nutrient guides have been developed to meet nutrition and health needs of Americans. Their design has reflected social, political, and economic events of the times, as well as a rapidly developing nutritional science and its relation to human health.[12] For example, they have addressed needs during wars and emergencies and economic depression. And now, with our changing economics and modern health problems, their focus has shifted from preventing primary deficiency diseases caused by insufficient nutritional intake to controlling chronic diseases and excessive intake. In current use, there are three general types of nutritional guides: (1) nutrient standards, (2) food guides, and (3) dietary guidelines. Each one serves different needs. Note them carefully here, for you will be making frequent reference to them throughout your study and practice.

Nutrient Standards: The Recommended Dietary Allowances (RDAs)
U.S. Standards

Most of the developed countries of the world have set up standards by age and sex groups for intake of major nutrients by healthy persons. They serve as guidelines for maintaining healthy populations. They are not intended to indicate individual requirements, for these are highly variable, nor do they set clinical needs, which are determined by individual health problems. However, they do serve as a reference base from current nutrition research for intake levels of the essential nutrients judged to be adequate for meeting the known nutritional needs of healthy population groups. In the United States these nutrient and energy standards are called the *Recommended Dietary Allowances (RDAs)*. Such standards are similar in different countries but may vary a little according to their purpose and use.

Development of the RDAs

The first RDA standards grew out of a national nutrition conference for defense held in 1941 during World War II.[12] A summary background followed in 1943 as a guide for nutrition workers in planning and obtaining food supplies for national defense and general population needs for good nutrition. Since this first edition of the RDAs, a new edition has been published about every 4 or 5 years based on expanding current nutrition research. Through edition 9 in 1980 the RDAs continued to be developed and maintained by groups of leading nutrition scientists and practitioners working with the National Academy of Sciences in Washington, D.C. The Academy has numerous divisions of councils and is supported by the National Institutes of Health. The working groups responsible for the RDAs make up the Food and Nutrition Board of the National Research Council.

Current Status of RDAs Development

Edition 9 of the RDAs in 1980 gave evidence of increasing knowledge in nutrition and expanding social concerns about nutrition and health.[13] However, edition 10, planned for publication in 1985, was not issued because the study group of scientists and the Academy director could not reach full agreement about changes to be made.[14] This fact reflects our rapidly changing society and the difficult issues facing us in relating nutrition to broader standards for positive health promotion. Now, a newly appointed study group has completed the new 1989 report for edition 10.[15,15a] You will find these current RDA tables here inside the book covers for quick reference.

Other Standards

Canadian and British standards are similar to U.S. standards. In less developed countries where such factors as quality of available protein foods must be considered, nutrition workers look to standards such as those set by the Food and Agriculture Organization (FAO) of the World Health Organization (WHO). Nonetheless, all of these standards provide nutrient and energy guidelines for health workers in a variety of population groups to promote good health through sound nutrition.

Food Guides

To interpret and apply sound nutrient standards, health workers also need practical food guides for nutrition education and meal/snack planning with individuals and families. Two such food guides, very different in nature and serving different needs, are the Basic Four Food Groups Guide and the Food Exchange Lists Guide.

Basic Four Food Groups

Probably the most familiar food guide is the long-used but limited version issued by the U.S. Department of Agriculture (USDA), the Basic Four Food Groups. This guide reflects in its origin agricultural commodity concerns, as well as nutritional ones. Over the years the USDA has issued a succession of basic food guides. Their first guide in 1917 showed the limited nutritional knowledge of the time. Its main concern was adequate energy intake and contained five food groups: flesh foods, starchy foods, fat foods, watery fruits and vegetables, and sweets. A 1933 revision was concerned about newly discovered vitamins and minerals, as well as a depressed economy, in its 12 food groups on four different cost levels. Wartime editions in the early 1940s, known as the Basic Seven Food Groups, contained the basic milk, meat, and cereal groups, with three fruit and vegetable groups and a fat group. This seven-group scheme was used extensively.

In 1958 the three groups of fruits and vegetables were combined into a single group, the fat group was eliminated, and the guide was reissued as the Basic Four Food Groups.[12] In 1979 the guide was revised by adding a fifth group—fats, sweets, and alcohol—and was called the "Hassle-Free Guide to Better Diet." However, the guide soon returned to its initial four-group form, which continues in use today (see Table 1-2 on p. 18). But there are limits to the use of this simple guide. It has been criticized for its heavy emphasis on animal protein and limited value in ensuring micronutrient needs. Nonetheless, until a new basic food groups guide can be constructed, it fills a need for simple guidance.

The Exchange Lists Food Guide

In 1950 the American Diabetes Association and the American Dietetic Association introduced a quite different food guide, the Food Exchange Lists, as a meal-planning tool for managing diets for persons with diabetes. It was based on the unique concept of food exchange groups, with foods grouped on the basis of equivalent food values. In this exchange system of dietary management, since foods within each group are equal to one another in the portions indicated, group items could be freely exchanged within a given individual group and the planned diet in food values could be maintained. The freedom to exchange group foods also gave more variety of food choices. Since its introduction and initial follow-up revision in 1976, this food-groups guide has been widely used as a nutrition tool for diet calculations, meal planning, education, and counseling for many forms of diets.

In 1986 a major revision of the food exchange lists was published to reflect current nutrition and health promotion guidelines.[16] The basic six food groups have been completely reorganized: (1) starch/bread, (2) meat in three subgroups: lean, medium fat, and high fat, (3) vegetables, (4) fruits, (5) milk in three subgroups to reduce fat, and (6) fat in subgroups of unsaturated and saturated food sources. Three expanded lists were added: free foods and seasonings, combination foods, and foods for occasional use. In all groups, values for dietary fiber and sodium were identified and flagged. An interesting illustrated text accompanies the food lists in booklet form.[17] In both substance and style, this revised nutrition education tool combines current scien-

Table 1-2

Daily Food Guide—The
Basic Four Food Groups

Food group	Main nutrients	Daily amounts*
Milk Milk, cheese, ice cream, or other products made with whole or skimmed milk	Calcium Protein Riboflavin	Children under 9: 2-3 cups Children 9 to 12: 3 or more cups Teenagers: 4 or more cups Adults: 2 or more cups Pregnant women: 3 or more cups Nursing mothers: 4 or more cups (1 cup = 8 oz fluid milk or designated milk equivalent†)

Meats
 Beef, veal, lamb, pork, poultry, fish, eggs
 Alternates: dry beans and peas, nuts, peanut butter
	Protein
	 Iron
	 Thiamin
	 Niacin
	 Riboflavin
		2 or more servings
		 Count as 1 serving:
		   2-3 oz lean, boneless, cooked meat, poultry or fish
		   2 eggs
		   1 cup cooked dry beans or peas
		   4 tbsp peanut butter

Vegetables and fruits	Vitamin A
	 Vitamin C (ascorbic acid)
	 Smaller amounts of other vitamins and minerals
		4 or more servings
		 Count as 1 serving:
		   ½ cup vegetable or fruit or a portion such as 1 medium apple, banana, orange, potato, or half a medium grapefruit or melon
		 Include:
		   1 dark green or deep yellow vegetable or fruit rich in vitamin A, at least every other day
		   1 citrus or other fruit or vegetable rich in vitamin C daily
		   Other vegetables and fruits, including potatoes

Bread and cereals	Thiamin
	 Niacin
	 Riboflavin
	 Iron
	 Protein
		4 or more servings of whole-grain, enriched, or restored
		 Count as 1 serving:
		   1 slice bread
		   1 oz (a cup) ready-to-eat cereal, flake or puff varieties
		   ½-¾ cup cooked cereal
		   ½-¾ cup cooked pasta (macaroni, spaghetti, noodles)
		   Crackers: 5 saltines, 2 squares graham crackers, and so forth

*Use additional amounts of these foods or added butter, margarine, oils, sugars, and so forth as desired or needed.

†Milk equivalents: 1 oz cheddar cheese, 3 servings cottage cheese, 1 cup fluid skimmed milk, 1 cup buttermilk, ¼ cup dry skimmed milk powder, 1 cup ice milk, 1⅔ cup ice cream, ½ cup evaporated milk.

tific knowledge and practical diet planning. You will find these revised food exchange lists in the Appendix for your reference and use.

Health Promotion Guidelines

In recent years in the United States, several dietary guidelines for health promotion that reflect growing health concerns of government, professional groups, and the public have been issued. Three significant ones are given here: a general set of statements concerning a healthy diet and two specific sets of guidelines relating in turn to heart disease and cancer risks. Each of these guidelines has stimulated discussion of important nutrition and health issues. Each has been useful in nutrition education and counseling.

U.S. Dietary Guidelines

This basic set of dietary guidelines developed from increasing public interest in nutrition and health beginning in the 1960s and the resulting Senate investigations in the 1970s of hunger and nutrition in the United States. They are based on a growing concern about chronic health problems in an aging population and a rapidly changing food environment. The initial "U.S. Dietary Goals" of 1977 were revised somewhat and reissued jointly in 1985 by the U.S. Departments of Agriculture and of Health and Human Services under the title "Nutrition and Your Health: Dietary Guidelines for Americans." These seven statements (see the box on p. 20) emphasize health promotion through risk reduction and relate current scientific thinking to America's leading health problems.[18-20] Of course, no guideline can guarantee health, and people differ in their food needs. But these general statements can lead persons to evaluate their food habits and move toward basic improvements.

Dietary Guidelines for Heart Disease Prevention

Following the general dietary guidelines above, the nutrition committee of the American Heart Association published an initial report in 1982 outlining modifications in the American diet that, based on current research, would help reduce identified risk factors for coronary heart disease.[21] Subsequent reports have reinforced this diet-heart connection. From its beginning, these six guidelines have provided the basis for a "prudent diet," the name that has remained ever since:

1. **Total energy intake.** Adjust dietary kilocalorie (kcalorie) value sufficiently to maintain ideal body weight.
2. **Fats.** Reduce the total dietary fat kcalories to no more than 30% to 35% of the total kcalories. Of these total fat kcalories, saturated fat should contribute 10% or less, monounsaturated 15%, and polyunsaturated 10%.
3. **Carbohydrates.** Increase carbohydrate kcalories to replace reduced fat, with 50% to 55% of the total kcalories coming from carbohydrates. Of these total carbohydrate kcalories, complex carbohydrates (starches) should contribute the majority of 30% to 35%, with simple carbohydrates (sugars) limited to 10%.
4. **Proteins.** Use protein foods in moderation, about 12% to 20% of the diet's total kcalories, with less use of animal protein, which carries more fat.

Clinical Application

**Dietary Guidelines
for Americans**

Eat a variety of foods

About 40 different known nutrients, and probably additional as yet unknown factors, are needed to maintain health. No single food can supply all the essential nutrients in the amounts needed. Thus the greater the variety of foods used, the less likely a person is to develop either a deficiency or an excess of any single nutrient. One way to ensure variety, and with it a balanced diet, is to select foods each day from all the major food groups.

Maintain ideal weight

Excessive fatness is associated with some chronic disorders such as hypertension and diabetes, which in turn relate to heart disease. The "ideal" body weight, however, must be determined individually, for many factors are involved, such as body composition, body metabolism, genetics, and physical activity.

Avoid too much fat, saturated fat, and cholesterol

Americans as a population have traditionally consumed a high-fat diet. In some persons, excess fat leads to high levels of blood fats and cholesterol carried in lipoprotein compounds. Elevated serum levels of these fats and cholesterol are associated with a higher risk of coronary heart disease. Thus it is wise to cut down on fats in general, using them only in moderation.

Eat foods with adequate starch and fiber

Complex carbohydrate foods (starches) are better fuel sources for energy than are simple carbohydrates (sugars) and fats. Starches also contain many essential nutrients and kcalories needed for energy. With an increased use of processed and refined foods, the modern American diet is relatively low in dietary fiber. Increasing the use of less refined complex carbohydrates will help increase dietary fiber. Evidence exists that certain types of dietary fiber may help control chronic bowel diseases, contribute to improved blood glucose management for persons with diabetes mellitus, and bind dietary lipids such as cholesterol. Starches, especially forms with more dietary fiber, may therefore be sustained for some of the fats and sugars as energy sources.

Avoid too much sugar

The major health hazard from eating too much sugar is tooth decay (dental caries). Contrary to popular opinion, however, too much sugar does not in itself cause diabetes. It can only contribute to poor control of diabetes in persons who have inherited the disease. Most Americans consume a relatively large amount of sugar, over 100 pounds per person per year. Much of this sugar occurs in processed food products. Again, moderation is the key.

Avoid too much sodium

Excessive sodium is not healthy for anyone and certainly not for persons who have high blood pressure. In general, since many processed food products contain considerable sodium or salt and since most Americans eat more sodium than they need, it is wise to limit the use of these products, especially "salty" ones, and reduce added salt in food preparation. These practices will lower individual salt tastes, which are learned habits and not biologic necessities. There is ample sodium as a natural mineral in foods to meet usual needs.

If you drink alcohol, do so in moderation

Alcoholic beverages tend to be high in kcalories and low in other nutrients. Limited food intake may accompany large alcohol intake. Also, heavy drinking contributes to chronic liver disease and some neurologic disorders, as well as some throat and neck cancers. Thus moderation is the key, if alcohol is used at all.

5. **Cholesterol.** Limit dietary cholesterol to 300 mg or less per day, which is about half to one-third the amount in the usual American diet. Since cholesterol occurs *only* in animal food sources, mainly with fat tissues, this means fewer egg yolks, well-trimmed leaner meat in small portions, limited use of organ meats or processed meats, and use of nonfat dairy products.
6. **Sodium.** Limit the use of salt and salty foods. A reasonable limit of 2 to 3 g of sodium a day can be achieved by using salt only lightly in cooking, adding none at the table, and avoiding highly salted processed foods.

The American Heart Association provides a number of leaflets and booklets based on these prudent diet guidelines for use in diet counseling and meal planning. These principles have also been incorporated into a wide variety of "light cooking" recipe books and even restaurant menus.

Dietary Guidelines for Cancer Prevention

In the same year, 1982, the Committee on Diet, Nutrition, and Cancer also published its initial report based on what it called "interim" guidelines for reducing cancer risks.[22] Later reports by the American Cancer Society have reinforced these initial findings.[23,24] The following revised set of statements issued in 1985 comprises the American Cancer Society's current guidelines:

1. **Fats.** Reduce fat intake from its present level (approximately 40%) to 30% of the total diet's kcalories, and avoid obesity.
2. **Dietary fiber.** Include fruits, vegetables, and whole-grain cereals in the daily diet.

3. **Vitamins A and C.** Include foods rich in vitamins A and C in your daily diet.
4. **Cruciferous vegetables.** Include cruciferous vegetables frequently in your diet.
5. **Preserved food.** Limit use of food preserved by salt-curing (including salt pickling), smoking, or nitrite-curing.
6. **Alcohol.** Use alcoholic beverages in moderation, if at all.

The National Cancer Institute and the American Cancer Society have published a number of helpful materials based on these guidelines for use in nutrition education and counseling.

Plan of Study

Basic Objective

Throughout your beginning study of nutrition here, you will find that the basic objective of this book is twofold: (1) to provide a sound and concise introduction to the science of human nutrition and (2) to translate these principles into clear concepts and apply them to person-centered health care in everyday living and in clinical care.

Organization of Material

Part One—Introduction to Human Nutrition

In this first section of the text, the basic elements of the science of nutrition—the essential nutrients and their functions in the body—are introduced. These functions are developed around three fundamental problems of sustaining human life that nutrition solves: energy, tissue building, and regulation and control.

Part Two—Community Nutrition: the Life Cycle

Here the changing food environment and the web of factors that controls it are considered. These factors include influences on individual choices from available foods, cultural food patterns and nutrition education, age group needs throughout the life cycle, and health maintenance through physical fitness and weight management, as well as stress management.

Part Three—Introduction to Diet Therapy

Here the hospitalized patient, nutrition assessment and care-planning, including observations and patient education concerning some basic drug-nutrient interactions, are discussed. Then the person-centered approach applies basic principles of diet therapy and nutritional support in various disease situations.

Learning Tools for Study

To aid your study of human nutrition and its multiple applications in our lives both in health and disease, a number of learning tools are used throughout the text. Look for these study guides in each chapter as you proceed.

Chapter Preview and Learning Objectives

At the beginning of each chapter, a brief preview and some key learning objectives help set the scene, and visual attention is focused by a chapter theme photograph.

Concepts and Terms

Each idea is considered first in terms of basic principles or **concepts** involved, which are then applied to specific situations to help clarify meaning. Diagrams and line drawings further illustrate basic concepts. Words are important vehicles for communicating ideas in any body of knowledge. Here you will find many key words analyzed along with their derivations and meanings in practice. Many of these terms are pulled out into the margins for emphasis; a reference glossary is included at the book's end.

Concept
Combined ideas forming a whole.

Boxes: Further Probes and Clinical Applications

Abstract theory is of little practical value until it can be understood by examples and applications. It finds meaning only as it is related to key needs and problems. To extend your learning, then, numerous boxes—To Probe Further and Clinical Application—are inserted in each chapter text to guide your learning. Look for these nuggets of nutritional science applied to specific situations and needs.

Chapter Summaries and Review

At the end of each chapter you will find a brief succinct summary of the material presented. Using these To Sum Up sections and the following Questions for Review, you may review what you have read and organize your understanding of the principal concepts discussed.

Chapter References and Further Readings

Many specific current references from research, clinical work, conferences, and reviews are given at the end of each chapter to indicate source materials. These may stimulate your interest in going to the primary source for an even broader base of background knowledge of the topic discussed. In like manner, the Further Readings section provides an annotated listing of a few selected materials for additional reading.

Issues and Answers

Nutritional science is often controversial because it is constantly growing and developing. At the end of each chapter, the section Issues and Answers addresses questions or controversies related to the chapter topic in a pertinent article. This focus may help you seek current applications in your own experience, in your community, and in clinical situations and perhaps find some related answers and activities.

Reference Tools

At the end of the book's text, in addition to the glossary, more tools for reference are included in the various appendixes. Finally, an index is provided for quick location or cross-referencing of desired topics for study.

Results of this Approach to the Study of Nutrition

Growing evidence of linkages between diet and disease continue to bring increased awareness of the importance of nutrition in health care. Nutrition is playing a large role in the management of health problems and in the control of rising health care costs through its emphasis on health promotion and risk reduction and its extended work in team practice. Recognizing the importance of food and nutrition in health care will deepen and facilitate care of your own health and that of your families, clients, or patients.

To Sum Up

Basic issues in nutrition and health center on world nutrition needs, major U.S. health problems and their relation to nutrition, and methods of organizing effective health care systems to meet these problems.

World nutrition needs are inevitably linked to our own in the United States, since food security in underdeveloped countries is interrelated with world food markets, import-export policies, and our own food production and storage systems. The Food and Agriculture Organization (FAO) of the United Nations has a major responsibility in helping to coordinate work in many nations toward meeting world food security problems.

Our own major U.S. health problems include heart disease, cancer, and complications of diabetes and renal disease. All of these problems relate closely to nutrition. Wise approaches to health care must be person-centered, seeking to meet the needs of the whole person, both physical and psychosocial. This can best be done with a team approach that pursues the goal of health promotion and personal well-being.

Tools for use in building sound nutritional practices involve nutrient standards for populations, food guides for individual use, and specific dietary guidelines for reducing health risks. U.S. tools involve the RDAs, food groups and exchange lists for meal planning, and dietary guidelines for making wise food choices to promote health and reduce health risks.

Questions for Review

1. Name some major causes of world food problems. What is the work of the FAO in helping to solve some of the food security problems of poorer nations? How effective do you think this work is?
2. What are some of the main world health problems resulting from lack of food? How do you think these problems can be solved? What role do you think we have, on both a national and personal level, in dealing with these problems?
3. What are the major U.S. health problems? What do you know about the possible relationships of nutrition to these problems?
4. What values do you see in the health team approach to patient care?
5. Compare the various nutritional guides for health in terms of nature and development, purpose, and appropriate use in health care.

References

1. Monsen ER: The dietitian as the nutrition counselor, J Am Diet Assoc 89(1):43, 1989.
2. Haan M, Kaplan GA, and Camacho T: Poverty and health: prospective evidence from the Alameda County Study, Am J Epidemiol 125:989, June 1987.
3. Hogue CJR and others: Overview of the National Infant Mortality Surveillance (NIMS) project—design, methods, results, Pub Health Reports 102:126, March/April 1987.
4. Physician Task Force on Hunger in America: The growing epidemic, Cambridge, Mass, 1985, Harvard University Press.
5. American Dietetic Association: Hunger—worldwide problem, J Am Diet Assoc 86(10):1414, 1986.
6. Miller SA and Stephenson MG: The 1990 national nutrition objectives: lessons for the future, J Am Diet Assoc 87(12):1665, 1987.
7. Shields M: A portrait of America, Newsweek, p 20, Jan 17, 1983.

8. Report: DRGs and the Prospective Payment System: a guide for physicians, Chicago, 1984, American Medical Association.

9. Stern RS and Epstein AM: Institutional responses to prospective payment based on diagnosis-related groups: implications for cost, quality, and access, N Engl J Med 312:621, 1985.

10. Huyck NI and Fairchild MM: Provision of clinical nutrition services by diagnosis-related groups (DRGs) and major diagnostic categories (MDCs), J Am Diet Assoc 87(1):69, 1987.

11. Blackburn SA and Himburg SP: Nutrition care activities and DRGs, J Am Diet Assoc 87(11):1535, 1987.

12. Haughton B, Gussow JD, and Dodds JM: An historical study of the underlying assumptions for United States food guides from 1917 through the Basic Four Food Groups Guide, J Nutr Ed 19(4):169, 1987.

13. Food and Nutrition Board, National Academy of Sciences—National Research Council: Recommended dietary allowances, ed 9, Washington, DC, 1980, The Academy Press.

14. Marshall E: The Academy kills a nutrition report, Science 230:420, Oct 25, 1985.

15. Food and Nutrition Board, National Research Council: Recommended dietary allowances: scientific issues and process for the future, J Nutr 116:482, March 1986.

15a. Food and Nutrition Board, National Academy of Sciences—National Research Council: Recommended dietary allowances, ed 10, Washington, DC, 1989, The Academy Press.

16. Franz MJ and others: Exchange lists: revised 1986, J Am Diet Assoc 87(1):28, 1987.

17. Exchange lists for meal planning, Chicago, 1986, American Dietetic Association and American Diabetes Association.

18. Dietary Guidelines Advisory Committee reports, Nutr Today 20(3):8, 1985.

19. Miller SA and Stephenson MG: Scientific and public rationale for the dietary guidelines for Americans, Am J Clin Nutr 42:739, 1985.

20. ADA Reports: Statement on nutrition and your health: dietary guidelines for Americans, J Am Diet Assoc 86(1):107, 1986.

21. American Heart Association Nutrition Committee: Rationale of the diet-heart statement of the AHA, Arteriosclerosis 4:177, 1982.

22. Committee on Diet, Nutrition and Cancer: diet, nutrition and cancer, Washington, DC, 1982, National Academy Press.

23. Newell GR: Cancer prevention: update for physicians, four years later, Cancer Bull 37:103, 1985.

24. 1986 Cancer facts and figures, New York, 1986, American Cancer Society.

Further Readings

Bright-See E: Diet and prevention of cancer: the state of knowledge and current dietary recommendations, J Can Diet Assoc 48:13, Feb 1987.
This author compares dietary guidelines for cancer prevention in Canada, the United States, and Europe, and finds general agreement among them. Background research supporting these guidelines is reviewed, and the issue of whether recommendations should be made in the current state of knowledge is examined.

Califano JA: America's health care revolution: health promotion and disease prevention, J Am Diet Assoc 87(4):437, 1987.
This former Secretary of Health and Human Services describes the background of changing health care in the United States and the role of nutrition in these changing practices.
Dietary Guidelines Advisory Committee reports, Nutr Today 20(3):8, 1985.

This is the full report of the Advisory Committee appointed to review and revise the U.S. dietary guidelines, with extensive references for each one.

Kline K: Breast cancer: the diet-cancer connection, Nutr Today 21(3):11, 1986.

This author uses breast cancer to make the case for widely held views concerning the relationships between food, nutrition, and cancer, with a special focus on high-fat diets.

Neville J and Catakis A: ADA and Foundation command strong presence in international dietetics, J Am Diet Assoc 88(7):785, 1988.

This report of expanding activities between the American Dietetic Association and nutrition organizations in different countries indicates the need for strengthening the network of international dietetics to help solve some of the current world nutrition problems.

Pennington JAT: Associations between diet and health: the use of food consumption measurements, nutrient databases, and dietary guidelines, J Am Diet Assoc 88(10):1221, 1988.

This nutritionist-scientist at the Center for Food Safety and Applied Nutrition of the U.S. Food and Drug Administration describes approaches used to study possible relationships between diet and the health of Americans.

Stephenson MG: The 1990 national objectives for improved nutrition, J Nutr Ed 19(4):155, 1987.

This nutritionist with the Food and Drug Administration, the leading U.S. Public Health Service agency designated to coordinate work in the area of improved nutrition, reviews current progress toward each nutrition objective in the 1990 national health goals and outlines the work underway for developing objectives for the year 2000.

Wodarski LA, Bundschuk E, and Forbus WR: Interdisciplinary case management: a model for intervention, J Am Diet Assoc 88(3):323, 1988.

These authors use the model of Prader-Willi syndrome, a complex multisystem disorder of childhood, to describe the team approach to comprehensive and continuing health care and the role of nutrition in this team care.

If You're Not Healthy, It's Your Own Fault!

Some critics of the current health promotion/self-care movement, concerned with maintaining the traditional medical model of patient care, are once again blaming the victim for health problems. This is a misplaced accusation. It apparently started in the 1970s, when the public and practitioners alike became increasingly alarmed at the soaring costs of health care and sought ways in which individuals could cut their chances of being ill. The result was the now-growing field of preventive health care.

Many preventive health care practitioners are sensitive, skilled professionals who have used different methods of sharing their knowledge and skills with the public:

- Identification of risks
- Patient education regarding special illnesses
- Medical self-care
- Alternatives to traditional medical care (e.g., holistic health)
- Promotion of "wellness" as a state of mind or an attitude

Their task has not been easy because (1) their recommendations are often taken over and redefined by business opportunists; (2) there are no guarantees that every recommendation will achieve the same results (e.g., everyone who jogs 10 miles a day does not escape heart disease); (3) our culture stresses "antihealth" habits (e.g., availability of high-sodium convenience foods, high alcohol use, and overeating promoted by the media); and (4) health activists are viewed as attempting to impose their personal value system on others.

However, recommendations of some of these practitioners are not based on solid research and tend to yield inconsistent results. Because these "opinions" almost always involve the personal habits of the client, the "wellness" promoter *is* in effect telling persons that it's their fault if they're sick—they don't eat the "right" foods, they aren't keeping their weight down, they smoke/drink too much, they even *think* too

much. In doing so they may be confusing the issue:

- Is it really the 16-year-old's fault that he eats too much when, in his lifetime, he's seen over 300,000 television commercials, most of which advertise readily available food?
- Is it the fault of the working woman that she relies on high-sodium/high-fat convenience foods to feed her family?
- Is the low-income patient with no recreation available other than meal preparation totally at fault for obesity?

Health professionals who have improved their own health because of wellness practices can contribute to the wellness of their patients. They can teach those same health-promoting ideas nonjudgmentally, rather than concentrating *only* on the "challenge" of illness. Otherwise, if the "victim" role is reinforced, circumstances that created vulnerability to poor health are perpetuated and legitimized, and further attempts to help are often turned down. To avoid this type of situation:

Examine personal value systems Is my own work designed to point a finger at the victim or to truly help the client help himself?

Consider every aspect of the client Is it really within my client's power to control food intake at home? What social, financial, or other factors may be limiting choice of foods or activities other than eating?

Be realistic If current research is not conclusive, do I avoid presenting recommendations as being "failure-proof"?

Practitioners may benefit in their health promotion activities by determining which persons may be open to such approaches and which may not. Researchers have used a health-promoting life-style profile to investigate patterns of health behavior and the effects of efforts to change these behaviors. They identified six

Continued.

If You're Not Healthy, It's Your Own Fault—cont'd

areas involved in these behaviors that should be considered in working with each client: (1) degree of health responsibility, (2) capacity for self-fulfillment, (3) exercise capacity and amount, (4) nutritional status and problems, (5) interpersonal support, and (6) capacity for coping with stress. As a result of these studies, a useful checklist of positive health behaviors was constructed. Items concerned with nutrition focused on meal patterns and food choices.

REFERENCES

Dismuke SE and Miller ST: Why not share the secrets of good health? JAMA 249(23):3181, 1983.

Walker SN, Sechrist KR, and Pender NJ: The health-promoting lifestyle: development and psychometric characteristics, Nurs Res 36:76, March/April 1987.

2 Digestion, Absorption, and Metabolism

After studying this chapter, the student should be able to:

1. Identify the processes by which food is prepared for the body's use and determine why this preparation is necessary.

2. Describe integrated work of specific muscles and secretions in this task.

3. Relate the roles of the nervous and endocrine systems to this work.

4. Relate specific intestinal structures to the task of nutrient absorption.

5. Identify basic cell processes and agents that yield fuels and building materials to sustain and nourish the whole body.

Chapter Objectives

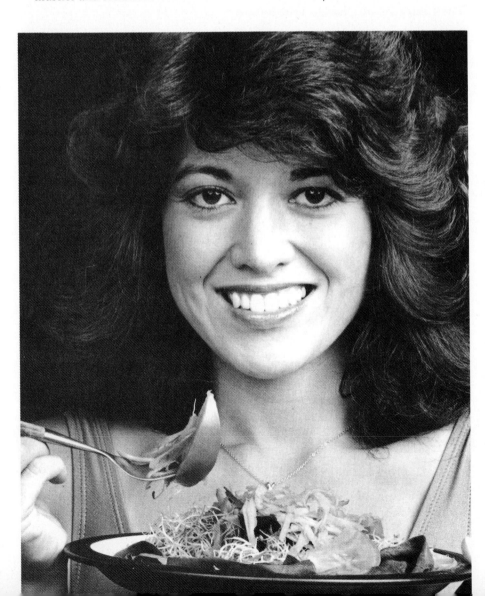

PREVIEW

■

A health worker's knowledge of the process of breaking down the food we eat and carrying its vital nutrients to all the body cells can be an important foundation for conveying scientifically sound information about nutrition. Thus here at the beginning of your study of the nutrients we will use this framework for introducing the individual nutrients and look first at the integrated overall body system that handles them.

This unique system of organ structures and functions uses the fuels we consume in our food to energize and empower our bodies. This marvelous physiologic process consists of three integrated events: digestion, absorption, and metabolism. But here, as you review these three processes separately, remember that they are highly interrelated. They are not functioning singly but as one continuum—a *dynamic whole* that gives us life.

The Human Body as a Dynamic Whole

The Concepts of Change and Balance

Through a successive interrelated system of balanced change, the foods we eat must be transformed into simpler substances and then into other, still simpler, substances that our cells can use to sustain life. All these many changes prepare food for use by the body. Together they constitute the overall digestion-absorption-metabolism process.

The Concept of Wholeness
Body Integrity

The parts of this overall process of change do not exist separately. Rather they comprise one continuous *whole*. Look carefully at the respective components of the gastrointestinal tract and their relative position in this overall body system (Figure 2-1). In your review here, follow the fate of food components as they travel *together* through the successive parts of the gastrointestinal tract and into the body cells. This fundamental body system has indeed rightly been called "the portal to nutrient utilization."[1]

Reasons for Human Life Systems

Why is this intricate complex of activities so necessary to human life? Two reasons are apparent: (1) *Food* as it naturally occurs and as we eat it is not a single component but a mixture of substances. If these substances are to release their stored energy and building materials for use, they must be separated into their respective components so that the body may handle each one as a separate unit. (2) *Nutrients* released from food may still remain unavailable to the body, and some additional means of changing their forms must follow. The intermediate units must be broken down, simplified, regrouped, and rerouted. This complex chemical work must take place because the human being, whose life is developed and sustained in a dynamic internal chemical environment, is the most highly organized and intricately balanced of all organisms. This view of the human body as an integrated physiochemical organism is basic to an understanding of human nutrition, both in health and in disease.[2]

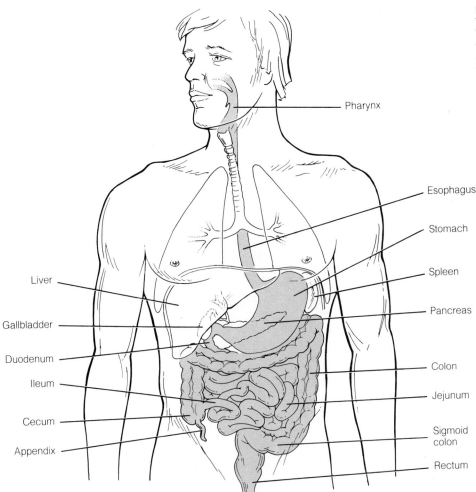

Figure 2-1
The gastrointestinal system. Through the successive parts of the system, multiple activities of digestion liberate and re-form food nutrients to our use.

Pharynx

Esophagus

Stomach

Spleen

Pancreas

Liver

Gallbladder

Duodenum

Ileum

Cecum

Appendix

Colon

Jejunum

Sigmoid colon

Rectum

Digestion initially prepares the food for the body's use. Two basic types of action are involved: (1) *mechanical* or muscular activity and (2) *chemical* or enzymatic activity.

Gastrointestinal Motility

Mechanical digestion takes place through a number of neuromuscular, self-regulating processes. These actions work together to move the food mass along the alimentary tract at the best rate for digestion and absorption of the nutrients to occur.

Types of Muscles

Four types of muscle in the stomach and intestine contribute to this necessary motility:
1. **Contractile rings.** A layer of circular contractile muscle rings break up, mix, and churn the food particles.
2. **Longitudinal muscles.** Long, smooth muscles help propel the food mass along the tract.

Basic Principles of Digestion

Digestion
Process by which food is broken down chemically in the gastrointestinal tract through the action of secretions containing specific enzymes. Digestion separates complex food structures into their simpler parts, which are the chemicals needed by the body to sustain life.

3. **Sphincter muscles.** Muscle rings at strategic points act as valves—pyloric, ileocecal, and anal—to control passage of materials to the next segments of the intestine.
4. **Mucosal muscles.** A thin layer of smooth muscle raises intestinal folds to increase the absorbing surface area.

Types of Muscle Action

The interaction of these four types of muscles produces two basic types of movement: (1) a general muscle tone or tonic contraction that ensures continuous passage and valve control and (2) periodic, rhythmic contractions that mix and propel the food mass. These alternating muscular contractions and relaxations that force the contents forward are known as *peristalsis.*

Nervous System Control

Specific nerves regulate these muscular actions. An interrelated network of nerves within the gastrointestinal wall, called the **intramural nerve plexus** (Figure 2-2), extends from the esophagus to the anus. This network controls muscle tone of the gastrointestinal wall, regulates the rate and intensity of muscle contractions, and coordinates the various movements.

Gastrointestinal Secretions

Food is digested chemically by the combined action of a number of secretions. Generally these secretions are of four types:
1. **Enzymes.** Specific kind and quantity break down specific nutrients.
2. **Hydrochloric acid and buffer ions.** These agents produce the necessary pH for the activity of given enzymes.
3. **Mucus.** This agent lubricates and protects the inside wall tissues of the gastrointestinal tract and facilitates food mass passage.
4. **Water and electrolytes.** These agents provide a balanced solution base in sufficient volumes to circulate the organic substances released.

Special cells in the mucosal tissue of the gastrointestinal tract or in adjacent accessory organs, especially the pancreas, produce these secretions. The secretory action of these cells or glands is stimulated by the intake of food, by the sensory nerve network, or by hormones specific for certain nutrients.

Intramural nerve plexus
Network of interwoven nerve structures within a particular organ. The action of smooth muscle layers comprising the gastrointestinal wall is controlled by such a network of nerve fibers.

Digestion in the Mouth and Esophagus

Mechanical Digestion
Mastication

Initial biting and chewing begins the breaking up of food into smaller particles. The teeth and other oral structures are particularly suited for this function. The incisors cut; the molars grind. Tremendous force is supplied by the jaw muscles. Mastication makes possible an enlarged surface area of food for constant enzyme action. Also, the fineness of the food particles eases the continued passage of material through the gastrointestinal tract.

Swallowing

The mixed mass of food particles is swallowed and passes down the esophagus largely by perstaltic waves controlled by nerve reflexes. Muscles at the base of the tongue aid the process of swallowing and, in the upright position, gravity aids the movement of food down the esophagus.

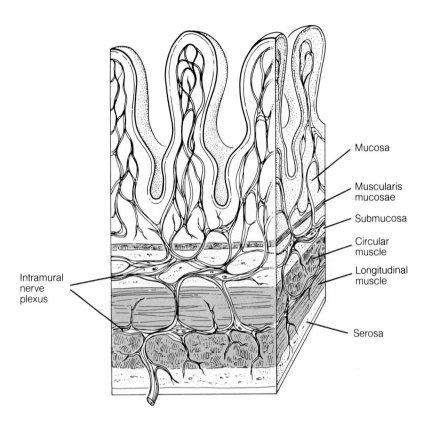

Figure 2-2
Innervation of the intestine by intramural nerve plexus.

Mucosa

Muscularis mucosae

Submucosa

Circular muscle

Longitudinal muscle

Serosa

Intramural nerve plexus

Entry into the Stomach

At the point of entry into the stomach, the *gastroesophageal constrictor muscle* relaxes to allow food to enter. Then it contracts again to prevent regurgitation of stomach contents up into the esophagus. When regurgitation does occur, through failure of this mechanism, the person feels it as "heartburn." Two clinical problems may hinder normal food passage at this point: (1) *cardiospasm,* caused by failure of the constrictor muscle to relax properly or (2) *hiatal hernia,* caused by protrusion of the upper part of the stomach into the thorax through an abnormal opening of the diaphragm.

Chemical or Secretory Digestion

In the mouth, three pairs of salivary glands—*parotid, submaxilary,* and *sublingual*—secrete serous material containing *salivary amylase (ptyalin).* This is an enzyme specific for starches. Mucus is also secreted to lubricate and bind the food particles. Stimuli such as sight, smell, taste, and touch—and even thoughts of likes and dislikes in food—greatly influence these secretions. Food remains in the mouth only a short time, so starch digestion here by ptyalin is brief and is terminated by the more acid medium of the stomach.

Salivary secretions: 1000 to 1500 mL/day; pH range around neutral or 6.0 to 7.0.

Mechanical Digestion

The major parts of the stomach are shown in Figure 2-3. Muscles in the stomach wall provide three basic motor functions: storage, mixing, and controlled emptying. As the food mass enters the stomach, it lies against the stomach walls, which can stretch outward to store as much as 1 L. Gradually

Digestion in the Stomach

Gastric secretions: 2000 mL/day; acid pH around 2.0.

Figure 2-3
Stomach.

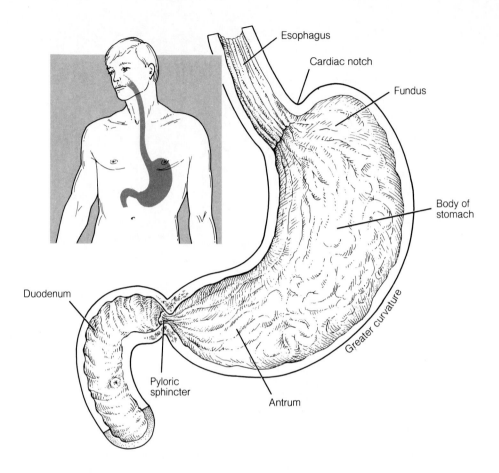

local tonic muscle waves increase their kneading and mixing action as the mass of food and secretions moves on toward the pyloric valve at the distal end of the stomach. Here waves of peristaltic contractions reduce the mass to a semifluid *chyme*. Finally, with each wave, small amounts of chyme are forced through the pyloric valve. This sphincter muscle constricts and periodically relaxes then constricts again to control the emptying of the stomach contents into the duodenum. This control releases the acid chyme slowly enough to be buffered by the alkaline intestinal secretions. The caloric density of a meal, in addition to its particular volume and composition, influences the rate of stomach emptying.[1]

Chemical or Secretory Digestion
Types of Secretion

Stomach secretions contain three basic types of materials: acid, mucus, and enzymes:

1. **Acid.** Hydrochloric acid is produced to prepare certain enzymes and materials for digestion and absorption by creating the necessary degree of acidity for given enzymes to work.
2. **Mucus.** Special mucous secretions protect the stomach lining from the eroding effect of the acid. This **mucus** also binds and mixes the food mass and helps move it along.

Mucus
Viscid fluid secreted by mucous membranes and glands, consisting mainly of mucin (a glycoprotein), inorganic salts, and water.

3. **Enzymes.** The main enzyme in the stomach is *pepsin,* which begins the breakdown of protein. It is first secreted in the inactive form *pepsinogen,* which is then activated by the hydrochloric acid present. A small amount of *gastric lipase (tributyrinase)* is present and works on emulsified fats such as butterfat. This is a relatively minor activity, however. In childhood an enzyme called *rennin* (not to be confused with the vital lifelong renal enzyme *renin*) is also present in gastric secretions to aid in the coagulation of milk. However, in adults rennin is absent.

Control of Secretions

Stimuli for these gastric secretions come from two sources:

1. **Nerve stimulus** is produced in response to the senses, ingested food, and emotions. For example, anger and hostility increase secretions. Fear and depression decrease secretions and inhibit blood flow and motility as well.
2. **Hormonal stimulus** is produced in response to the entrance of food into the stomach. Certain stimulants, especially caffeine, alcohol, and meat extractives, cause the release of a local hormone **gastrin** from mucosal cells in the antrum, which in turn stimulates the secretion of more hydrochloric acid. When the pH reaches 2.0, a feedback mechanism stops further secretion of the hormone to prevent excess acid formation. Another local hormone, **enterogastrone,** produced by glands in the duodenal mucosa, counteracts excessive gastric activity by inhibiting acid and pepsin secretion and gastric motility.

Mechanical Digestion

Intestinal Muscle Layers

Note the exquisite structural arrangement of the intestinal wall shown in Figure 2-4. Finely coordinated intestinal motility is achieved by the three basic

Gastrin
Hormone secreted by mucosal cells in the antrum of the stomach that stimulates the parietal cells to produce hydrochloric acid.

Enterogastrone
Hormone produced by glands in the duodenal mucosa that counteracts excessive gastric activity by inhibiting acid and pepsin secretion and gastric motility.

Digestion in the Small Intestine

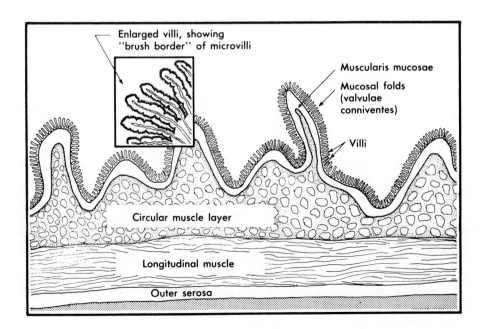

Enlarged villi, showing "brush border" of microvilli

Muscularis mucosae

Mucosal folds (valvulae conniventes)

Villi

Circular muscle layer

Longitudinal muscle

Outer serosa

Figure 2-4
Intestinal wall. Note the arrangement of muscle layers and structures of mucosa that increase surface area for absorption—mucosal folds, villi, and microvilli.

layers of muscle: (1) the thin layer of smooth muscle, the mucosa or *muscularis mucosa,* with fibers extending up into the villi; (2) the circular muscle layer; and (3) the longitudinal muscle next to the outer serosa.

Types of Intestinal Muscle Actions

Under the control of the nerve plexus, wall-stretch pressure from food, or hormonal stimuli, these muscles produce several different types of movement to aid digestion:

1. **Segmentation contractions** of circular muscle rings progressively chop the food into successive **boluses,** mixing food and secretions.
2. **Longitudinal rotation** of the long muscle running the length of the intestine rolls the slowly moving food mass in a spiral motion, mixing it and exposing new surfaces for absorption.
3. **Pendular movements** of small local muscle contractions sweep back and forth and stir the chyme at the mucosal surface.
4. **Peristalsis** produces waves by contracting deep circular muscle, propelling the food mass slowly forward. The intensity of the wave may be increased by food intake or by the presence of irritants, causing in some cases long sweeping waves over the entire intestine.
5. **Villi motions** constantly sweep the mucosal surface with alternating contractions and extensions of mucosal muscle fibers. This action agitates the mucosal surface, stirring and mixing chyme in contact with the intestinal wall and exposing additional nutrient material for absorption.

Chemical Digestion

Major Role of Small Intestine

More than any other part of the entire gastrointestinal tract, the small intestine carries the major burden of chemical digestion. Thus this area secretes a large number of enzymes, each specific for some member of the macronutrients—carbohydrates, fats, and proteins. These specific enzymes are secreted from both the intestinal glands and the pancreas. They are summarized in Table 2-1.

Types of Secretions

Four basic types of digestive secretions complete this final process of chemical breakdown in the small intestine:

1. **Enzymes.** A number of specific enzymes, as indicated in Table 2-1, act on specific nutrients to bring the final breaking down of the nutrient materials in food to forms the body can absorb and use.

2. **Mucus.** Intestinal glands located immediately inside the duodenum secrete large quantities of mucus. This secretion protects the mucosa from irritation and digestion by the highly acid gastric juices at this point. Additional mucous cells on the intestinal surface continue to secrete mucus when touched by the moving food mass. This secretion lubricates and protects the tissues.

3. **Hormone.** In response to the presence of acid in the entering food mass, mucosal cells in the upper part of the small intestine produce a hormone called **secretin.** In turn, secretin then stimulates the pancreas to send alkaline pancreatic juices into the duodenum to buffer the entering gastric acid chyme. The unprotected intestinal mucosa alone at this point could not withstand this high degree of acidity.

Bolus
Rounded mass of food ready to swallow or a mass passing through the gastrointestinal tract.

Combined secretions of the mucous glands of the intestine and pancreas total about 2400 mL daily.

Secretin
Hormone produced in the mucous membrane of the duodenum in response to the entrance of the acid contents of the stomach into the duodenum.

Table 2-1
Summary of Digestive Processes

Nutrient	Mouth	Stomach	Small intestine
Carbohydrate	Starch $\xrightarrow{\text{Ptyalin}}$ Dextrins		**Pancreas** Starch $\xrightarrow{\text{Amylase}}$ (Disaccharides) Maltose and sucrose **Intestine** Lactose $\xrightarrow{\text{Lactase}}$ (Monosaccharides) Glucose and galactose Sucrose $\xrightarrow{\text{Sucrase}}$ Glucose and fructose Maltose $\xrightarrow{\text{Maltase}}$ Glucose and glucose
Protein		Protein $\xrightarrow[\text{Hydrochloric acid}]{\text{Pepsin}}$ Polypeptides	**Pancreas** Proteins, Polypeptides $\xrightarrow{\text{Trypsin}}$ Dipeptides Proteins, Polypeptides $\xrightarrow{\text{Chrymotrypsin}}$ Dipeptides Polypeptides, Dipeptides $\xrightarrow{\text{Carboxypeptidase}}$ Amino acids **Intestine** Polypeptides, Dipeptides $\xrightarrow{\text{Aminopeptidase}}$ Amino acids Dipeptides $\xrightarrow{\text{Dipeptidase}}$ Amino acids
Fat		Tributyrin $\xrightarrow{\text{Tributyrinase}}$ Glycerol (butterfat) Fatty acids	**Pancreas** Fats $\xrightarrow{\text{Lipase}}$ Glycerol Glycerides (di-, mono-) Fatty acids **Intestine** Fats $\xrightarrow{\text{Lipase}}$ Glycerol Glycerides (di-, mono-) Fatty acids **Liver and Gallbladder** Fats $\xrightarrow{\text{Bile}}$ Emulsified fat

4. **Bile.** Another important aid to digestion and absorption in the small intestine is bile, since it is an emulsifying agent for fats (see the box on p. 39). A large volume of bile is produced in the liver as a dilute watery solution. It is then concentrated and stored by the gallbladder. When fat enters the duodenum, the hormone *cholecystokinin* is secreted by glands in the intestinal mucosa and stimulates the gallbladder to contract and release the needed bile.

Factors Influencing Secretions

Here in the small intestine, as well as in other sections of the system, many factors influence various secretions. These factors include controls by hormones and nerve plexus, stimulated by physical contact with the food materials and by emotions. These influencing factors are summarized in Figure 2-5.

Figure 2-5
Summary of factors influencing secretions of the gastrointestinal tract.

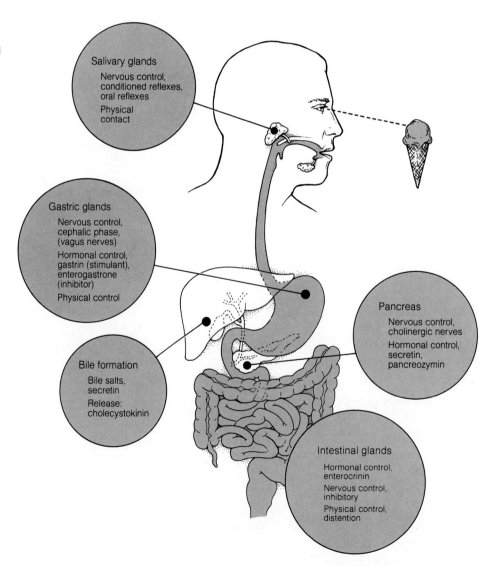

Salivary glands

Nervous control, conditioned reflexes, oral reflexes

Physical contact

Gastric glands

Nervous control, cephalic phase, (vagus nerves)

Hormonal control, gastrin (stimulant), enterogastrone (inhibitor)

Physical control

Bile formation

Bile salts, secretin

Release: cholecystokinin

Pancreas

Nervous control, cholinergic nerves

Hormonal control, secretin, pancreozymin

Intestinal glands

Hormonal control, enterocrinin

Nervous control, inhibitory

Physical control, distention

To Probe Further

The efficiency of the enterohepatic circulation of bile salts between the small intestine and the liver demonstrates the body's amazing ability to conserve materials needed for its basic functions. These built-in conservation systems, because they maintain their own balance, are called *homeostatic mechanisms.* They are specifically designed to sustain life in a relatively stable state of equilibrium among the multitude of interdependent elements and subsystems that make up the human organism.

For example, of the 20 to 30 g of bile acids circulated daily in the body to aid in the digestion and absorption of fats, only about 0.8 g is lost in the feces. Therefore only this small amount needs to be replaced daily by newly synthesized bile. After its tasks in digestion and absorption of fat—emulsifying and transporting—are completed, the bile is separated from its fat complex, returned to the liver, and recirculated again and again.

The Enterohepatic Circulation of Bile

End Products of Digestion

After digestion of the food nutrients is complete, the simplified end products are ready for **absorption,** aided by a number of transport mechanisms. The end products include the *monosaccharides* glucose, fructose, and galactose from carbohydrates; *fatty acids* and *glycerides* from fats; and *amino acids* from proteins. In some cases, incompletely digested nutrients, such as lactose in the absence of lactase, remain in the intestine and cause problems. (See Issues and Answers on p. 50.) Some small peptides may be absorbed intact and finally broken down to amino acids within the mucosal absorptive cells. Vitamins and minerals are also liberated. Finally, with a water base for solution and transport plus necessary electrolytes, the total fluid food mass is now prepared for absorption as part of the large gastrointestinal circulation (Table 2-2).

Absorption in the Small Intestine
Surface Structures

Viewed from the outside, the intestine appears smooth, but the inner mucosal surface lining is quite different. Refer again to Figure 2-4, and note the three types of convolutions and projections that greatly enhance the absorbing surface area: (1) *mucosal folds* similar to hills and valleys in a mountain range, which are easily seen by the naked eye; (2) *villi* or finger-like projections on these folds, which can be seen through a simple microscope; and (3) *microvilli* or extremely small projections on each villus, which can be seen only with an electron microscope. The array of **microvilli** covering the edge of each villus is called the *brush border* because it looks like bristles on a brush. Each villus has an ample network of blood capillaries and a central lymph vessel called a *lacteal* because the fat substances it absorbs have a creamy, milk-like appearance at this point.

Absorption

Absorption
Process by which digested food materials pass through epithelial cells of the alimentary canal (mainly of the small intestine) into the blood or lymph.

Microvilli
Minute surface projections that cover the edge of each intestinal villus, visible only though the electron microscope. This vast array of microvilli on each villus is called the "brush border." The microvilli add a tremendous surface area for absorption.

Table 2-2

Daily Absorption Volume in Human Gastrointestinal System

	Intake (L)	Intestinal absorption (L)	Elimination (L)
Food ingested	1.5		
Gastrointestinal secretions	8.5		
TOTAL	10.0		
Fluid absorbed in small intestine		9.5	
Fluid absorbed in large intestine		0.4	
TOTAL		9.9	
Feces			0.1

Absorbing Surface Area

The three structures of the small intestine—mucosal folds, villi, and microvilli—increase the inner absorbing surface area some 600 times over that of the outside serosa. These special structures, plus the contracted length of the live organ (630 to 660 cm, or 21 to 22 ft), produce a tremendously large absorbing surface. This inner surface of the small intestine, if stretched out flat, would be as large or larger than half a basketball court. All three of these mucosal structures serve as a unit for the absorption of nutrients. Although the intestine is popularly known as the lowly "gut," it is actually one of the most highly developed, exquisitely fashioned, specialized tissues in the human body.

Mechanisms of Absorption

Absorption is accomplished through the wall of the small intestine by means of a number of transport processes. These include passive diffusion and osmosis, active carrier-mediated diffusion, energy-driven active transport, and penetration by engulfment or pinocytosis. Some transport mechanisms are often called "pumps" (see the box on the facing page). For example, glucose is absorbed largely by a so-called sodium-potassium pump mechanism of active transport.

Routes of Absorption

After their absorption by these various processes, the nutrients from carbohydrates and proteins, being water soluble, enter the portal blood stream directly and travel to the liver and other body tissues. Only fat, not being water-soluble, is unique in its route. After being carried in a bile complex into the cells of the intestinal wall, and enzyme-processed there to human lipid compounds, fats are largely converted to a complex with protein as a carrier, packaged as *lipoproteins*. These packages flow into the lymph, empty into the **cisterna chyli,** then travel upward into the chest through the thoracic duct, and finally flow into the venous blood at the left subclavian vein. Then these

Cisterna chyli
Dilated sac at the origin of the thoracic duct, which is the common trunk that receives all the lymphatic vessels.

To Probe Further

"Pumping" Mechanisms for Absorbing Nutrients

Various nutrients cross absorbing membranes by biologic devices called *pumps*. The use of the word *pump* for this type of absorbing mechanism may be confusing at first. But it is a helpful term when you think about it.

Remember that what makes a pump pump is the *threat of vacuum*, a situation that cannot exist in biologic organisms. A pump pulls material from one place to another by the exercise of negative pressure. The pump is able to "suck" material from one place to another because the new site *cannot endure the absence of material*.

It is from this characteristic of nature that biochemists and physiologists have adapted the name *pump*. The empty site's absolute necessity for something to fill its space provides the impetus to move molecules across membranes. A biochemical "pumping mechanism" is one that works by pulling a fresh molecule in to fill a place that has been emptied by the removal of a molecule that was formerly present.

---

initial lipoproteins, called *chylomicrons* from their large fat load just absorbed, are rapidly cleared from the blood by a special fat enzyme, *lipoprotein lipase*. Current research is beginning to unfold the structure and function of this unique and vital enzyme in the body's handling of fat.[3] Exceptions to this route of fat absorption are the medium-chain and short-chain fatty acids, which are more water soluble and hence absorbed directly into blood circulation. However, most of the fats in the human diet are made of long-chain fatty acids, are not water soluble, and must travel the lacteal lymphatic route described.

Absorption in the Large Intestine (Colon)
Water Absorption

Absorption of water is the main task remaining for the large intestine. Related nutrient factors are involved, such as minerals, vitamins, amino acids, intestinal bacteria, and nondigestible dietary fiber. Within a 24-hour period about 500 ml of the remaining food mass leaves the *ileum*, the last portion of the small intestine, and enters the *cecum*, the pouch at the start of the large intestine. Here the *ileocecal valve* controls passage of the semiliquid chyme. Normally the valve remains closed, but each perstaltic wave relaxes the valve and squirts a small amount of chyme into the cecum. This mechanism holds the food mass in the small intestine long enough to ensure digestion and absorption of vital nutrients.

The watery chyme continues to move slowly through the large intestine, aided by mucous secretion from mucosal glands and muscle contractions. The major portion of the water in the chyme, 350 to 400 ml, is absorbed in the first half of the colon. Only about 100 to 150 ml remains to form the feces.

This food residue mass now begins to slow its passage. Usually a meal, having traveled the 630 to 660 cm (21 to 22 ft) of the small intestine, starts to enter the cecum about 4 hours after it is consumed. About 8 hours later it reaches the sigmoid colon, having traveled about 90 cm (3 ft) through the large intestine. In the sigmoid colon the residue descends still more slowly toward the anus. Even 72 hours after a meal, as much as 25% of it may still remain in the rectum.

Mineral Absorption

Iron from meat sources is absorbed more readily than iron from plant foods.

Electrolytes, mainly sodium, are transported into the blood stream from the colon. Intestinal absorption is a major balance control point for many of the minerals, and much of the dietary intake remains unabsorbed for elimination in the feces. For example, 20% to 70% of the ingested calcium is eliminated here and 80% to 85% of the iron.

Vitamin Absorption and Bacterial Action

Intestinal absorption also serves as a balance control point for some of the vitamins, determining how much the body will keep and how much it will excrete.[4] In addition, colon bacteria are closely associated with a number of vitamins. For example, colon bacteria synthesize vitamin K and some vitamins of the B-complex, which are then absorbed from the colon to help meet daily needs. At birth the colon is sterile, but very shortly intestinal bacterial flora become well established. The adult colon contains large numbers of bacteria, and great masses of them are passed in the stool.

Other Bacterial Action

Intestinal bacteria also affect the color and odor of the stool. The brown color represents bile pigments that are formed by the colon bacteria from *bilirubin*. In conditions where the bile flow is hindered, the stools may become clay colored or even white. The characteristic odor results from amines, especially *indole* and *skatole*, which are formed by bacterial enzymes from amino acids.

Intestinal gas, or flatus, contains hydrogen sulfide or methane produced by the bacteria. Gas formation, a common complaint, is often caused not so much by specific foods as the state of the body that receives them (see the box on p. 43). Many foods have been labeled "gas formers," but in reality these effects are highly variable from one person to another and such classifications have little or no scientific basis.

Dietary Fiber

Since humans have no microorganisms or enzymes to break down fiber, this plant carbohydrate remains after nutrient digestion and absorption as residue. However, pectin, one of the soluble fibers, is degraded in the large intestine. Undigested fiber contributes important bulk to the diet and helps form the feces. Fully formed and ready for elimination, the normal feces contain about 75% water and 25% solids. The solids include fiber, bacteria, inorganic matter such as minerals, a small amount of fat and its derivatives, some mucus, and sloughed off mucosal cells.

Some major features of nutrient absorption are summarized in Table 2-3.

Clinical Application

A common complaint of many persons after eating a meal or certain foods is the discomfort, and sometimes embarrassment, of "gas." This gas is a normal byproduct of digestion, but when it becomes painful or apparent to others it may become a physical and social problem.

The gastrointestinal tract normally holds about 3 oz of gas, moving along with the food mass and silently absorbed into the bloodstream. Sometimes extra gas collects in the stomach or intestine, creating an embarrassing, though usually harmless, situation.

Stomach gas

Gas in the stomach results from uncomfortable air bubbles trapped there. It occurs when a person eats too fast, drinks through a straw, or otherwise takes in extra air while eating. Burping relieves it. But these tips may help to avoid this social slip:

- Avoid carbonated beverages
- Don't gulp
- Chew with your mouth closed
- Don't drink from a can or through a straw
- Don't eat when you're nervous

Intestinal gas

The passing of gas from the intestine is usually a social embarrassment. This gas is formed in the colon, where bacteria attack nondigested items, causing them to decompose and produce gas. Carbohydrates release hydrogen, carbon dioxide, and in people with certain types of bacteria in the gut, *methane*. All three of these products are odorless (though noisy) gases. Protein produces *hydrogen sulfide* and such volatile amines as *indole* and *skatole*, which add a distinctive aroma to the expelled air. However, these suggestions may help control the problem:

- Cut down on simple carbohydrates—sugars. Especially observe milk's effect because *lactose intolerance* may be the real culprit. Substitute cultured forms such as yogurt or use milk treated with a lactase product such as LactAid or Lactrace.
- Eliminate all known food offenders. These vary among individuals, but beans, onions, cabbage, and high fiber wheat are among the most common.

Once relief is achieved, you may add more complex carbohydrates and high fiber foods to the diet—slowly. Once small amounts are tolerated, somewhat greater amounts can be tried. If there is still no relief, a medical examination may be needed to rule out or treat an overactive gastrointestinal tract.

REFERENCES

Biller JA and others: Efficacy of lactase-treated milk for lactose-intolerant pediatric patients, J Pediatr 111:91, July 1987.

Martini MC, and Savaiano DA: Reduced intolerance symptoms from lactose consumed during a meal, Am J Clin Nutr 47:57, Jan 1988.

Digestion's Sometimes Embarrassing Effects

Table 2-3
Intestinal Absorption of Some Major Nutrients

Nutrient	Form	Means of absorption	Control agent or required cofactor	Route
Carbohydrate	Monosaccharides (glucose and galactose)	Competitive	—	Blood
		Selective	—	
		Active transport via sodium pump	Sodium	
Protein	Amino acids	Selective	—	Blood
	Some dipeptides	Carrier transport systems	Pyridoxine (pyridoxal phosphate)	Blood
	Whole protein (rare)	Pinocytosis	—	Blood
Fat	Fatty acids	Fatty acid-bile complex (micelles)	Bile	Lymph
	Glycerides (mono-, di-)		—	Lymph
	Few triglycerides (neutral fat)	Pinocytosis	—	Lymph
Vitamins	B_{12}	Carrier transport	Intrinsic factor (IF)	Blood
	A	Bile complex	Bile	Blood
	K	Bile complex	Bile	From large intestine to blood
Minerals	Sodium	Active transport via sodium pump	—	Blood
	Calcium	Active transport	Vitamin D	Blood
	Iron	Active transport	Ferritin mechanism	Blood (as transferritin)
Water	Water	Osmosis	—	Blood, lymph, interstitial fluid

The various absorbed nutrients, including water and electrolytes, are carried to the cells to produce many substances the body needs to sustain life. Cell **metabolism** encompasses the total continuous complex of chemical changes that determine the final use of the individual nutrients.

Carbohydrate Metabolism
Sources of Blood Glucose

Both carbohydrate and noncarbohydrate substances provide sources of blood glucose:

1. **Carbohydrate sources.** Three carbohydrate sources provide blood glucose: (1) dietary starches and sugars, (2) glycogen stored in liver and muscle tissue (the hydrolysis of glycogen to form glucose is called **glycogenolysis** or simply **glycolysis**), and (3) products of intermediary carbohydrate metabolism, such as lactic acid and pyruvic acid.

2. **Noncarbohydrate sources.** Both protein and fat provide additional indirect sources of glucose. Certain amino acids from protein are called *glucogenic amino acids* because they form glucose after they are broken down. About 58% of the protein in a mixed diet is composed of such glucogenic amino acids. Thus more than half of dietary protein may ultimately be used for energy if sufficient carbohydrate and fat are not available for fuel. After the breakdown of fat into fatty acids and *glycerol*, the small glycerol portion (about 10% of the fat) can be converted to glycogen in the liver and made available for glucose formation. The production of glucose from protein, fat, and intermediary carbohydrate metabolites is called **gluconeogenesis.**

Uses of Blood Glucose

Three uses of glucose serve to regulate the blood sugar within a normal range of 70 to 120 mg/dL (3.9 to 6.6 mmol/L):

1. **Energy production.** The primary function of glucose is to supply energy to meet the body's constant demand. A vast array of interacting metabolic pathways employing many specific successive cell enzymes accomplish this task in a highly efficient manner.

2. **Energy storage.** Two storage forms may be used for glucose: (1) *Glycogen*—glucose may be converted to glycogen and stored in limited amounts in the liver and muscle tissue. Only a small supply of glycogen is present at any one time and it turns over rapidly. (2) *Fat*— after energy demands have been fulfilled, any excess glucose is converted to fat and stored as adipose tissue.

3. **Glucose products.** Small amounts of glucose are used in the production of various carbohydrate compounds, which have significant roles in overall body metabolism. Examples include DNA and RNA, galactose, and certain amino acids.

These sources and uses of glucose act as checks and balances to maintain normal blood sugar levels by adding sugar to the blood or removing it as needed.

Hormonal Controls

A number of hormones directly and indirectly influence the metabolism of glucose and regulate the blood sugar level.

Metabolism

Metabolism
Sum of all physical and chemical changes that take place within an organism, by which it maintains itself and produces energy for its functioning.

Glycogenolysis
Specific term for conversion of glycogen into glucose in the liver; the chemical process of enzymatic hydrolysis or breakdown by which this conversion is accomplished.

Glycolysis
Catabolism of carbohydrate (glucose and glycogen) by enzymes with release of energy and production of pyruvic acid or lactic acid.

Gluconeogenesis
Formation of glucose from non-carbohydrate sources (protein or fat).

Blood sugar-lowering hormone. Only one hormone, *insulin*, acts to lower blood sugar. It is produced by special beta cells in the pancreas. These cells are scattered in cell clusters forming "islands" in the pancreatic tissue, thus they are called *islets of Langerhans*, named for the scientist Paul Langerhans, who, as a young German medical student, first discovered and studied them. Insulin regulates blood sugar through several actions: (1) *glycogenesis* stimulates conversion of glucose to glycogen in the liver for constant energy reserve; (2) *lipogenesis* stimulates conversion of glucose to fat for storage in adipose tissue; and (3) *cell permeability* to glucose is increased, allowing it to pass into the cells for oxidation to supply needed energy.

Blood sugar-raising hormones. A number of hormones effectively raise blood sugar levels: (1) *Glucagon*, produced by pancreatic islet alpha cells, acts opposite to insulin, increasing breakdown of liver glycogen to glucose and maintaining blood glucose during fasting sleep hours. (2) *Somatostatin*, produced in the pancreatic delta cells and in the hypothalamus, suppresses insulin and glucagon and acts as a general modulator of related metabolic activities. (3) *Steroid hormones*, originating from the adrenal cortex, release glucose-forming carbon units from protein and act as insulin antagonists. (4) *Epinephrine*, originating from the adrenal medulla, stimulates the breakdown of liver glycogen and a quick release of immediate glucose. (5) *Growth hormone (GH)* and *adrenocorticotropic hormone (ACTH)*, released from the anterior pituitary gland, act as insulin antagonists. (6) *Thyroxine*, originating from the thyroid gland, influences the rate of insulin breakdown, increases glucose absorption from the intestine, and liberates epinephrine.

Lipid Metabolism
Fat Synthesis and Breakdown

Two organ tissues, the liver and adipose tissue, form an overall balanced axis of fat metabolism. Both function in fat synthesis and breakdown. The fatty acids released from fat are used by body cells as concentrated fuel to produce energy.

Lipoproteins

These lipid-protein complexes provide the major transport form of fat in the blood circulation. An excess amount in the blood produces a clinical condition called *hyperlipoproteinemia*. Lipoproteins are produced in the intestinal wall after initial absorption of dietary fat and in the liver for constant recirculation to and from cells.

Hormonal Controls

Since fat and carbohydrate metabolism are closely interrelated, the same hormones are involved: (1) *GH, ACTH,* and *thyroid-stimulating hormone (TSH)*, all from the pituitary gland, increase the release of free fatty acids from stored body fat by imposing energy demands. (2) *Cortisone* and *hydrocortisone*, from the adrenal gland, cause release of free fatty acids. (3) *Epinephrine* and *norepinephrine* stimulate breakdown of fat. (4) *Insulin*, from the pancreas, promotes fat synthesis, whereas *glucagon* has the opposite effect of breaking fat tissue to release free fatty acids. (5) *Thyroxine*, from the thyroid gland, stimulates fat tissue release of free fatty acids and also lowers blood cholesterol levels.

Protein Metabolism
Anabolism or Tissue Building

Protein metabolism centers on the essential balance between anabolism, tissue building, and catabolism, tissue breakdown. The process of anabolism builds protein tissue through the synthesis of new protein. This build-up is specifically governed by a definite pattern—a specific "blueprint" provided by DNA in the cell nucleus—that requires specific amino acids. Specific selection and supply of amino acids are necessary. Control agents include specific cell enzymes and coenzymes. Also, specific hormones—growth hormone, gonadotropins, and thyroxine—control or stimulate the building of tissue protein.

Catabolism or Tissue Breakdown

Amino acids released by tissue breakdown, if not reused in new tissue synthesis, are further broken down and used for other purposes. Two main parts of these amino acids result: the nitrogen-containing group and the remaining nonnitrogen residue.

1. **Nitrogen group.** The nitrogen portion is first split off the amino acid, a process called **deamination.** The nitrogen is converted to ammonia and excreted in the urine or retained for use in making other nitrogen compounds.
2. **Nonnitrogen residue.** The nonnitrogen residues are called **keto acids.** They may be used to form either carbohydrates or fats. They may also be reaminated to form a new amino acid.
3. **Control agents.** As in the case of tissue building, cell enzymes and coenzymes as well as hormones influence tissue catabolism. In health, there is a dynamic equilibrium between the two processes of anabolism and catabolism to sustain growth and maintain sound tissue.

Metabolic Interrelationships

Each of the chemical processes of overall body metabolism is purposeful, and all are interdependent. They are designed to fill two essential needs: to produce energy and to grow and maintain healthy tissue. The controlling agents in the cells for all of these intricately balanced processes to proceed in an orderly fashion are the cell enzymes, their coenzymes (many of which involve key vitamins and minerals), and special hormones. Overall human metabolism is an exciting biochemical process, designed to develop, sustain, and protect our most precious possession—life itself.

Deamination
Initial step in the metabolic breakdown (catabolism) of amino acids in which the amino group (NH_2) is split off. Deamination takes place chiefly in the liver.

Keto acid
Amino acid residue left after deamination. Glycogenic keto acids are used to form carbohydrates. Ketogenic keto acids are used to form fats.

To Sum Up

Nutrients are converted into usable forms by means of digestion and absorption. Metabolism is the means by which the body uses these nutrients to produce energy, build and rebuild body tissues, and maintain normal body functions.

Digestion consists of two basic activities: muscular and chemical. Muscular activity is responsible for food's mechanical breakdown by such means as mastication and movement of food along the gastrointestinal tract by such motions as peristalsis. Chemical activity involves enzymatic action that degrades food into smaller and smaller components for absorption.

Absorption involves the passage of food's nutrients from the gut into the blood stream across the intestinal wall. It occurs mainly in the small intestine by means of a number of efficient mechanisms.

Cell metabolism handles the absorbed nutrients. This metabolic work is accomplished by a large number of biochemical reactions that result in energy and maintain a dynamic balance between tissue breakdown and rebuilding.

Questions for Review

1. Describe five types of movement involved in mechanical digestion.
2. Identify digestive enzymes and any cofactors secreted by the following glands or organs: salivary, mucosal, pancreas, liver. What activity do they perform on fats, proteins, and carbohydrates? What stimulates their release? What inhibits their activity?
3. Describe four mechanisms of nutrient absorption from the small intestine. Describe the routes taken by the breakdown products of fats, proteins, and carbohydrates after absorption. Why must fat follow a different initial route?
4. Describe in detail two major activities that occur in the large intestine.

References

1. Wilson PC and Greens HL: The gastrointestinal tract: portal to nutrient utilization. In Shils ME and Young VR, editors: Modern nutrition in health and disease, ed 7, Philadelphia, 1988, Lea & Febiger.
2. Cashman MD: Principles of digestive physiology for clinical nutrition, Nutr Clin Pract 1(5):241, 1986.
3. Wion KL and others: Human lipoprotein lipase complementary DNA sequence, Science 235:1638, March 1987.
4. Sauberlich HE: Vitamins—how much is for keeps? Nutr Today 22(1):20, 1987.

Cashman MD: Principles of digestive physiology for clinical nutrition, Nutr Clin Pract 1(5):241, 1986.

This clinician presents a succinct, updated review of the physiology of digestion and absorption, especially as it relates to clinical problems.

Hattner JAT: The dietitian's role in the treatment of common gastrointestinal problems, Topics Clin Nutr 2(1):62, 1987.

The author, a clinical nutritionist, describes the two most common GI problems in the care of children, relating them to GI function, individual needs, and guides for therapy. A set of multiple-choice questions provides review.

Imes S, Pinchbeck BC, and Thomason ABR: Diet counseling modifies nutrient intake of patients with Crohn's disease, J Am Diet Assoc 87(4):457, 1987.

This article illustrates how an inflammatory bowel disease can interfere with the normal process of absorption in the small intestine and require individual diet modifications to meet nutrient needs.

Further Readings

Lactose Intolerance—Common Problem Worldwide

Picture this: a natural disaster strikes a poor nation, leaving thousands homeless and with very little food. CARE, UNICEF, and other international organizations work quickly to collect and ship foodstuffs to the area. Yet, the people find it difficult to be grateful: since the shipments began, they have found themselves not only without shelter but also in distress—gastrointestinal distress.

One of the most common foodstuffs shipped to impoverished areas is milk. One of the most common problems throughout the world is *lactose intolerance*—a condition that results in abdominal cramps, nausea, bloating, or diarrhea when milk is consumed. The problem stems from a deficiency in *lactase*, a digestive enzyme found in the microvilli of the small intestine that by **hydrolysis** converts marginal milk sugar (lactose) into its component monosaccharides, glucose and galactose, for absorption. All mammals are born with sufficient amounts of lactase to accommodate very high lactose levels in "mother's milk." In animal species the amount of enzyme activity drops off significantly shortly after birth; in most humans, this occurs after age 5. A few among the human species do not experience this problem. Northern Europeans, a few African cattle-raisers, and residents of the northwestern sector of India manage to digest lactose very easily throughout adulthood. The remaining majority of the world's population experience symptoms on drinking as little as a half pint of milk.

Symptoms are similar to those seen in other food sensitivities. When there is any doubt regarding the cause, lactose intolerance tests are usually performed:

Lactose loading A 50-g dose of lactose (approximately the amount provided by 4 cups of milk) is administered and symptoms evaluated.

Breath-hydrogen assay Hydrogen levels in the breath after a lactose load are measured to indicate the degree of intolerance.

Lactase assay Lactase levels in a jejunal biopsy are measured.

Once lactose intolerance has been identified and other clinical conditions with which it is associated are ruled out, treatment consists simply of cutting down on milk consumption. Most lactose-intolerant individuals digest fermented milk products (cheese, buttermilk, yogurt) very well and can use them as their primary source of calcium instead of milk. But these foods carry problems of transportation, storage, and cost. And yet the nutritional benefits of lactose-rich foods may become crucial in offsetting deficiency signs among those in dire need. A possible solution to this problem is the use of recently developed low-lactose milk, sweet acidophilus milk. Sweeter than regular milk, this lactose-hydrolyzed product has been quite acceptable and effectively reduces symptoms. The necessary processing increases the cost by a mere 2 to 3 cents/L, keeping it inexpensive enough to be considered for mass distribution.

Hydrolysis
Process by which a chemical compound is split into other compounds by taking up the elements of water. Common examples are the reactions of digestion in which the nutrients are split into simpler compounds by the digestive enzymes; that is, the conversion of starch to maltose, of fat to fatty acids and glycerol, and so on.

REFERENCES
Mankind, calcium, and milk, Gastroenterology 92:260, Jan 1987.
Rosado JL, Allen LH, and Solomans NW: Milk consumption, symptom response, and lactose digestion in milk intolerance, Am J Clin Nutr 45:1457, June 1987.

3 Carbohydrates

Chapter Objectives

After studying this chapter, the student should be able to:

1. Identify practical reasons for the prime position of carbohydrates in the human diet worldwide and name its two main dietary forms, giving examples of each.

2. Define carbohydrate in terms of its basic chemical components and identify some of its major forms and functions that are important in human metabolism.

3. Describe the processes by which food carbohydrates are changed to a usable refined fuel form and then carried to the cells for energy production.

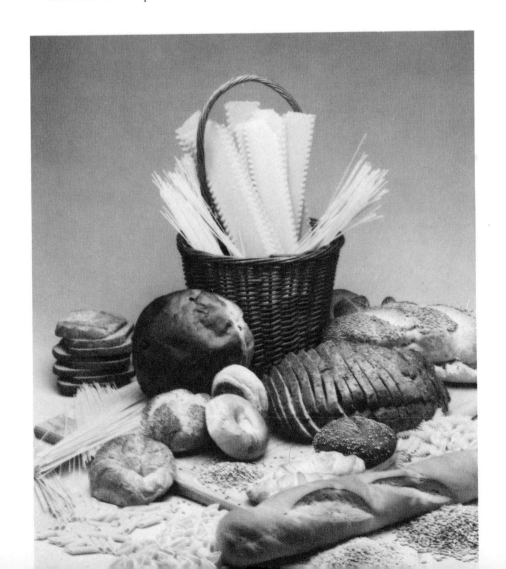

PREVIEW

The human body has been uniquely designed and developed to solve three basic survival problems: (1) energy to do its work, (2) materials to build and maintain its form, and (3) agents to control these processes efficiently. Key nutrients in the food we eat have provided sensitive life-sustaining solutions.

All three of these problems are interrelated, but we will look at them one at a time. In this chapter, we consider the first of these basic problems—*energy production*—and the body's primary fuel—*carbohydrates*.

Carbohydrates as Basic Body Fuel

The Nature of Carbohydrates
The Problem of Energy

Energy is a primary necessity for life. It is the power an organism must have to do its work. Any energy system, to be successful, must provide four basic components: (1) a basic fuel, (2) a means of changing this basic fuel to a refined fuel that the machine is designed to use, (3) a means of carrying this refined fuel to the energy production sites, and (4) a means of burning the fuel at the production sites to produce energy. In the human energy system, this major basic fuel comes from carbohydrates.

Starches and Sugars

The basic fuel forms of carbohydrates are starches and sugars that occur naturally in our foods. Energy on the planet Earth comes ultimately from the sun and its tremendous nuclear reactions. In the presence of this life-giving sunlight, plants use their internal process of **photosynthesis** to transform the sun's energy into the stored plant fuel form of carbohydrates. In this important process, plants use carbon dioxide from the air and water from the soil, along with *chlorophyll* in their green leaves as a chemical catalyst, to manufacture starches and sugars. Since the human body can rapidly break down these starches and sugars to yield body energy, carbohydrates are called "quick energy" foods. They provide our major source of energy.

Photosynthesis
Process by which plants containing chlorophyll are able to manufacture carbohydrate by combining carbon dioxide from the air and water from the soil. Sunlight is used as energy and chlorophyll is the catalyst.

Dietary Importance

There are practical reasons for the large quantities of carbohydrates in diets all over the world. First, carbohydrates are widely available, easily grown in plants such as grains, vegetables, and fruits. In some countries, carbohydrate foods make up almost the entire diet of the people. In the American diet about half of the total kilocalories is in the form of carbohydrates. Second, carbohydrates are relatively low in cost. And third, they may be stored easily. Compared with other types of foods, carbohydrate foods can be kept in dry storage for relatively long time periods without spoilage. Modern processing and packaging further extend the shelf life of carbohydrate products almost indefinitely.

Definition

The name *carbohydrate* comes from its chemical nature. It is composed of the elements carbon, hydrogen, and oxygen, with the hydrogen/oxygen ratio usually that of water—CH_2O.

Classification of Carbohydrates

Carbohydrates are classified according to the number of basic sugar, or *saccharide*, units making up their structure:

Monosaccharides

The simplest form of carbohydrate is the **monosaccharide,** often called a simple (single) sugar. The three main monosaccharides important in human nutrition are glucose, fructose, and galactose.

   1. **Glucose.** A moderately sweet sugar, glucose is found naturally preformed in only a few foods, such as corn syrup. Mainly it is created in the body from starch digestion. In human metabolism all other types of sugar are converted into glucose. It is the form, sometimes called **dextrose,** in which sugar circulates in the blood stream. The normal blood sugar range is about 3.9 to 6.1 mmol/L (70 to 110 mg/dL). The term *hyperglycemia* refers to an elevated blood glucose level. *Hypoglycemia* results from blood glucose levels below the normal range. In recent years public controversy has developed concerning the condition of hypoglycemia (see the box on p. 54). Glucose is the ultimate common refined body fuel that is oxidized in the cells to give energy.

   2. **Fructose.** The sweetest of the simple sugars, fructose is found in fruits and other substances such as honey. In human metabolism fructose is converted to glucose to be burned for energy.

   3. **Galactose.** The simple sugar galactose is not found free in foods but is produced in human digestion from lactose (milk sugar) and is then changed to glucose for energy. This reaction is reversible, and during lactation glucose may be reconverted to galactose for use in milk production. In the genetic disease *galactosemia* the enzyme for this change to glucose is missing, and galactose accumulates.

Disaccharides

The **disaccharides** are simple (double) sugars composed of two monosaccharides linked together. The three main disaccharides of physiologic importance are sucrose, lactose, and maltose.

   1. **Sucrose.** Sucrose is the common "table sugar" made commercially from sugar cane and sugar beets. It is the most prevalent disaccharide. With the increasing use of processed foods, sucrose contributes some 30% to 40% of the total kilocalories in the American diet (see Issues and Answers on p. 73). Sucrose can be found in all forms of common sugar, in molasses, and in some fruits and vegetables such as pineapple and carrots.

   2. **Lactose.** The sugar in milk is called *lactose* because of its source. It is formed in the body from glucose to supply the needed sugar component of milk during lactation. It is the least sweet of the disaccharides, about one sixth as sweet as sucrose. When milk sours, as in the initial stages of cheese making, the lactose changes its form and separates out in the liquid whey from the solid curd. The curd is then processed for cheese. Thus, although milk has a relatively high carbohydrate content in the form of lactose, one of its main products—cheese—has very little or none.

   3. **Maltose.** Maltose occurs in commercial malt products of starch breakdown and in germinating cereal grains. As such, it is a negligible *dietary* carbohydrate. But it is a highly significant *metabolic* carbohydrate as an intermediate product of starch digestion.

Monosaccharide
Class of simple sugars composed of one saccharide (sugar) unit. Common members are glucose, fructose, and galactose.

Dextrose
Another name for glucose.

Disaccharides
Class of compound sugars composed of two molecules of monosaccharide. The three common members are sucrose (table sugar), lactose (milk sugar), and maltose (grain sugar).

Clinical Application

Hypoglycemia: Fact or Fiction?

Recent controversy has developed concerning *hypoglycemia,* the condition of low blood sugar. Is it fact or fiction? Probably some of both. The lay public associates hypoglycemia with an excessive amount of sugar in the diet and at various times has attributed a number of symptoms to this condition ranging from hunger and headaches to depression and crime. On the other hand, members of the medical community have fueled the problem with statements about "nonhypoglycemia" as a "nondisease."

Clinicians and consumers alike, however, agree on some of the symptoms, for example, nervousness, anxiety, hunger, palpitations, and headaches. But they disagree about causes of the problem, methods of diagnosis, and treatment.

Cause. While consumers have generally named excess dietary sugar as the culprit, clinicians have specifically identified two types of hypoglycemia and their known causes:

- **Reactive hypoglycemia** occurs after a meal and most frequently affects persons who have recently had abdominal surgery or who have diabetes.
- **Fasting hypoglycemia** occurs after extended periods without adequate food or from poor eating habits. It may also be caused by several drugs: (1) alcohol, which blocks glucose production by the liver; (2) hypoglycemic medications used to treat diabetes; and (3) salicylate in aspirin. More serious conditions that may cause this effect include (1) tumors of the pancreas that stimulate excessive insulin secretion and (2) adrenal insufficiency, a rare condition, that prevents the adrenal glands from responding to certain body needs, especially under stress. Unrelieved general stress, whatever the cause, increases metabolic demands on the body and can contribute to hypoglycemia.

Diagnosis. A normal blood glucose range is about 3.9 to 6.1 mmol/L (70 to 110 mg/dL). The traditional basis for medical diagnosis has been the oral glucose tolerance test. The patient drinks a beverage containing 75 to 100 g of glucose, and the blood glucose levels are measured at half-hour intervals for up to 5 hours. But this very test situation is unrealistic and induces the abnormal response itself. So, more recently, physicians have used blood tests at the time the person is having the characteristic symptoms to obtain a more realistic measure.

Treatment. In general, the lay public believes that hypoglycemia should be treated with a very low-carbohydrate, high-protein diet. However, a very low-carbohydrate diet will make it difficult for the body to obtain sufficient amounts of glucose to achieve and maintain normal blood sugar levels. It is evident now from current carbohydrate research, that a diet of frequent small meals, rich in complex carbohydrates and a good dietary fiber content, with fewer simple carbohydrates and sugars, will maintain a more stable blood sugar level without dipping periods of low blood sugar.

Sound approaches. The simple procedure for home blood glucose monitoring developed for persons with diabetes can be used by persons with hypoglycemic symptoms to test their own blood sugar levels at the time they are having symptoms and to record results. This record will then provide an accurate profile of the blood glucose levels in the free home environment. This procedure can provide a therapeutic tool for use in counseling and teaching. If the record shows no documented hypoglycemic periods, a sensitive counselor can help the person gain more insight into the problem, exploring other reasons for the symptoms. On the other hand, if the record documents actual hypoglycemia, further diagnostic evaluation is required. This technique is simple, accurate, and effective for persons being evaluated for reactive or postprandial hypoglycemia.

REFERENCE

Andreani D, Marks V, and Lefebvre PJ, editors: Hypoglycemia, Serono Symposia Publications, vol 38, New York, 1987, Raven Press.

Polysaccharides

These much more complex carbohydrates are called **polysaccharides** because they are made up of *many* single sugar (saccharide) units. The most important polysaccharide in human nutrition is starch. Other forms are glycogen and dextrins. The nondigestible forms of dietary fiber—cellulose and other noncellulose polysaccharides—provide important bulk in the diet.

1. **Starch.** In human nutrition starch is by far the most significant polysaccharide. It is a relatively large complex compound made up of many coiled or branching chains of simple sugar (glucose) units. It yields only glucose on digestion. The cooking of starch not only improves its flavor but also softens and ruptures the starch cells, which makes digestion easier. Starch mixtures thicken when cooked because the portion that encases the starch granules has a gel-like quality that thickens the mixture the same way that pectin causes jelly to set.

Starch is also by far the most important source of dietary carbohydrate worldwide. It is recognized as a significant factor in human nutrition and health. For example, standards of U.S. dietary guidelines, as outlined in Chapter 1, recommend that about 50% to 60% of the total kilocalorie value of the diet come from carbohydrates, with a greater portion of that allowance coming from complex carbohydrate forms of starch. In many other countries, where starch is the staple food material, it makes up an even greater portion of the diet. The major food sources of starch include cereal grains, legumes, potatoes, and other vegetables.

2. **Glycogen.** The animal storage compound comparable to starch in plants is **glycogen.** It is formed during cell metabolism and stored in relatively small amounts in the liver and muscle tissues. These stores help sustain normal

Polysaccharides
Class of complex carbohydrates composed of many monosaccharide units. The common members are starch, dextrins, dietary fiber, and glycogen.

Glycogen
Polysaccharide of animal body. It is formed in the body from glucose and stored in liver and muscle tissue.

blood glucose levels during fasting periods such as sleep hours and provide immediate fuel for muscle action. Dietary carbohydrate is essential to maintain these needed glycogen stores and prevent the symptoms of low carbohydrate intake—fatigue, dehydration, and energy loss, as well as other undesirable metabolic effects such as ketoacidosis (see Chapter 21) and excessive protein breakdown. Sometimes a process of "glycogen-loading" is used by athletes to provide added fuel stores (see Chapter 14), but this diet manipulation can cause problems if used too often.

3. **Dextrins.** Dextrins are polysaccharide compounds formed as intermediate products in the breakdown of starch. This starch breakdown occurs constantly in the process of digestion.

Dietary Fiber

Based on current research, dietary fiber may be classed into three major groups according to structure and properties, with one of these groups having five different members[1]:

1. **Cellulose.** This dietary fiber is the chief constituent of the framework of plants. Humans cannot digest cellulose because they lack the necessary digestive enzymes. Therefore it remains in the digestive tract and contributes important bulk to the diet. This bulk helps move the food mass along and stimulates peristalsis, as described in Chapter 2. Cellulose makes up the principal structural material in plant cell walls and provides most of the substance labeled "crude fiber" (see the box on the facing page). The main food sources are stems and leaves of vegetables, seed and grain coverings, skins, and hulls.

2. **Noncellulose.** This group of dietary fiber polysaccharides includes five types of compounds: (1) hemicellulose, (2) pectins, (3) gums, (4) mucilages, and (5) algal substances. They absorb water and slow gastric emptying time. All of them except hemicellulose are gum-like water soluble substances that aid in binding cholesterol and controlling its absorption. They also prevent colon pressure by providing bulk for normal intestinal muscle action.

3. **Lignin.** This substance is the only noncarbohydrate type of dietary fiber. It is a large compound that forms the woody part of plants. In the intestine it combines with bile acids to form insoluble compounds, thus preventing their absorption.

A summary of these dietary fiber classes is given in Table 3-1. Some main food sources of the various types of dietary fiber are indicated in Table 3-2.

In general, dietary fiber produces various effects on the food mix consumed and its fate in the body. Most of these effects are caused by its physiologic properties: (1) *Water absorption,* which contributes to its bulk-forming laxative effect, influences the transit time of the food mass through the digestive tract and consequent absorption of the various nutrients. (2) *Binding effect,* characteristic of certain fibers such as the noncellulose substances, influences blood lipid levels through their capacity to bind cholesterol and bile salts and prevents their absorption. However, excessive dietary fiber can have the undesirable effect of binding minerals such as iron, zinc, or calcium,[2] thus preventing needed absorption. (3) *Colon bacteria effect* on fermentation substrates for bacterial action produces volatile fatty acids and gas.[3] Current research concerning various clinical applications has centered largely on diabetes mellitus, coronary heart disease, colon cancer, and other intestinal

To Probe Further

The Semantics of Fiber: A Question of Definition

Much of the confusion concerning fiber in the human diet has centered on semantics. No term has seemed fully acceptable to cover all the different types of fiber or the various meanings involved. The older word *roughage* and the current general term *fiber* denote a rough abrasive material of the physical nature observed in plant cellulose, a woody type of material. However, a number of the undigestible materials in food have a soft amorphous gel-like character, more soluble in physical nature and hence having different properties and functions.

This difference in physical properties adds to the problem nutritionists and clinicians have had in determining a more precise nutritional and clinical significance for fiber in the human diet and in defining the variety of food substances involved. Further problems have surrounded methods of accurately analyzing and measuring these substances in their variety of food sources.

The general term *fiber* was initially applied to a variety of nondigestible carbohydrate and noncarbohydrate substances for which specific hydrolytic enzymes are lacking in the human digestive system. Confusion has resulted mainly from the erroneous interchange of the two terms *dietary fiber* and *crude fiber*.

Dietary fiber refers to the total amount of naturally occurring material in foods, mostly plants, that is not digested. This includes (1) plant dietary fiber from such foods as whole grains, legumes, vegetables, fruits, seeds, and nuts; (2) undigested animal tissue polysaccharides; (3) undigested pharmaceutical products; and (4) undigested biosynthetic polysaccharides. Refined diets in Western countries usually contain little fiber in the energy foods starches, sugars, and fats. Diets in rural communities of other developing countries contain much more fiber. Research suggests that these higher-fiber diets protect against a wide variety of Western civilization diseases.

Crude fiber is the material remaining after vigorous treatment of the food sources with acid and alkaline agents in the laboratory. These were the initial results given in most food value tables. These strong laboratory processes remove a good portion of the total dietary fiber that cannot withstand such treatment. Since the proportion of total dietary fiber and crude fiber varies widely among specific foods, depending on the fiber composition of a particular food, the fiber values given in earlier food value tables have had limited usefulness. However, as new laboratory procedures are developed, better information is being provided.

Thus the term *crude fiber* is of little value in current usage. The term of choice, though not perfect, is *dietary fiber*. It refers to the nondigestible residues of plant foods: (1) cellulose; (2) noncellulose polysaccharides, including hemicellulose, pectins, gums, mucilages, and algal substances; and (3) the single noncarbohydrate member, lignin. All resist digestion by any human digestive enzymes, but all are valuable in nutrition and related disease.

REFERENCES

Lanza E and Butrum RR: A critical review of food fiber analysis and data, J Am Diet Assoc 86(6):732, 1986.

Slavin JL: Dietary fiber: classification, chemical analysis, and food sources, J Am Diet Assoc 87(9):1164, 1987.

Table 3-1

Summary of Dietary Fiber Classes

Dietary fiber class	Plant parts	Functions
Cellulose	Main cell wall constituent	Insoluble; holds water, laxative; reduces elevated colonic intraluminal pressure; binds minerals
Noncellulose polysaccharides		
Hemicellulose	Secretions, cell wall material	Mostly insoluble; holds water, increases stool bulk; reduces colonic pressure; binds bile acids
Pectins	Intracellular cement material	Soluble, binds cholesterol and bile acids
Gums	Special cell secretions	Soluble; binds cholesterol and bile acids; slows gastric emptying; provides fermentable material for colonic bacteria with production of volatile fatty acids and gas
Mucilages	Cell secretions	Soluble; slows gastric emptying time; fermentable substrate for colonic bacteria; binds bile acids
Algal substances	Algae, seaweeds	Soluble; slows gastric emptying time; fermentable substrate; binds bile acids
Noncarbohydrate		
Lignin	Woody part of plants	Insoluble; antioxidant; binds bile acids and metals

problems such as diverticulosis.[2-6] About 15 to 20 g/day of dietary fiber is wise for health. Some of these clinical associations between dietary fiber and various health problems are summarized in Table 3-3.

Functions of Carbohydrates

Energy

As indicated, the primary function of carbohydrate in human nutrition is to provide fuel for energy production. Fat is also a fuel, but the body needs only a small amount of dietary fat, mainly to supply the essential fatty acids. To function properly, however, the body tissues require a daily dietary supply of carbohydrate providing 50% to 60% of the total kilocalories.

The amount of carbohydrate in the body, though relatively small, is important to maintain energy reserves. For example, in an adult male about 300 to 350 g are stored in the liver and muscle tissues as glycogen, and about 10 g are present in circulating blood glucose. This total amount of available glycogen and glucose provides energy sufficient for only about half a day of moderate activity. Thus carbohydrate foods must be eaten regularly and at moderately frequent intervals to meet the constant energy demands of the body.

Dietary fiber class	Grains	Fruits	Vegetables
Cellulose	Bran Whole wheat Whole rye	Apples Pears	Beans, peas Cabbage family Root vegetables Tomato, fresh
Noncellulose polysaccharides			
Hemicellulose	Bran Cereals Whole grains		
Pectins		Apples Citrus fruits Berries, especially strawberries	Green beans Carrots
Gums	Oatmeal	Food products thickener, stabilizer	Dried beans, other legumes Vegetable gums used in food pro- cessing
Mucilages		Food products thickener, stabilizer	
Algal substances		Food products thickener, stabilizer	
Noncarbohydrate			
Lignins	Whole wheat Whole rye	Strawberries Peaches Pears Plums	Mature vegetables

Table 3-2

Selected Food Sources of Various Classes of Dietary Fiber

Special Functions of Carbohydrates in Body Tissues

As part of their general function as the body's main energy source, carbohydrates serve special functions in many body tissues.

Glycogen Reserves

As indicated, the liver and muscle glycogen reserves provide a constant interchange with the body's constant overall energy balance system. Thus this reserve protects cells from depressed metabolic function and injury.

Protein-Sparing Action

Carbohydrate helps regulate protein metabolism. The presence of sufficient carbohydrate for energy demands of the body prevents the channeling of too much protein for this purpose. This protein-sparing action of carbohydrate allows the major portion of protein to be used for its basic structural purpose of tissue building.

Table 3-3

Relationship Between Fiber and Various Health Problems

Problem	Effect of fiber	Possible mode of action	Future research needs
Diabetes mellitus	Reduces fasting blood sugar levels Reduces glycosuria Reduces insulin requirements Increases insulin sensitivity	Slows carbohydrate absorption by Delaying gastric emptying time Forming gels with pectin or guar gum in the intestine, thus impeding carbohydrate absorption "Protecting" carbohydrates from enzymatic activity with a fibrous coat Allowing "protected" carbohydrates to escape into large colon where they are digested by bacteria	Influence of short-chain fatty acid (SCFA) production on metabolism of glucose and fats in the liver Exact mechanisms by which fiber influences glucose metabolism
	Inhibits postprandial (after meals) hyperglycemia	Alters gut hormones (for example, glucagon) to enhance glucose metabolism in the liver	
Obesity	Increases satiety rate	Prolongs chewing and swallowing movements	Cause of increased satiety rate reported by subjects
	Reduces nutrient bioavailability	Increases fecal fat content	Effect on nutrient binding on nutritional status
	Reduces energy density	Inhibits absorption of carbohydrate in high fiber foods	Studies based on food composition and caloric density instead of fiber content alone
		Increases transit time	Effects of different types of fiber on gastric, small intestine, and colonic emptying time
	Alters hormonal response	Alters action of insulin, gut glucagon, and other intestinal hormones	
	Alters thermogenesis		
Coronary heart disease	Inhibits recirculation of bile acids	Alters bacterial metabolism of bile acids	Influence of fiber on cholesterol content of specific lipoprotein fractions (see Chapter 20)

*This effect is based on epidemiologic studies, usually observed in combination with reduced fat intake.

†Insulin is required for fat synthesis.

‡Preventive effect of fiber is assumed from epidemiologic studies that associate low-fiber, high-fat diets with an *increased* incidence of disease.

§Segmentation increases pressure and weakness along the wallls of the intestinal tract.

Table 3-3
Relationship Between Fiber and Various Health Problems—cont'd

Problem	Effect of fiber	Possible mode of action	Future research needs
		Alters bacterial flora, resulting in a change in metabolic activity	Influence on production of short-chain fatty acids
		Forms gels that bind bile acids	Role of dietary fiber as an independent variable in reducing risk of heart disease
		Alters the function of pancreatic and intestinal enzymes	
	Reduces triglyceride and cholesterol levels*	Reduces insulin levels†	Relationship between lipoprotein turnover and glucose turnover/sensitivity to insulin
		Binds cholesterol, preventing absorption	Effect of higher concentration of bile salts on colon function
		Slows fat absorption by forming gel matrices in the intestine	
Colon cancer	Reduces incidence of disease‡	Bile acids or their bacterial metabolites may affect the structure of the colon, its cell turnover rate, and function	Testing of current hypotheses regarding the effects of dietary factors on the structure of the colon and cell turnover rate
Other gastrointestinal disorders	Reduces pressure from within the intestinal lumen	Increases transit time	
Diverticular disease Constipation Hiatal hernia Hemorrhoids	Increases diameter of the intestinal lumen, thus allowing intestinal tract to contract more, propelling contents more rapidly, and inhibiting segmentation§	Increases water absorption, resulting in a larger, softer stool	

Antiketogenic Effect

Carbohydrate also relates to fat metabolism. The amount of carbohydrate present in the diet determines how much fat will be broken down, thus affecting the formation and disposal rates of *ketones*. Ketones are intermediate products of fat metabolism, which normally are produced at a low level during fat oxidation. However, in extreme conditions such as starvation or uncontrolled diabetes, as well as the unwise use of very low carbohydrate diets, carbohydrate is inadequate or unavailable for energy needs, so too much fat is oxidized. Ketones accumulate and the result is *ketoacidosis* (see Chapter 21). Sufficient carbohydrate consumption prevents damaging ketone excess.

Heart Action

Heart action is a life-sustaining muscular exercise. Although fatty acids are the preferred regular fuel for the heart muscle, the glycogen reserve in cardiac muscle is an important emergency source of contractile energy. In a damaged heart poor glycogen stores or low carbohydrate intake may cause cardiac symptoms and angina.

Central Nervous System Function

A constant supply of carbohydrate is necessary for the proper functioning of the central nervous system (CNS). The CNS regulatory center, the brain, contains no stored supply of glucose and is therefore especially dependent on a minute-to-minute supply of glucose from the blood. Sustained and profound hypoglycemic shock may cause irreversible brain damage. In all nerve tissue, carbohydrate is indispensable for functional integrity.

Digestion: Changing Basic Fuel into Usable Refined Fuel

Most carbohydrate foods, starches and sugars, cannot immediately be used by the cells to make energy available. They must first be changed into the refined fuel for which the cell is designed—*glucose*. The process by which these vital changes are made is *digestion*. The digestion of carbohydrate foods proceeds through the successive parts of the gastrointestinal tract, accomplished by two types of actions: (1) mechanical or muscle functions that render the food mass into smaller particles and (2) chemical processes in which specific enzymes break down food nutrients into smaller usable metabolic products.

Mouth

Mastication breaks food into fine particles and mixes it with saliva. During this process, a salivary amylase (ptyalin) is secreted by the parotid gland. It acts on starch to begin its breakdown into dextrins and maltose.

Stomach

Successive wavelike contractions of the muscle fibers of the stomach wall continue the mechanical digestive process. This action is called *peristalsis*. It further mixes food particles with gastric secretions to allow chemical digestion to take place more readily. The gastric secretion contains no specific enzyme for the breakdown of carbohydrate. The hydrochloric acid in the stomach stops the action of salivary amylase. But before the food mixes completely with the acid gastric secretion, as much as 20% to 30% of the starch may have been changed to maltose. Muscle actions continue to bring the food mass to the lower part of the stomach. Here the food mass is now a thick creamy *chyme*, ready for its controlled emptying through the *pyloric valve* into the duodenum, the first portion of the small intestine.

Small Intestine

Peristalsis continues to aid digestion in the small intestine by mixing and moving the chyme along the **lumen** in the length of the tube. Chemical digestion of carbohydrate is completed in the small intestine by specific enzymes from two sources: pancreas and intestine.

Lumen
Space within a tube; e.g., gastrointestinal tract or a blood vessel.

Pancreatic Secretions

These secretions from the pancreas enter the duodenum through the common bile duct. They contain a pancreatic amylase, which continues the breakdown of starch to maltose.

Intestinal Secretions

These secretions contain three disaccharidases: *sucrase, lactase,* and *maltase.* These specific enzymes act on their respective disaccharides to render the monosaccharides—glucose, galactose, fructose—ready now for absorption. These specific disaccharidases are integral proteins of the brush border of the small intestine that break down the disaccharides as absorption takes place. The digestive products, the monosaccharides, are then immediately absorbed into the portal blood circulation.

A summary of the major aspects of carbohydrate digestion through these successive parts of the gastrointestinal tract is given in Table 3-4.

Lactose intolerance, a condition causing gastrointestinal problems, results from a deficiency of the enzyme lactase.

The refined fuel glucose is now ready to be carried to the individual cells to be "burned" or stored to produce energy. The process by which the body transports this basic end product of carbohydrate digestion to the cells throughout the body is called *absorption.* The major glucose absorption mechanism is an active transport "pumping" system requiring sodium as a carrier substance.

Absorption: Carrying Refined Fuel to Energy Production Sites—Cells

Absorbing Structures

The absorbing surface area of the small intestine is uniquely enhanced by its three basic structures: mucosal folds, villi, and microvilli, which are described in detail in the previous chapter (see Figure 2-4). Together, these structures provide a greatly increased absorbing surface that allows 90% of the digested food material to be absorbed in the small intestine. Only water absorption remains for the large intestine.

Route of Absorption

By way of the capillaries of the villi, the simple sugars enter the **portal** circulation and are transported to the liver. Here fructose and galactose are con-

Portal
Entryway, usually referring to the portal circulation of blood through the liver. Blood is brought into the liver by the portal vein and out by the hepatic vein.

Table 3-4
Summary of Carbohydrate Digestion

Organ	Enzyme	Action
Mouth	Ptyalin	Starch → Dextrins → Maltose
Stomach	None	(Above action continued to minor degree)
Small intestine	Pancreatic amylopsin	Starch → Dextrins → Maltose
	Intestinal:	
	Sucrase	Sucrose → Glucose + Fructose
	Lactase	Lactose → Glucose + Galactose
	Maltase	Maltose → Glucose + Glucose

verted to glucose, and glucose in turn is either used immediately for fuel or converted to glycogen for brief storage. Then glycogen is constantly being reconverted to glucose as needed by the body.

Metabolism: Burning Refined Fuel at Production Sites to Produce Energy

Cell Metabolism

Cells are the functional units of life in the human body. In cell nutrition the most important end product of carbohydrate digestion is glucose, since the other two monosaccharides, fructose and galactose, are eventually converted to glucose. The liver is the major site of the intricate metabolic machinery that handles glucose. However, energy metabolism in general goes on in all cells. In these individual cells glucose is burned to produce energy through a series of chemical reactions involving specific cell enzymes. The final energy produced is then available to the cell to do its work. Extra glucose not immediately needed for energy may also be changed to fat and stored as a reserve fuel.

Metabolism

Metabolism
Sum of all chemical changes that take place within an organism, by which it maintains itself and produces energy for its functioning.

Metabolite
Any substance that forms as a result of the breakdown (catabolism) or growth or maintenance (anabolism) of living tissue.

The general term **metabolism** refers to the sum of the various chemical processes in a living organism by which energy is made available for the functioning of the whole organism. It also includes processes by which basic structures of cells and tissues are built, maintained, or broken down to be rebuilt. Products of specific metabolic processes are called **metabolites.**

Metabolic Concept of Unity

Here and in following discussions of other nutrients, a central significant scientific principle will emerge—*the unity of the human organism.* The human body is a whole made up of many parts and processes that possess unequaled specificity and flexibility. Intimate metabolic relationships exist among all the basic nutrients and metabolites. Thus it is impossible to understand any one of the body's many metabolic processes without viewing it in relationship to the whole.

Therefore, in all your study and work with patients and clients, you should remember this important fact: **All nutrients do their best work in partnership with other nutrients.** From this fundamental fact you can draw two practical conclusions: (1) the emphasis in health teaching and nutrition education should be on achieving a sound balanced nutritional basis for any dietary program, and (2) some deficiency states may be *iatrogenic* (induced by medical treatment), or may have their origin in a fad, or may be caused by long-term, overzealous emphasis on one particular nutrient to the exclusion of other equally essential ones.

Carbohydrate supplies most of the world's population with its primary source of energy. A product of photosynthesis, it is widely distributed in nature and its food products are easy to store and generally low in cost.

There are two basic types of carbohydrates: simple and complex. *Simple carbohydrates* consist of single and double sugar units (monosaccharides and disaccharides) that are easily digested and provide quick energy. *Complex carbohydrates*, or polysaccharides, are less easily prepared for use. Though their effect on blood sugar varies somewhat, generally they provide energy more slowly and prevent large fluctuations in blood glucose levels.

In addition to providing general body energy, carbohydrates maintain liver, heart, brain, and nerve tissue function. They also prevent the breaking down of fats and proteins for energy, which results in excessive production of toxic metabolic byproducts. *Dietary fiber,* a complex carbohydrate that forms the undigestible part of plants, also affects the digestion and absorption of foods in ways that have proved beneficial to good health.

1. Refer to the RDA table to determine the daily caloric need of a 25-year-old woman who is 5 ft 4 in tall and weighs 125 lbs. How many kilocalories should be provided by carbohydrate in her diet? How much fiber is recommended?
2. Give a general description of the clinical effects of fiber in each of the following disease states: diverticular disease, hyperlipidemia, diabetes mellitus, and colon cancer.
3. Your client, Mr. Brown, wants desperately to lose 20 lbs before meeting his future in-laws next month. He purchased a month's worth of liquid protein and takes multivitamins daily. He seems adamant about not eating any starches or sweets. Based on your readings, how would you explain the effects of a very low carbohydrate diet on carbohydrate functions so that he will know why carbohydrates are important even in a weight-loss program?

1. Slavin JL: Dietary fiber: classification, chemical analyses and food sources, J Am Diet Assoc 87(9):1164, 1987.
2. Klurfeld DM: The role of dietary fiber in gastrointestinal disease, J Am Diet Assoc 87(9):1172, 1987.
3. Ink SL and Hurt HD: Nutritional implications of gums, Food Technol 41:77, Jan 1987.
4. Anderson JW and others: Dietary fiber and diabetes: a comprehensive review and practical application, J Am Diet Assoc 87(9):1189, 1987.
5. Anderson JW and Gustafson NJ: Dietary fiber and heart disease: current management concepts and recommendations, Top Clin Nutr 3(2):21, 1988.
6. Greenwald P, Lanza E, and Eddy GA: Dietary fiber in the reduction of colon cancer risk, J Am Diet Assoc 87(9):1178, 1987.

Further Readings

Andon SA: Applications of soluble dietary fiber, Food Technol 41:74, Jan 1987.

This article provides interesting information about the use of soluble fiber in various gums as a thickener and stabilizer in such common food products as applesauce, chocolate pudding, iced tea mix, strawberry and orange drinks, chicken and mushroom soups, and noodle soup.

Hannigan KJ: The sweetener report 1982-1987, Food Eng 54:75, July 1982.

This article provides interesting information about the use of soluble fiber in various gums as a thickener and stabilizer in such common food products as applesauce, chocolate pudding, iced tea mix, strawberry and orange drinks, chicken and mushroom soups, and noodle soup.

Lanza E, and Butrum RR: A critical review of food fiber analysis and data, J Am Diet Assoc 86(6):732, 1986.

These authors clarify the problems related to accurate food fiber analysis and provide a useful table of dietary fiber in selected foods.

Skinner S and Martens RA: The milk sugar dilemma: living with lactose intolerance, East Lansing, Mich, 1985, Medi-Ed Press.

These authors, a registered dietitian and a gastroenterologist, provide much helpful information for persons with lactose intolerance, including practical guidelines for the lactose-restricted diet.

The Sugar Phobia Syndrome

The Puritan "pleasure is evil" ethic has probably done as much as nutrition misinformation in popular media to promote Americans' general fear of sweets. Actually, carbohydrate-rich foods have provided people with one of their primary sources of nutrients—and pleasure—since the beginning of time. And because of our inborn taste for sweets, the greater the pleasure it has often provided. Yet the idea has persisted, "If it's good tasting, it must be bad for you."

Whatever the cause, it is becoming increasingly obvious that America has developed a fear of carbohydrates, especially in one of the simplest forms—sugar. This fear appears in an obsession with weight control, to be achieved mainly through elimination of sweets and the large number of kilocalories they add to the average diet, and the use instead of sugar substitutes. It also surfaces in beliefs that sugar is responsible for many ills such as heart disease, diabetes, hypoglycemia, hyperactivity, and dental caries. But only in the case of dental caries is the evidence indisputable. Consider these fears and beliefs in turn.

Kilocalories. Approximately 20% of the total caloric intake of the average American diet is provided by sugar, often through pies, cakes, ice cream, and other rich desserts high in fat. Since fat provides more than twice the number of kilocalories per serving as sugar, the dieter should be primarily concerned with reducing this nutrient as well. In fact, the intelligent dieter should be concerned with reducing the overall excessive caloric intake.

Heart disease. Sucrose has been associated in past research with various dietary factors related to heart disease, such as cholesterol, low-density lipoproteins (LDLs), and plasma triglycerides. However, current research does not support these earlier associations, and a direct cause and effect relationship has not been shown.

Diabetes mellitus. Sugar and other simple carbohydrates can contribute to elevated blood glucose levels in persons with diabetes. But contrary to popular opinion, sugar does *not* cause diabetes. It is only one of many variables, such as caloric intake and stress, that can trigger a rise in blood sugar in persons with diabetes.

Hypoglycemia. Sugar intake first brings hyperglycemia, which in turn triggers the release of insulin. The insulin output, which may exceed the need, then reduces the blood sugar level, and in some sensitive persons these levels may become abnormally low. The popular press has often recommended a very low-carbohydrate, high-protein diet to counteract this effect while condemning the use of sugar entirely. However, current research indicates that a diet low in simple sugars, whatever their form, and more liberal in complex carbohydrates and dietary fiber is effective in raising the blood glucose to a normal level, even in persons with diabetes.

Hyperactivity. Some practitioners have observed changes in the behavior of certain children consuming a high-sugar diet and have noted greater activity, ease of stimulation, and other signs suggesting an association between sugar intake and hyperactivity. But a number of problems have clouded the issue, including the absence of reliable methods for measuring a child's behavior, the possibility of environmental factors such as stress contributing to the changed behavior, and the lack of conclusive controlled studies relating sugar intake to hyperactivity.

Dental caries. Here is the one definitive sugar-associated problem. Dental caries is the only health problem that has been proved to be "caused" by sugar. However, the effect of sugar has been waning because of the widespread practice of fluoridation, which together with better dental care has greatly reduced the incidence of caries.

Continued.

Issues and Answers

Sugar substitutes

Despite sugar's questionable contribution to major health problems, the "fear of sugar" has led the public to increase its demand for alternative sweeteners. These agents include both nonnutritive sweeteners, such as saccharin, and nutritive factors such as lactose or fructose, as well as amino acids (aspartame: NutriSweet and Equal), that contribute both kilocalories and specific nutrient factors to the diet. But these sweeteners have not solved the dieter's dilemma. For example, although consuming enough saccharin, and now aspartame, to replace 150 kilocalories' worth of sugar every day, Americans still have failed to make a dent either in the total amount of sugar they consume—as much as 63 kg (140 lb) per person per year—or in the average body weight of the population. In two ways, these sugar substitutes do not fill the need:

■ **Physiologic response differences.** Artificial sweeteners do not replace the desire for sugar because they do not trigger the same physiologic responses mediated by neurotransmitters in the brain, induced by sugar, to produce **satiety**. Although for many persons the level of natural sweetness provided by vegetables, fruits, and milk often satisfies the need for a sweet taste, the average user of nonnutritive sweeteners may find that the desire for "something sweet" is even greater than that of the average sugar user.

■ **Increased fat intake.** Often users of artificial sweeteners try to achieve satiety by increasing their intake of fats. This excess fat only adds to their health problems and sabotages their weight-loss efforts.

Thus the use of artificial sweeteners may help some persons reduce their excessive sugar intake, but it is wise to temper the use of these products in the light of current knowledge:

■ Artificial sweeteners cannot satisfy the need for satiety or the physiologic experience of a sweet taste. In fact, they may even increase the desire for "real" sweets.

■ Excessive amounts of artificial sweeteners can also cause real problems, such as diarrhea in the case of sorbitol. Saccharin, through approved for use by the general public, is still considered a weak carcinogen. Aspartame (Equal, NutriSweet), approved for widespread use in soft drinks and other commercial products, enjoys a large consumer market, but because it is made from two amino acids, phenylalanine and aspartic acid, it cannot be used freely by children with the genetic disease phenylketonuria.

So what is the answer? Even though there is growing evidence that sugar may not be the dangerous food item some people seem to believe, sugar-eaters may benefit from a little pseudo-Puritanical advice: too much of *anything* can be harmful. Summing up, then, consumers should become aware of the benefits of moderate sugar use, as well as the hazards of excessive amounts of sugar and its substitute sweeteners. In this way they can make intelligent decisions regarding their use.

Satiety
Feeling of fullness or satisfaction as after a meal or quenching one's thirst.

REFERENCES

Bennett W: The taste that failed, Am Health 2(4):49, 1983.

Cohen SM: Saccharin: past, present, and future, J Am Diet Assoc 86(7):929, 1986.

Crapo PA, Kolterman OG, and Henry RR: Metabolic consequences of two-week fructose feeding in diabetic subjects, Diabetes Care 9:111, March/April 1986.

Report: Sweeteners—nutritive and nonnutritive, Food Technol 40:195, Aug 1986.

4 Fats

Chapter Objectives

After studying this chapter, the student should be able to:

1. Identify forms of fat and other lipids essential in the human diet and describe their nature and functions in the human body.

2. Determine how much and what type of fats are necessary in our diet and in our bodies to maintain good health.

3. Identify sound guidelines to ensure the appropriate dietary use of fats to promote health.

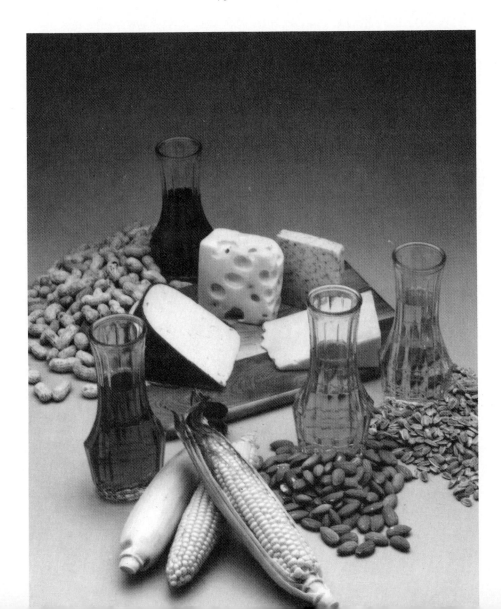

PREVIEW

In addition to carbohydrate, to further solve its energy problem, the body turns to fat as another basic fuel source. Fat is a valuable fuel because it is highly concentrated, having about twice the energy value of carbohydrate.

Traditionally fat has held a prominent place in the American diet. We have maintained a relatively rich fare in our basic food patterns with approximately 45% of our total caloric intake coming from fat, more than that of any other developed country.

However, spurred by our justified health concerns, our attitudes and habits regarding fat have begun to change. Our general goal in this chapter is to help achieve some balance in our food habits and our attitudes toward fat and health, based on our current knowledge of the nature of fat and its related compounds, its fate in our bodies, and its role in human nutrition.

Fats as Basic Fuel for Energy

Lipids
Group name for organic substances of fatty nature. The lipids include fats, oils, waxes, and related compounds.

Backup Fuel Storage

Fats provide a concentrated storage form of basic fuel for the human energy system. They include substances such as fat, oil, and related compounds that are greasy to the touch and insoluble in water. Substances of this class are called **lipids.** Some basic food fuel forms of fat are easily seen as fat: butter, margarine, oil, salad dressings, bacon, cream. Other food forms of fat are more hidden: egg yolk, meat fats, olives, avocados, nuts, seeds.

Relation of Fats to Health

Dietary Fat

Many Americans eat a relatively large amount of fat, about 45% or more of the total kilocalories in their diet. However, questions are being raised about the amount and kind of fat we eat in relation to our health.

Health Needs for Fat

We need fat in our food and in our bodies to keep us healthy. This need is indicated by the number of functions fat performs in nutrition, both in our diets and in our overall body metabolism.

Food fats

Linoleic acid
Major essential fatty acid. It is polyunsaturated.

1. **Fuel source.** Food fats supply a basic continuing source of fuel for the body to store and burn as needed for energy. Food fat yields 9 kcal/g when oxidized in the body, whereas carbohydrate yields 4 kcal/g.
2. **Essential nutrient supply.** Food fats supply the essential fatty acids, especially **linoleic acid,** and cholesterol as needed to supplement the body's endogenous supply.
3. **Food satiety.** Fats in the diet supply flavor to food, which contributes to a feeling of satisfaction that lasts longer after eating than does the feeling of satisfaction after eating carbohydrates. This satiety is enhanced by the fuller texture and body that fat contributes to food mixtures and the slower gastric emptying time it brings.

Body fats

1. **Energy.** A major function of fat in nutrition is to supply an efficient fuel to all tissues except the central nervous system and brain, which depend on glucose.
2. **Thermal insulation.** The layer of fat directly underneath the skin controls body temperature within the range necessary for life.
3. **Vital organ protection.** A web-like padding of **adipose** fat surrounds vital organs such as the kidneys, protecting them from mechanical shock and providing a supporting structure.
4. **Nerve impulse transmission.** Fat layers surrounding nerve fibers provide electrical insulation and transmit nerve impulses.
5. **Tissue membrane structure.** Fat serves as a vital constituent of the cell membrane structure, helping transport nutrient materials and metabolites across cell membranes.
6. **Cell metabolism.** Combinations of fat and protein, **lipoproteins** carry fat in the blood to all cells.
7. **Essential precursor substances.** Fat supplies necessary components such as fatty acids and cholesterol for synthesis of many materials required for metabolic functions and tissue integrity.

Adipose
Fat present in cells of adipose or fatty tissue.

Health Problems with Fat

From the lists above it is evident that fat is an essential nutrient. But if fat is as vital to human health as indicated, what is the problem about fat in the diet? As with so many things, and certainly with fat, the old maxim still holds true: you need what you need, but you don't need more than you need. Specifically, health problems with fat focus on two main issues: too much dietary fat, reflected in too much body fat, and too much of the dietary fat coming from animal food sources.

Lipoproteins
Noncovalent complexes of fat with protein. The lipoproteins probably function as major carriers of lipids in the plasma, since most of the plasma fat is associated with them. Such a combination makes possible the transport of fatty substances in a predominantly aqueous medium such as plasma.

Amount of Fat

Too much fat in the diet provides excessive kilocalories, more than required for immediate energy needs. The excess is stored as increasing adipose tissue and body weight. How much fat is in your own diet? You might try figuring it out for a day (see the box on p. 72). This increased body weight (more precisely, the increased proportion of body fat making up the total body composition) has been associated with health problems such as diabetes, hypertension, and heart disease. Look for specific relationships in later chapters on these topics.

Kind of Fat

An excess of saturated fat and cholesterol in the diet, which comes from animal sources, has been clearly related by current research to *atherosclerosis*, the underlying blood vessel disease characterized by fatty plaques on interior vessel walls that can eventually fill the vessel and cut off blood circulation at that point (see Chapter 20). This disease process contributes to heart attacks and strokes (see Issues and Answers on p. 84).

Fatty Acids

The class name for fats and fat-related compounds is *lipids*. These are compounds that have in common a relationship to the fatty acids. The same basic

The Nature of Lipids

Clinical Application

How Much Fat Are You Eating?

Keep an accurate record of everything you eat or drink for 1 day. Be sure to estimate and add amounts of all fat or other nutrient seasonings used with your foods. (If you want a more representative picture and have a computer available with nutrient analysis software, keep a 1-week record and calculate an average of the 7 days.)

Calculate the total kilocalories (kcal) and grams of each of the energy nutrients (carbohydrate, fat, and protein) in everything you eat. Multiply the total grams of each energy nutrient by its respective fuel value:

$$\text{carbohydrate}\underline{\hspace{1cm}}g \times 4 = \underline{\hspace{1cm}}\text{kcal}$$
$$\text{fat}\underline{\hspace{1cm}}g \times 9 = \underline{\hspace{1cm}}\text{kcal}$$
$$\text{protein}\underline{\hspace{1cm}}g \times 4 = \underline{\hspace{1cm}}\text{kcal}$$

Calculate the percentage of each energy nutrient in your total:

$$\text{Fat kcal} \div \text{total kcal} \times 100 = \% \text{ fat kcal in diet}$$

Compare with fat in American diet (45%); with the U.S. dietary guidelines (25% to 30%).

---

chemical elements that make up carbohydrate—carbon, hydrogen, and oxygen—also make up the fatty acids and their related fats. Fatty acids are also refined fuel forms of fat that some cells such as heart muscle prefer over glucose.

Saturation of Fatty Acids

Saturation
To cause to unite with the greatest possible amount of another substance through solution, chemical combination, or the like.

This state of **saturation** or unsaturation gives fats varying textural characteristics. Saturated fats are harder, less saturated ones are softer, and unsaturated ones are usually liquid oils. This differing state results from the ratio of hydrogen to carbon in the structures of the respective fatty acids that make up a particular fat. If a given fatty acid is filled with as much hydrogen as it can take, the fatty acid is said to be completely *saturated* with hydrogen. If, however, the fatty acid has less hydrogen it is obviously less saturated. Three terms designate the varying degree of saturation:

1. **Saturated.** Food fats composed of such saturated fatty acids are called *saturated fats*. These fats are of animal origin.
2. **Monounsaturated.** Food fats composed mainly of fatty acids with one less hydrogen atom creating one double bond are called *monounsaturated fats*. These fats are mostly from plant sources, for example, olive oil.
3. **Polyunsaturated.** Food fats composed mainly of unsaturated fatty acids with two or more places unfilled with hydrogen creating double bonds are called *polyunsaturated fats*. These fats are from plant sources. Notable exceptions are coconut oil, palm oil, and cocoa butter, which are saturated.

Essential Fatty Acids

The term *essential* or *nonessential* is applied to a nutrient according to its relative necessity in the diet. The nutrient is essential if its absence creates a specific disease and the body cannot manufacture it so must obtain it from the diet. If fat makes up only 10% or less of the diet's daily kilocalories, the body cannot obtain adequate amounts of the essential fatty acids. Three fatty acids—linoleic, linolenic, arachidonic—are the only ones known to be essential for the complete nutrition of humans. Actually only linoleic acid is a *true* **essential fatty acid (EFA),** since the other two may be naturally synthesized from it. These fatty acids, linoleic acid, along with linolenic and arachidonic acids, serve important body functions:

1. **Membrane structure.** Linoleic acid strengthens cell membranes, helping prevent a damaging increase in skin and membrane permeability. A linoleic acid deficiency leads to a breakdown in skin integrity, resulting in characteristic eczema and skin lesions. A similar effect also occurs in other tissue membranes throughout the body.

2. **Cholesterol transport.** Like other fatty acids, linoleic acid combines with cholesterol to form cholesterol esters for transport in the blood.

3. **Serum cholesterol.** As do other unsaturated fatty acids, linoleic acid helps lower serum cholesterol levels. It plays a key role in both transport and metabolism of cholesterol.

4. **Blood clotting.** With its closely associated metabolic products arachidonic acid and linolenic acid, linoleic acid helps prolong blood clotting time and increase fibrinolytic activity.

5. **Local hormone-like effects.** Linoleic acid is a major metabolic precursor of a group of physiologically and pharmacologically active compounds known as *prostacyclins, prostaglandins, thromboxanes,* and *leukotrienes,* which are called *eicosanoids* (from Greek *eicosa,* twenty) because of their structure, long 20-carbon chain polyunsaturated fatty acids (see the box on p. 74). These eicosanoid compounds have extensive local hormone-like effects.[1] They are synthesized in the body from arachidonic acid, which is derived from essential linoleic acid. The synthesis of these highly active important compounds is diagrammed in Figure 4-1, which also shows some of their significant physiologic functions and sites.

Prostaglandins

Of these groups of *eicosanoid* compounds related to the omega-3 long-chain fatty acids, perhaps the most familiar is the group of **prostaglandins** because of their extensive functions. They were first discovered by Swedish investigators in their study of reproductive physiology, identified initially in human semen, and named prostaglandins because they were thought to originate in the prostate gland. They are now known to exist in virtually all body tissues, acting as local "hormones" to direct and coordinate important biologic functions. For example, they have been shown to be powerful modulators of vascular smooth muscle tone and platelet aggregation and hence have a significant relationship to cardiovascular disease.[2]

Chain Length of Fatty Acids

Another characteristic of fatty acids, important in their absorption, is the length of the carbon chain composing their structure. The long-chain fatty

Essential fatty acid (EFA)
Fatty acid that is (1) necessary for body metabolism or function and (2) cannot be manufactured by the body and must therefore be supplied in the diet. The major essential fatty acid is linoleic acid ($C_{17}H_{31}COOH$). It is found principally in vegetable oils. Two other fatty acids usually classified as essential are linolenic acid and arachidonic acid.

Prostaglandins
Group of naturally occurring long-chain fatty acids having local hormone-like actions of widely diverse forms.

To Probe Further

Omega-3 Fatty Acids: Health or Hype?

Often with new nutrition research findings comes a heavy dose of hype and a new diet fad. This is especially true when the research holds promise for combating heart disease and its dreaded fatty arteries, as well as other chronic health problems. Such is the case with the *omega-3* fatty acids and their rich presence in fatty fish.

Currently, several major brands of omega-3 fish oil capsules are competing for an estimated $100-million to $200-million market, twice the number of brands in 1986, when sales were $30 million. And despite warnings from many medical scientists and nutritionists about their safety, effectiveness, and cost, these fish oil capsules are being touted as the "nutritional breakthrough" of the decade.

But if you can get past the commercial hype and maintain perspective, you'll find some remarkable scientific data accumulating. Scientific interest was first sparked by earlier observations among Greenland Eskimos, who eat a diet rich in fish oils but have a low incidence of heart disease. These fish oils contain high levels of the class of long-chain polyunsaturated fatty acids called *omega-3* fatty acids. [Omega (ω) is the last letter in the Greek alphabet, used by scientists for naming fatty acid classes by the structure of their carbon chain, counting from the end of the chain.] There is an especially high level of one of these omega-3 fatty acids in fish oils, **eicosa-pentaenoic acid (EPA)** (from Greek *eicosa-*, twenty; *penta-*, five). The name designates its structure, abbreviated $20:5\omega3$, meaning a long-chain polyunsaturated fatty acid of 20 carbons with 5 double bonds (unsaturated points), the first double bond located at carbon 3 counting from the omega end of the carbon chain.

Accumulating evidence supports the potential nutritional and clinical relevance of these omega-3 fatty acids, and research budgets have increased. The National Institutes of Health (NIH), for example, is currently studying both synthesis and comparative effects of these fatty acids. The human body obtains omega-3 EPA mainly from fatty fish in the diet but can synthesize it from linolenic acid. The other two essential fatty acids, linoleic and arachidonic, are omega-6 fatty acids, closely related in their metabolic pathways and functions. In fact, the two precursor essential fatty acids, linolenic (omega-3) and linoleic (omega-6) acids, compete for the same metabolic enzyme systems in the body in producing their *eicosanoid* substances. A focus of current research is the optimal dietary balance of omega-3 and omega-6 fatty acids and the metabolic balance effects of their differing forms of the eicosanoids.

The eicosanoids—*leukotrienes, thromboxanes, prostacyclines,* and the more familiar *prostaglandins*—are highly active hormone-like substances produced and acting locally in various body tissues (Figure 4-1). They have highly significant physiologic effects in helping to modulate and balance cardiovascular functions.

Current research has begun to clarify these eicosanoid effects and their relationships to health and disease. On the basis of results thus far, successful applications to major diseases of our times affecting vascular function, inflammatory reactions, and immune response are highly probable. In any event, wherever these intensified studies take us, they are certain to be important to health professionals and the public alike.

REFERENCES

Anderson PA and Sprecher HW: Omega-3 fatty acids in nutrition and health, Dietetic Currents 14(2):7, 1987.

Kinsella JE: Dietary fish oils, Nutr Today 21(6):7, 1986.

acids are more difficult to absorb and require a helping carrier. The medium- and short-chain fatty acids are more soluble in water and hence easier to absorb directly into the blood stream. In intestinal malabsorption disease, when the absorbing mucosal surface is inflamed or infected, short- or medium-chain fat products are preferred. A commercial product called MCT (medium-chain triglycerides) is an oil made of medium- and short-chain fatty acids that can be used in the diet just as any ordinary vegetable oil.

Triglycerides

Structure

Fats are **glycerides** composed of **glycerol** and fatty acids. When glycerol is combined with one fatty acid it is called a *monoglyceride,* with two fatty acids a *diglyceride,* and with three fatty acids a *triglyceride.* Whether in food or in the body, fatty acids combine with glycerol to form glycerides. Most natural fats, whether from animal or plant sources, are triglycerides. These fats, the **triglycerides,** occur in body cells as oily droplets. They circulate in water-based blood serum encased in a covering of water-soluble protein. These fat-protein complexes are called *lipoproteins.* They serve multiple functions throughout the body.

Nature of Food Fats

Food fats, as well as body fats, are composed of saturated and unsaturated fatty acids. If the food fat is made up mainly of saturated fatty acids, it is called a saturated fat. Foods from animal sources such as meat, milk, and eggs contain saturated fats. Conversely, food from plant sources such as the vegetable oils are unsaturated fats. A general saturated-unsaturated spectrum of food fats is shown in Figure 4-2. The animal food fats on the saturated end of the spectrum are solid; those toward the center become somewhat less saturated and are softer. The plant fats on the unsaturated end are free-flowing oils that do not solidify even at low temperatures. Exceptions

Glycerides
Group name for fats, any of a group of esters obtained from glycerol by the replacement of one, two, or three hydroxyl (OH) groups with a fatty acid. Glycerides are the principal constituent of adipose tissue and are found in animal and vegetable fats and oils.

Glycerol
Colorless, odorless, syrupy, sweet liquid; a constituent of fats usually obtained by the hydrolysis of fats. Chemically, glycerol is an alcohol; it is esterified with fatty acids to produce fats.

Triglycerides
Compound of three fatty acids esterified to glycerol. A neutral fat, synthesized from carbohydrate, stored in adipose tissue. It releases free fatty acids into the blood after being hydrolyzed by enzymes.

Figure 4-1
Synthesis, sites, and functions of eicosanoids.

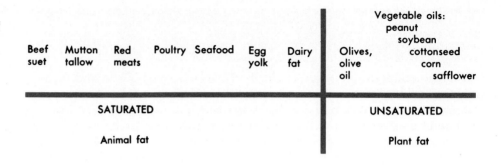

| Beef suet | Mutton tallow | Red meats | Poultry | Seafood | Egg yolk | Dairy fat | Olives, olive oil | Vegetable oils: peanut soybean cottonseed corn safflower |

SATURATED   UNSATURATED

Animal fat   Plant fat

Figure 4-2
Spectrum of food fats according to degree of saturation of component fatty acid.

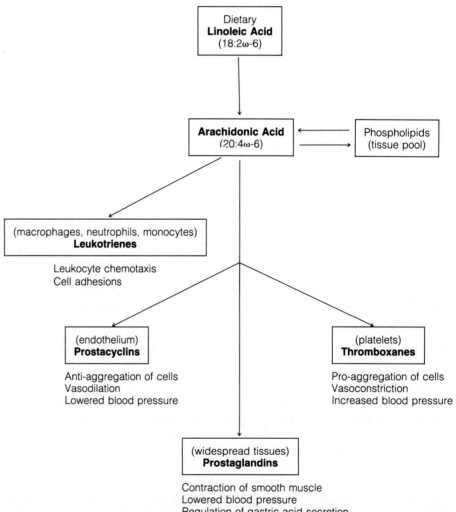

Dietary
Linoleic Acid
(18:2ω-6)

Arachidonic Acid
(20:4ω-6) ⟷ Phospholipids (tissue pool)

(macrophages, neutrophils, monocytes)
Leukotrienes

Leukocyte chemotaxis
Cell adhesions

(endothelium)
Prostacyclins

Anti-aggregation of cells
Vasodilation
Lowered blood pressure

(platelets)
Thromboxanes

Pro-aggregation of cells
Vasoconstriction
Increased blood pressure

(widespread tissues)
Prostaglandins

Contraction of smooth muscle
Lowered blood pressure
Regulation of gastric acid secretion
Regulation of body temperature
Regulation of platelet aggregation
Control of inflammation, vascular permeability

are coconut oil, palm oil, and cocoa butter, which are saturated fats. Since these saturated plant fats are used extensively in commercial products because they are usually cheaper oils, it is important to read product labels carefully. More label information about fat composition is needed. This distinction in saturation, as shown in Figure 4-2, is helpful in explaining to persons on modified fat diets the correct choices of food fats. Also, the unsaturated oils can be hardened commercially into products such as margarine and shortening by injection of hydrogen gas to saturate them, a process called **hydrogenation.**

Visible and Hidden Food Fat

As indicated, food fats are sometimes called "visible" or "hidden" fats according to how obvious they are in food. In most cases the food fat is quite evident, such as in butter, margarine, oil, salad dressing, bacon, and cream, which account for about 40% of the fat in the American diet. However, less obvious hidden fats in foods such as meat, milk (unless it is a nonfat form), eggs (only in the yolk; the white is pure protein), nuts, seeds, olives, and avocados contribute more to our fat intake. A large part of this fat comes from our relatively high consumption of meats. Even when all the fat is trimmed off a cut of meat, its lean portion still contains 4% to 12% hidden fat. Higher grades of meat, both prime and choice, have considerable "marbling," tiny fat deposits within the muscle tissue. This is especially true of beef, the major meat on the American market for many years. Thus the meat and milk food groups together contribute about half the fat in the American diet. And considering all sources, about 45% of the total kilocalories come from fat, an excessive amount.

Yet even with increasing health concerns about their fat intake, Americans still seem ambivalent. They cut down in some areas, but at the same time purchase larger amounts of red meats with considerable nonseparable fat, such as ground beef and hamburgers. This conflicting pattern of meat fat consumption, termed "meat fat madness" by one research team, suggests that such contradictory choices are made by an ill-informed public.[3] But the meat industry, challenged by health-conscious consumers, is now developing leaner breeds through genetic engineering, the so-called Lite or Ultra label for meat containing 25% less fat, and promoting leaner cuts in smaller portions for low-fat cooking.[4]

Cholesterol
Structure

Although **cholesterol** is often discussed in connection with dietary fat, it is not a fat (triglyceride) itself. Many people confuse cholesterol with saturated fat. It is a fat-related compound that is quite different from triglycerides in structure. Generally, cholesterol travels in the blood stream attached to long-chain fatty acids, forming cholesterol **esters.**

Functions

Cholesterol is a vital substance in human metabolism. It belongs to a family of substances called **steroids,** or sterols, and is a precursor to all steroid hormones. A compound in the skin, *7-dehydrocholesterol,* a derivative of cholesterol, is irradiated by sunlight's ultraviolet rays to produce vitamin D hor-

Hydrogenation
Process of adding hydrogen to unsaturated fats to produce a solid, saturated fat. This process is used to produce vegetable shortening from vegetable oils.

Cholesterol
Fat-related compound, a sterol ($C_{27}H_{45}OH$). It is a normal constituent of bile and a principal constituent of gallstones. In body metabolism, cholesterol is important as a precursor of various steroid hormones, such as sex hormones and adrenal corticoids.

Ester
A compound produced by the reaction between an acid and an alcohol with elimination of a molecule of water. For example, a triglyceride is an ester.

Steroids
Any of a large group of fat-related organic compounds, including sterols, bile acids, sex hormones of the adrenal cortex, and D vitamins.

mone. It is also essential in the formation of bile acids, which emulsify fats for enzymatic digestion and then serve as a carrier for fat absorption. Cholesterol is widely distributed in all cells of the body and is found in large amounts in brain and nerve tissue. It is an essential component of cell membranes. It is small wonder therefore that a constant supply of so vital a material for body processes would be made in body tissues, mainly in the liver. If a person consumed *no* cholesterol at all, the body would still synthesize a needed supply.

Food Sources

Cholesterol occurs naturally in all animal foods. There is none in plant foods. Its main food sources are egg yolks and organ meats such as liver and kidneys. In fact, cholesterol occurs *only* in animal fats and animal tissues, *not* in plant fats or tissues. Therefore vegetable oils do not contain cholesterol. Plant oils may vary in degree of saturation, but *none* of them contain cholesterol.

Health Concerns

Cholesterol has now been strongly implicated in vascular disease as a large risk factor in the development of *atherosclerosis,* the underlying pathology in coronary heart disease, in which cholesterol-containing fatty plaques build up in blood vessel walls. Current research has strengthened the association of this process with elevated serum cholesterol levels.[5,6] As a result, the U.S. Department of Health and Human Services through its National Institutes of Health is currently conducting a National Cholesterol Education Program to help physicians screen and treat persons with high blood cholesterol levels, working first with nutritionists to improve food habits and adding drug therapy as needed.[7,8] The various U.S. dietary guidelines (see Chapter 1) recommend that Americans reduce their dietary cholesterol intake to about 300 mg/day. An increase in soluble types of dietary fiber, described in the previous chapter, is also recommended because these fibers bind bile acids and dietary cholesterol, helping to eliminate excess cholesterol from the body.

Lipoproteins
Function

The lipoproteins are important combinations of fat with protein and other fat-related components that are highly significant in human nutrition. They are complexes of lipids and **apoproteins** that serve as the major vehicle for fat transport in the blood stream.

Fat Transport

Fat is insoluble in water. This simple fact poses a problem in carrying fat to cells in a water-based circulatory system. The body has solved this problem through the development of the *lipoproteins,* packages of fat wrapped in water-soluble protein. These plasma lipoproteins contain fatty acids, triglycerides, cholesterol, **phospholipids,** and traces of other materials such as fat-soluble vitamins and steroid hormones. The high or low density of the lipoprotein is determined by its relative loads of fat and protein. The higher the protein ratio, the higher the density:

Apoprotein
Protein part of a compound, as of a lipoprotein. For example, apoprotein C II, an apoprotein of HDL and VLDL that functions to activate the enzyme, lipoprotein lipase.

Phospholipids
Any of a class of fat-related substances that contain phosphorus, fatty acids, and a nitrogenous base. The phospholipids are essential elements in every cell.

1. **Chylomicrons,** formed in the intestinal wall following a meal and carrying a high ratio of fat (90%) with a small amount of protein, have the lowest density. They deliver diet fat to liver cells for initial conversion to other transport lipoproteins.
2. **Very low-density lipoproteins (VLDLs)** deliver endogenous triglycerides to tissue cells.
3. **Intermediate low-density lipoproteins (ILDLs)** continue the delivery of endogenous triglycerides to tissue cells.
4. **Low-density lipoproteins (LDLs)** deliver cholesterol to the peripheral tissue cells.
5. **High-density lipoproteins (HDLs)** transfer free cholesterol from tissues to the liver for catabolism and excretion.

The lipoproteins are related to lipid disorders and vascular disease, so look for details of their structures and functions in Chapter 20.

The basic fat fuel—various animal and plant fats (triglycerides) that naturally occur in foods—are then taken into the body with the diet. Then the task is to change these basic fuel fats into a refined fuel form of fat that the cells can burn for energy. This key refined fuel form is the individual **fatty acid.** The body accomplishes this task through the process of fat digestion.

Mouth

No chemical fat breakdown takes place in the mouth. In this first portion of the gastrointestinal tract, fat is simply broken up into smaller particles through chewing and moistened for passage into the stomach with the general food mass.

Stomach

Little if any chemical fat digestion takes place in the stomach. General peristalsis continues the mechanical mixing of fats with the stomach contents. No significant amount of enzymes specific for fats is present in the gastric secretions except a *gastric lipase* (tributyrinase), which acts on emulsified butterfat. As the main gastric enzymes act on other specific nutrients in the food mix, fat is separated from them and made readily accessible to its own specific chemical breakdown in the small intestine.

Small Intestine

Not until fat reaches the small intestine do the chemical changes necessary for fat digestion occur, with agents from three major sources: a preparation agent through the biliary tract (liver and gallbladder) and specific enzymes from the pancreas and the small intestine itself.

Bile From the Liver and Gallbladder

The presence of fats in the duodenum stimulates the secretion of **cholecystokinin,** a local hormone from glands in the intestinal walls. In turn, cholecystokinin causes contraction of the gallbladder, relaxation of the sphincter muscle, and subsequent secretion of **bile** into the intestine by way of the common bile duct. The liver produces a large amount of dilute bile, then the gallbladder concentrates and stores it, ready for use with fat as needed. Its function is that of an **emulsifier.** *Emulsification* is not a chemical digestive

Digestion: Changing Basic Fuel to Usable Refined Fuel

Fatty acid
Structural components of fats. See *glycerides*, p. 75.

Cholecystokinin
Hormone that is secreted by the mucosa of the duodenum in response to the presence of fat. It causes the gallbladder to contract, which propels bile into the duodenum, where it is needed to emulsify the fat.

Bile
Greenish yellow to golden brown alkaline fluid secreted by the liver and concentrated in the gallbladder. Made of bile salts, cholesterol, phospholipid, bilirubin diglucuronide, and electrolytes.

Emulsifier
An agent that breaks down large fat globules to smaller, uniformly distributed particles.

process itself, but is an important first preparation step for fat's chemical digestion by its specific enzymes. This preparation process accomplishes two important tasks: (1) it breaks the fat into small particles, or globules, which greatly enlarges the total surface area available for action of the enzyme, and (2) it lowers the surface tension of the finely dispersed and suspended fat globules, which allows the enzymes to penetrate more easily. This process is similar to the wetting action of detergents. The bile also provides an alkaline medium for the action of the fat enzyme lipase.

Enzymes From the Pancreas

Lipase
Any of a class of enzymes that break down fats.

Pancreatic juice contains an enzyme for fat and one for cholesterol. First, *pancreatic* **lipase,** a powerful fat enzyme, breaks off one fatty acid at a time from the glycerol base of fats. One fatty acid plus a diglyceride, then another fatty acid plus a monoglyceride, are produced in turn. Each succeeding step of this breakdown occurs with increasing difficulty. In fact, separation of the final fatty acid from the remaining monoglyceride is such a slow process that less than one third of the total fat present actually reaches complete breakdown. The final products of fat digestion to be absorbed are fatty acids, diglycerides, monoglycerides, and glycerol. Some remaining fat may pass into the large intestine for fecal elimination. Second, the enzyme *cholesterol enterase* acts on free cholesterol to form cholesterol esters by combining free cholesterol and fatty acids in preparation for absorption.

Enzyme From the Small Intestine

The small intestine secretes an enzyme in the intestinal juice called *lecithinase.* As its name indicates, it acts on lecithin, a *phospholipid,* to break it down into its components for absorption.

A summary of fat digestion in the successive parts of the gastrointestinal tract is given in Table 4-1 for review.

Absorption: Carrying Refined Fuel to Energy Production Sites—Cells

The task of fat absorption is not easy. The problem is that fats are not soluble in water, and blood is basically water. Hence fat always requires some type of solvent carrier. To accomplish this task of transporting fat from the small intestine into the blood stream, the body has three basic stages of operation.

Stage I: Initial Fat Absorption

Micellar bile-fat complex
A particle formed by the combination of bile salts with fat substances (fatty acids and glycerides) to achieve the absorption of fat across the intestinal mucosa. Bile salt micelles act as detergents to prepare lipids for digestion and absorption.

In the small intestine, bile combines with products of fat digestion in a **micellar bile-fat complex.** This unique carrier system, shown in Figure 4-3, then takes fat along its initial passage into the intestinal wall.

Stage II: Absorption Within the Intestinal Wall

Once inside the wall of the small intestine, the bile separates from the fat complex and returns in circulation to accomplish its task over and over again. Two important actions on the fat products occur inside the intestinal wall: (1) *enteric lipase action*—an enteric lipase within the cells of the intestinal wall completes the digestion of the remaining glycerides, and (2) *triglyceride synthesis*—with the resulting fatty acids and glycerol, new human triglycerides are formed as body fats, ready now for final absorption and circulation.

Table 4-1
Summary of Fat Digestion

Organ	Enzyme	Activity
Mouth	None	Mechanical, mastication
Stomach	No major enzyme	Mechanical separation of fats as protein and starch digested out
	Small amount of gastric lipase tributyrinase	Tributyrin (butterfat) to fatty acids and glycerol
Small intestine	Gallbladder bile salts (emulsifier)	Emulsifies fats
	Pancreatic lipase (steapsin)	Triglycerides to diglycerides and monoglycerides in turn, then fatty acids and glycerol

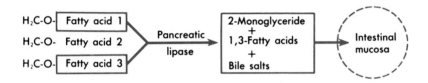

Figure 4-3
Micellar complex of fats with bile salts for transport of fats into intestinal mucosa.

Stage III: Final Absorption and Transport of Fat

These newly formed human fats—triglycerides—and other fat materials present are combined with a small amount of protein covering to form lipoproteins called **chylomicrons.** These packages of fat, in a milk-like liquid called *chyle,* cross the cell membrane intact into the lymphatic system and then into the portal blood. Here a final fat-clearing enzyme, *lipoprotein lipase,* helps clear the large meal load of dietary fat from circulation. In the liver the fat is converted to other lipoproteins for transport to the body cells for energy and other structural functions.

In the body cells, fatty acids are "burned" as concentrated fuel to produce energy. These derived units of fat have about twice the energy value of glucose products. As indicated in Chapter 2, cell metabolism of fat is closely interrelated with that of the other nutrients.

Chylomicrons
Particles of fat—lipoproteins—appearing in the lymph and blood after a meal rich in fat.

Metabolism: Burning Refined Fuel at Production Sites to Produce Energy

To Sum Up

Fat is an essential nutrient which, in addition to supplying the highest density of energy among the energy nutrients, insulates the body against low temperatures and protects vital organs from damage. It also aids in the transmission of nerve impulses, production of metabolic precursors, formation of cell membrane structure, and transport of other molecules such as protein.

Fats are composed of glycerol and attached fatty acids of varying lengths and degrees of saturation. Essential fatty acids are long-chain unsaturated fatty acids that cannot be manufactured by the body. The major one is *linoleic acid*. Its functions include improving skin integrity, lowering serum cholesterol levels, prolonging blood clotting time, and developing a group of special substances called *eicosanoids*, including *prostaglandins*, that are involved in many tissue activities including maintaining smooth muscle tone of blood vessels and platelet aggregations.

The type and amount of dietary fat can affect health. Large amounts of saturated fat and cholesterol add risk factors for cardiovascular disease and other general health problems. Too small an amount of fat can result in a deficiency of the essential fatty acid, linoleic acid. Americans get about 45% of their total kilocalories from fat; the U.S. dietary guidelines recommend 30% to 35%. When fat provides 10% or less of total kilocalories, deficiency symptoms occur.

Questions for Review

1. Two persons with strong family histories of cardiovascular disease are concerned about avoiding heart problems. Both reduce their cholesterol intake and avoid butter. The first person replaces butter with stick margarine made from corn oil, the second with corn oil itself. Which person might have more success with avoiding heart disease? Identify and describe two characteristics of a dietary lipid component that may affect this rate of success.
2. A woman runner concerned about her health dropped her total fat intake to an amount supplying about 10% of her total caloric intake. What health problems would you expect her to encounter?

References

1. Anderson PA and Sprecher HW: Omega-3 fatty acids in nutrition and health, Dietetic Currents 14(2):7, 1987.
2. Knapp HR and others: In vivo indexes of platelet and vascular function during fish-oil administration in patients with atherosclerosis, N Engl J Med 314:937, 1986.
3. Ratje WL and Ho EE: Meat fat madness: conflicting patterns of meat fat consumption and their public health implications, J Am Diet Assoc 87(10):1357, 1987.
4. Report: genetic engineering produces low-fat Ultra Beef, Food Engineering 59:48, July 1987.
5. Report: the lipid research clinics coronary primary prevention trial results. II. The relationship of reduction in incidence of coronary heart disease to cholesterol lowering, JAMA 251(3):365, 1984.
6. Report: Council for Agricultural Science and Technology: diet and coronary heart disease, Nutr Today 21(2):26, 1986.
7. Report: Lowering blood cholesterol to prevent heart disease, Consensus Conference, JAMA 253:2080, 1985.
8. Cleeman JI and Lenfant C: New guidelines for the treatment of high blood cholesterol in adults from the National Cholesterol Education Program: from controversy to consensus, Circulation 76:960, 1987.

Further Readings

Brewer ER, et al: Food group system of analysis with special attention to type and amount of fat—methodology, J Am Diet Assoc 87(5):584, 1987.

This report of 5640 participants in the Lipid Research Clinics Prevalence Study indicates that the amounts and types of dietary fats being consumed by this large population sample of children and adults frequently exceed the recommendations of the dietary guidelines.

Hepburn FN, Exler J, and Weihrauch JL: Provisional tables on the content of omega-3 fatty acids and other fat components of selected foods, J Am Diet Assoc 86(6):788, 1986.

This article provides useful reference tables for omega-3 fatty acid content of a wide variety of seafood, as well as selected foods in other commonly used food groups.

Kolata G: Cholesterol tests: what your blood will tell, Am Health 7(1):41, 1988.

Roberts L: Measuring cholesterol is as tricky as lowering it, Science 238:482, Oct 23, 1987.

Both of these articles describe laboratory inaccuracies in cholesterol tests and give suggestions for improving these procedures.

Report: Council for agricultural science and technology, diet and coronary disease, Nutr Today 21(2):26, 1986.

This official report reviews current knowledge about the nature and function of lipids, fat intake, cholesterol, and the role of fat in coronary heart disease. Many helpful tables and references are provided.

Dietary Fat and Cholesterol: From Controversy to Consensus

Our initial question remains. What about fat in our diets? How much? What kind? Over the past years, experts and consumers alike have not always agreed. They have drawn differing conclusions from the developing body of research. It is small wonder that the public has often been confused. Now, however, the weight of current research is moving scientists and clinicians from years of controversy to an emerging broad international consensus: elevated serum cholesterol *is* a major contributor to vascular disease, and dietary fat, especially saturated fat, *can* affect the serum cholesterol level. Consider this emergence of basic consensus over the past decade of developing research and recommendations.

1977 The controversy began gathering steam, fanned by a government report. The U.S. Senate Committee on Nutrition and Human Health, justly alarmed by the extent of major chronic disease in the gradually aging population, developed a plan that included strategies for attacking the leading killer—coronary heart disease. Its approach was direct and apparently simple: it would advise millions of Americans to reduce their intake of total fats, cholesterol, and saturated fats. These recommendations were based on research showing that people who eat large amounts of fat, as Americans do, tend to develop heart disease more than people who follow leaner diets. This sounds reasonable. But it it is not as simple as it sounds. The fat-disease link was still tenuous. Moreover, Americans seem to love their fat, and a great many sources of vested interests would like to keep it that way and whet those appetites further. On the other hand, many concerned groups of health professionals and consumers remained uneasy about fat.

In the first place, getting Americans to reduce their fat intake is not easy for several reasons:

- Fats make foods more tasteful and give them a pleasing texture. This is a taste cultivated over the past years by our marketplace and is probably why some 45% of the kilocalories in the U.S. diet is made up of fats.

- Meats, milk, eggs, and cheese provide about half of the fat consumed in the U.S., making the task of reducing such animal fat components as cholesterol and saturated fats *very* challenging, to say the least.

In the second place, the task of making any dietary recommendations for the United States is further complicated by two additional concerns:

- Our population is such a heterogeneous group, with a wide variety of food preferences dictated by culture, religion, food availability, and personal likes and dislikes that change is extremely difficult.

- We are such a large group, with persons requiring a wide range of dietary fat, depending on individual health and energy needs, that a "flat rate" for all wouldn't fit for all. So the initial guidelines were simple and general: (1) reduce total fat consumption to 30% of energy intake, (2) reduce saturated fats and increase unsaturated fats instead, and (3) reduce cholesterol consumption.

These initial guidelines also recommended that meat consumption be reduced to meet the general recommendations. Obviously, this conflicts with the interests of meat-producing and marketing concerns. Many organizations were not comfortable with the initial dietary recommendations. The Senate committee, bombarded with comments ranging from considered reflections to angry replies initiated by a wide variety of organizations in both the scientific and medical communities and their adherents, was discontinued after 1978.

1978 A majority of nutrition experts serving on the American Society of Clinical Nutrition panels agreed that there was a real association between fats and heart disease but could not agree on its importance.

1979 The American Medical Association declared that it could not accept the idea of specific amounts of fats, saturated fats, and cholesterol being ideal for the entire country but did suggest that healthy Americans use fat "in moderation."

1980 The Food and Nutrition Board of the National Research Council/ National Academy of Sciences stated that the fat content of the American diet only needs to be adjusted to meet the individual's need for energy and not limited to any specific amount.

In essence, these organizations stated that dietary guidelines must provide for a three-way balance between:

- Individual *need* for dietary fat
- Effects of *excess* dietary fat
- Public *need* for education and guidance regarding basic preventive health issues

Apparently, these suggestions were taken to heart. New guidelines were issued: (1) eat a variety of foods, (2) maintain an ideal weight, and (3) avoid too much fat, saturated fat, and cholesterol.

The government has developed a booklet that explains these and other revised U.S. dietary guidelines to the public, identifying food sources of nutrients, recommended weights for heights, and other general nutrition information. Advice to persons wanting more specific information, such as answers to the question "How much fat and cholesterol are all right for *me*?", is to contact their physician or clinical nutritionist-dietitian for personal counsel.

1985-1988 During these years movement toward consensus became more rapid. Continuing research and expert reports further strengthened the preventive-care approach to health maintenance and vascular disease.

1985 A 30-member expert task force of the Council for Agricultural Science and Technology reviewed current research concerning the role of dietary fat and cholesterol in coronary heart disease and concluded in their 1986 report that the evidence indicated a strong relation, especially in high-risk individuals.

1985 Based on results of the Coronary Primary Prevention Trials, the NIH began the National Cholesterol Education Program on a broad basis.

1986 The International Life Sciences Institute's 1986 Conference on Diet and Health: Scientific Concepts and Principles, involving some 200 scientists from various disciplines forming the basis of nutritional science, stated in its 1987 report of the panel on fat and cholesterol that serum cholesterol concentration was now so consistently correlated with coronary heart disease as to be a strong causative factor. Lowering of fat and saturated fat, as well as weight control, were considered important factors also, and there was agreement that the current research on omega-3 polyunsaturated fatty acids was strong and exciting.

1987 Various published reports of a study at the University of Southern California indicated that a low-fat, low-cholesterol diet, assisted by drugs only in certain cases after vigorous diet therapy, lowered serum cholesterol and reversed coronary disease. Many experts believed that this study provided strong evidence linking cholesterol to heart disease.

1987 A panel of experts convened by the National Heart, Lung, and Blood Institute of NIH, working with more than 20 health agencies, issued its report outlining for physicians important steps in the control of serum cholesterol as a major attack on heart disease. The report emphasized cholesterol monitoring and diet.

1988 Interim reports of the Bogalusa Heart Study, a longitudinal study now in its sixteenth year of monitoring the health and lifestyle of children growing into adulthood in this Louisiana town, reinforced the finding that the fatty changes in arteries underlying heart disease begin early in life in genetically predisposed individuals and are enhanced by elevated serum cholesterol levels. These researchers stated that preventive practices should start early in life, especially in high-risk children, instilling principles of a "prudent" diet to control excess fat, cholesterol, and energy intake, together with the value of exercise and an active life.

Continued.

Dietary Fat and Cholesterol: From Controversy to Consensus—cont'd

1988 U.S. Surgeon General C. Everett Koop issued a strong report focused on dietary fat, saturated fat, and cholesterol as major factors in coronary heart disease and outlining a preventive approach to health promotion and risk reduction through improved dietary patterns.

So firm answers seem to be in. We stand now on firmer ground for developing programs to help people move toward more prudent diets in relation to amount of fat, saturated fat, and cholesterol. Our current U.S. dietary guidelines, along with the more specific guidelines of the American Heart Association, as outlined in Chapter 1, provide us with sound reasonable bases for general nutrition counseling, applied with concern for each individual's life situation. It is possible to *enjoy* food and still exercise considered judgment and selection within whatever variety of food may be available to us.

REFERENCES

Byrne G: Surgeon general takes aim at saturated fats, Science 241:651, Aug, 1988.

Cleeman JI and Lenfant C: New guidelines for the treatment of high blood cholesterol in adults from the National Cholesterol Education Program: from controversy to consensus, Circulation 76:960, 1987.

Grundy SM and Nestel PJ: Fat and cholesterol, in diet and health: scientific concepts and principles, Am J Clin Nutr 45 (suppl):1035, May 1987.

Report: Council for agricultural science and technology: diet and coronary disease, Nutr Today 21(2):26, 1986.

Report of National Cholesterol Education Program, National Heart, Lung, and Blood Institute: Cholesterol counts, Washington, 1986, NIH.

Shell ER: Kids, catfish, and cholesterol, Am Health 7(1):52, 1988.

5 Energy Balance

After studying this chapter, the student should be able to:

1. Define energy and metabolism in terms of dynamic change and balance.

2. Identify and compare the basic units used in measuring human energy.

3. Describe the body's energy sources and means of control.

4. Determine individual energy needs and calculate own total energy balance.

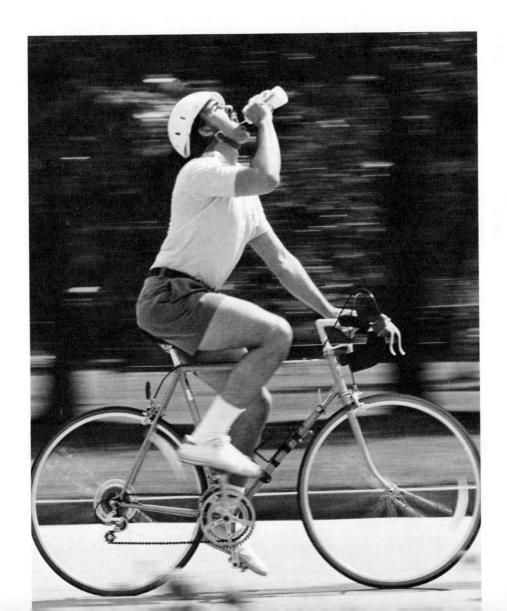

■

In human nutrition the fundamental question is, "How do our efficiently designed bodies transform the elements in food we eat to energy?"
This is basic, for energy is our power to do all that we do. Carbohydrates
and fats, as we have seen, provide the major fuel supply for power in the
human energy system.

Here we look at this remarkable overall energy transformation process
from fuel to power. It is overall *energy metabolism* that deals with the many
dynamic body processes underlying all life, in essence processes of *change*
and *balance*, that produce this power within us. These many constant
changes and balances in the food we eat and the body's physiologic constituents—nutrients and their metabolites—produce energy for the body's
work.

In fact, our study of energy metabolism reminds us that we really live
in two worlds. We discover anew that we exist in both a large energy cycle
in the Earth's environment and a microscopic one within our own body
cells. Here in this inner warm, watery chemical environment, fuel is ig-
nited and "burned" or stored briefly for continuous turnover use as
needed, all the while yielding energy for all our pursuits, both work and
play.

Measurement of Energy

Here, in our brief overview of human energy balance, we look first at the
units we use for measuring energy in our fuel foods and how these food energy values are derived. Then we will apply these units in our general review
of balance in our remarkably efficient human energy system and our energy
requirements for maintaining this system.

Unit of Measure: Kilocalorie (kcal)

Calorie
Measure of heat. The *energy*
required to do the work of the
body is measured as the amount
of *heat* produced by the body's
work.

Since the body can perform work only as energy is released and since all
work takes the form of heat production, energy may be measured in terms of
heat equivalents. Such a heat measure is the **calorie.** In practice, however, to
avoid using large numbers professional nutritionists and scientists use the
term *kilocalorie* (kcalorie, kcal: 1000 calories). By definition, this is the
amount of heat required to raise 1 kg of water 1° C. The international unit
for energy measure is the *joule* (J): one kilocalorie (kcal) equals 4.184 kilo-
joules (kJ); one *megajoule* (MJ) equals 239 kcal. Presently food and energy tables are given in kilocalories, and this measure will be used throughout this
book. However, as America moves toward joining the rest of the world in using the metric system and an international system of units, energy values will
begin to involve these other measures and it is good now to recognize their
names.

Food Energy Measure

The fuel energy in various foods we eat is generally measured in two basic
ways: calorimetry and proximate composition.

Calorimetry

The caloric values of various foods listed in food value tables have usually been determined by the use of a *calorimeter*. This is a measuring instrument made of two parts: an inner part that holds the measured food sample to be tested and a larger outer part that holds surrounding water. As an electric spark burns the food, the surrounding water takes up the heat produced, and the food's caloric value is then measured by the rise in the water temperature. Remember when you use food value tables, however, that these values are actually averages of a number of samples of a given food tested and that a particular serving of that food will vary around that figure. According to nutrient composition, foods have varying degrees of **caloric density.**

Proximate Composition

Another way of measuring food energy is by computing the approximate nutrient composition of a given food using food value tables or data bases. Today such analysis is done rapidly by a computer using a variety of programs and data bases.

Fuel Factors

These food values are based on the average kilocalorie value of each of the energy nutrients. These caloric values are known as the energy nutrient's respective **fuel factor**: 1 g of carbohydrate yields 4 kcal, 1 g of protein yields 4 kcal, 1 g of alcohol yields 7 kcal, and 1 g of fat yields 9 kcal. These basic values are used constantly in general nutrient-energy calculations.

Energy Cycle and Transformation
Forms of Human Energy

It is clear that in our physical world **energy,** like matter, is neither created nor destroyed. When we speak of energy "production," what we really mean is that it is being *transformed.* It is being changed in form and cycled throughout a system. In the human body the various metabolic processes convert stored chemical energy in our food to other forms of energy for the body's work. In our bodies energy is available in four basic forms for life processes: *chemical, electrical, mechanical,* and *thermal.* Our ultimate source of power is the sun with its vast reservoir of nuclear reactions, as diagrammed in Figure 5-1. Then through the process of photosynthesis, using water and carbon dioxide as raw materials, plants transform the sun's energy into food storage forms of chemical energy. In the body these stored food fuels are converted to the basic energy unit glucose, which together with fatty acids is "burned" to release its energy to be transformed and cycled through body systems. Water and carbon dioxide, the initial materials used by plants, are retrieved as end products of this process of oxidation in the body. And so the cycle goes on and on.

Transformation of Energy

Through the many processes of metabolism, after stored chemical energy in food is taken into the body, it is converted further to chemical energy in other metabolic products to do the body's work. This chemical energy is then changed still further to other forms of energy as this work is performed. For

Calorimetry
Measurement of heat loss.

Caloric density
Higher concentration of energy (kilocalories) in smaller amount of food.

Fuel factor
The kcal value (energy potential) of food nutrients; that is, the number of kcals 1 g of a nutrient yields when oxidized.

The Human Energy System

Energy
Capacity of a system for doing work; power to affect changes in self and surroundings.

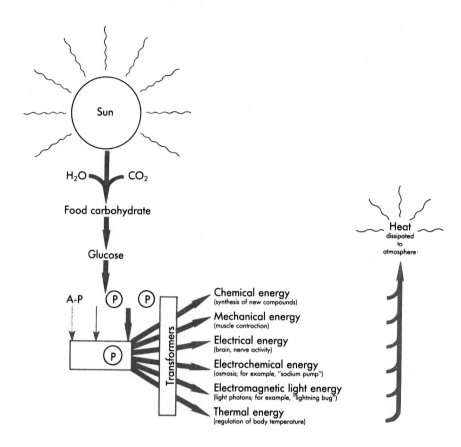

Figure 5-1
Transformation of energy from its primary source (the sun) to various forms for biologic work by means of metabolic processes ("transformers").

example, chemical energy is changed to electrical energy in brain and nerve activity. It is changed to mechanical energy in muscle contraction. It is changed to thermal energy in the regulation of body temperature. It is changed to still other types of chemical energy in the synthesis of new compounds. In all these work activities of the body, heat is given off to the surrounding atmosphere and larger biosphere.

Metabolism
Sum of all the chemical and physical processes that sustain life.

In human **metabolism** as in any energy system, energy is always present as either *free energy* or *potential energy*. Free energy is the energy involved at any given moment in the performance of a task. It is unbound and in motion. Potential energy is the energy that is stored or bound in various chemical compounds, available for conversion to free energy as needed for work. For example, energy stored in sugar is potential energy. When we eat it and it is burned, free energy is released and work results. As work is done, energy in the form of heat is released.

Energy Balance: Input and Output

Whether the energy system is electrical, mechanical, thermal, or chemical, in the course of the many reactions that comprise its operation, free energy is decreased and the reservoir of potential energy is secondarily diminished.

Therefore the system must constantly be refueled from some outside source. In the human energy system this basic input of fuel is our food.[1]

The energy demands of the body require a constant supply of available energy. These energy needs support the body's total basic metabolic needs, as well as its additional physical activity requirements.[2] In the human energy system this physical energy output is evident in our activities. But energy output to an even larger degree is also going on internally at all times to meet our basal metabolic needs.

Energy Control in Human Metabolism

In the human body the energy produced in its many chemical reactions, if "exploded" all at once, would be destructive. There must be some mechanism therefore by which energy is controlled in the human system so that it may support life and not destroy it. Several basic means of control are used to accomplish this task.

Chemical Bonding

The main mechanism by which energy is controlled in the human system is **chemical bonding.** The chemical bonds that hold elements of compounds together consist of energy. As long as the compound remains constant, energy is being exerted to maintain it. When the compound is taken into the body and broken into its parts, this energy is released and available for body work. Three basic types of chemical bonds transfer energy in the body. First are *covalent bonds* such as those that hold carbon atoms together in the core of an organic compound. Second are *hydrogen bonds,* which are weaker than covalent bonds but significant because they can be formed in large numbers. Also, the very fact that they are less strong and can be broken easily makes them important because they can be transferred or passed readily from one substance to another to help form still another substance. Third are the strong *high-energy phosphate bonds,* the main example of which is **adenosine triphosphate (ATP).** This is the unique compound the human body uses to store energy for its cell work. Like storage batteries for electrical energy, these bonds become the controlling force for ongoing energy needs.

Chemical bonding
Mutual attachment of various chemical elements to form chemical compounds.

Adenosine triphosphate (ATP)
A high-energy phosphate compound important in energy exchange for cellular activity.

Controlled Reaction Rates

The many chemical reactions that make up the body's energy system must also have controls. Some of the reactions that break down proteins, for example, if left to themselves (as in sterile decomposition), would span several years. Such reactions must be accelerated or else getting the needed energy from a meal would take years. At the same time, they must be regulated so that too fast a reaction will not produce a burst of energy in a single "explosion." Enzymes, coenzymes, and hormones are the control agents regulating these cell activities.

1. **Enzymes.** Many specific **enzymes** in every cell control specific reactions there. All enzymes are protein compounds. They are produced in the cells under control of specific genes. One specific gene controls the making of one specific enzyme, and there are thousands of enzymes in each cell. Each enzyme works on its own particular substance, which is called its **substrate.** The enzyme and its substrate lock together to produce a new reaction product, and the original enzyme remains unchanged, ready to do its specific work over and over again (Figure 5-2).

Enzyme
Complex organic substance originating in living cells and capable of producing certain chemical changes in other organic substances by catalytic action.

Substrate
Specific organic substance on which a particular enzyme acts.

Figure 5-2
Lock and key concept of the action of enzyme, coenzyme, and substrate to produce a new reaction product.

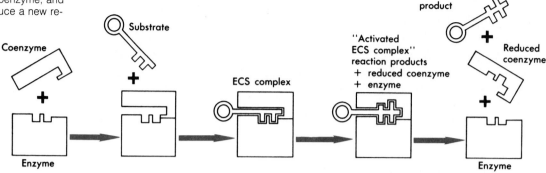

Coenzymes
Enzyme-activators required by some enzymes to produce their reactions.

Hormone
A compound produced in an endocrine organ (an organ of internal secretion; a ductless gland), secreted by the endocrine organ into the bloodstream, and transported by body fluids to a specific receptor or target organ whose function the hormone controls.

2. **Coenzymes.** Many reactions require a partner to assist the enzyme in completing the reaction. These coenzymes in many instances involve several of the vitamins, especially the B vitamins, and some of the minerals. It may be helpful to think of the coenzyme as another substrate, for in receiving the material transferred, the coenzyme is changed or reduced.

3. **Hormones.** In energy metabolism **hormones** act as messengers to trigger or control enzyme action. For example, the rate of oxidative reactions in the tissues, the body's metabolic rate, is controlled by the *thyroid-stimulating hormone (TSH)* from the anterior pituitary gland. Another familiar example is the controlling action of insulin from the pancreas islet cells on the rate of glucose utilization in the tissues. Steroid hormones also have the capacity to regulate the cell's ability to synthesize enzymes.

Types of Metabolic Reaction

The two types of reaction constantly going on in energy metabolism are anabolism and catabolism. Each requires energy. The processes of *anabolism* synthesize new and more complex substances. Energy is required to generate this synthesis. The processes of *catabolism* break down more complex substances to simpler ones. These processes release free energy but also use up some free energy in the work. Therefore there is a constant energy deficit, which must be supplied by food.

Sources of Stored Energy

When food is not available, as in periods of fasting or starvation, the body must draw on its own stores for energy:

1. **Glycogen.** Only a 12- to 48-hour reserve of glycogen exists in liver and muscle and is quickly depleted.
2. **Muscle mass.** Storage of energy as protein exists in limited amounts in muscle mass, but in greater volume than glycogen stores.
3. **Adipose fat tissue.** Although fat storage may be larger, the supply varies from person to person and from circumstance to circumstance.

Energy Requirements

A major portion of an individual's energy needs are based on requirements to maintain the body's internal work. This requirement is a measure of *basal metabolism energy needs*. Also, to these basal needs should be added the needs for food intake's effect and for physical activities to determine the person's *total energy requirements*.

Basal Metabolism Energy Needs

Basal Metabolic Rate (BMR)

The term **basal metabolism** refers to the sum of all internal chemical activities that maintain the body at rest. The basal metabolic rate (BMR) is a measure of the energy required by these activities of resting tissue, sometimes referred to as *resting energy expenditure* (REE). Certain small but vitally active tissues—brain, liver, gastrointestinal tract, heart, kidney—together make up less than 5% of the total body weight, yet they contribute about 60% of the total basal metabolic needs. Although resting muscle and adipose fat tissues are far larger in mass, they contribute much less to the body's BMR.

Measuring BMR

Both direct and indirect methods have been used to measure BMR. In direct methods, a room large enough for a person to enter is used and the body's heat production at rest is measured. But this instrument is large and costly, so it is limited to research studies. Indirect calorimetry is seldom used now in clinical practice but is applied mainly in research. This method measures the exchange of gases in respiration (**respiratory quotient**—CO_2:O_2) while the subject is at rest.[3] Energy (BMR) calculated in this manner is equivalent to the body heat given off.

Today, however, in clinical practice newer methods employ measurements of glandular activities such as that of the thyroid gland. These tests serve as indirect measures of BMR. They include measures of serum protein-bound iodine (PBI), radioactive iodine uptake tests, and serum thyroxine levels. The free thyroxine index (FTI) is a common clinical measure, which is based on the product of T_3 (triiodothyronine) and T_4 (thyroxine). These two compounds are produced in the final two stages of thyroid hormone synthesis in the thyroid gland. This product ($T_3 \times T_4$) reflects the relative functioning of the thyroid gland and the amount of circulating hormone activity influencing the BMR.

Factors Influencing BMR

A number of factors influence the BMR and should be considered when interpreting test results.

1. **Lean body mass.** The major influencing factor of BMR is lean body mass because the metabolic activity in lean tissues is greater than that in less active tissues such as bones and fat. Other factors such as surface area, sex, and age are only influencing factors as they relate to the lean body mass. Energy requirement per unit of body weight is higher when the weight is made up of a higher proportion of muscle mass (see Issues and Answers on p. 99). It is lower when body weight is made up of a higher proportion of fat or bone. Differences, for example, in metabolic requirements for women are primarily related to differences in lean body mass.

2. **Growth.** During growth periods the growth hormone stimulates cell metabolism and raises BMR 15% to 20%. Thus the BMR slowly rises during the first 5 years of life, levels off, rises again just before and during puberty, and then declines into old age. During *pregnancy*, a rapid growth period, the BMR rises 20% to 25% because of the accelerated tissue growth process and

Basal metabolism
Amount of energy needed by the body for maintenance of life when the person is at digestive, physical, and emotional rest

Respiratory quotient =
$$\frac{CO_2 \text{ produced}}{O_2 \text{ consumed}}$$

increased work of heart and lungs. The *lactation* period following pregnancy also increases the BMR about 60%, or 1000 kcal, to meet the energy demands of milk production.

3. **Fever and disease.** For each .83° C (1° F) rise in body temperature, the BMR increases about 7%. Also, diseases involving increased cell activity such as cancer, certain anemias, cardiac failure, hypertension, and respiratory problems such as emphysema usually increase the BMR. In the abnormal states of starvation and malnutrition, the BMR is lowered, since the lean body mass is diminished.

4. **Cold climate.** BMR rises in response to lower temperatures as a compensatory mechanism to maintain body temperature.

Table 5-1

Energy Expenditure/Hour During Various Activities*

Light activities: 120-150 kcal/hr	Light-moderate activities: 150-300 kcal/hr	Moderate activities: 300-420 kcal/hr	Heavy activities: 420-600 kcal/hr
Personal care	Domestic work	Yard work	Yard work
Dressing	Making beds	Digging	Chopping wood
Washing	Sweeping floors	Mowing lawn (not motorized)	Digging holes
Shaving	Ironing	Pulling weeds	Shoveling snow
Sitting	Washing clothes	Walking	Walking
Rocking	Yard work	3½-4 mph on level surface	5 mph
Typing	Light gardening	Up and down small hills	Upstairs
Writing	Mowing lawn (power mower)	Recreation	Up hills
Playing cards	Light work	Badminton	Climbing
Peeling potatoes	Auto repair	Calisthenics	Recreation
Sewing	Painting	Ballet exercises	Bicycling 11-12 mph or up and down hills
Playing piano	Shoe repair	Canoeing 4 mph	Cross-country skiing
Standing or slowly moving around	Store clerk	Dancing (waltz, square)	Jogging 5 mph
Billiards	Washing car	Golf (no cart)	Swimming
	Walking	Ping-Pong	Tennis (singles)
	2-3 mph on level surface or down stairs	Tennis (doubles)	Water-skiing
	Recreation	Volleyball	
	Archery		
	Bicycling 5½ mph on level surface		
	Bowling		
	Canoeing 2½-3 mph		

*Energy expenditure will depend on the physical fitness (that is, amount of lean body mass) of the individual and continuity of exercise. Note that some of these activities can be used as aerobic activities to promote cardiovascular fitness. For more information, see Chapter 14.

Food Intake Effect

Food intake stimulates metabolism and requires energy to meet the many activities of digestion, absorption, and transport of the nutrients. This overall stimulating effect of food is called its *specific dynamic action (SDA),* or, more recently, *dietary thermogenesis.*[4] About 10% of the body's total energy needs for metabolism is attributed to activities related to handling the food we eat.

Physical Activity Needs

Exercise involved in work and recreation accounts for wide individual variation in energy requirement (see Chapter 14). Some representative kilocalorie expenditures in various types of physical activity are given in Table 5-1. Any mental effort, such as in studying, demands few, if any, kilocalories. Fatigue following periods of study is caused by various amounts of muscle tension or moving about. Heightened emotional states alone do not increase energy needs, but they may bring additional needs because of increased muscle tension, restlessness, and agitated movements.

Total Energy Requirements

The energy demands of basal metabolism combined with the effect of food intake and the variable requirements of physical activity make up an individual's total energy requirement (Table 5-2). The energy requirement for the physical activity part may be measured by a 3-day activity record. To maintain daily energy balance, a person's total energy requirement is the total

Table 5-2

Recommended Daily Energy Intake*

Category	Age (years) or Condition	Weight kg	lb	Height cm	in	REE[a] (kcal/day)	Multiples of REE	Average Energy Allowance (kcal)[b] Per kg	Per day[c]
Infants	0.0-0.5	6	13	60	24	320		108	650
	0.5-1.0	9	20	71	28	500		98	850
Children	1-3	13	29	90	35	740		102	1,300
	4-6	20	44	112	44	950		90	1,800
	7-10	28	62	132	52	1,130		70	2,000
Males	11-14	45	99	157	62	1,140	1.70	55	2,500
	15-18	66	145	176	69	1,760	1.67	45	3,000
	19-24	72	160	177	70	1,780	1.67	40	2,900
	25-50	79	174	176	70	1,800	1.60	37	2,900
	51+	77	170	173	68	1,530	1.50	30	2,300
Females	11-14	46	101	157	62	1,310	1.67	47	2,200
	15-18	55	120	163	64	1,370	1.60	40	2,200
	19-24	58	128	164	65	1,350	1.60	38	2,200
	25-50	63	138	163	64	1,380	1.55	36	2,200
	51+	65	143	160	63	1,280	1.50	30	1,900
Pregnant	1st trimester								+0
	2nd trimester								+300
	3rd trimester								+300
Lactating	1st 6 months								+500
	2nd 6 months								+500

[a]Resting energy expenditure (REE)

[b]In the range of light to moderate activity, the coefficient of variation is ±20%.

[c]Figure is rounded.

*Food and Nutrition Board, National Research Council, National Academy of Sciences: Recommended dietary allowances, ed 10, Washington, DC, 1989, Academy Press.

Clinical Application

Estimate Your Own Daily Energy Requirement

Basal metabolism (BMR)

Use general formula: Women—0.9 kcal/kg/hr
Men—1.0 kcal/kg/hr
Convert weight (lb) to kg: 1 kg = 2.2 lb
Multiply by formula: 1 (or 0.9) × kg × 24 (hours in day)

Physical activity

Estimate your general average level of physical activity (Table below).
Find energy cost of activity (% of BMR) and add it to BMR.

Average Activity Level	Energy Cost: % of BMR
Sedentary	20%
Very light	30%
Moderate	40%
Heavy	50%

Example: if you are sedentary (mostly sitting): BMR + (20% × BMR)

Specific dynamic action (SDA) of food

Record food intake for day and calculate approximate energy value (kcal).
Find energy cost of food effect (10% of kcal in food consumed).

Total energy output

BMR + physical activity + SDA

number of kilocalories necessary to replace daily basal metabolic cost plus cost of exercise and other physical activities. Obesity represents an energy imbalance from excess energy input (food) over energy output (exercise). Extreme weight loss as in anorexia nervosa is also a state of energy imbalance but a different state from a different cause—an energy deficit from inadequate energy input from food to meet the body's demands, exhausting energy reserves stored in body tissues.

Where do you stand in your own energy balance? Try estimating your own energy requirement using the steps indicated here (see the box above). Compare your estimate with your general energy needs as indicated in the RDA standards.

Energy is that force or power that enables the body to carry out its life-sustaining metabolic activities and physical activities. The energy provided by foods is measured in *kilocalories (kcal)* or *joules.*

Energy exists in various basic forms such as chemical, electrical, mechanical, and thermal. *Metabolism* is the body's way of changing *chemical* energy in food into *electrical* energy of brain and nerve activity, *mechanical* energy of muscle contraction, *thermal* energy of body temperature control, and other forms of chemical energy in the body. Throughout the cycling of these energy forms, two types of balancing metabolic reactions constantly occur: *anabolism,* in which substances are synthesized and energy is stored, and *catabolism,* in which substances are broken down and energy is released.

When food is not available, the body draws on its own stores to meet energy needs. *Carbohydrate* stores (glycogen) are most easily depleted and thus the first to undergo catabolism. *Fat* stores (adipose tissue) are larger and catabolized once glycogen stores are depleted. *Protein* stores (body tissue) contain a fair amount of potential energy and are catabolized also after carbohydrate is depleted, along with fat stores.

Total energy needs are based on basal (maintenance) and nonbasal (exercise) requirements. The *basal metabolic rate (BMR)* reflects the amount of energy required to maintain the body at rest. The best indicator of BMR is body composition, especially *lean body mass. Nonbasal requirement* for energy includes physical exercise and food intake.

1. What are the fuel factors of protein, carbohydrate, fat, and alcohol?
2. Define "basal metabolism." What factor(s) influence basal energy needs? Which body tissues contribute most of the body's basal metabolic needs?
3. Which health conditions usually bring about a reduction in BMR? Which bring about a rise in BMR?
4. What factors influence nonbasal energy needs?
5. Calculate your own energy balance for 1 day, based on your energy input (food) and your energy output (BMR + SDA + physical activity).

Martin RJ and Mullen BJ: Control of food intake: mechanisms and consequences, Nutr Today 22(5):4, 1987.

Wright ED and Paige DM: Physical exercise and energy requirements, Clin Nutr 7(1):9, 1988.

Ireton-Jones CS and Turner WW Jr: The use of respiratory quotient to determine the efficacy of nutrition support regimens, J Am Diet Assoc 87(2):180, 1987.

Woo R, Daniels-Kush R, and Horton ES: Regulation of energy balance, Ann Rev Nutr 5:411, 1985.

Further Readings

Martin RJ and Mullen BJ: Control of food intake: mechanisms and consequences, Nutr Today 22(5):4, 1987.
With many helpful tables and diagrams, these authors provide insight concerning energy balance and regulations, especially states of energy imbalance such as obesity or anorexia.
Nash JD: Eating behavior and body weight: physiologic influences, Am J Health Promotion 1:5, Winter 1987.
This article gives a comprehensive review of physiologic influences on eating behavior, including set point theory and genetics, that relate to satiety and consequent energy balance.
Wright ED and Paige DM: Physical exercise and energy requirements, Clin Nutr 7(1):9, 1988.
This article provides details of current energy balance studies, especially in relation to physical exercise, with many practical applications to both recreational and competitive athletics.

The Difference Between Sam and Joe

Sam and Joe are both healthy, 35-year-old accountants who are 5 ft 10 in tall, weigh 165 lb, and jog 2 miles a day. They need the same number of kcal to get through the day—right? Not necessarily.

Tradition dictates that energy requirements are based on basal needs plus physical activity. Since basal requirements are said to depend on the three factors of sex, age, and body composition, Sam and Joe should have the same basal needs.

However, current researchers have taken a second look at an old study that concluded that these three factors could predict basal energy needs and found that only one—body composition—really makes a difference. After analyzing data about the original 223 subjects, the current investigators found *lean body mass (LBM)* to be the *only* predictor of BMR.

Sam and Joe may weigh the same, but if Sam's weight is made up of more fatty tissue than lean, his requirements may be lower. But suppose that Sam and Joe have the same amount of LBM, which you may suspect because of their similar activity levels. Would their energy levels be the same? Again, not necessarily. The assumptions that energy needs for physical activity are the same among individuals or stay the same within the same individual over time have both now been questioned.

As far back as 1947, a study showed that workers performing similar tasks had a wider range of energy intake (kcal) than energy output, which means that some persons burn their kcal more efficiently than others. The same study, whose results have been repeated over the years by other researchers, also showed that individuals varied widely in the amount of energy spent doing the same work over a week's time, *even when changes in weight were accounted for,* which means that the individual might be more energy efficient at certain times than at others. One study suggests that the differences might result from the body's attempt to regulate the amount of energy stored in the body. Answers to this metabolic puzzle, as continuing study seems to reinforce, point to strong genetic influence on individual differences in energy balance.

Joe always seems to eat more than Sam. Sam wonders about this difference when they seem so much alike in their size and activity. But Sam does not know about the internal gene-governed metabolism of his energy-efficient friend. Old and new energy balance studies are now helping to provide some of the answers.

REFERENCES

Cunningham JJ: An individualization of dietary requirements for energy in adults, J Am Diet Assoc 80:335, 1982.

Harris RBS, and Martin RJ: Lipostatic theory of energy balance: concepts and signals, Nutr Beh 1:253, 1984.

Nash JD: Eating behavior and body weight: physiologic influences, Am J Health Promotion 1:5, Winter 1987.

6 Proteins

Chapter Objectives

After studying this chapter, the student should be able to:

1. Describe the general process by which tissue protein is built.

2. Identify and compare the building units that structure proteins.

3. Identify the types and amounts of food proteins needed in our diets.

4. Describe the fate of dietary protein in our bodies.

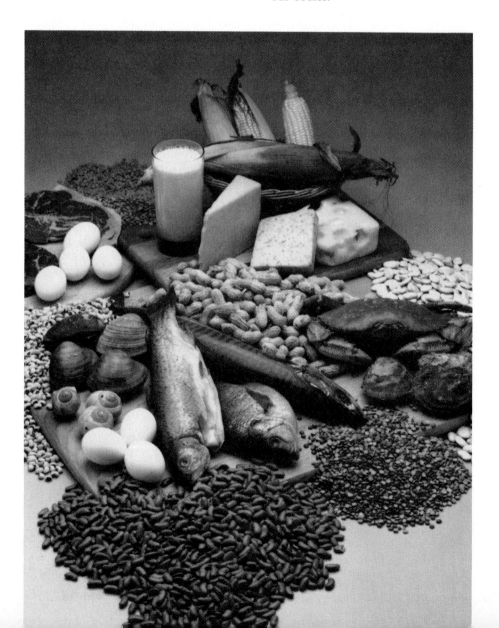

There are myriads of proteins in the human body whose tremendous diversity makes life possible. The body contains thousands upon thousands of specific proteins, each one different, designed to do its special job.

How can these proteins do their complex jobs? They accomplish their assigned tasks by their unique structure and packaging. But where do we get the necessary raw building materials to construct all these thousands of specific proteins that make up our bodies?

We get these essential building units—the *amino acids*—from the variety of food proteins we eat each day. Our bodies then break these food proteins down to their unit-building materials, specific amino acids, and use them to build the multitude of specific structures we need—the tissue proteins. It is this very *specificity* throughout the process that builds and maintains each person's unique individual body.

The Nature of Amino Acids

The story of protein must begin with its unique building materials, the **amino acids.** A major life-sustaining task of the human body is the constant building and rebuilding of all its body tissues (see box on p. 104). The name of these building units, the amino acids, indicates that they have a dual nature. The word *amino* refers to base (alkaline) substance, so we at once confront a paradox. How can a chemical material be both a base and an acid at the same time and why is this important here? Consider the significance of this fact as you first examine the structure of amino acids.

General Pattern and Specific Structure

A general fundamental pattern holds for all amino acids. It is the unique side group attached to the common baseline pattern that makes each of the amino acids that make up protein different. Amino acids are made of the same three elements—carbon, hydrogen, oxygen—that make up carbohydrates and fats. But amino acids and their proteins have an additional important element—*nitrogen*—as the base (alkaline, NH_2) portion of their structure. There are some 22 amino acids, all of which are important in the body's metabolism. They all have the same basic core pattern, but each is unique because it has a specific different side group attached.

Amphoteric Nature

This dual chemical structure of amino acids, combining both acid and base (amino) factors, gives them a unique *amphoteric* nature. As a result, an amino acid in solution can behave either as an acid or a base, depending on the pH of the solution. This means that amino acids have a *buffer capacity,* which is an important clinical characteristic.

Essential Amino Acids

Eight of the amino acids are vital in our diets and have been termed **essential amino acids.** Note these eight amino acids carefully in Table 6-1. They

Amino Acids: Basic Tissue-Building Material

Amino acid
These compounds form the structural units of protein. Out of a total of 20 or more, eight are considered *dietary essentials,* indispensable to life. (See *essential amino acid,* below.) The various food proteins, when digested, yield their specific constituent amino acids. These amino acids are then available for use by the cells as the cells synthesize specific tissue proteins.

Essential amino acid
Amino acid that is indispensable to life and growth and that the body cannot manufacture; it must be supplied in the diet.

are significant in our diets because they're the only ones that we cannot make. Over the years of human development, we have apparently lost the ability to synthesize these eight amino acids, so we must get them in our foods. Thus the label "essential" means that they are *dietary* essentials. The remaining amino acids, some 14 of them, which we can synthesize in our own bodies, are then labeled "nonessential" amino acids. Actually, this is a poor choice of label in the sense that all of the amino acids are necessary for building the various body tissue proteins. However, the concept of *dietary essentiality* for these so-designated eight amino acids is important to remember in assessing food protein quality and protein-controlled diets such as vegetarian food patterns.

The Nature of Proteins

The building units, amino acids, are used by the body to construct specific tissue proteins. This process is made possible by the nature of amino acids, which enables them to form peptide linkages and arrange themselves into peptide chains.

Tissue Protein Structure

Peptide linkage
Characteristic joining of amino acids to form proteins. Such a chain of amino acids is termed a "peptide."

The dual chemical nature of amino acids—the presence of a base (amino, NH_2) group containing nitrogen on one end and an acid (carboxyl, COOH) group on the other—enables them to join in the characteristic chain structure of proteins. The end amino group of one amino acid joins the end carboxyl group of another amino acid beside it. This characteristic joining of specific amino acids in a specific sequence to make a specific protein is called a **peptide linkage.** Long chains of amino acids linked in this manner form proteins and are called *polypeptides*. To make a compact structure, the long polypeptide chains then coil or fold back on themselves in a spiral shape called a *helix* or in a "pleated sheet" arrangement.

Types of Proteins

The proteins illustrate a huge diversity of compounds produced by specific amino acid linkages. As a result, according to their varied specific structures, tissue proteins perform many vital roles in body structure and metabolism. Some of these examples include structural proteins such as collagen, contractile proteins such as muscle fibers, antibodies such as gammaglobulin, blood proteins such as albumin and fibrinogin, some hormones such as insulin, and all the enzymes.

Complete and Incomplete Food Proteins

Complete protein
Protein that contains the essential amino acids in quantities sufficient for maintenance of the body and for a normal rate of growth; includes egg, milk, cheese, and meat.

According to the amounts of essential amino acids that given protein foods contain, food proteins are generally classified as complete or incomplete. **Complete proteins** are those that contain all the essential amino acids (Table 6-1) in sufficient quantity and ratio to meet the body's needs. These proteins are of animal origin: egg, milk, cheese, and meat. *Incomplete proteins* are those deficient in one or more of the essential amino acids. These proteins are mostly of plant origin: grains, legumes, nuts, and seeds. In a mixed diet, however, animal and plant proteins supplement one another. Even a mixture of plant proteins is planned carefully, especially to cover the "limiting" essential amino acid—the one occurring in the smallest amount and most

Essential amino acids	Semiessential amino acids*	Nonessential amino acids
Isoleucine	Arginine	Alanine
Leucine	Histidine	Asparagine
Lysine		Aspartic acid
Methionine		Cystine (cysteine)
Phenylalanine		Glutamic acid
Threonine		Glutamine
Tryptophan		Glycine
Valine		Hydroxyproline
		Hydroxylysine
		Proline
		Serine
		Tyrosine

Table 6-1
Amino Acids Required in Human Nutrition, Grouped According to Nutritional (Dietary) Essentiality

*These are considered semiessential because the rate of synthesis in the body is inadequate to support growth; therefore these are essential for children. Recent studies indicate that some histidine may also be required by adults.

likely to be deficient. The value of *variety* in the diet is therefore quite evident.

Functions of Protein

To sum up, proteins function in three main ways: building tissue, performing various specific additional physiologic roles, and sometimes providing energy.

Growth and Tissue-Building Maintenance

The primary function of dietary protein is to supply building material for growth and maintenance of body tissue. It does this by furnishing amino acids in appropriate numbers and types for efficient synthesis of specific cellular tissue proteins. Also, protein supplies amino acids for other essential nitrogen-containing substances such as enzymes and hormones.

Specific Physiologic Roles

All amino acids supplied by dietary protein participate in growth and tissue maintenance. But some also perform other important physiologic and metabolic roles. For example, *methionine* is an agent in the formation of choline, which is a precursor of acetylcholine, one of the major neurotransmitters in the brain. In addition, methionine is not only the precursor of the nonessential amino acid cystine, but also of the lesser known ones carnitine and taurine, which are now known to have widespread metabolic functions.[1,2] *Tryptophan* is the precursor of the B vitamin niacin and of the neurotransmitter serotonin. *Phenylalanine* is the precursor of the nonessential amino acid tyrosine, which leads to formation of the hormones thyroxine and epinephrine. In addition, protein antibodies provide essential components of the body's immune system, and plasma proteins guard water balance.

Clinical Application

The Problem of Building Tissue

As you have discovered thus far in your study of nutrition, the first major problem of the body, securing a fuel source and converting it into a refined fuel we can burn to supply energy, is solved by using carbohydrates and fats for this purpose. These food nutrients provide the fuel, and the body provides a balanced system of chemical changes to get energy from them.

The second major problem the body must solve to survive and maintain health is that of *building tissue*. Any successful construction system requires four basic components:

- Basic building materials
- A means of changing the basic building materials to ready-to-use construction units
- A means of carrying the finished construction units to the site for building
- A plan ("blueprint") and process for building and maintaining the specifically designed structures at the construction site

Body growth and maintenance require constant building and rebuilding of body tissues to maintain its form and structure and function. Healthy tissue is necessary for strength, vigor, and body functioning. The building material in food that enables us to accomplish this task is *protein* and its special building units, the *amino acids*. The necessary components for any successful construction system can be applied to the body's use of protein for this vital task.

Available Energy

Protein also contributes to the body's overall energy metabolism. This occurs as needed in the fasting state or in extended physical effort such as marathon running, but not in the fed state. After the removal of the nitrogen-containing portion of the constituent amino acid, the amino acid residue, its carbon "skeleton," called a *keto-acid*, may be converted either to glucose or to fat. On the average, 58% of the total dietary protein may become available when needed to be burned for energy. Thus sufficient amounts of nonprotein kilocalories from carbohydrate are always needed to spare protein for its primary building purpose and to prevent unnecessary protein breakdown in the process of providing energy.

Digestion: Changing Basic Building Material to Usable Building Units

After the source of basic body building materials—the food protein—is secured, it must be changed into the needed ready-to-use building units, the amino acids. This work is done through the successive parts of the gastrointestinal tract by the mechanical and chemical processes of digestion.

Mouth

In the mouth only mechanical breaking up of the protein foods by chewing occurs. Here the food particles are mixed with saliva and passed on as a semisolid mass into the stomach.

Stomach

Because proteins are such large complex structures, a series of enzymes is necessary to finally break them down to produce the amino acids. These chemical changes, through a system of enzymes, begin in the stomach. In fact, the stomach's chief digestive function in relation to all foods is the initial partial enzymatic breakdown of protein. Three agents in the gastric secretions help with this task: pepsin, hydrochloric acid, and rennin.

Pepsin

The main gastric enzyme, specific for proteins, is **pepsin.** It is first produced as an inactive **proenzyme (zymogen),** *pepsinogen,* by a single layer of cells (the chief cells) in the mucosa of the stomach wall. Pepsinogen then requires hydrochloric acid for activation to the enzyme pepsin. The active pepsin then begins splitting the peptide linkages between the protein's amino acids, changing the large polypeptides into successively smaller peptides. If the protein were held in the stomach longer, pepsin could continue the breakdown until individual amino acids resulted. However, with normal gastric emptying time, only the beginning stage is completed by the action of pepsin.

Hydrochloric Acid

Gastric hydrochloride is an important catalyst in gastric protein digestion. It provides the acid medium necessary to convert pepsinogen to pepsin. Clinical problems result from lack of the normal secretion of hydrochloric acid.

Rennin

This gastric enzyme (not to be confused with the renal enzyme *renin*) is present only in infancy and childhood and disappears in adulthood. It is especially important in the infant's digestion of milk. Rennin and calcium act on the casein of milk to produce a curd. By coagulating milk, rennin prevents too rapid a passage of the food from the child's stomach.

Small Intestine

Protein digestion begins in the acid medium of the stomach and is completed in the alkaline medium of the small intestine. A number of enzymes, from secretions of both the pancreas and the intestine, take part.

Pancreatic Secretions

Three enzymes produced by the pancreas continue breaking down proteins to simpler and simpler substances:

1. **Trypsin** is secreted first as inactive trypsinogen and is then activated by the hormone enterokinase, which is produced by glands in the duodenal wall. The active enzyme **trypsin** then acts on protein and large polypeptide fragments carried over from the stomach, producing smaller polypeptides and dipeptides.
2. **Chymotrypsin** is produced by special cells in the pancreas as inactive chymotrypsinogen and then activated by the trypsin already present. **Chymotrypsin** continues the same protein-splitting action of trypsin.
3. **Carboxypeptidase,** as its name indicates, attacks the carboxyl end (acid, COOH) of the peptide chain. It produces in turn smaller peptides and some free amino acids.

Pepsin
Main gastric enzyme specific for proteins that begins breaking large protein molecules into shorter chain polypeptides, proteoses, and peptones.

Proenzyme
Inactive form of an enzyme as it is initially secreted. See *zymogen.*

Zymogen
Inactive precursor converted to the active enzyme by the action of an acid, another enzyme, or other means. Also called proenzyme.

Trypsin
Protein-splitting (proteolytic) enzyme secreted by the pancreas that acts in the small intestine to reduce proteins to shorter chain polypeptides and dipeptides.

Chymotrypsin
Protein-splitting (proteolytic) enzyme produced by the pancreas that acts in the intestine. Together with trypsin, it reduces proteins to shorter chain polypeptides and dipeptides.

Intestinal Secretions

Glands in the intestinal wall produce two more protein-splitting enzymes in the peptidase group:

1. **Aminopeptidase** releases amino acids one at a time from the nitrogen-containing amino end (base, NH_2) of the peptide chain. Through this cleavage, it produces smaller short-chain peptides and free amino acids.
2. **Dipeptidase,** final enzyme in this protein-splitting system, breaks the remaining dipeptides into their two, now free, amino acids.

Through this total system of protein-splitting enzymes, the large complex proteins are broken down into progressively smaller peptide chains and finally into free amino acids, now ready for absorption by the intestinal mucosa. A summary of these steps in protein digestion is given in Table 6-2.

Absorption: Carrying Building Units to Construction Sites in the Cells

The construction sites in the body for building necessary specific tissue proteins are in the *cells.* Each cell, depending on its particular nature and function, has a specific job to do. Thus its proteins must be specifically structured.

Absorption of Amino Acids

The end products of protein digestion are the amino acids. They are water soluble, so their absorption directly into the water-based blood stream poses

Table 6-2
Summary of Protein Digestion

Organ	Inactive precursor	Activator	Active enzyme	Digestive action
Mouth			None	Mechanical only
Stomach (acid)	Pepsinogen	Hydrochloric acid	Pepsin	Protein→polypeptides
			Rennin (infants) (calcium necessary for activity)	Casein→coagulated curd
Intestine (alkaline)				
Pancreas	Trypsinogen	Enterokinase	Trypsin	Protein, polypeptides→polypeptides, dipeptides
	Chymotrypsinogen	Active trypsin	Chymotrypsin	Protein, polypeptides→polypeptides, dipeptides
			Carboxypeptidase	Polypeptides→simpler peptides, dipeptides, amino acids
Intestine			Aminopeptidase	Polypeptides→peptides, dipeptides, amino acids
			Dipeptidase	Dipeptides→amino acids

no problem. These building units are rapidly absorbed from the small intestine into the portal blood system through the fine network of villus capillaries.

Active Transport System

Most of the amino acid absorption takes place in the first section of the small intestine, the duodenum. An energy-dependent active transport, using pyridoxine (vitamin B_6) as carrier, absorbs the amino acids into the blood circulation, delivering them into the cells for eventual metabolism.

Competition for Absorption

When we eat a mixed diet containing a variety of different amino acids, the amino acids compete with each other for absorption. The amino acid present in the largest quantity retards the absorption of the others. In plasma, competition also exists among circulating amino acids for entry receptor sites for transport across cell membranes into the cell.

Absorption of Peptides and Whole Proteins

A few larger fragments of short-chain peptides or smaller intact proteins are absorbed as such, and then by **hydrolysis** within the absorbing cells they yield their amino acids. These whole protein molecules may play a part in the development of immunity and sensitivity. For example, antibodies in the mother's colostrum, the premilk breast secretion, are passed on to her nursing infant.

In human nutrition the amino acids are the "metabolic currency" of protein. It is with the fate of these vital compounds that the metabolism of protein is ultimately concerned. Protein's fascinating complex metabolic activities are intricately interwoven with those of carbohydrates and fats. Here we will look briefly at the fundamental metabolic concept of protein and nitrogen balance. This will provide a base for relating the tissue-building processes of **anabolism** with those of the breaking-down processes of **catabolism** to maintain these important protein balances.

The Concept of Balance
Homeostasis

Many interdependent checks and balances exist throughout the body to keep it in its fine working order. There is a constant ebb and flow of materials, a building up and breaking down of parts, and a depositing and taking up of components. The body has built-in controls that operate as finely tuned co-ordinated responses to meet any situation that tends to disturb its normal condition or function. This resulting state of dynamic equilibrium is called **homeostasis,** and the various mechanisms designed to preserve it are called *homeostatic mechanisms*. This highly sensitive balance between body parts and functions is life-sustaining.

Dynamic Equilibrium

As more and more is learned about human nutrition and physiology, older ideas of a rigid body structure are giving way to this important concept of *dynamic equilibrium*—balance amid constant change. All body constituents are

Hydrolysis
Splitting of a compound into fragments by the addition of water, the hydroxyl group (OH) being incorporated in one fragment and the hydrogen atom (H) in the other.

Metabolism: Building and Maintaining Specific Body Tissues

Anabolism
Constructive metabolic processes that build up the body substances by synthesizing more complex substances from simpler ones; the opposite of catabolism.

Catabolism
Breaking-down phase of metabolism, the opposite of anabolism.

Homeostasis
State of equilibrium of the body's internal environment.

in a constant state of flux, although some tissues are more actively engaged than others. This dynamic concept can be seen in all metabolism. It is especially striking in protein metabolism.

Protein Balance

Protein Turnover

For a number of years the use of radioactive isotopes has clearly demonstrated that the body's protein tissues are continuously being broken down into amino acids and then resynthesized into tissue proteins. When "labeled" amino acids are fed, they can be traced as they are rapidly incorporated into various body tissue proteins. The rate of this protein turnover varies in different tissues. It is highest in the intestinal mucosa, liver, pancreas, kidney, and plasma. It is lower in muscle, brain, and skin. It is much slower in structural tissues such as collagen and bone.

Protein Compartments

Body protein exists in a balance between two compartments, tissue protein and plasma protein. These stores are further balanced with dietary protein intake. Protein from one compartment may be drawn to supply need in the other. For example, during fasting, resources from the body protein stores may be used for tissue synthesis. But even when the intake of protein and other nutrients is adequate, the tissue proteins are still being constantly broken down, reshaped, and reformed according to body need. Such a dynamic state is necessary to life and growth because the body is an open system. It must sustain a dynamic balance not only within its own internal environment but also with its larger and extended external environment.

The body's state of stability is the result then of a **protein balance** between the rates of protein breakdown and resynthesis. In periods of growth the synthesis rate is higher so that new tissue can be formed. In conditions of starvation, wasting disease, and more gradually as aging continues in the elderly, tissue breakdown exceeds that of synthesis, and the body gradually deteriorates.

Protein balance
The word *balance* refers to relation between intake and output of a substance. Negative balance = output greater than intake. Positive balance = intake greater than output.

Metabolic Amino Acid Pool

Amino acids derived from tissue breakdown and amino acids from dietary protein digestion and absorption both contribute to a common collective metabolic "pool" of amino acids throughout the body available for use (Figure 6-1). A balance of amino acids is thus maintained to supply the body's constant needs. Shifts in balances between tissue breakdown and dietary protein intake ensure a balanced mixture of amino acids. From this reserve pool, specific amino acids are supplied to synthesize specific body proteins.

Nitrogen Balance

Another useful reference for indicating a person's state of protein balance is **nitrogen balance.** Total nitrogen balance involves all sources of nitrogen in the body— protein nitrogen and nonprotein nitrogen present in other compounds such as urea, uric acid, ammonia, and in other body tissues and fluids. It is the net result of all nitrogen gains and losses in all the body protein. A person is in a harmful state of negative nitrogen balance when the loss of body protein exceeds the input of food protein. Such a state exists in condi-

Nitrogen balance
Difference between intake and output of nitrogen in the body. If intake is greater, a positive nitrogen balance exists. If output is greater, a negative nitrogen balance exists.
6.25 g protein = 1 g nitrogen

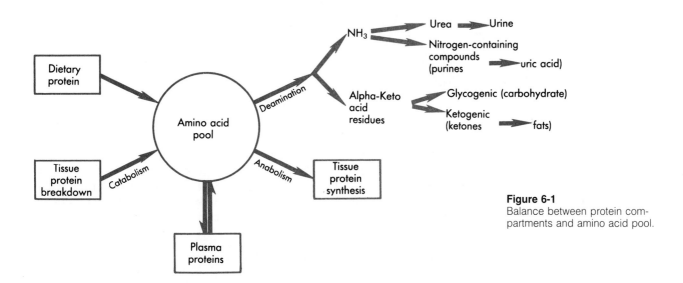

Figure 6-1
Balance between protein compartments and amino acid pool.

tions such as long-term illness, a hypermetabolic wasting disease, or starvation.

It is clear that protein is an essential nutrient. But just how much and what kind do we actually need? We know that some people get far less than they need. On a worldwide basis, protein-energy malnutrition is a major health concern, especially in underdeveloped countries. In contrast, however, in America and most other Western societies protein deficiency is not a problem. Actually most persons in America eat two or three times as much protein as they really need, largely because of the extensive role of meat and dairy products in cultural food habits. But such excess protein intake often creates other problems. First, excessive intake of animal protein foods, which carry animal fat, can contribute to obesity and vascular health problems.[3] Second, the excessive nitrogen load can place a cumulative burden on the kidneys for nitrogen excretion. Clinicians have begun to raise questions about the long-term effects of habitual excess protein intake on the human kidney designed in earlier ages to handle a different supply of protein.

Factors Influencing Protein Requirements
Tissue Growth

The primary purpose of protein in the diet is to supply amino acids in the quantity and quality necessary for growth and maintenance of tissue. Thus any period of growth increases the need for protein. Growth-related factors include age, body size, and general physical state. For example, elderly men and women may need more protein than other adults.[4] Also, special periods of rapid growth, such as the growth of the fetus and maternal tissue during pregnancy, require added protein.

Diet

Other factors include the nature of the protein in the diet and its ratio or pattern of amino acids. There must be sufficient nonprotein foods in the diet

Protein Requirements

to have a protein-sparing effect, so that the total amount of protein will not be diminished for energy requirements. Also, the digestibility and absorption of the protein is affected by the cooking of the food, and time intervals between eating protein foods lowers the competition for absorption sites and enzymes.

Illness or Disease

Any illness or disease will usually increase the requirement for protein. Diseases accompanied by fever usually increase the need for protein because of the increase in basal metabolic rate and the general breaking down of tissue. Traumatic injury requires extensive tissue rebuilding. Postsurgical states require protein for wound healing and to replenish losses. Extensive tissue destruction as in burns requires considerable increase in protein intake for the healing process.

Measurement of Protein Requirements

It is evident, then, that two basic measures of protein requirement must be considered: quantity and quality.

Protein Quantity

The quantity of protein needed is the basis for establishing the total protein requirement. The RDA standard for adults is 0.8 g/kg (2.2 lb) of body

Table 6-3

Recommended Amounts of Protein Per Day*

Individuals	g/kg	g/day
Men (79 kg)	0.8	63
Women (63 kg)	0.8	50
Pregnancy, last 4½ mo		(+ 10)
Lactation		(+ 15)
Infants		
0 to 6 mo	2.2	13
6 to 12 mo	1.6	14
Children		
1 to 3 yr	1.2	16
4 to 6 yr	1.1	24
7 to 10 yr	1.0	28
Boys		
11 to 14 yr	1.0	45
15 to 18 yr	0.9	59
Girls		
11 to 14 yr	1.0	46
15 to 18 yr	0.8	44

*From Food and Nutrition Board: Recommended dietary allowances, ed. 9, Washington, D.C., 1980, National Academy of Sciences.

weight. This amounts to about 63 g/day for a man weighing 79 kg and 50 g/day for a woman weighing 63 kg. Increased protein is indicated during pregnancy and lactation (see Table 6-3). Requirements for infants and children vary according to age and growth patterns.

Protein Quality

Since the value of a protein depends on its content of essential amino acids, in the final analysis the measure of protein need must be based on its amino acid quality. Guidelines for protein needs, based on nitrogen balance studies determining specific amino acid requirements, have been developed (Table 6-3).

Comparative Quality of Food Proteins

The nutritive value of a food protein is often expressed in terms of its *chemical score*, a value derived from its amino acid composition. Using the amino acid pattern of a high-quality protein food such as egg and giving it a value of 100, other foods are compared according to their ratios of essential amino acids. Other measures also determine aspects of protein quality:

1. **Biologic value (BV)** based on nitrogen balance.
2. **Net protein utilization (NPU)** based on biologic value and degree of digestibility.
3. **Protein efficiency ratio (PER)** based on weight gain of a growing test animal divided by its protein intake.

A comparison of the scores of various protein foods with their nutritive values based on these measures is shown in Table 6-4. A sound diet is the best way to obtain needed protein. There is no need for amino acid supplements. They are both costly and inefficient.

Table 6-4

Comparative Protein Quality of Selected Foods According to Chemical (Amino Acid) Score, Biologic Value (BV), Net Protein Utilization (NPU), and Protein Efficiency Ratio (PER)*

Food	Chemical score	BV	NPU	PER
Egg	100	100	94	3.92
Cow's milk	95	93	82	3.09
Fish	71	76	—	3.55
Beef	69	74	67	2.30
Unpolished rice	67	86	59	—
Peanuts	65	55	55	1.65
Oats	57	65	—	2.19
Polished rice	57	64	57	2.18
Whole wheat	53	65	49	1.53
Corn	49	72	36	—
Soybeans	47	73	61	2.32
Sesame seeds	42	62	53	1.77
Peas	37	64	55	1.57

*Data adapted from Guthrie H: Introductory Nutrition, ed. 7, St Louis, 1989, The CV Mosby Co, and Food and Nutrition Board: Recommended dietary allowances, ed 9, Washington, DC, 1980, National Academy of Sciences.

Vegetarian Diets: Complementary Food Proteins

Protein requirements in various vegetarian diets may be met by applying the principle of combining complementary plant proteins to achieve the necessary balance of essential amino acids. There are three basic types of vegetarian diets: (1) lactoovovegetarian (including dairy foods and eggs), (2) lactovegetarian (including dairy foods), and (3) pure vegan (no animal protein). Each must be planned carefully to secure needed essential amino acids (see Issues and Answers on p. 114). Guidelines for vegetable protein combinations and interesting recipes for preparing these foods are now widely available owing to increased public interest.[5,6] In general, in relation to animal protein sources, larger amounts of vegetable protein foods must be consumed to obtain comparable amounts of complete protein.

Questions for Review

1. What is the difference between *essential* and *nonessential* amino acids? List the names of the essential amino acids.
2. Explain the term "protein-sparing effect." Which nutrients have this effect?
3. List and describe factors that affect dietary protein needs.
4. Calculate your own protein intake for a day and compare it with your general need according to the RDA allowances.
5. A vegetarian couple decides to raise their 2-year-old daughter on a strict vegan diet. As expected, the child does not often finish meals and snacks on fruits and whole grain biscuits. Eventually, they notice that she is falling behind in her growth rate and becoming thin. What food patterns would you expect in this family? What dietary factor may be involved in the child's poor growth? What advice would you offer these parents to improve their child's nutritional status? Plan 1 day's meals for this family, indicating amounts for the child that would meet her dietary protein need, while still adhering to a typical vegan meal pattern.

Proteins build tissue, perform various physiologic roles, and provide energy. Amino acids are the structural components of proteins. There is a total of 22, 8 of which the body cannot synthesize in adequate amounts. These 8 are called essential amino acids (EAAs). Food proteins are considered "complete" when they contain all 8 EAAs. Animal proteins are complete. Vegetable proteins are incomplete but can be mixed with complete proteins or with each other to provide all 8 EAAs during the day.

Amino acids participate in protein building (anabolism) or breakdown (catabolism). Both processes are dictated by genetic information and hormonal influences. *Anabolism* occurs when specific amino acids required for each protein are present. If one is missing, the protein is not formed—the law of "all or none." *Catabolism* occurs when the body tissues are broken down. The amino acid splits into its nitrogen group, which helps to form amino acids or other nitrogen compounds, and its nonnitrogen residue, which can form carbohydrates for energy or fat storage. In the unfed state, proteins are broken down for energy. Thus dietary carbohydrates have a protein-sparing effect.

Protein requirements are influenced by growth needs and rate of protein synthesis, food protein quality, and dietary carbohydrate and fat levels. Clinical factors affecting protein needs include fever, disease, surgery, or other trauma to body tissues.

To Sum Up

References

1. Borum PR: Carnitine—who needs it? Nutr Today 21(6):4, 1986.
2. Picone TA: Taurine update: metabolism and function, Nutr Today 22(4):16, 1987.
3. Carpenter KJ: The history of enthusiasm for protein, J Nutr 116:1364, July 1986.
4. Hautvast J: Proteins and selected vitamins. In Diet and health: scientific concepts and principles, Am J Clin Nutr 45(suppl):1044, May 1987.
5. Shulman MR: The vegetarian good life, Health 19(7):36, 1987.
6. Hasselbring B: Subtle and savory, Med Self-Care 43:40, Nov/Dec 1987.

Further Readings

Carpenter KJ: The history of enthusiasm for protein, J Nutr 116:1364, July 1986.
This author describes the interesting roots of our high regard for protein, especially meat, in early frontier America, which led to the 1890s USDA recommendation of over 110 g/day of protein for working men, based on the now-disproved nutritional science of the time. Then more recent views of the "World Protein Gap" led to inappropriate attempts to transfer modern protein technology to more primitive communities.
Madison D, and Brown E: The Greens cookbook, New York, 1987, Bantam Books.
This little book presents a wide selection of gourmet vegetarian recipes from dishes made famous by Greens' Restaurant in San Francisco, drawn from a wide variety of traditions—Mediterranean cooking from southern France, Italy, and Greece, foods of Asia, Mexico, and the American Southwest.
Ratto T: Protein, Med Self-Care 37:24, Nov/Dec 1986.
This author, a registered dietitian, explains in a popular style the truth about dietary protein—the real problem of most Americans' getting too much—and provides practical guides for calculating your own need.

Vegetarian Food Patterns: Harm or Health?

At least 7 million Americans have become vegetarians, replacing meats as a main entree item with legumes, grains, and vegetables. Their meals follow a variety of patterns. Some groups call themselves "true" vegetarians because they allow no animal products in their diets. But their highly restrictive "dietary laws" have caused serious malnutrition problems. These problems are found among:

Zen macrobiotics, who eat only brown rice and herb tea to achieve a perfect balance of yin and yang in order to fend off disease.

Vegans, who rely on fruits, vegetables, nuts, and seeds, refusing any source of animal protein, fortified foods, or nutritional supplements.

Fruitarians, who eat only fresh and dried fruits, nuts, honey, and sometimes olive oil.

Other vegetarian diets, however, if well planned can be very nutritious. These include the "animal-product" vegetarians:

Lactovegetarians, who allow milk, cheese, yogurt, and other milk products as the only animal protein in their diets.

Ovovegetarians, who use eggs as their only source of animal protein.

Lactoovovegetarians, who consume milk and eggs, but no other animal products.

Pescovegetarians, who permit fish as their only animal product.

Pollovegetarians, who allow poultry.

"Red-meat abstainers," who eat any animal product except red meat and consider themselves to be vegetarians, too.

Reasons people give for becoming vegetarian are as varied as these diets:

Religion Religious communities, such as the Seventh-Day adventists, use vegetarianism as a means of self-discipline, as well as promoting good health. Other vegetarians may or may not be religious but feel it is "sinful" to kill a living animal for food.

Ecology Approximately half of the world's grain output is used to feed livestock. Some vegetarians feel it could be better used to feed people so that less land would be used to meet the world's protein needs. Some also feel that using less land would result in a reduction in the use of pesticides now used to ensure large crops.

Economics Beans, grains, and vegetables are cheaper than meat. Some vegetarians are not only concerned with saving money for themselves but also finding a way to meet food shortages in poor nations throughout the world.

Health Another common reason for selecting vegetarianism is to achieve good health. By avoiding animal products, vegetarians manage to reduce their intake of cholesterol and saturated fats, thus perhaps gaining some protection against heart disease.

Does a vegetarian diet offer other important nutrients besides protein?
Yes. Vegetarians can meet the recommended dietary allowance for most major nutrients without taking supplements. However, a few key nutrients create problems if the vegetarian is not careful:

Vitamin B_{12} This vitamin is found only in animal products. People who follow veganism or the macrobiotic diets are at the greatest risk for a deficiency. Vegans may be at special risk because they take in a large amount of folacin, another B vitamin that can mask signs of B_{12} deficiency. A deficiency can be avoided, however, by including fortified foods or taking a B_{12} supplement along with sufficient complete protein from complementary amino acids to ensure synthesis of the intrinsic factor (a mucoprotein) necessary for B_{12} absorption.

Vitamin A Vegetarians tend to get more provitamin A, carotene, than they need. This usually isn't a problem—unless they are also taking supplements that include vitamin A. One study shows that 85% of vegetarians take supplements. These may include as much as 10 times the RDA for vitamin A! As a fat-soluble vitamin, vitamin A can build up in body tissues and reach toxic levels. The result could be anorexia, irritability, dry skin, hair loss.

Iron Grains and legumes have iron but much of it is poorly absorbed from the gut. Absorption can be enhanced, however, by including a good source of vitamin C (p. 131) in the same meal.

Can vegetarian women get enough protein for a successful pregnancy?
Yes, though including animal products, as in lactoovovegetarianism, may become essential to meet extra nutritional needs. Supplements are recommended also for such hard-to-get nutrients as iron.

Is the vegetarian diet safe for children?
Children manage to grow and develop fairly well on a vegetarian diet that includes the nonmeat animal proteins milk, cheese, and eggs. They tend to be a little shorter than average but this may be the result of other genetic or environmental factors. Vegetarian children also tend to be mildly anemic, probably because of the poor availability of iron from grains and legumes. Again, including a source of vitamin C with meals may be helpful. The vegan and macrobiotic diets are too poor in required nutrients to sustain childhood growth needs.

Can you lose weight on a vegetarian diet?
Yes, definitely. Eliminating meats automatically removes a major source of fat in the diet. Since fats provide more than twice the number of kilocalories per gram than carbohydrates or protein, the vegetarian diet is usually much lower in kilocalories than the "meat-and-potatoes" diet. In fact, some vegetarians, especially pregnant women, children, and athletes, have to be careful to get *enough* kilocalories.

Thus the well-planned vegetarian diet can be nutritious. If used wisely, especially in its lactoovo forms, it can offer many advantages in terms of health, economy, and ecology.

REFERENCES

Havala S and Dwyer J: Position of the American Dietetic Association: vegetarian diets—technical support paper, 88(3):352, 1988.

Wagner M: Ten years after *Diet for a Small Planet*, Med Self-Care 21:60, Summer 1983.
Yanez E and others: Long-tern validation of 1 gram protein per kilogram body weight from a predominantly vegetable mixed diet to meet the requirements of young adult males, J Nutr 116:865, May 1986.

7 Vitamins

Chapter Objectives

After studying this chapter, the student should be able to:

1. Define *vitamin* and describe the general nature of each one.
2. Identify the functions of each vitamin.
3. Relate each vitamin's requirement to problems of deficiency and excess.
4. Identify each vitamin's food sources and any situations requiring possible supplementation.

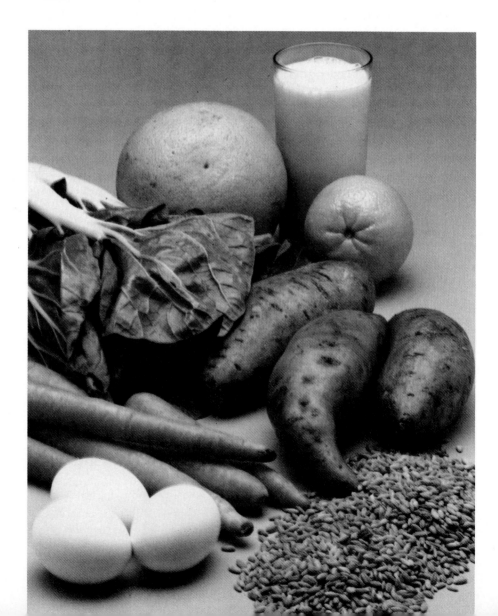

PREVIEW

Probably no other group of nutritional elements has so captured the interest of scientists, health professionals, and the general public as has the vitamin group. Attitudes toward vitamins have varied widely. Concern about them has run the gamut from wise functional use to wild flagrant abuse.

From 1900 to 1950 the discovery of vitamins formed a fascinating chapter in nutrition history. During this time the list of vitamins grew one by one. Some were first discovered in the search for the causes of age-old diseases such as scurvy, beriberi, pellagra, and rickets. Others were discovered later as a result of studies of various body functions.

In general, in cases of malnutrition, not just one but a number of vitamins may be lacking. And in the case of one vitamin at least, current knowledge indicates that the organic substance we have been calling vitamin D was initially misassigned to the vitamin group. It is now known to behave as a hormone and is rightly called vitamin D hormone. In this chapter we will look at both fat- and water-soluble vitamins. We will focus on why we need them and how we may obtain them.

General Nature and Classification

The Study of Vitamins

During the five decades of vitamin discovery in the first half of the 1900s, the remarkable nature of these vital agents became more and more apparent. Three key characteristics were evident: (1) they were not "burned" to yield energy as were the energy nutrients carbohydrate, fat, and sometimes protein; (2) they were vital to life; and (3) often not a single substance but a group of related substances turned out to have the particular metabolic activity. The name *vitamin* developed during initial research years when one of the early scientists working with a nitrogen-containing chemical substance called an **amine** thought that this was the common nature of these vital agents. So he named his discovery *vitamine (vital-amine)*. Later the final "e" was dropped when other similarly vital substances turned out to be a variety of organic compounds. The name *vitamin* has been retained to designate compounds of this class of essential substances. At first letter names were given to individual vitamins discovered. But as the number of them increased rapidly, this practice created confusion. So in recent years more specific names based on structure or function have developed. Today these scientific names are preferred and commonly used.

Amine
Organic compound containing nitrogen, formed from ammonia.

Definition of a Vitamin

As the vitamins were discovered one by one and the list of them grew, two basic characteristics clearly emerged to define a compound as a vitamin:

1. It must be a vital organic dietary substance that is not an energy-producing carbohydrate, fat, or protein, and is usually necessary in only very *small* quantities to perform a particular metabolic function or to prevent an associated deficient disease.
2. It cannot be manufactured by the body and therefore must be supplied in food.

Classification

Vitamins are usually grouped and distinguished according to their solubility in either fat or water:

Fat-Soluble

The fat-soluble vitamins are A, D, E, and K. They are closely associated with lipids in their fate in the body. They can be stored, and their functions are generally related to structural activities.

Water-Soluble

The water-soluble vitamins are the B-complex ones and C. These have fewer problems in absorption and transport. They cannot be stored except in the general "tissue saturation" sense. The B vitamins function mainly as coenzyme factors in cell metabolism. Vitamin C is a vital structural agent.

Current Concepts and Key Questions

To clarify current concepts concerning each known vitamin, consider these key questions as basis for your study:

Nature. What is the vitamin's general structural nature?

Absorption and transport. How does the body handle this particular vitamin?

Function. What does this vitamin do? This is, perhaps, the most significant question.

Requirement and sources. How much of this vitamin do we need and where can we obtain it?

Here, then, we will briefly review each of the vitamins in turn—four fat-soluble (A, D, E, and K) and nine water-soluble (C and 8 B). In each case we will identify the specific chemical name, a more common usage now, and review answers to the key questions above. In some cases, a group of similar substances have the vitamin activity, not just the single substance bearing the specific name.

Fat-Soluble Vitamin A

General Nature of Vitamin A
Chemical and Physical Nature

Vitamin A is a generic term for a group of compounds having similar biologic activity. These compounds include retinol, retinal, and retinoic acid. The term *retinoids* refers to both the natural forms of retinol and its synthetic analogs. Because this main substance has a specific function in the retina of the eye and is an alcohol, vitamin A has been given the specific chemical name *retinol*. It is soluble in fat and in ordinary fat solvents. Because it is insoluble in water, it is fairly stable in cooking.

Forms

There are two basic dietary forms of vitamin A. One of these is *preformed vitamin A—retinol*. This substance, in its natural form, is found only in animal food sources and is usually associated with fats. It is deposited primarily in the liver but also in small amounts in kidney and fat tissue. In this form, its dietary sources are mainly the fat portion of dairy products, egg yolk, and storage organs such as liver. The other basic dietary form of vitamin A is *provitamin A—beta-carotene*. The original source of retinol is this plant pigment, beta-carotene, which animals eat then convert to retinol and store. It was first called carotene because one of the main plant sources of this pigment was found to be carrots. Beta-carotene is the most common precursor of vitamin A and supplies about two thirds of the vitamin supply in human nutrition.

Absorption and Storage

Substances that Aid Absorption

Vitamin A enters the body in the two forms, preformed vitamin A from animal sources and the precursor carotene from plant sources. Several substances aid in the absorption of vitamin A and carotene by the body:

1. **Bile.** As with fat and other fat-related compounds, bile serves as a vehicle of vitamin A transport through the intestinal wall. Clinical conditions affecting the biliary system, such as obstruction of the bile ducts, infectious hepatitis, and liver cirrhosis, hinder absorption.
2. **Pancreatic lipase.** This fat-splitting enzyme is necessary for initial hydrolysis in the upper small intestine of fat emulsions or oil solutions of the vitamin. In diseases of the pancreas where secretion of pancreatic lipase is curtailed, the water-soluble analog would have to be used.
3. **Dietary fat.** Some fat in the food mix, simultaneously absorbed, stimulates bile release for effective absorption.

Carotene Conversion

In the intestinal wall during absorption some of the carotene is converted to vitamin A. The remainder is absorbed and transported as such, dissolved in the fat part of lipoproteins.

Transport and Storage

The route of absorption of both vitamin A and carotene parallels that of fat. In the intestinal mucosa all the retinol, from both natural preformed animal sources and from plant carotene conversion, is incorporated into the chylomicrons. In this form it enters the bloodstream by way of the lymphatic system and is carried to the liver for storage and distribution to the cells. The liver, by far the most efficient storage organ for vitamin A, contains about 90% of the body's total quantity. This amount is sufficient to supply the body's needs for about 6 to 12 months, and some persons have been known to store as much as a 4-year supply. These stores are reduced, however, during infectious disease, especially in childhood infections such as measles. For example, among malnourished nonimmunized children in many parts of the world, measles has become a leading killer disease and is now designated by the WHO Expanded Program on Immunization as a target for both vitamin A supplementation and immunization.[1,2] Age is also a factor in absorption. For example, in the newborn, especially the premature infant, absorption is poor. With advancing age, elderly persons may have increasing difficulties with absorption. Chronic use of mineral oil as a laxative hinders vitamin A absorption.

Functions of Vitamin A

Vitamin A's role in visual adaption to light and dark has been well established. It also has a number of more generalized functions that influence epithelial tissue integrity, growth, and reproductive functions.

Vision

The eye's ability to adapt to changes in light depends on a light-sensitive pigment, **rhodopsin,** commonly known as visual purple, in the rods of the retina (Figure 7-1). Rhodopsin is composed of the vitamin A substance, retinal, and the protein, opsin. When the body is deficient in vitamin A, the normal rhodopsin cannot be made and the rods and cones of the retina become increasingly sensitive to light changes, causing *night blindness.* This condition can usually be cured in a half-hour or so by an injection of vitamin A (retinol), which is readily converted into retinal and then into rhodopsin.

Epithelial Tissue

Vitamin A is necessary to build and maintain healthy epithelial tissue, which provides our primary barrier to infections. The epithelium includes not only the outer skin but also the inner mucous membranes. This function of vitamin A is the basis for current study of retinoids and carotene in relation to cancers of epithelial origin.

Without vitamin A, the epithelial cells become dry and flat. They gradually harden to form keratin, a process called **keratinization.** Keratin is a protein that forms dry, scale-like tissue, normal in the case of nails and hair but abnormal in the case of skin and mucosal membranes. When the body is deficient in vitamin A, many such abnormal epithelial tissue changes may occur:

1. **Eye.** The cornea dries and hardens, a condition called *xerophthalmia.* In extreme deficiency the process may progress to blindness. This progressive blindness resulting from vitamin A deficiency is a serious public health problem; it affects the health and sight of a staggering number of persons in many parts of the world.[3] The tear ducts dry, robbing the eye of its cleansing and lubricating means, and infection follows easily.
2. **Respiratory tract.** Ciliated epithelium in the nasal passages dries and the cilia are lost, thus removing a barrier to entry of infection. The salivary glands dry, and the mouth becomes dry and cracked, open to invading organisms.
3. **Gastrointestinal tract.** Mucosal membrane secretions decrease so that tissues dry and slough off, affecting digestion and absorption.
4. **Genitourinary tract.** As epithelial tissue breaks down, problems such as urinary tract infections, calculi, and vaginal infections increase.
5. **Skin.** As skin becomes dry and scaly, small pustules or hardened, pigmented, papular eruptions appear around hair follicles, a condition called **follicular hyperkeratosis.**
6. **Tooth formation.** Specific epithelial cells surrounding tooth buds in fetal gum tissue that normally become specialized cup-shaped organs called **ameloblasts** may not develop properly. These little organs form the enamel of the developing tooth.

Growth

Vitamin A is essential for the growth of skeletal and soft tissues. This effect is probably caused by the vitamin's influence on protein synthesis, mitosis (cell division), or stability of cell membranes.

The vision cycle: light-dark adaptation role of vitamin A.

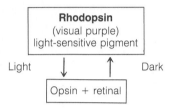

Rhodopsin
(visual purple)
light-sensitive pigment

Light   ↓   ↑   Dark

Opsin + retinal

Keratinization
Process occurring in vitamin A deficiency states in which the epithelial cells either slough off or become dry and flattened, then gradually harden and form rough, horny scales.

Follicular hyperkeratosis
Vitamin A deficiency condition in which the skin becomes dry and scaly and small pustules or hardened, pigmented, papular eruptions form around the hair follicles.

Ameloblasts
Special epithelial cells surrounding tooth buds in gum tissue, which form cup-shaped organs for producing the enamel structure of the developing teeth.

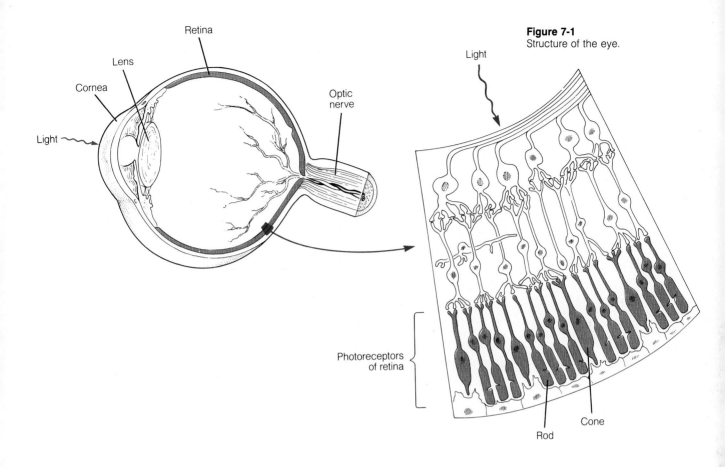

Retina

Lens

Cornea

Light

Optic nerve

Figure 7-1
Structure of the eye.

Light

Photoreceptors of retina

Cone

Rod

Reproduction

The retinoids are necessary to support normal function of the reproductive system in both males and females. In tests with animals the lack of retinol and retinal produces sterility, testicular degeneration in males, and aborted or malformed offspring in females.

Vitamin A Requirement
Influencing Factors

A number of variables modify vitamin A needs. Although the vitamin is generally ample in most diets, many factors may alter need in a given individual: (1) amount stored in the liver, (2) form in which it is taken (carotene or vitamin A), (3) illness, and (4) gastrointestinal or hepatic defects. Vitamin A deficiency may occur for three basic reasons: (1) inadequate dietary intake, (2) poor absorption resulting from lack of bile or defective absorbing surface, and (3) inadequate conversion of carotene because of liver or intestinal disease.

Units of Measure

To cover such variables, the RDA standard recommends a margin of safety above minimal needs. Traditionally, vitamin A has been measured in inter-

Retinol equivalent (RE)
Measure of vitamin A activity currently adopted by FAO/WHO and U.S. National Research Council's Food and Nutrition Board, replacing the term International Unit (IU). The measure accounts for dietary variances in preformed vitamin A (retinol) and its precursor, carotene. One retinol equivalent (RE) equals 3.33 IU or 1 mg retinol.

national units (IU). Currently, the RDA uses the term **retinol equivalents (RE)** (see RDA Tables inside front cover). This is a more accurate measure. It accounts for individual absorption and conversion variances. All other countries and international agencies have also adopted the retinol equivalent (RE) measure.

Hypervitaminosis A

Because the liver can store large amounts of vitamin A, and many persons take additional megadose supplements, it is clearly possible to consume a potentially toxic quantity. Hypervitaminosis A is manifested by joint pain, thickening of long bones, loss of hair, and jaundice. Excess vitamin A may also cause liver injury with resulting portal hypertension and ascites.

Food Sources of Vitamin A

There are few animal sources of natural preformed vitamin A: liver, kidney, cream, butter, and egg yolk. Our main dietary sources are the yellow and green vegetable and fruit sources of carotene, such as carrots, sweet potatoes, squash, apricots, cantaloupe, spinach, collards, broccoli, and cabbage. In addition, commercial products such as margarine are fortified with vitamin A.

Fat-Soluble Vitamin D

General Nature of Vitamin D
Chemical and Physical Nature

Early investigators wrongly classed this substance as a vitamin. But it is now clear that it is really a *prohormone* of a sterol type and should be viewed as a hormone. The term *vitamin D activity* is sometimes useful in talking about the several substances that the body makes from untraviolet irradition of steroids, collectively known as vitamin D. Since the precursor base in human skin is the lipid material *7-dehydrocholesterol,* all forms of these compounds with vitamin D activity are soluble in fat but not in water. They are heat stable and are not easily oxidized.

Forms

Two compounds with vitamin D activity are involved in human nutrition: *ergocalciferol (vitamin D_2)* and *cholecalciferol (vitamin D_3).* The much more significant one of these two is D_3, so its name **cholecalciferol** is the chemical name usually given to vitamin D in common usage. It is formed by the sun's ultraviolet irradiation of 7-dehydrocholesterol in the skin. D_3 occurs also in fish liver oils.

Absorption, Transport, and Storage
Absorption

The absorption of dietary vitamin D_3 occurs in the small intestine with the aid of bile. It mixes with the intestinal bile-fat complex and is absorbed in these fat packets. Malabsorption diseases such as celiac syndrome and Crohn's disease hinder vitamin D absorption.

Active Hormone Synthesis

1,25-Dihydroxycholecalciferol
Physiologically active hormone form of vitamin D.

The synthesis of the active hormonal form of **1,25-dihydroxycholecalciferol [1,25 $(OH)_2$ D_3]** is accomplished by the combined action of skin, liver, and kidneys, an overall process now called the vitamin D endocrine system:

1. **Skin.** In the skin, 7-dehydrocholesterol, the precursor cholesterol compound, is irradiated by the sun's ultraviolet rays to produce vitamin D_3. The amount of D_3 produced by this irradiation in the skin depends on a number of variables, including length and intensity of sunlight exposure and color of the skin. For example, heavily pigmented skin can prevent up to 95% of ultraviolet radiation from reaching the deeper layer of the skin for adequate synthesis of the steroid hormone. Also, persons who lack exposure to sunlight—house-bound elderly persons or those living in crowded city areas with high air pollution rates—would fail to receive adequate skin irradiation (see the box on p. 125).

2. **Liver.** After synthesis in the skin, vitamin D_3 is transported by its special globulin protein carrier to the liver. Here a special liver enzyme converts D_3 to the intermediate product 25-hydroxycholecalciferol, which is then transported by the same serum protein carrier to the kidney for final activation.

3. **Kidneys.** In the kidney special cell enzymes form the physiologically active vitamin D hormone, 1,25-dihydroxycholecalciferol.

Functions of Vitamin D
Absorption of Calcium and Phosphorus

In balance with the *parathyroid hormone* and the thyroid hormone *calcitonin*, the vitamin D hormone stimulates the active transport of calcium and phosphorus from the small intestine.

Bone Mineralization

After it has aided calcium and phosphorus absorption, vitamin D hormone continues to work with these minerals to form bone tissue. It directly increases the rate of mineral deposit and resorption in bone, the process by which bone tissue is built and maintained. A deficiency of vitamin D causes *rickets*, a condition characterized by malformation of skeletal tissue in growing children (Figure 7-2).

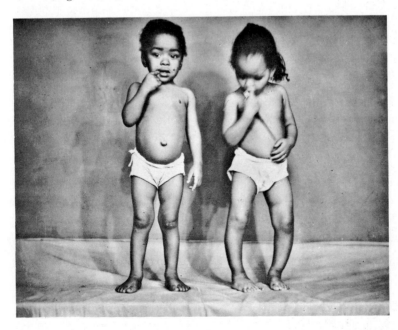

Figure 7-2
Rachitic children. Note knock-knees of child on left and bow-legs of child on right.
(From Therapeutic notes, Parke, Davis & Co, Detroit. Courtesy Dr. Tom Spies and Dr. Orson D. Bird.)

Basic Cell Processes

Beyond this role in bone and mineral metabolism, evidence is growing that the vitamin D hormone system is involved in widespread basic cell processes with targets in a number of organ tissues such as brain, kidney, liver, skin, reproductive tissue, hormone-secreting glands, and certain cells of the immune system.[4] Investigators suggest that these expanded metabolic activities probably relate to an active hormonal role in controlling basic cell functions such as cell reproduction and spread, as well as cell differentiation. This ongoing work may lead to possible use of the vitamin D analogs in treatment of such clinical problems as certain leukemias and the persistent skin disorder psoriasis.[5]

Vitamin D Requirement
Influencing Factors

Difficulties exist in setting requirements for vitamin D. Variables arise from numerous sources: a limited number of food sources available, lack of knowledge of precise body needs, and differing degrees of skin synthesis by irradiation. Needs vary between winter and summer in northern climates. Also, a person's living situation and occupation determine the degree of sunlight exposure. For example, a city dweller living in a high-rise apartment or tenement building and working indoors needs more than a farmer. Growth demands in childhood and in pregnancy and lactation necessitate increased intake.

RDA Standard

The RDA standard is 10 μg of cholecalciferol (400 IU) daily for children and for women during pregnancy and lactation. The daily allowance for young adults is 10 μg and for older adults, 5.0 μg.

Hypervitaminosis D

As with vitamin A, it is possible to ingest excess vitamin D and so produce toxicity. Intakes of vitamin D above 50 μg cholecalciferol (2000 IU/day), which is 5 times the recommended daily allowance, for prolonged periods can produce hypercalcemia in infants and nephrocalcinosis in infants and adults. Infant feeding poses a special caution. Excess intake is possible in infant feeding practices where fortified milk, fortified cereal, plus variable vitamin supplements are used. The infant needs only 10 μg (400 IU) daily, whereas the amount in all the items cited can easily total 100 μg (4000 IU) or more. The symptoms of toxicity include calcification of soft tissues, such as lungs and kidneys, and bone fragility. Renal tissue is particularly prone to calcify, affecting glomerular filtration and overall function.

Food Sources and Vitamin D

Few natural food sources of vitamin D exist. The two basic substances with vitamin D activity, D_2 and D_3, occur only in yeast and fish liver oils. The main food sources are those to which crystalline vitamin D has been added. Milk, because it is a common food, has proved to be the most practical carrier (see the box on the facing page). It is now a widespread commercial practice to standardize the added vitamin content of milk at 400 IU/qt. Milk is also a good carrier for the vitamin because it contains calcium and phosphorus as well. Butter substitutes, different forms of margarine, are also fortified.

Sunlight, Milk, and Cholecalciferol

Sunlight and milk are our two primary sources of vitamin D. But can we rely on them to supply our need? And do we really need fortified milk? Consider the differences in these two sources:

Sunlight

Sunlight is often discussed as a major source of vitamin D. Milk is considered more a source of other nutrients it contains naturally, especially calcium. Actually, however, of these two primary sources of vitamin D, sunlight is the least constant because of numerous factors that can affect its absorption into the skin and ability of these ultraviolet rays to transform the skin's precursor cholesterol compound, 7-dehydrocholesterol, into provitamin D_3 for the body's vitamin D hormone system to convert to the active vitamin.

▪ **Season of the year.** Ultraviolet exposure varies by season, depending on the type of activity, especially indoor versus outdoor, of the individual and the type of clothing worn. Age and mobility also interfere. For example, older persons immobilized by fractures or illness get very little exposure to sunshine.

▪ **Body composition.** Gross obesity, which also reduces the person's mobility and confines one indoors, in addition to presenting more layers of adipose tissue to be penetrated, decreases exposure to ultraviolet light, even to the point of increasing the risk of vitamin D deficiency.

Milk

Milk remains the most reliable source of vitamin D, especially for persons at risk for deficiency problems, for example, postmenopausal women, especially those who must spend much of their time indoors, and infants. The milk must be *fortified* with vitamin D, however, to provide necessary amounts with reasonable intake. Unfortified cow's milk does provide some vitamin D compounds, but many of them contribute little or nothing to its biologic activity. A liter provides only 40 IU of *active* vitamin D, as compared with 422 IU/L (400 IU/qt) of fortified cow's milk. The adult need is about 200 IU/day. Thus a woman 23 to 50 years of age with limited exposure to sunlight would have to drink 5 L (5 1/4 qt) of unfortified milk vs only 2 cups of whole fortified milk to meet her daily need for vitamin D. Along with the volume of unfortified milk, if it were whole milk, she would be getting 10 times as much fat, cholesterol, and kilocalories.

Remember this comparison when talking with milk-drinking persons, in case they are tempted to use nonfortified milks to reduce their intake of "over-processed" foods. This is one case in which that philosophy backfires.

REFERENCES

DeLuca HF: The vitamin D story: a collaborative effort of basic science and clinical medicine, FASEB J 2:224, March 1988.

Lips P and others: Determinants of vitamin D status in patients with hip fracture and in elderly control subjects, Am J Clin Nutr 46:1005, 1987.

Reeve LE, Jorgenson NA, and DeLuca HF: Vitamin D levels in unfortified cow's milk, J Nutr 112:667, April 1982.

Fat-Soluble Vitamin E

General Nature of Vitamin E
Chemical and Physical Nature

Vitamin E was discovered in connection with studies concerning the reproductive responses of rats and was identified as an alcohol. Because of this rat reproductive function and its chemical nature as an alcohol, it was named **tocopherol** from the Greek word *tokos* meaning "child-birth." Since then, tocopherol has come to be commonly known as the antisterility vitamin, but this effect has been demonstrated only in rats and not in humans, despite all advertising claims for its contribution to sexual powers.

Forms

Vitamin E is the generic name for a group of compounds with similar physiologic activity. One of these, *alpha-tocopherol,* is the most significant in human nutrition. It is a pale yellow oil, stable to acids and heat and insoluble in water. It oxidizes very slowly, which gives it an important role as an **antioxidant** with widespread clinical application.

Absorption, Transport, and Storage

Vitamin E is absorbed with the aid of bile. With other lipids in the chylomicrons, it is transported out of the intestinal wall into body circulation in the blood plasma lipoproteins. It is stored in different body tissues but especially in fat tissue.

Functions of Vitamin E
Antioxidant

Vitamin E acts as nature's most potent fat-soluble antioxidant. The polyunsaturated fatty acids in the structural lipid membranes of cells are particularly vulnerable to oxidative breakdown by free radicals in the cell. The tocopherols can interrupt this oxidation process, protecting the cell membrane fatty acids from the oxidative damage.

Selenium Relationship

Even with adequate vitamin E intake, some damaging cell peroxides may be formed, so a second line of defense is needed to destroy them before they can damage the cell membrane. The agent providing this added defense is a selenium-containing enzyme. Thus the trace element selenium spares vitamin E by reducing the vitamin's requirement. Similarly, in this partnership role, vitamin E helps reduce the selenium requirements.

Vitamin E Requirement
RDA Standard

The requirements for vitamin E vary with the amount of polyunsaturated fatty acids in the diet. The RDA standard for adults in *alpha-tocopherol equivalents (a-TE)* is 10 mg for men and 8 mg for women. Needs during childhood growth years range from 3 to 10 mg.

Special Clinical Needs

Since vitamin E protects cellular and subcellular membranes and hence tissue integrity, it is an important nutrient in the diets of pregnant and lactating women and especially for newborn infants. Two medical problems found

---

Tocopherol
Vitamin E; from two Greek words meaning "childbirth" and "to bring forth"; so named because of its association with reproduction in rats.

Antioxidant
Substance added to a product to delay or prevent its breakdown by oxygen.

in infants, particularly premature ones, have responded positively to vitamin E therapy: (1) *retrolental fibroplasia,* a condition causing severely limited vision or complete blindness from the effect of excess oxygen therapy following birth, and (2) *hemolytic anemia,* a condition in which fragile erythrocyte membranes break down because of high cell peroxide levels and the induced deficiency of vitamin E.[6] Also, older persons may require more vitamin E. It has been proved effective for those suffering circulatory disturbances such as pain in the legs after walking has begun, but it is of no help in varicose veins. Its effectiveness has not been supported in relation to treatment of coronary heart disease. However, in a large population study of men over a 10-year period, a high serum alpha-tocopherol level was associated with a reduced risk of cancer, even after adjustment for other confounding factors was made.[7]

Food Sources of Vitamin E

The richest dietary sources of vitamin E are the vegetable oils. Curiously enough, these are also the richest sources of polyunsaturated fatty acids, which vitamin E protects from oxidation. Other food sources include milk, eggs, muscle meats, fish, cereals, and leafy vegetables.

General Nature of Vitamin K

Chemical and Physical Nature

Fat-Soluble Vitamin K

The studies of a biochemist at the University of Copenhagen working with a hemorrhagic disease in chicks fed a fat-free diet led to the discovery of vitamin K. He found that the absent factor responsible was a fat-soluble, blood-clotting vitamin. Because of its blood clotting function, he called it "koagulationsvitamin" or vitamin K, from this Swedish word for its physiologic action. Later he succeeded in isolating and identifying the compound from alfalfa, for which he received the Nobel Prize in physiology and medicine. This major form of the vitamin found in plants has been named **phylloquinone** for its chemical structure. This is our dietary form of vitamin K; its name is generally used as the vitamin's basic chemical name.

Forms

As with most of the vitamins, several forms of vitamin K comprise a group of substances with similar biologic activity in blood-clotting. There are three main forms of vitamin K:

1. K_1, which is the major form found in plants.
2. K_2, which is synthesized by intestinal bacteria, so vitamin K is not required directly in the diet.
3. K_3, a water-soluble analog, which does not require bile for absorption and goes directly into the portal blood system.

Absorption, Transport, and Storage

K_1 and K_2 require bile for absorption as with other fat-related products. They are packaged in the intestinal chylomicrons and travel by means of the abdominal lacteals into the lymphatic system and then into the portal blood for transport to the liver. In the liver, vitamin K is stored in small amounts, though its concentration there declines rapidly. It is excreted in considerable quantity after administration of therapeutic doses.

Function of Vitamin K

The one basic function of vitamin K is to catalyze the synthesis of blood-clotting factors in the liver. Vitamin K produces the active form of several precursors, mainly **prothrombin** (factor II), which combines with calcium (factor IV) to help produce the clotting effect. In the absence of functioning liver tissue, vitamin K cannot act. When liver damage has caused decreased blood levels of prothrombin, and this problem in turn has led to hemorrhage, vitamin K is ineffective as a therapeutic agent.

Clinical Problems

Several clinical problems relate to vitamin K:

1. **Neonatology.** The sterile intestinal tract of the newborn can supply no vitamin K during the first few days of life until normal bacterial flora develop. During this immediate postnatal period, *hemorrhagic disease of the newborn* can occur. To prevent this disease, a prophylactic dose of vitamin K is usually given to the infant soon after birth.

2. **Malabsorption disease.** Any defect in fat absorption will cause a failure in vitamin K absorption, resulting in prolonged blood clotting time. For example, patients with bile duct obstruction are usually given vitamin K before surgery. Also, after a cholecystectomy, which hinders normal bile release, vitamin K, which requires bile and fat for normal absorption, is not readily absorbed. The water-soluble analog K_3—*menadione* may be used instead.

3. **Drug therapy.** Several drug-nutrient interactions involve vitamin K. An anticlotting drug such as *bishydroxycoumarin* (Dicumerol) acts as an antimetabolite or **antagonist,** thus inhibiting the action of vitamin K. When such drugs are used as anticoagulants for treating conditions such as vascular problems, vitamin K may be used as a balancing "antidote" to the drug in the management of blood clotting time. Also, in extended use of antibiotics, the intestinal bacterial flora may be diminished, thus reducing the body's main source of vitamin K.

4. **Generalized coagulopathy.** Severely ill, malnourished, hospitalized patients have been misdiagnosed sometimes as having a spreading intravascular coagulation disease when the true underlying problem is vitamin K deficiency.[8] Contributory factors in patients studied have included malabsorption, antibiotic therapy, hepatic dysfunction, and recent major surgery. Supplements of vitamin K can prevent such deficiency problems in ill patients who are not eating adequately.

Vitamin K Requirement

Until 1989, in edition 10, no specific recommendation for vitamin K had been stated in the RDA standards because there was less information on which to base allowances, since highly sensitive testing methods are needed to detect the very small normal tissue amounts. In one study of healthy adults, for example, the median serum value of phylloquinone was only 1.1 ng/mL.[9] Dietary need is based on two factors: (1) about half our daily need is supplied by intestinal bacteria synthesis, and (2) our body reserves are small and turn over rapidly.[10] The new RDA standard for adults has been stated as 80 μg/day, with relatively smaller amounts for children. A deficiency of vitamin K is unlikely except in the clinical conditions indicated.

Food Sources of Vitamin K

Dietary vitamin K is found in green leafy vegetables such as cabbage, spinach, kale, and cauliflower. Lesser amounts are found in tomatoes, cheese, egg yolk, and liver. However, the main source remains bacterial synthesis.

A summary of the fat-soluble vitamins is given in Table 7-1.

General Nature of Vitamin C
Chemical and Physical Nature

The recognition of vitamin C is associated with the history of an unrelenting search for the cause of the ancient hemorrhagic disease **scurvy.** Early observations, mostly among British sailors and explorers, led to the American discovery of an acid in lemon juice that prevented or cured scurvy. The specific chemical name of vitamin C is *ascorbic acid,* given to this substance because of its antiscorbutic, or "antiscurvy," properties. The structure of vitamin C is similar to that of glucose, its metabolic precursor in most animals, but humans lack a specific enzyme needed to change glucose to ascorbic acid. Thus human scurvy can really be called a disease of distant genetic origin, an inherited metabolic defect.

Care in Handling Food Sources

Vitamin C is an unstable, easily oxidized acid. It can be destroyed by oxygen, alkalis, and high temperatures. Therefore cook vitamin C foods in as little water as possible for brief periods and keep them covered. Never add soda as a coloring agent during cooking. Do not cut vegetables into small pieces until time of use, to curtail cut surface exposure to the air. Keep juices tightly closed.

Absorption, Transport, and Storage

Vitamin C is easily absorbed from the small intestine. But this absorption is hindered by a lack of hydrochloric acid or by bleeding from the gastrointestinal tract. Vitamin C is not stored in single tissue deposits as is vitamin A. Rather it is more generally distributed throughout the body tissues, maintaining a tissue saturation level. Any excess is excreted in the urine. The tissue levels relate to intake, and the size of the total body pool adjusts to maintain balances. The total amount in adults varies from about 0.3 g to 4.0 g. Tissue levels diminish slowly, so with no intake deficiency symptoms would not appear for approximately 3 months. This explains why generally healthy people in more isolated living situations can survive the winter without eating many fresh fruits and vegetables. Sufficient vitamin C for early infancy needs is present in breast milk if the mother has a good lactation diet. Cow's milk, however, contains very little vitamin C; remember that these animals have the enzymes to make their own vitamin C from glucose. Because of this, human infant formulas made from cow's milk are supplemented with ascorbic acid.

Functions of Vitamin C
Intercellular Cement Substance

We require vitamin C to build and maintain body tissues in general, including bone matrix, cartilage, dentin, collagen, and connective tissue. When vitamin C is absent, the important ground substance does not develop into col-

Water-Soluble Vitamin C

Scurvy
Hemorrhagic disease caused by lack of vitamin C.

Table 7-1
Summary of Fat-Soluble Vitamins

Vitamin	Physiologic functions	Results of deficiency	Requirement	Food sources
Vitamin A Provitamin: beta-carotene Vitamin: retinol	Production of rhodopsin and other light-receptor pigments Formation and maintenance of epithelial tissue Growth Reproduction Toxic in large amounts	Poor dark adaptation, night blindness, xerosis, xerophthalmia Keratinization of epithelium Growth failure Reproductive failure	Adult male: 1000 μg RE Adult female: 800 μg RE Pregnancy: 800 μg RE Lactation: 1300 μg RE Children: 400-1000 μg RE	Liver, cream, butter, whole milk, egg yolk Green and yellow vegetables, yellow fruits Fortified margarine
Vitamin D Provitamins: ergosterol (plants); 7-dehydrocholesterol (skin) Vitamins: D_2 (ergocholecalciferol) and D_3 (cholecalciferol)	1,25-dihydroxycholecalciferol, a major hormone regulator of bone mineral (calcium and phosphorus) metabolism Calcium and phosphorus absorption Toxic in large amounts	Faulty bone growth: rickets, osteomalacia	Adult: 5-10 μg cholecalciferol Pregnancy and lactation: 10 μg Children: 10 μg	Fortified milk Fortified margarine Fish oils Sunlight on skin
Vitamin E Tocopherols	Antioxidation Hemopoiesis Related to action of selenium	Anemia in premature infants	Adults: 8-10 mg αTE Pregnancy and lactation: 10-12 mg αTE Children: 3-10 mg αTE	Vegetable oils
Vitamin K K_1 (phylloquinone) K_2 (menaquinone) Analog: K_3 (menadione)	Activation of blood-clotting factors (for example, prothrombin) by α-carboxylating glutamic acid residues Toxicity can be induced by water-soluble analogs	Hemorrhagic disease of the newborn Defective blood clotting Deficiency symptoms, which can be produced by coumarin anticoagulants and by antibiotic therapy	Adult: 65-80 μg Children: 15-65 μg Infants: 5-10 μg	Cheese, egg yolk, liver Green leafy vegetables Synthesized by intestinal bacteria

lagen. When the vitamin is given, formation of cartilaginous tissue follows quickly. **Collagen** is a protein substance that exists in many body tissues, such as the white fibers of connective tissue. Blood vessel tissue particularly is weakened without the "cementing" substance from vitamin C's metabolic action that helps provide firm capillary walls. Thus vitamin C deficiency is characterized by fragile capillaries, easily ruptured by blood pressure or trauma, resulting in diffuse tissue bleeding. Deficiency signs include easy bruising, pinpoint hemorrhages of the skin, bone and joint hemorrhages, easy bone fracture, poor wound healing, and soft bleeding gums with loosened teeth, or *gingivitis.*

> The word collagen is derived from two Greek words that mean "glue" and "to produce."

General Body Metabolism

The concentration of vitamin C is greater in the more metabolically active tissue such as the adrenal glands, brain, kidney, liver, pancreas, thymus, and spleen than in less active tissues. More vitamin C is also present in a child's actively multiplying tissue than in adult tissue. Vitamin C helps in the formation of hemoglobin and the development of red blood cells in two ways: (1) it aids in the absorption of iron and (2) it influences the removal of iron from its transport complex so that it is available to tissues producing the hemoglobin.

Clinical Problems and Normal Growth

Some basic clinical problems, as well as normal growth, require additional vitamin C:

1. **Wound healing.** The significant role of vitamin C in cementing the ground substance of supportive tissue makes it an important agent in wound healing. This creates added demands for vitamin C in traumatic injury or surgery, especially where extensive tissue regeneration is involved.

2. **Fevers and infections.** Infectious processes deplete tissue stores of vitamin C. Optimal tissue stores help maintain resistance to infection. Just how large an amount may be required to maintain this protection is not known.

3. **Growth periods.** Additional vitamin C is required during the growth periods of infancy and childhood. It is also needed during pregnancy to supply demands for rapid fetal growth and development of maternal tissues.

> Controversial claims have been made that massive doses of vitamin C have various therapeutic effects such as prevention of the common cold or treatment of cancer. Controlled studies have failed to support these claims.

Vitamin C Requirement

Difficulties in establishing requirements for vitamin C involve questions about individual tissue needs and whether minimum or optimum intakes are desired. Studies indicate that an intake of 30 to 40 mg/day is sufficient to maintain a suitable body pool of vitamin C in healthy adults.[10] The RDA standard is 60 mg/day for an optimal margin to cover variances in tissue demand.

Food Sources of Vitamin C

Vitamin C can be oxidized easily. Thus the handling, preparation, cooking, and processing of any food source of the vitamin should be considered in evaluating that food's contribution of the vitamin to the diet. Well-known sources include citrus fruit and tomatoes. Less regarded, but good additional sources include white potatoes, sweet potatoes, cabbage, broccoli, and other

Table 7-2
Summary of Vitamin C
(Ascorbic Acid)

Physiologic functions	Clinical applications	Requirement	Food sources
Antioxidation	Scurvy (deficiency)	60 mg	Fresh fruits, especially citrus
Collagen biosynthesis	Wound healing, tissue formation	Vegetables, such as tomatoes, cabbage, potatoes, chili peppers, and broccoli	
General metabolism	Fevers and infections		
Makes iron available for hemoglobin synthesis	Stress reactions		
Influences conversion of folic acid to folinic acid	Growth		
Oxidation-reduction of the amino acids, phenylalanine and tyrosine			

green and yellow vegetables. Other sources are seasonal, local, or regional foods such as berries, melons, chili peppers, guavas, pineapple, chard, kale, turnip greens, and asparagus.

A summary of vitamin C and its role in the body is given in Table 7-2. Some guidelines for vitamin supplementation are provided to help in nutrition counseling (see Issues and Answers on p. 149).

Water-Soluble B Vitamins

Deficiency Disease and Vitamin Discoveries

The story of the B vitamins is a compelling one. It tells of persons dying of a puzzling, age-old disease for which there was no cure. It was eventually learned that common, everyday food held the answer. The paralyzing disease was **beriberi,** which had plagued the Orient for centuries and caused many men in high places to search for its solution. Early observations and studies provided important clues, but application of the "vitamine" connection to the creeping human sickness was needed. This was finally achieved when an American chemist with the Philippine Bureau of Science used extracts of rice polishings and cured the epidemic infantile beriberi. The food factor was named *water-soluble B* because it was thought to be a single vitamin. Now we know it to be a large group of different individual vitamins, all water-soluble but each having a variety of significant metabolic functions in human health. Because of this developing knowledge, the original letter-naming scheme has long since become confusing and meaningless and we are now accustomed to calling them by their familiar specific chemical names as you see them discussed here.

Beriberi
Disease of the peripheral nerves caused by a deficiency of thiamin (vitamin B_1).

Vital Coenzyme Role

The B vitamins, originally believed to be important only in preventing the deficiency diseases that led to their discovery, have now been identified in relation to many important metabolic functions. As vital control agents, they serve in many specific reactions as **coenzyme** partners with key cell **enzymes** in energy metabolism and tissue building.

Here we will review briefly the eight basic vitamins in this group of water-soluble compounds. First we will look at the three classic deficiency disease factors: thiamin, riboflavin, and niacin. Then we will explore more recently discovered coenzyme factors: pyridoxine, pantothenic acid, and biotin. Finally, we will examine the blood-forming factors: folic acid and cobalamin.

General Nature of Thiamin
Deficiency Disease Relation

The search of many persons for the cause of *beriberi* led eventually to a successful conclusion with the identification of thiamin as the control agent involved. Its basic nature and metabolic function were then clarified in the early 1930s.

Chemical and Physical Nature

Thiamin is a water-soluble, fairly stable vitamin. However, it is destroyed by alkalis. The name "thiamin" comes from its chemical ringlike structure. One of its major parts is a thiazole ring: *thi*(o + vit)*amin*.

Absorption and Storage

Thiamin is absorbed more readily in the acid medium of the first section of the small intestine, the duodenum. In the lower duodenum the acidity of the food mass is buffered by the alkaline intestinal secretions. Thiamin is not stored in large quantities in the tissues. The tissue content is highly relevant to increased metabolic demand, as in fever, increased muscular activity, pregnancy, and lactation. The tissue stores also depend on the adequacy of the diet and on its general composition. For example, carbohydrate increases the need for thiamin, whereas fat and protein spare thiamin. Any unused thiamin is constantly excreted in the urine.

Function of Thiamin
Basic Coenzyme Role

The main function of thiamin as a metabolic control agent is related to energy metabolism. It serves as a coenzyme in key reactions that produce energy from glucose or that convert glucose to fat for tissue energy storage. Thus the symptoms of beriberi—muscle weakness, gastrointestinal disturbances, and neuritis—can be traced to problems related to these basic functions of thiamin.

Clinical Problems

Inadequate thiamin to provide the key energizing coenzyme factor in the cells produces broad clinical effects:

1. **Gastrointestinal system.** Various symptoms such as anorexia, indigestion, constipation, gastric atony, and deficient hydrochloric acid secretion may result from thiamin deficiency. When the cells of the smooth muscles and the secretory glands do not receive sufficient energy from glucose, they cannot do their work in digestion to provide still more glucose. A vicious cycle ensues as the deficiency continues.

Coenzyme
Compound or molecule that must be present with an enzyme for a specific reaction to occur.

Enzyme
Protein that acts as a catalyst by accelerating the chemical reactions of its often specific substrate.

Thiamin

One of thiamin's major parts is a thiazole ring: *thi*(o + vit)*amin*.

2. **Nervous system.** The central nervous system depends on glucose to do its work. Without sufficient thiamin to help provide this constant fuel, neuronal activity is impaired, alertness and reflex responses are diminished, and general apathy and fatigue result. If the deficiency continues, lipogenesis is hindered and damage or degeneration of *myelin sheaths* (lipid tissue covering the nerve fibers) follows. This causes increasing nerve irritation, pain, and prickly or deadening sensations. Paralysis results if the process continues unchecked, as demonstrated in the classic thiamin deficiency disease beriberi.

3. **Cardiovascular system.** With continuing thiamin deficiency, the heart muscle weakens and cardiac failure results. Also, smooth muscle of the vascular system may become involved, causing dilation of the peripheral blood vessels. As a result of cardiac failure, edema appears in the lower legs.

Thiamin Requirement

RDA Standard

The thiamin requirement in human nutrition is sometimes stated in terms of carbohydrate and energy needs, as expressed in caloric intake. By this measure daily adult thiamin needs may range from 0.3 to 0.5 mg/1000 kcal. The RDA adult standard is stated as 0.5 mg/1000 kcal with a minimum of 1 mg for any intake between 1000 to 2000 kcal, or 1.1 to 1.5 mg/day.

Special Needs

Several important factors influence thiamin requirements:

1. **Alcoholism.** Thiamin is most important in nutritional therapy for persons with alcoholism. Both a primary (lack of adequate diet) and a conditioned (effect of alcohol itself) malnutrition may develop and bring serious neurologic disorders.

2. **Other disease.** Fevers and infections increase cellular energy requirements. Geriatric patients and those with chronic illness require particular attention to prevent deficiencies.

3. **Growth and development.** About a 50% increase in thiamin requirement accompanies pregnancy and lactation, demanded by the rapid fetal growth, the increased metabolic rate during pregnancy, and the production of milk. Continued growth during infancy, childhood, and adolescence requires more thiamin. At any point in the life cycle, the larger the body and its tissue volume, the greater its cellular energy requirements and thus its thiamin needs.

Food Sources of Thiamin

Although thiamin is widespread in almost all plant and animal tissues commonly used as food, the content is usually small. Deficiency of thiamin is a distinct possibility when kilocalories are markedly curtailed, as in alcoholism, and when persons are following some highly inadequate special diet. In general, good food sources include lean pork, beef, liver, whole and enriched grains (flour, bread, cereals), and legumes. Eggs, fish, and a few vegetables are fair sources.

Riboflavin

General Nature of Riboflavin

Discovery

As early as 1897 a London chemist first observed in milk whey a water-soluble pigment with peculiar yellow-green fluorescence. But it was not until

1932 that riboflavin was actually discovered by researchers in Germany. The vitamin was given the chemical group name *flavins* from the Latin word for *yellow.* Later, because the vitamin was found also to contain a sugar named *ribose,* the name *riboflavin* was officially adopted.

Chemical and Physical Nature

Riboflavin is a yellow-green fluorescent pigment that forms yellowish brown, needle-like crystals. It is water-soluble and relatively stable to heat but easily destroyed by light and irradiation. It is stable in acid media and is not easily oxidized. However, it is sensitive to strong alkalis.

Absorption and Storage

Absorption of riboflavin occurs readily in the upper section of the small intestine, assisted by combination with phosphorus in the intestinal mucosa. Studies indicate that long-term laxative use of some bulk fiber supplements such as psyllium gum, especially when taken with milk or near meals, can hinder riboflavin absorption and contribute to its deficiency in body metabolism.[11] Storage is limited, although small amounts are found in liver and kidney. Day-to-day tissue turnover needs must be supplied in the diet.

Functions of Riboflavin
Basic Coenzyme Role

The cell enzymes of which riboflavin is an important part are called *flavoproteins.* Riboflavin enzymes operate at vital reaction points in the process of energy metabolism and in *deamination.* This is the key reaction that removes the nitrogen-containing amino group from certain amino acids. Thus riboflavin acts as a control agent in both energy production and tissue building.

Clinical Problems

Problems associated with riboflavin deficiency include the following:

1. **Ariboflavinosis.** A deficiency of riboflavin, or **ariboflavinosis,** brings a combination of symptoms, which centers on tissue inflammation and breakdown and poor wound healing. Even minor injuries easily become aggravated and do not heal easily. The lips become swollen, cracking easily, and characteristic cracks develop at the corners of the mouth, a condition called *cheilosis.* Cracks and irritation develop at nasal angles. The tongue becomes swollen and reddened—a condition called **glossitis.** Extra blood vessels develop in the cornea—*corneal vascularization*—and the eyes burn, itch, and tear. A scaly, greasy skin condition—*seborrheic dermatitis*—may develop, especially in skin folds. Since nutritional deficiencies are usually multiple rather than single, riboflavin deficiencies seldom occur alone. They are especially likely to occur in conjunction with deficiencies of other B vitamins.

2. **Deficiency in newborns.** Because riboflavin is light sensitive, newborn infants with elevated blood levels of bilirubin treated with phototherapy have shown signs of riboflavin deficiencies even when supplements were provided.

Riboflavin Requirement
Influencing Factors

The body's riboflavin requirement is related to total energy needs, level of exercise, body size, metabolic rate, and rate of growth.

Ariboflavinosis
Riboflavin deficiency state.

Glossitis
Swollen, reddened tongue; riboflavin deficiency symptom.

RDA Standard

For practical purposes the general RDA standard for riboflavin is based on 0.6 mg/1000 kcal for healthy persons, or an adult range of 1.2 to 1.7 mg/day.

Risk Groups

Persons in certain risk groups or clinical situations may require increased riboflavin. These include persons living in poverty or following bizarre food habits. It also applies to those with gastrointestinal disease or chronic illness where appetite is poor and malabsorption exists. In addition, at risk are people who have poor wound healing and those persons in growth periods such as in childhood, pregnancy, and lactation.

Food Sources of Riboflavin

Lactoflavin
Form in which riboflavin occurs in milk.

The most important source of riboflavin is milk. One of the pigments in milk, **lactoflavin,** is the milk form of riboflavin. Each quart of milk contains 2 mg of riboflavin, which is more than the daily requirement. Other good sources are organ meats such as liver, kidney, and heart, whole or enriched grains, and vegetables. Since riboflavin is water soluble and destroyed by light, considerable loss can occur in open, excess-water cooking.

Niacin

Pellagra
Deficiency disease caused by a lack of niacin in the diet and an inadequate amount of protein containing the amino acid, tryptophan, which is a precursor of niacin.

General Nature of Niacin
Deficiency Disease Related

The age-old disease related to niacin deficiency is **pellagra.** It is characterized by a typical dermatitis and often has fatal effects on the nervous system. Pellagra was first observed in eighteenth century Europe, where it was endemic in populations subsisting largely on corn. Later observations by an American physician studying the problem in an orphanage gave further clues. He noticed that although the majority of the children had pellagra to some degree, a few of them did not. He discovered that the few who were free of pellagra were sneaking into the pantries at night and eating the orphanage's limited supply of milk and meat. His investigation established the relation of the disease to a certain food factor. But it was not until 1937 that a University of Wisconsin scientist definitely associated niacin with pellagra by using it to cure a related disease, black tongue in dogs.

Chemical and Physical Nature

Further study of niacin and pellagra made clear a close connection of niacin to the essential amino acid tryptophan:

Precursor
Something that precedes; in biology, a substance from which another substance is derived.

1. **Precursor role of tryptophan.** Curious observations were made by early investigators that raised puzzling questions. Why was pellagra rare in some population groups whose diets were actually low in niacin, whereas the disease was common in other groups whose diets were higher in niacin? And why did milk, which is low in niacin, cure or prevent pellagra? Further, why was pellagra so common in groups subsisting on diets high in corn? In 1945 workers at the University of Wisconsin finally made the key discovery—tryptophan can be used by the body to make niacin; it is a **precursor** of niacin. Milk prevents pellagra because it is high in tryptophan. Almost exclusive use of corn contributes to pellagra because it is low in tryptophan. And some populations with diets low in niacin may never have pellagra because they happen also to be consuming adequate amounts of tryptophan.

2. **Niacin equivalent.** This tryptophan-niacin relationship led to the development of a unit of measure called **niacin equivalent (NE).** In persons with average physiologic needs, approximately 60 mg of tryptophan produces 1 mg of niacin, the amount designated as a niacin equivalent. Dietary requirements are now given in terms of total milligrams of niacin and niacin equivalents.

Forms

Two forms of niacin exist. Niacin (nicotinic acid) is easily converted to its amide form, *nicotinamide,* which is water soluble, stable to acid and heat, and forms a white powder when crystallized.

Functions of Niacin
Basic Coenzyme Role

Niacin is a partner with riboflavin in the cellular coenzyme system that converts protein to glucose and oxidizes glucose to release controlled energy.

Drug Therapy

High doses of nicotinic acid, but not nicotinamide, act as vasodilators and cause skin-flushing, gastrointestinal distress, and itching. Such a dosage has been effective in lowering serum cholesterol, although the mechanisms for such action are unclear.

Clinical Problems

Generally, niacin deficiency appears as weakness, lassitude, anorexia, indigestion, and various skin eruptions. More specific symptoms involve the skin and nervous system. Skin areas exposed to sunlight are especially affected and develop a dark, scaly dermatitis. If deficiency continues, the central nervous system becomes involved, and confusion, apathy, disorientation, and neuritis develop.

Niacin Requirement
Influencing Factors

Factors such as age and growth periods, pregnancy and lactation, illness, tissue trauma, body size, and physical activity affect the niacin requirement.

RDA Standard

The RDA standard is 6.6 mg/1000 kcal and not less than 13 niacin equivalents at intakes of less than 2000 kcal. This is about 50 mg higher than the minimum requirements to provide a safety margin to cover variances in individual need. The adult standard is 15 to 19 mg/day. These recommendations also allow for the contribution of tryptophan in terms of niacin equivalents from the dietary protein sources.

Food Sources of Niacin

Meat is a major source of niacin. Other good sources include peanuts and dried beans and peas. Enrichment makes good sources of all grains. Otherwise, corn and rice are poor food sources of niacin, because they are low in tryptophan. Oats are also low in niacin. Fruits and vegetables generally are relatively poor sources.

Niacin equivalent (NE)
Measure of the total dietary sources of niacin equivalent to 1 mg of niacin. Thus, a niacin equivalent (NE) is 1 mg of niacin or 60 mg of tryptophan.

Pyridoxine

General Nature of Pyridoxine
Chemical and Physical Nature

The chemical structure of this vitamin, a pyridine ring, accounts for its specific name *pyridoxine*. It is water soluble, heat stable, but sensitive to light and alkalis.

Forms

Vitamin B_6 is a generic term for a group of vitamins with a similar function. Three forms occur in nature: pyridoxine, pyridoxal, and pyridoxamine. In the body all three forms are equally active as precursors of the potent pyridoxine coenzyme *pyridoxalphosphate (B_6-PO_4)*.

Absorption and Storage

Pyridoxine is easily absorbed in the upper portion of the small intestine. It is "stored" in the tissue saturation sense and found throughout the body tissues, evidence of its many essential metabolic activities.

Functions of Pyridoxine
Coenzyme in Protein Metabolism

In its active phosphate form, pyridoxine is a coenzyme in many types of amino acid reactions:
1. **Neurotransmitter.** Helps produce gamma-aminobutyric acid (GABA) and serotonin, vital regulatory substances in brain activity.
2. **New amino acids.** Transfers nitrogen from amino acids to form new ones and releases carbon residues for energy.
3. **Sulfur transfer.** Moves sulfur from an essential sulfur-containing amino acid (methionine) to form other sulfur compounds.
4. **Niacin.** Controls formation of niacin from tryptophan.
5. **Hemoglobin.** Incorporates amino acids into *heme,* the essential nonprotein core of hemoglobin.
6. **Amino acid transport.** Actively transports amino acids from the intestine into circulation and across cell walls into the cells.

Coenzyme in Carbohydrate and Fat Metabolism

The active phosphate coenzyme provides metabolites for energy-producing fuel. It also converts the essential fatty acid, linoleic acid, to another fatty acid, arachidonic acid.

Clinical Problems

It is evident from such an impressive list of metabolic activities—and these are only a few examples— that pyridoxine holds a key to a number of clinical problems.

1. **Anemia.** A hypochromic type of anemia relates to the role of pyridoxine in heme formation. It can occur even in the presence of a high serum iron level. A deficiency of pyridoxine has been demonstrated in such cases by a special test, and the anemia has been cured by supplying the deficient vitamin.

2. **Central nervous system problems.** Through its role in the formation of the two regulatory compounds in brain activity, serotonin and GABA, pyridoxine controls related neurologic conditions. In infants deprived of the vi-

tamin, as was the case when a batch of formula was mistakenly autoclaved at high temperature, there is increased irritability progressing to convulsions. The condition responds immediately to supplementation with the vitamin.

3. **Physiologic demands in pregnancy.** Pyridoxine deficiencies during pregnancy have been demonstrated by special tests and subsequently alleviated by supplementation. Fetal growth creates greater maternal metabolic needs and increases pyridoxine requirement.

4. **Oral contraceptive use.** Women taking estrogen-progesterone oral contraceptives require additional pyridoxine. An abnormal state of tryptophan metabolism contributes to the increased need.

5. **Drug therapy.** The drug isonicotinic acid hydrazide, or INH (Isoniazid), used as a chemotherapeutic agent for tuberculosis, is an antagonist to pyridoxine. Also, it inhibits the conversion of glutamic acid, the only amino acid the brain metabolizes, and causes a side effect of neuritis. Treatment with large doses of pyridoxine, 50 to 100 mg/day, prevents this effect.

Pyridoxine Requirement
RDA Standard

A deficiency of pyridoxine is unlikely because the amounts present in the general diet are large relative to the requirement. Since pyridoxine is involved in amino acids metabolism, the need varies with dietary protein intake. For adults approximately 1 mg/day is minimal. The RDA standard is 1.6 to 2.0 mg/day to ensure a safety margin for variances in need.

Toxic Effects

Pyridoxine abuse has been reported in which megadoses of 1 g/day or more were used (see the box on p. 140). Cases of pyridoxine abuse with megadoses up to 5 g/day have been reported, with primary symptoms resulting from severe nerve damage.[12]

Food Sources of Pyridoxine

Pyridoxine is widespread in foods, but many sources provide only very small amounts. Good sources include grains, seeds, and liver and kidney and other meats. There are limited amounts in milk, eggs, and vegetables.

General Nature
Discovery

Pantothenic acid was isolated and synthesized between 1938 and 1940. Because it occurs in all forms of living things and is an acid it was named **pantothenic acid.** True to its name, it is widespread in nature and in body functions. Intestinal bacteria synthesize considerable amounts. This source, together with its widespread natural occurrence, makes deficiencies unlikely.

Chemical and Physical Nature

Pantothenic acid is a white crystalline compound. It is readily absorbed in the intestine and combines with phosphorus to form the active coenzyme, *coenzyme A.* It is in this key controlling compound of coenzyme A that pantothenic acid has such widespread metabolic presence and use throughout the body. There is no known toxicity or a natural deficiency.

Pantothenic Acid

Pantothenic comes from a Greek word that means "in every corner" or "from all sides."

Clinical Application

Nutrient or Drug?

In 1954 researchers found out that large doses, 10 to 1000 times the RDA, of specific nutrients helped alleviate symptoms in certain genetic disorders. Twenty years later, the general public began to think that this would be helpful for healthy people, too. So they started using nutrients as drugs.

A similarity does exist. Both nutrients and drugs are used by the body in specific amounts to control or improve a physiologic condition or illness, to prevent a disease, or to relieve symptoms. But for many persons, the similarity seems to end there. They know that too much of any drug can be harmful, but they fail to apply this same wise logic to nutrients.

Some bad effects

Toxic effects of vitamin megadoses. Physicians may prescribe large doses of water-soluble vitamins, believing they are safe because they are not stored in the body. However, they have recently discovered the potential toxicity of at least one such vitamin—pyridoxine (B_6). Gynecologists have been prescribing this vitamin at levels that were 100 to 2700 times its RDA to help patients relieve the discomfort of edema during their menstrual cycle. The patients eventually developed unstable gaits, with such numbness in the hands that they were unable to walk or carry out their usual duties at work. To make matters worse, the prescription did nothing to relieve their discomfort.

"Artificially-induced" deficiency symptoms. These occur when blood levels of one nutrient rise above normal, resulting in an increased need for other nutrients with which it interacts. Deficiencies also occur when large doses are suddenly removed, creating a "rebound effect." This effect has been seen in infants born to mothers who took megadoses of vitamin C during pregnancy, yet developed scurvy after birth when their high nutrient supply was cut off.

Wise warnings

The megavitamin lesson is not easily taught. Megadose salespersons frequently have more time, money, and better "selling" techniques with which they can misinform the public. Nonetheless, for your clients' welfare, you will still want to warn them:

Vitamins, like drugs, can be harmful in large amounts. The only time megadoses are helpful is when the body already has a severe deficiency or is unable to absorb or metabolize the nutrient efficiently.

All nutrients work in harmony to promote good health. Adding large amounts of one only makes the body believe that it isn't getting enough of the others and increases the risk of developing deficiency symptoms.

Supplements should not be taken without first analyzing nutrient levels currently in the diet. This helps to avoid problems of excess, which may increase with an accumulative effect over time.

Food remains the best source of nutrients. Most food items provide a wide variety of nutrients, as opposed to the dozen or so found in a vitamin bottle. By itself a vitamin can do very little. Its action is catalytic and so it requires a substrate to work on. These necessary substrates are the energy nutrients—carbohydrate, protein, fat—and their metabolites. Food provides these necessities and a great deal of pleasure as well.

REFERENCES

Hartz SC and Blumberg J: Use of vitamin and mineral supplements by the elderly, Clin Nutr 5(3):130, 1986.

McDonald JT: Vitamin and mineral supplement use in the United States, Clin Nutr 5(1):27, 1986.

Rudman D: Megadose vitamins: use and abuse, N Engl J Med 309(8):489, 1983.

Functions of Pantothenic Acid

In its one basic role as an essential constituent of the body's key activating agent coenzyme A, pantothenic acid is vital to metabolic reactions involving carbohydrate, fat, and protein metabolism in all cells.

Pantothenic Acid Requirement

Since deficiency is unknown, a requirement for pantothenic acid has not been stated. The RDA's "estimated safe and adequate" range for adults is 4 to 7 mg. The daily intake in an average American diet of 2500 to 3000 kcal is about 10 to 20 mg, well above this estimated need. A deficiency is unlikely because of its widespread occurrence in food.

Food Sources of Pantothenic Acid

Sources of pantothenic acid are equally as widespread as its occurrence in body tissue. Rich sources include metabolically active tissue such as liver and kidney. Egg yolk and milk contribute more. Fair additional sources include other meat, cheese, legumes, and vegetables.

General Nature of Biotin

Biotin

The minute traces of biotin in the body perform multiple metabolic tasks. Its potency is great and natural deficiency is unknown. But some cases of induced deficiency have occurred in patients on long-term total parenteral nutrition (TPN), and several inborn errors of biotin metabolism have been defined according to the specific enzyme that is lacking.[13] There is no known toxicity.

Functions of Biotin

Biotin functions as a partner with acetyl-coenzyme A in reactions that transfer carbon dioxide from one compound and fix it onto another. Examples of this combination of cofactors at work include (1) initial steps in synthesis of some fatty acids, (2) conversion reactions involved in synthesis of some amino acids, and (3) carbon dioxide fixation in forming purines.

Biotin Requirements

Since the amount needed for metabolism is so small, the human requirement for biotin has not yet been established in specific terms. The RDA adult estimate is 30 to 100 µg/day. Most of the body's need is supplied from intestinal bacteria synthesis.

Food Sources of Biotin

Biotin is widely distributed in natural foods, but its bioavailability is highly variable in different foods. For example, the biotin of corn and soy meals is completely available, whereas that of wheat is almost unavailable. Excellent food sources include egg yolk, liver, kidney, and other animal tissues, as well as tomatoes and yeast.

Folic Acid

General Nature of Folic Acid
Discovery

Folic acid was identified and isolated in laboratory studies of anemias and growth factors in animals. In 1945 folic acid was obtained from liver and finally synthesized. The vitamin was given the name *folic acid* from the Latin word *folium*, meaning "leaf," because a major source of its extraction was dark-green leafy vegetables such as spinach. A reduced form of folic acid has since been discovered—*folinic acid*. The term *folate* is the salt form of folic acid and both terms are often used interchangeably for the vitamin.

Chemical and Physical Nature

Folic acid forms yellow crystals and is a conjugated substance made up of three acids, one of which is para-aminobenzoic acid (PABA). PABA is sometimes touted in nutrition supplements as a separate essential factor in human nutrition. It is not. Its only role in human nutrition is that of a component of the vitamin folic acid. Animal and human cells are not capable of synthesizing PABA nor of attaching it to the rest of the vitamin molecule. Only plants and certain bacteria can do this. Thus dietary folic acid, preformed by plants, is the essential substance in human nutrition, and the major source of this folic acid is green leafy vegetables.

Functions of Folic Acid
Basic Coenzyme Role

Folic acid coenzyme is a necessary agent in the important task of attaching single carbon to compounds. Several key compounds are examples:
1. **Purines.** Nitrogen-containing compounds essential to all living cells, involved in cell division and in the transmission of inherited traits.
2. **Thymine.** Essential compound forming a key part of deoxyribonucleic acid (DNA), the important material in the cell nucleus that controls and transmits genetic characteristics.
3. **Hemoglobin.** Heme, the iron-containing nonprotein portion of hemoglobin.

Clinical Problems

Some clinical problems associated with folic acid are:

1. **Anemia.** A nutritional **megaloblastic anemia** occurs in simple folic acid deficiency. Since tissue growth requires additional folic acid, this anemia is a special risk in pregnant women, growing infants, and young children.

2. **Sprue.** Folic acid is an effective agent in the treatment of sprue, the adult form of celiac disease, a gastrointestinal problem characterized by intestinal lesions, malabsorption defects, diarrhea, macrocytic anemia, and general malnutrition. The vitamin corrects both the blood-forming and the gastrointestinal defects of the disease.

3. **Chemotherapy.** The drug methotrexate (amethopterin), currently used in cancer chemotherapy, acts as a folic acid antagonist to reduce the tumor growth. The effect of this action is to prevent synthesis of DNA and purines in the cell.

4. **Growth and stress.** Increased folic acid is needed during periods of rapid growth, especially during fetal development.

Megaloblastic anemia
Anemia characterized by formation of large immature red blood cells that are deficient carriers of oxygen; caused by deficiency of folic acid and hence faulty synthesis of heme.

Folic Acid Requirement

The average American diet contains about 0.6 mg of total folic acid activity. The adult RDA standard is 180 to 200 µg/day. This amount covers variances in need. It also covers the limited bioavailability of folic acid in foods, which studies indicate is only about 50%.[14] An intake of 400 µg/day is recommended for women during pregnancy to meet increased fetal growth demands.

Food Sources of Folic Acid

Green leafy vegetables, liver, kidney, and asparagus are rich sources of folic acid. Relatively poorer sources are milk, poultry, and eggs.

General Nature of Cobalamin (B₁₂)
Discovery

Cobalamin

The discovery of vitamin B_{12} was associated with the search for the specific agent responsible for control of *pernicious anemia*. At first the disease was thought to be related to a deficiency of folic acid. However, although folic acid helped the initial red blood cell regeneration in persons with pernicious anemia, it was not permanently effective and did not control the nerve problems associated with the disease. When folic acid was found to be lacking in full effectiveness, the search continued for the remaining piece of the disease puzzle.

In 1948 two groups of workers, one in America and one in England, crystallized a red compound from liver, which they then numbered B_{12}. In the same year it was clearly shown that this new vitamin could control both the blood-forming defect and the neurologic involvement in pernicious anemia. Soon afterward, the working groups of scientists were able to produce the vitamin through a process of bacterial fermentation. This process remains the main source of commercial supply today. The scientists named their vitamin discovery *cobalamin* because of its unique structure with a single brilliant red atom of the trace element cobalt at its center.

Chemical and Physical Nature

Cobalamin is a complex red crystalline compound of high molecular weight, with a single cobalt atom at its core. It occurs as a protein complex in foods, so its food sources are mainly of animal origin. The ultimate source, however, may be designated as the synthesizing bacteria in the intestinal tract of herbivorous animals. Some synthesis is done by human intestinal bacteria.

Absorption, Transport, and Storage
Absorption

Intestinal absorption takes place in the ileum. Cobalamin is first split from its protein complex by the gastric hydrochloric acid and then bound to a specific glycoprotein called *intrinsic factor,* secreted by the gastric mucosal cells. This cobalamin−intrinsic factor complex then moves into the intestine where it is absorbed by special receptors in the ileal mucosa.

Storage

Cobalamin is stored in active body tissues. Organs holding the greatest amounts are the liver, kidney, heart, muscle, pancreas, testes, brain, blood, spleen, and bone marrow. These amounts are very minute, but the body holds them tenaciously and the stores are only slowly depleted. For example, a typical postgastrectomy anemia does not become apparent until 3 to 5 years after removal of the organ and subsequent loss of its secretions.

Functions of Cobalamin
Basic Coenzyme Role

As an essential coenzyme factor, cobalamin is closely related to amino acid metabolism and the formation of the heme portion of hemoglobin. Its requirement increases as protein intake increases.

Clinical Problems

Special needs for cobalamin occur in several problems related to blood-forming:

1. **Pernicious anemia.** In the absence of the intrinsic factor (specific component of gastric secretion required for cobalamin absorption), **pernicious anemia** develops. The vitamin is then not available for its key role in heme formation, and adequate hemoglobin cannot be synthesized.

Conversely, however, folic acid is not the primary agent for treating pernicious anemia. As indicated, although folic acid results in blood cell regeneration in persons with pernicious anemia, its effect is not permanent, nor does it control the degenerative neurologic problems. This is the critical distinction between cobalamin and folic acid in the diagnosis and treatment of this anemia. Therefore the American Medical Association and the U.S. Food and Drug Administration have recommended that no more than 0.4 mg of folic acid be included in multivitamin preparations, as this amount would suffice for common needs and not mask the development of pernicious anemia or prevent its diagnosis.

A person with defective cobalamin absorption, and hence pernicious anemia, can be given from 15 to 30 µg/day of cobalamin in intramuscular injections during a relapse and can be maintained afterward by an injection of

Pernicious anemia
Chronic, macrocytic anemia occurring most commonly in Caucasians after age 40. It is caused by the absence of the intrinsic factor normally present in gastric juice and necessary for the absorption of vitamin B_{12}. Pernicious anemia is controlled by intramuscular injections of vitamin B_{12}.

about 30 μg every 30 days. This treatment controls both the blood-forming disorder and the degenerative effects on the nervous system.

2. **Megaloblastic anemia.** Since cobalamin shares close metabolic relations with folic acid, a megaloblastic anemia develops when either of the vitamins is deficient. Cobalamin indirectly affects blood formation by providing an activated form of folate.

3. **Sprue.** Like folic acid, cobalamin is effective in the treatment of the intestinal syndrome of sprue. However, it is most effective when used in conjunction with folic acid, because its role is indirect activation of folic acid.

Cobalamin Requirement

The amount of dietary cobalamin needed for normal human metabolism is very small. Reported minimum needs have been from 0.6 to 1.2 μg/day, with a range upward to approximately 2.8 μg in individual cases. The ordinary diet easily provides this much and more. For example, one cup of milk, one egg, and 4 oz meat provide 2.4 mg. The RDA standard recommends an intake of 2 μg/day for adults. This amount allows a safety margin to cover variances in individual need, absorption, and body stores.

Food Sources of Cobalamin

Cobalamin is supplied by animal foods. The richest sources are liver and kidney, lean meat, milk, egg, and cheese. Natural dietary deficiency is rare. It has only been observed in some groups of strict vegetarians, who displayed symptoms of nervous disorders, sore mouth and tongue, neuritis, and amenorrhea.

A summary of the water-soluble B vitamins is given in Table 7-3.

Table 7-3

Summary of B-Complex Vitamins

Vitamin	Coenzymes: physiologic function	Clinical applications	Requirement/day	Food sources
Thiamin (B_1)	Carbohydrate metabolism Thiamin pyrophosphate (TPP): oxidative decarboxylation	Beriberi (deficiency) Neuropathy Wernicke-Korsakoff syndrome (alcoholism) Depressed muscular and secretory symptoms	1.1-1.5 mg	Pork, beef, liver, whole or enriched grains, legumes
Riboflavin (B_2)	General metabolism Flavin adenine dinucleotide (FAD) Flavin mononucleotide (FMN)	Cheilosis, glossitis, seborrheic dermatitis	1.2-1.7 mg	Milk, liver, enriched cereals

Continued.

Table 7-3

Summary of B-Complex Vitamins—cont'd

Vitamin	Coenzymes: physiologic function	Clinical applications	Requirement/day	Food sources
Niacin (nicotinic acid, nicotinamide)	General metabolism Nicotinamide adenine dinucleotide (NAD) Nicotinamide adenine dinucleotide phosphate (NADP)	Pellagra (deficiency) Weakness, anorexia Scaly dermatitis Neuritis	15-19 mg NE	Meat, peanuts, enriched grains (protein foods containing tryptophan)
Vitamin B_6 (pyridoxine, pyridoxal, pyridoxamine)	General metabolism Pyridoxal phosphate (PLP): transamination and decarboxylation	Reduced serum levels associated with pregnancy and use of oral contraceptives Antagonized by isoniazid, penicillamine, and other drugs	1.6-2.0 mg	Wheat, corn, meat, liver
Pantothenic acid	General metabolism CoA (coenzyme A): acetylation	Many roles through acyl transfer reactions (for example, lipogenesis, amino acid activation, and formation of cholesterol, steroid hormones, heme)	4-7 mg	Liver, egg, milk
Biotin	General metabolism N-carboxybiotinyl lysine: CO_2 transfer reactions	Deficiency induced by avidin (a protein in raw egg white) and by antibiotics Synthesis of some fatty acids and amino acids	30-100 μg	Egg yolk, liver Synthesized by intestinal microorganisms
Folic acid (folacin)	General metabolism Single carbon transfer reactions (for example, purine nucleotide, thymine, heme synthesis)	Megaloblastic anemia	Infants: 25-35 μg Children: 50-180 μg Adults: 150-180 μg	Liver; green leafy vegetables
Cobalamin (B_{12})	General metabolism Methylcobalamin: methylation reactions (for example, synthesis of amino acids, heme)	Pernicious anemia induced by lack of intrinsic factor Megaloblastic anemia Methylmalonic aciduria Homocystinuria Peripheral neuropathy (strict vegetarian diet)	2.0 μg	Liver, meat, milk, egg, cheese

A vitamin is an organic, noncalorigenic food substance that is required in small amounts for certain metabolic functions and cannot be manufactured by the body. Vitamins may be fat or water soluble, and their solubility affects their absorption and mode of transport to target tissues.

The fat-soluble vitamins are A, D, E, and K. Their metabolic tasks are mainly structural in nature, and their fate in the body is associated with lipids. The possibility of toxicity is enhanced for fat-soluble vitamins because the body can store them. Such toxicity is no longer rare, because of the current popularity of vitamin A supplements.

The remaining vitamins are water soluble: ascorbic acid (C) and the B-complex. These vitamins share three characteristics: (1) synthesis by plants and thus dietary supply by plant foods or animal foods (except vitamin B_{12}), (2) no stable "storage" form and thus must be provided regularly in the diet (except vitamin B_{12}), and (3) function as a coenzyme factor in cell metabolism (except vitamin C). Toxicity levels are usually not associated with water-soluble vitamins because excess is easily excreted in the urine. However, two vitamins have shown toxic effects when taken in megadoses (i.e., in gram amounts): pyridoxine (B_6), which can result in severe nerve damage, and ascorbic acid (C), which has been associated with gastrointestinal disturbances, renal calculi, and lowered resistance to infection. All water-soluble vitamins, especially vitamin C, are easily oxidized, and care must be taken in food storage and preparation practices.

To Sum Up

1. List and describe health problems caused by a vitamin A deficiency. Give three possible causes of a deficiency.
2. Describe the function of vitamin D endocrine system. Who would be at risk for developing a deficiency? Why?
3. What three characteristics are shared by most water-soluble vitamins? Identify an exception to each and explain the reason.
4. Which B vitamins play significant roles in blood formation? Describe their roles and interactions.

Questions for Review

References

1. Barclay AJC, Foster A, and Sommer A: Vitamin A supplements and mortality related to measles: a randomized clinical trial, Brit Med J 294:294, Jan 31, 1987.
2. Vitamin A for measles, Lancet 1:1067, May 9, 1987.
3. Bauernfeind JC: Vitamin A deficiency: a staggering problem of health and sight, Nutr Today 23(2): 34, 1988.
4. Vitamin D: New perspectives, Lancet 1:1122, May 16, 1987.
5. DeLuca HF: The vitamin D story: a collaborative effort of basic science and clinical medicine, FASEB (Federation of American Societies for Experimental Biology) 2:224, March 1, 1988.
6. Bieri JG, Corash L, and Hubbard VS: Medical uses of vitamin E, N Engl J Med 308(18):1063, 1983.
7. Knekt P and others: Serum vitamin E and risk of cancer among Finnish men during a 10-year follow-up, Am J Epidemiol 127:28, Jan 1988.
8. Alperin JB: Coagulopathy caused by vitamin K deficiency in critically ill hospitalized patients, JAMA 258: 1916, Oct 1987.
9. Mummah-Schendel LL and Suttie JW: Serum phylloquinone concentration in a normal adult population, Am J Clin Nutr 44:686, Sept 1986.
10. Olson JA: Recommended dietary intakes (RDI) of vitamin K in humans, Am J Clin Nutr 45:687, April 1987.

11. Roe DA, Kalkwarf H, and Stevens J: Effect of fiber supplements on the apparent absorption of pharmacological doses of riboflavin, J Am Diet Assoc 88(2):211, 1988.

12. Schaumburg H and others: Sensory neuropathy from pyridoxine abuse, N Engl J Med 309(3):445, 1983.

13. Marshall M: The nutritional importance of biotin—an update, Nutr Today 22(6):26, 1987.

14. Sauberlich HE and others: Folate requirement and metabolism in nonpregnant women, Am J Clin Nutr 46:1016, Dec 1987.

Further Readings

Bauernfeind JC: Vitamin A deficiency: a staggering problem of health and sight, Nutr Today 23(2):34, 1988.

This article describes in detail, with a number of illustrations, the function of vitamin A in vision and the worldwide extensive problem of blindness from a deficiency of the vitamin.

Belko AZ and others: Effects of exercise on riboflavin requirements of young women, Am J Clin Nutr 35:509, April 1983.

Casey V and Dwyer JT: Premenstrual syndrome: theories and evidence, Nutr Today 22(6):4, 1987.

van den Berg H and others: Vitamin B_6 status of women suffering from premenstrual syndrome, Human Nutr: Clin Nutr 40C:441, Nov 1986.

Weininger J and King JC: Effect of oral contraceptive agents on ascorbic acid metabolism, Am J Clin Nutr 35(6):1408, 1982.

This group of four articles explores the relation of specific vitamins to health concerns of women: evidence that exercising young women require more riboflavin, evidence that vitamin B_6 is no more effective than a placebo in relieving symptoms of PMS, but evidence that women using oral contraceptives do need more vitamin C.

Greger JL: Food, supplements, and fortified foods: scientific evaluations in regard to toxicology and nutrition bioavailability, J Am Diet Assoc 87(10):20, 1987.

Sauberlich HE: Vitamins—how much is for keeps? Nutr Today 22(1):20, 1987.

These two articles provide excellent background for the important concept of bioavailability and factors that explain why all the nutrients we consume by no means get into our body systems and cells to do their intended jobs.

Guidelines for Vitamin Supplementation

Conservative health workers often flatly declare that no one needs vitamin supplements. Pill-pushing, self-proclaimed "nutrition experts" push megadoses of everything from A through Z to cure anything.

Who's right? Probably someone who suggests something between these two extremist views. The Recommended Dietary Allowances (RDA) standards are based on the average needs of a healthy population, not on individual needs that can vary widely. But extremists may take these two concepts too far. Extreme "traditionalists" try to apply these standards rigidly to every individual. "Pill-pushers" recommend megadoses of everything "to cover all the bases" and increase their profits.

Biochemical individuality is a very real concept. It cannot be overlooked when assessing an individual client's nutritional needs. Since it is influenced by health status, personal habits, age, and other factors, the assessment process should consider *at least* the following conditions:

Pregnancy and lactation The RDA takes into account increased nutrient requirements for these situations. Meeting increased needs by diet alone may be difficult because of food preferences and availability. Reasonable supplements then ensure an adequate intake to meet the increased nutrient demands.

Oral contraceptive use This practice lowers serum levels of several B vitamins, including B_6 and niacin, as well as vitamin C. If nutrient intake levels are marginal, some supplements may be necessary. But the client should be encouraged to improve her diet or assisted in obtaining nutritious foods.

Aging Older adults often have decreased food intake and impaired nutrient absorption, storage, or usage. Marginal deficiencies of ascorbic acid, thiamin, riboflavin, and B_6 have been seen in the elderly, even among individuals using supplements. Current RDA standards may be too low to meet their particular needs.

Restricted diets Eternal "dieters" may find it difficult to meet any of the nutrient standards, particularly if their meals provide less than 1200 kcal/day. Very strict diets are not recommended. Anyone on a weight reduction regimen should be carefully assessed.

Exercise Exercise increases the need for riboflavin. The combination of a reducing diet and exercise increases this need and may indicate supplement use, especially in women who do not tolerate milk (the major source of riboflavin).

Smoking This unhealthful addictive habit can reduce vitamin C levels by as much as 30%. If dietary intake is marginal, a small supplement (100 mg/day) may help compensate. Of course, kicking the habit will help even more.

Alcohol Chronic or abusive use of alcohol impedes absorption and use of the B vitamins, especially thiamin, and even destroys folic acid. Supplements of multivitamins rich in B-complex vitamins will help. But alcohol reduction must accompany nutritional therapy to prevent recurrence of deficiency signs.

Caffeine In large quantities, caffeine will flush water-soluble vitamins out of the body faster than usual. Small supplements of B-complex vitamins and ascorbic acid may help. Reduced caffeine intake will help even more.

Continued.

Guidelines for Vitamin Supplementation—cont'd

Disease Carefully assess patients with disease, malnutrition, debilitation, or hypermetabolic demands to determine the degree of overall nutrient supplementation and diet modification needed for clinical purposes. These needs are particularly evident in long-term illness.

Once all of these conditions are carefully evaluated, help your client with a wise nutrition program. In many situations supplementation can be avoided by a change in personal habits. Best of all, the general public will be better served. They will be able to maintain good health while avoiding "artificially-induced" deficiencies and expensive health food store bills.

REFERENCES

ADA statement: Recommendations concerning supplement usage, J Am Diet Assoc 87(10):1342, 1987.

AMA Council on Scientific Affairs: Vitamin preparations as dietary supplements and as therapeutic agents, JAMA 257:1929, April 1987.

Callaway CW and others: Statement on vitamin and mineral supplements, J Nutr 117:1649, Oct 1987.

8 Minerals

Chapter Objectives

After studying this chapter, the student should be able to:

1. Identify the comparative amounts of the various body minerals and the forms in which they occur.
2. Describe the function of each mineral in the body and relate these functions to health and disease.
3. Compare the amount we need of each mineral and give some main food sources of each one.
4. Identify the role of minerals and other solutes in helping to maintain body water balance.

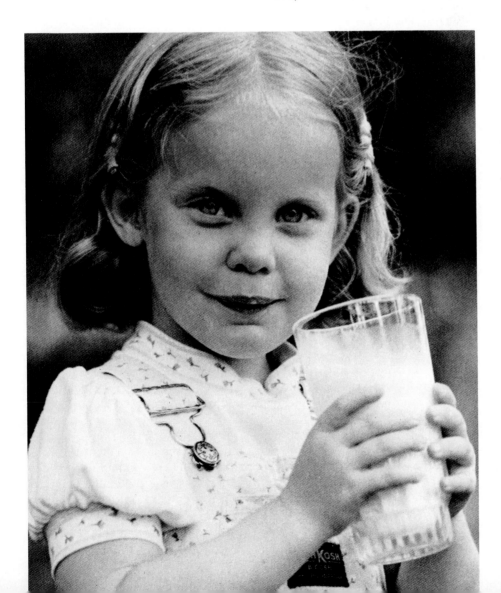

PREVIEW

▌ We live within an extended cycle of minerals essential to our existence. Over eons of time in our planet's development, shifting oceans and mountains have deposited an array of elements that move from rock to soil to plants to animals to humans.

These vital minerals may seem simple in comparison to the complex organic vitamin compounds. Nonetheless, in our bodies they fulfill an impressive variety of essential metabolic functions.

Elements for which the human dietary need is greater than 100 mg/day are usually called *major minerals*. Those needed in much smaller amounts are called *trace elements*.

Minerals in Human Nutrition

Metabolic Roles
Variety of Functions

Minerals are inorganic elements widely distributed in nature. They have vital roles in human metabolism that are as varied as are the minerals themselves. These substances, which appear so inert in comparison with the complex organic vitamin compounds, fulfill an impressive variety of metabolic functions: building, activating, regulating, transmitting, and controlling. For example, ionized sodium and potassium exercise all-important control over shifts in body water. Dynamic calcium and phosphorus provide structure for the body's framework. Oxygen-hungry iron gives a core to heme in hemoglobin. Brilliant red cobalt is the atom at the core of cobalamin (vitamin B_{12}). Iodine is the necessary constituent of the thyroid hormone, which in turn controls the rate of body metabolism. Far from being static and inert, minerals are active participants, helping to control many of the metabolic processes in the body.

Variety in Amount Needed

Minerals also differ from vitamins in another way. Vitamins, as you saw in the previous chapter, all require very small amounts of their complex organic compounds to do their metabolic jobs. Minerals, however, require varying amounts—from the relatively large amounts of the major minerals to the exceedingly small amounts of the trace elements. For example, the major mineral calcium forms a relatively large amount of body weight, about 2%. Most of this is in skeletal tissue. Thus an adult weighing 150 lbs has about 3 lb of calcium in the body. On the other hand, the trace element iron is present in very small amounts. This same adult has only about 3 g (about 1/10 oz) of iron in his body, mostly in the hemoglobin of red blood cells.

Classification

In your study here, you will find these important mineral elements grouped in three main sections, one major and two trace. These commonly used divisions are based on (1) how much of the mineral is required by the body and (2) how much we know at this point about its essentiality, in cases of some of the trace elements.

Major Minerals

Seven minerals present in the body in large amounts are called the *major minerals*. These include calcium, magnesium, sodium, potassium, phosphorus, sulfur, and chlorine.

Trace Elements

The remaining minerals are present in smaller amounts and are called *trace elements*. The essential nature of 10 of these has been determined; the precise functioning of the remaining 8, is as yet not entirely clear.

In Table 8-1, as a study guide, you will find a listing of the minerals in each group. We will briefly review each in turn, looking at (1) balance controls maintaining the body's needed amount, (2) physiologic function, (3) clinical problems associated, (4) the body's requirement, and (5) food sources.

Calcium

Of all the minerals in the body, calcium occurs in the largest amount by far. The total amount of body calcium is in constant balance with food sources from the outside and with tissue calcium within the body among its various parts. A number of dynamic balance mechanisms are constantly at work to maintain these levels within normal ranges. The balance concept, therefore, can be applied at three basic levels: (1) the intake-absorption-output balance, (2) the bone-blood balance, and (3) the calcium-phosphorus blood serum balance.

Intake-Absorption-Output Balance

Calcium Intake

The average adult American diet contains about 700 to 1200 mg of calcium. Most of this comes from dairy products and some from green leafy vegetables and grains. However, the absorption of minerals in general is less efficient than that of the vitamins and macronutrients. Not all of the food intake

Table 8-1

Major Minerals and Trace Elements in Human Nutrition

Major minerals (required intake over 100 mg/day)	Trace elements	
	Essential (required intake under 100 mg/day)	Essentiality unclear
Calcium (Ca)	Iron (Fe)	Silicon (Si)
Phosphorus (P)	Iodine (I)	Vanadium (V)
Magnesium (Mg)	Zinc (Zn)	Nickel (Ni)
Sodium (Na)	Copper (Cu)	Tin (Sn)
Potassium (K)	Manganese (Mn)	Cadmium (Cd)
Chloride (Cl)	Chromium (Cr)	Arsenic (As)
Sulfur (S)	Cobalt (Co)	Aluminum (Al)
	Selenium (Se)	Boron (B)
	Molybdenum (Mo)	
	Fluorine (Fl)	

Bioavailability
Degree to which the amount of a nutrient ingested actually gets absorbed and is available to the body.

of minerals is necessarily available. The term **bioavailability** refers to the degree to which the body uses a particular nutrient, such as calcium in this case, which depends on many factors that influence its absorption-excretion balance or its balance in body tissues.[1] This is one of the basic facts that makes the setting of precise requirements for minerals difficult. Stated requirements for many of these elements are given as estimated ranges of need rather than as precise figures.

Absorption of Calcium

Only about 10% to 30% of the calcium in an average diet is absorbed. Most food calcium occurs in complexes with other dietary components. These complexes must be broken down and the calcium released in a soluble form before it can be absorbed. Absorption takes place in the small intestine, chiefly in the first section, the duodenum, where the gastric acidity is still effective rather than being buffered as the food mass moves along.

Factors Increasing Calcium Absorption

The following factors increase calcium absorption:

1. **Vitamin D hormone.** An optimum amount of this control agent is necessary for calcium absorption. This agent controls the synthesis of a calcium-binding protein carrier in the duodenum that transports the mineral into the mucosal cells and blood circulation.

2. **Body need.** During periods of greater body demand, such as growth or depletion states, more calcium is absorbed. Physiologic states in the life cycle—growth, pregnancy and lactation, and old age—have a strong influence on the amount of absorption needed to meet body requirements. In elderly persons in general and in postmenopausal women in particular, the ability to absorb calcium is reduced.[2]

3. **Dietary protein and carbohydrate.** A greater percentage of calcium is absorbed when the diet is high in protein. However, this larger amount absorbed results in increased renal excretion, with a negative calcium balance following. Thus, in essence, high protein diets only induce increased calcium requirements to maintain calcium balance. Lactose enhances calcium absorption through the action of the lactobacilli, which produce lactic acid and lower intestinal pH. Nature's packaging of both lactose and calcium in milk makes a fortunate combination. Unfortunately, however, this relation of lactose and calcium absorption no longer holds in postmenopausal women with osteoporosis.[3]

4. **Acidity.** Lower pH (increased acidity) favors solubility of calcium and consequently its absorption.

Each of the following food items contributes about 300 mg of calcium:
1 cup milk
1 ounce cheese
1 cup dark greens (except spinach, chard, beet greens)
1 serving of oysters
1 serving of salmon (with bones)
2 servings of ice cream

Factors Decreasing Calcium Absorption

The following factors decrease calcium absorption:

1. **Vitamin D deficiency.** Vitamin D hormone, along with parathyroid hormone, is essential for calcium absorption.

2. **Dietary fat.** Excess dietary fat or poor absorption of fats results in an excess of fat in the intestine. This fat combines with calcium to form insoluble soaps. These insoluble soaps are excreted, with consequent loss of the incorporated calcium.

3. **Fiber and other binding agents.** An excess of dietary fiber binds calcium and hinders its absorption. Other binding agents include oxalic acid, which

combines with calcium to produce calcium oxalate, and phytic acid, which forms calcium phytate. Oxalic acid is a constituent of green leafy vegetables, but the amount of oxalates in them varies, making some of them better sources of calcium than others. Phytic acid is found in the outer hull of many cereal grains, especially wheat.

4. **Alkalinity.** Calcium is insoluble in an alkaline medium and consequently poorly absorbed.

Calcium Output

The overall body calcium balance is maintained first, therefore, at the point of absorption. A large unabsorbed amount—some 70% to 90%, varying according to body need—remains to be eliminated in the feces. A small amount of calcium may be excreted in the urine, about 200 mg/day, to maintain normal levels in the body fluids.

Bone-Blood Balance

Calcium in the Bones

In a healthy state the body maintains a constant turnover of the calcium in the bone tissue, which is the major site of calcium storage. Calcium in the bones and teeth is about 99% of that in the entire body. However, this is not a static storage. Bone tissue is constantly being built and reshaped according to various body needs and stresses (Figure 8-1). As much as 700 mg calcium

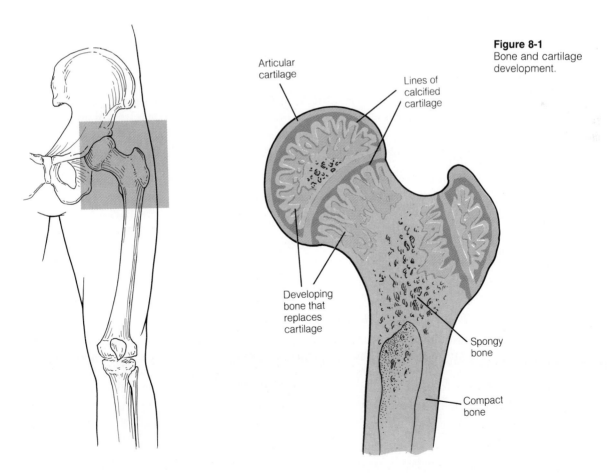

Figure 8-1
Bone and cartilage development.

Articular cartilage

Lines of calcified cartilage

Developing bone that replaces cartilage

Spongy bone

Compact bone

enters and leaves the bones each day. And all the while the body maintains a dynamic equilibrium. But in certain conditions or diseases, withdrawals may exceed deposits and a state of calcium imbalance occurs. For example, conditions such as immobility from a body cast or diseases such as osteoporosis would cause such excess bone calcium withdrawals.

Calcium in the Blood

The remaining small amount of calcium not in bone tissue, about 1%, circulates in the blood and other body fluids. Despite its small amount, however, this serum calcium plays a vital role in controlling body functions. This calcium in the blood occurs in two main forms:

1. **Bound calcium.** About half the calcium in the blood is bound in the plasma proteins and hence is not free or diffusable, that is, able to move about or to enter into other activities.

2. **Free ionized calcium.** Free particles of calcium, carrying electrical charges and hence in an active ionized form, move freely about and diffuse through membranes to control a number of body functions. These functions include blood clotting, transmission of nerve impulses, muscle contraction and relaxation, membrane permeability, and enzyme activation. This is a good illustration of a small amount of a nutrient doing a great deal of metabolic work because it is in an activated form.

Calcium-Phosphorus Serum Balance

Calcium-to-phosphorus (Ca:P) ratio
Inverse ratio affecting the absorption rate of each mineral. The *dietary ratio* of 1:1 is ideal for periods of rapid growth, 1:1½ for normal adult functions.

A final level of calcium balance is that which calcium maintains with phosphorus in the blood serum. Amounts of these two minerals in the blood are normally maintained in a definite relationship because of their relative solubility. This relationship is called the **serum calcium-to-phosphorus (Ca:P) ratio.** This ratio is the solubility product of calcium × phosphorus, expressed in milligrams of each mineral per deciliter (mg/dL) of serum. This is an important ratio in the blood. Normal serum calcium level is 10 mg/dL; for phosphorus it is 4 mg/dL for adults and 5 mg/dL for children. So the normal serum calcium-phosphorus ratios are 10 × 4 = 40 for adults and 10 × 5 = 50 for children. Any situation that causes an increase in the serum phosphorus level would cause a resulting decrease in the serum calcium level to hold the calcium-phosphorus solubility product constant. In such a case, the decreased serum calcium may bring on signs of *tetany* from lack of neuromuscular controls. To help maintain the normal serum Ca:P ratio, the ideal **dietary calcium-to-phosphorus ratio** is 1.0 to 1.5 for children and women during pregnancy and lactation. Other adults require a 1:1 dietary ratio, meaning equal amounts of dietary calcium and phosphorus, for ideal absorption and utilization.

Control Agents for Calcium Balance

Synergism is an important biologic concept. It is the cooperative action of two or more factors acting together to produce a total effect greater than the sum of their separate effects.

Two main control agents work together to maintain these vital levels of calcium balance in the body: *parathyroid hormone (PH)* and *vitamin D hormone.* The cooperative action of these two factors is a good example of the **synergistic** behavior of metabolic controls. Consider the interdependent relationship of these agents:

1. **Parathyroid hormone.** The parathyroid glands, lying adjacent to the thyroid glands, are particularly sensitive to changes in the circulating blood

level of free ionized calcium. When this level drops, the parathyroid gland releases its hormone, which then acts in three ways to restore the normal blood calcium level: (1) stimulates intestinal mucosa to absorb more calcium, (2) withdraws more calcium rapidly from the **bone compartment,** and (3) causes kidneys to excrete more phosphate. These combined activities then restore calcium and phosphorus to their correctly balanced ratio in the blood.

2. **Vitamin D hormone.** In general, along with parathyroid hormone, vitamin D hormone controls absorption of calcium. However, still with parathyroid hormone, it also affects the deposit of calcium and phosphorus in bone tissue. Thus these two agents balance each other, with vitamin D hormone acting more to control calcium absorption and bone deposit and parathyroid acting more to control calcium withdrawal from bone and kidney excretion of its partner serum phosphorus.

A third hormonal agent, **calcitonin,** is also involved in calcium balance. Produced by special C cells in the thyroid glands, it prevents abnormal rises in serum calcium by modulating release of bone calcium. Thus its action counterbalances that of parathyroid hormone to help regulate serum calcium at normal levels in balance with bone calcium.

The overall balance relationship of the various factors involved in calcium metabolism is illustrated in the diagram in Figure 8-2.

Bone compartment
Body's total content of skeletal tissue. The bone compartment contains 99% of the body's total metabolic calcium pool.

Calcitonin
Quick-acting hormone secreted by the parathyroids in response to hypercalcemia; it acts to induce hypocalcemia.

Figure 8-2
Calcium metabolism. Note the relative distribution of calcium in the body.

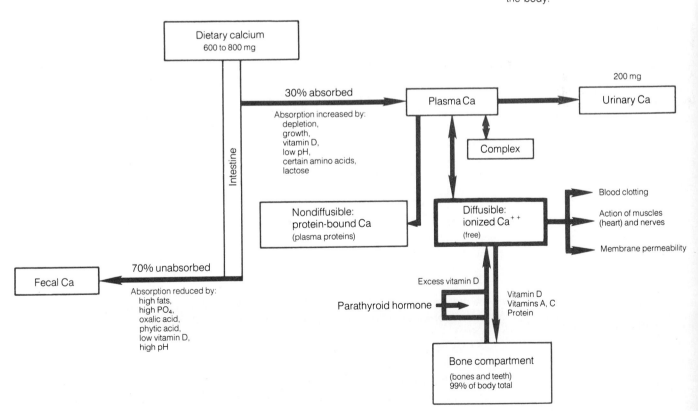

Physiologic Functions of Calcium
Bone Formation

The physiologic function of 99% of the body calcium is to build and maintain skeletal tissue. This is done by special types of cells that are in constant balance between depositing and withdrawing bone calcium.

Tooth Formation

Special tooth-forming organs in the gums deposit calcium to form teeth. The mineral exchange continues as in bone. This exchange in dental tissue occurs mainly in the dentin and cementum. Very little deposit occurs in the enamel once the tooth is formed.

General Metabolic Functions

The remaining 1% of the body's calcium performs a number of vital physiologic functions:

1. **Blood clotting.** In the blood clotting process, serum calcium ions are required for cross-linking of fibrin, giving stability to the fibrin threads.
2. **Nerve transmission.** Normal transmission of nerve impulses along axons requires calcium. A current of calcium ions triggers the flow of signals from one nerve cell to another and on to the waiting target muscles.
3. **Muscle contraction and relaxation.** Ionized serum calcium helps initiate contraction of muscle fibers and control of contraction following. This catalyzing action of calcium ions on the muscle protein filaments allows the sliding contraction between them to occur (see Chapter 14). This action of calcium is particularly vital in the constant contraction-relaxation cycle of the heart muscle.
4. **Cell membrane permeability.** Ionized calcium controls the passage of fluids and solutes through cell membranes by affecting membrane permeability. It influences the integrity of the intercellular cement substance.
5. **Enzyme activation.** Calcium ions are important activators of specific cell enzymes, especially ones that release energy for muscle contraction. They play a similar role with other enzymes, including lipase, which digests fat, and with some members of the protein-splitting enzyme system.

Clinical Problems

A number of clinical problems may develop from imbalances that interfere with the various physiologic and metabolic functions of calcium.

Tetany

Tetany
Disorder caused by abnormal calcium metabolism.

A decrease in ionized serum calcium causes **tetany,** a state marked by severe, intermittent spastic contractions of the muscle and by muscular pain.

Rickets

A deficiency of vitamin D hormone causes *rickets.* When there is inadequate exposure to sunlight or deficient dietary intake of the vitamin precursor, proper bone formation cannot take place.

Osteoporosis

The usual form of **osteoporosis,** which is characterized by bone mineral loss, occurs mainly in older persons, especially in postmenopausal women. In women affected the most rapid rate of loss occurs in the first 5 years after menopause. There is a negative calcium balance of about 40 to 120 mg/day, indicating loss from both the outer bone layer—*cortex*—and the small developing needle-like projections of bone—*trabecula* (L. *trabs,* "little beam")—into the central marrow forming the calcium anchoring network of bone matrix. Afterward the rate of bone loss is about 1% a year.[4] The cause is not entirely clear. In most patients it is not corrected by increased calcium alone but is often improved by exercise coupled with supplements. Current approaches to stimulate new bone growth involve hormonal therapy with both vitamin D hormone and estrogen.[5,6] An idiopathic osteoporosis occurring in young adults does not respond to calcium therapy.

Osteoporosis
Abnormal thinning of bone tissue caused by calcium loss.

Resorptive Hypercalciuria and Renal Calculi

Two conditions can tilt the usually fine-tuned calcium deposition-mobilization balance maintained by the controlling hormones. When this normal balance is disturbed, resorption of calcium from bone and subsequent increased urinary calcium excretion occurs. One condition that causes this imbalance is prolonged immobilization from a full body cast after orthopedic surgery, spinal cord injury, or back injury. In such cases, normal muscle tension on bones that is necessary for calcium balance is lessened, and the risk of renal stones from increased urinary calcium is increased. A second example is the hypercalciuria observed in astronauts, a problem that may pose a barrier to their prolonged space flights of the future.

Calcium Requirement
RDA Standard

To meet these varied body functions of calcium, the RDA standard for adults is set at 800 mg/day, with increases to 1200 mg/day for women during pregnancy and lactation. The recommendation for infants is 400 to 600 mg and for children, 800 to 1200 mg.

Older Adults

There is growing evidence that recommended amounts of calcium for older adults are insufficient. Actually, a wide variance exists among individuals in the efficiency of calcium absorption, and some studies indicate that as much as 1500 mg/day may be needed by some middle-aged and older adults.[7] Clinicians and investigators no longer accept the former general assumptions that calcium absorption easily adapts to lower calcium intakes of older adults and that the issue of optimum intake and bioavailability is of little concern in these persons. A majority of studies have found calcium supplementation for postmenopausal women to delay or treat osteoporosis to be beneficial.[8]

Calcium supplements should be monitored carefully. The ground dolomite popular in health food circles has been found to contain lead, mercury, arsenic, and aluminum. Elevated concentrations of these metals have been found in the hair of neurologic patients who had been taking large amounts of dolomite.

Food Sources of Calcium

Dairy products provide the bulk of dietary calcium. For example, 1 qt milk or about 4 oz brick-type cheese contains about 1 g calcium. Other nondairy sources, including eggs, green leafy vegetables, broccoli, legumes, nuts, and whole grains, contribute smaller amounts.

Phosphorus

Phosphorus makes up about 1% of total body weight. It is closely associated with calcium in human nutrition and has been called its "metabolic twin." However, it has some unique characteristics and functions of its own.

Absorption-Excretion Balance

Absorption

In the typical feedback mechanism of hormone action, when the serum phosphate level is low, the kidney is stimulated to produce vitamin D hormone, which in turn increases phosphorus absorption from the intestine.

The same factors that control calcium absorption also regulate phosphorus. Free phosphate is absorbed in the jejunum of the small intestine in relation to calcium and is also regulated by active vitamin D hormone although the hormonal effect is greater on calcium absorption than on phosphorus.[9] Equal amounts of calcium and phosphorus should exist in the diet in an optimal ratio. Since phosphate occurs in food as a phosphate compound, mainly with calcium, the first step for its absorption is its splitting off as the free mineral. Factors similar to those that influence calcium absorption also affect phosphorus absorption. For example, an excess of calcium or other binding material, such as aluminum or iron, inhibits phosphorus absorption.

Excretion

Renal threshold for phosphate means that the amount of phosphate excreted by the kidney is relative to the serum phosphorus level.

The kidneys provide the main excretion route for regulation of the serum phosphorus level. Usually, 85% to 95% of plasma phosphate is filtered at the renal glomeruli and largely reabsorbed at the tubules, along with calcium, under the influence of vitamin D hormone. But when increased phosphate excretion is needed to maintain the normal serum Ca:P ratio, parathyroid hormone acts to override the effect of vitamin D hormone. The amount of phosphorus excreted in the urine of a person ingesting an average diet is 0.6 to 1.8 g/day.

Bone-Blood-Cell Balance

Bone

From 80% to 90% of the body's phosphorus is in the skeleton, including the teeth, compounded with calcium. This bone compartment of phosphorus is in constant interchange with the rest of the body's phosphorus, which is circulating in the blood and other body fluids.

Blood

The serum phosphorus level normally ranges from 3 to 4.5 mg/dL in adults and somewhat higher, 4 to 7 mg/dL, in children. The higher range in growth years is a significant clue to its role in cell metabolism.

Cells

In its active phosphate form phosphorus plays a major role in the structure and function of all living cells. Here it works with proteins, lipids, and carbohydrates to produce energy, build and repair tissues, and to act as a buffer.

Hormonal Controls

Since calcium and phosphorus work closely together, phosphorus balance is under the direct control of the same two hormones controlling calcium—vitamin D hormone and parathyroid hormone. A deficiency or depletion of phosphate occurs from dietary lack, diminished absorption from the intestine, or excessive wasting through the kidney.

Physiologic Functions of Phosphorus
Bone and Tooth Formation

From 80% to 90% of the body phosphorus helps make bones and teeth. As a component of calcium phosphate, it is constantly being deposited and reabsorbed in the process of bone formation.

General Metabolic Activities

Far out of proportion to the relatively small remaining amount, the rest of the phosphorus is intimately involved in overall human metabolism in every living cell. It has several vital roles:

1. **Absorption of glucose and glycerol.** Phosphorus combines with glucose and glycerol to assist in their intestinal absorption. It also promotes renal tubular reabsorption of glucose to return this sugar to the blood.
2. **Transport of fatty acids.** Phospholipids provide a form of fat transport.
3. **Energy metabolism.** Phosphorus-containing compounds, for example, adenosine triphosphate (ATP), are key cell substances in energy metabolism.
4. **Buffer system.** The phosphate buffer system of phosphoric acid and phosphate helps control acid-base balance in the blood.

Physiologic Changes

Situations involving physiologic and clinical changes in serum phosphorus level include the following:

1. **Recovery from diabetic acidosis.** Active carbohydrate absorption and metabolism use much phosphorus, depositing it with glycogen and causing temporary hypophosphatemia.
2. **Growth.** Growing children usually have higher serum phosphate levels, resulting from high levels of growth hormone.
3. **Hypophosphatemia.** Low serum phosphorus levels occur in intestinal diseases such as sprue and celiac disease, which hinder absorption; in bone disease such as rickets or osteomalacia, which upset the calcium/phosphorus serum ratio; and in primary hyperparathyroidism, in which the excess secretion of parathyroid hormone causes excess renal tubular excretion of phosphorus. Symptoms of hypophosphatemia include muscle weakness, because the cells are deprived of phosphorus essential for energy metabolism.
4. **Hyperphosphatemia.** Both renal insufficiency or hypoparathyroidism cause excess accumulation of serum phosphate. As a result, the calcium side of the serum calcium to phosphorus ratio is low, causing tetany.

Phosphorus Requirement
Dietary Ratio

During growth, pregnancy, and lactation, the ratio of dietary phosphorus to calcium should ideally be 1:1. In ordinary adult life the intake of phosphorus is about 1.5 times that of calcium. In general, since these two minerals are found in the same food sources, if calcium needs are met, adequate phosphorus will be ensured.

RDA Standard

The RDA standard for phosphorus is the same as that of calcium for all ages—800 to 1200 mg—except for the young infant, for whom the proportion of phosphorus is lower than that for calcium—300 to 500 mg.

Food Sources of Phosphorus

Milk and milk products are the most significant sources of phosphorus as they are for calcium. However, because phosphorus plays such a large role in cell metabolism, it is also found in lean meats. There is a growing concern that we may be getting an excess of phosphorus in our diet because of its increasing use in processed foods and especially in soft drinks.

Sodium

Sodium is one of the most plentiful minerals in the body. About 120 mg (4 oz) is in the body of an adult, with one third in the skeleton as inorganic bound material. The remaining two thirds is free ionized sodium, the major electrolyte in body fluids outside the cells.

Absorption-Excretion Balance
Absorption

Sodium intake is readily absorbed from the intestine; normally only about 5% remains for elimination in the feces. Larger amounts are lost in abnormal states such as diarrhea.

Excretion

The major route of excretion is through the kidney, under the powerful hormonal control of **aldosterone,** the sodium-conserving hormone from the adrenal glands.

Aldosterone
Potent hormone secreted by the cortex of the adrenal glands, which acts on the distal renal tubule to cause reabsorption of sodium in an ion exchange with potassium.

Physiologic Functions of Sodium
Water Balance

Ionized sodium is the major guardian of body water outside of cells. Variations in its body fluid concentrations largely determine the distribution of water by **osmosis** from one body area to another.

Osmosis
Passage of a solvent such as water through a membrane that separates solutions of different concentrations. The water passes through the membrane from the area of lower concentration of solute to the area of higher concentration, which tends to equalize the concentrations of the two solutions.

Acid-Base Balance

In association with chloride and bicarbonate ions, ionized sodium helps regulate acid-base balance.

Cell Permeability

The sodium pump in all cell membranes helps exchange sodium and potassium and other cellular materials. A major substance carried into cells by this active transport system is glucose.

Muscle Action

Sodium ions play a large part in transmitting electrochemical impulses along nerve and muscle membranes and help maintain normal muscle action. Potassium and sodium ions balance the response of nerves to stimulation, the travel of nerve impulses to muscles, and the resulting contraction of the muscle fibers.

Sodium Requirement
RDA Standard

The body can function on a rather wide range of dietary sodium by mechanisms designed to conserve or excrete the mineral. Thus there is no specific stated requirement. The estimated adequate daily intake for adults is 1100 to 3300 mg.

General Dietary Intake

Sodium in the average American diet far exceeds the RDA estimate of adequate intake. About 4 g sodium is in the average 10 g of table salt consumed daily. A wiser adult intake of about 2 g sodium would equal about 5 g salt.

Food Sources of Sodium

The main dietary source of sodium is common salt used in cooking, seasoning, and processing of foods. Natural food sources include milk, meat, eggs, and certain vegetables such as carrots, beets, leafy greens, and celery.

Potassium is about twice as plentiful as sodium in the body. An adult body contains about 270 mg (9 oz, 4000 mEq). By far the greater portion is found inside the cells, since potassium is the major guardian of the body water inside cells. However, the relatively small amount in fluid outside cells has a significant effect on muscle activity, especially heart muscle.

Absorption-Excretion Balance

Absorption

Dietary potassium is easily absorbed in the small intestine. Potassium also circulates in the gastrointestinal secretions, being reabsorbed in the digestive process. However, diseases such as prolonged diarrhea cause dangerous losses.

Excretion

Urinary excretion is the principal route of potassium loss. Since maintenance of serum potassium within the narrow normal range is vital to heart muscle action and electrolyte balance, the kidneys guard potassium carefully. However, they cannot guard potassium as effectively as sodium. In the renal aldosterone mechanism for sodium conservation, potassium is lost in exchange for sodium. The normal obligatory loss is about 160 mg/day.

Physiologic Functions of Potassium

Water and Acid-Base Balance

As the major guardian of cell water, potassium balances with sodium outside cells to maintain normal osmotic pressures and water balance to protect cellular fluid. Potassium also works with sodium and hydrogen to maintain acid-base balance.

Muscle Activity

Potassium plays a significant role in the activity of skeletal and cardiac muscle. Together with sodium and calcium, potassium regulates neuromuscular stimulation, transmission of electrochemical impulses, and contraction of muscle fibers. This effect is particularly notable in the action of the *heart muscle*. Even small variations in serum potassium concentration are reflected in electrocardiographic (ECG) changes. Variations in serum levels or low serum potassium may cause muscle irritability and paralysis. The heart may even develop a gallop rhythm and finally cardiac arrest.

Carbohydrate Metabolism

When blood glucose is converted to glycogen for storage, 0.36 mmol of potassium is stored for each 1 g glycogen. When a patient in diabetic acidosis is

Potassium

Continuous use of some *diuretic drugs* (though not all) increases potassium loss, requiring adequate replacement, primarily in food sources. Heart failure and subsequent depletion of ionized potassium in heart muscle make the myocardial tissue more sensitive to *digitalis toxicity* and *arrhythmia,* or irregular contractions. Recent studies indicate that inadequate intake of potassium contributes to the development of essential hypertension whereas a high potassium intake may lower blood pressure, probably because potassium antagonizes the biologic effects of sodium.

treated with insulin and glucose, rapid glycogen production draws potassium from the serum. Serious hypokalemia can result unless adequate potassium replacement accompanies treatment.

Protein Synthesis

Potassium is required for the storage of nitrogen in muscle protein and general cell protein. When tissue is broken down, potassium is lost together with the nitrogen. Amino acid replacement includes potassium to ensure nitrogen retention.

Potassium Requirement

No specific dietary requirement is given for potassium. The RDA standard estimates a minimum daily intake for healthy adults of 2000 mg. The usual diet contains from 2000 to 4000 mg/day, which is ample for common need.

Food Sources of Potassium

Potassium is widely distributed in natural foods. Legumes, whole grains, fruits such as oranges and bananas, leafy green vegetables, broccoli, potatoes, and meats supply considerable amounts. Most other foods are supplementary sources.

Other Major Minerals

Three additional minerals are assigned to the major minerals group because of the extent of their occurrence in the body. These are magnesium, chloride, and sulfur.

Magnesium

Magnesium has widespread metabolic functions and is present in all body cells. An adult body contains about 25 g of magnesium or a little less than an ounce. About 70% of this small but vital amount is combined with calcium and phosphorus in the bone. The remaining 30% is distributed in various tissues and body fluids, where it has widespread metabolic use in all cells as a control agent. It acts as an enzyme activator for energy production and building tissue protein. It also aids in normal muscle action. The RDA standard is 350 mg/day for men and 280 mg for women. Magnesium is relatively widespread in nature. Its main food sources are nuts, soybeans, cocoa, seafood, whole grains, and dried beans and peas.

Chlorine (chloride)

Chloride accounts for about 3% of the body's total mineral content, mainly as part of fluid outside of cells, where it helps control water and acid-base balances. Spinal fluid has the highest concentration. A relatively large amount of ionized chloride is found in gastrointestinal secretions, especially gastric hydrochloric acid (HCl). An estimated need for healthy adults is 700 mg/day.

Sulfur

Sulfur is present in all body cells, usually as a constituent of cell protein. Elemental sulfur occurs in sulfate compounds with sodium, potassium, and magnesium. Organic forms occur mainly with other protein compounds: (1) sulfur-containing amino acids, such as methionine and cystine; (2) glycoproteins in cartilage, tendons, and bone matrix; (3) detoxification products

Decreased serum potassium of a dangerous degree may be caused by prolonged wasting disease with tissue destruction and malnutrition. This condition may also result from prolonged gastrointestinal loss of potassium such as occurs in diarrhea, vomiting, or gastric suction.

formed in part by bacterial activity in the intestine; (4) other organic compounds such as heparin, insulin, coenzyme A, lipoic acid, thiamin, and biotin; and (5) keratin in hair and nails.

The major minerals are summarized in Table 8-2 for review.

Table 8-2

Summary of Major Minerals (required intake over 100 mg/day)

Mineral	Metabolism	Physiologic functions	Clinical applications	Requirement/day	Food sources
Calcium (Ca)	Absorption according to body need; requires Ca-binding protein and regulated by vitamin D, parathyroid hormone, and calcitonin; absorption favored by protein, lactose, acidity Excretion chiefly in feces: 70%-90% of amount ingested Deposition-mobilization in bone tissue constant, regulated by vitamin D and parathyroid hormone	Constituent of bones and teeth Participates in blood clotting, nerve transmission, muscle action, cell membrane permeability, enzyme activation	Tetany (decrease in serum Ca) Rickets, osteomalacia Osteoporosis Resorptive hypercalcinuria, renal calculi Hyperthyroidism and hypothyroidism	Adults: 800 mg Pregnancy and lactation: 1200 mg Infants: 400-600 mg Children: 800-1200 mg	Milk, cheese Green leafy vegetables Whole grains Egg yolk Legumes, nuts
Phosphorus (P)	Absorption with Ca aided by vitamin D and parathyroid hormone as above; hindered by binding agents Excretion chiefly by kidney according to serum level, regulated by parathyroid hormone Deposition-mobilization in bone compartment constant	Constituent of bones and teeth, ATP, phosphorylated intermediary metabolites Participates in absorption of glucose and glycerol, transport of fatty acids, energy metabolism, and buffer system	Growth Recovery from diabetic acidosis Hypophosphatemia: bone disease, malabsorption syndromes, primary hyperparathyroidism Hyperphosphatemia: renal insufficiency, hypothyroidism, tetany	Adults: 800 mg Pregnancy and lactation: 1200 mg Infants: 300-500 mg Children: 800-1200 mg	Milk, cheese Meat, egg yolk Whole grains Legumes, nuts

Continued.

Table 8-2
Summary of Major Minerals (required intake over 100 mg/day)—cont'd

Mineral	Metabolism	Physiologic functions	Clinical applications	Requirement/day	Food sources
Magnesium (Mg)	Absorption according to intake load; hindered by excess fat, phosphate, calcium, protein Excretion regulated by kidney	Constituent of bones and teeth Coenzyme in general metabolism, smooth muscle action, neuromuscular irritability Cation in intracellular fluid	Low serum level following gastrointestinal losses Tremor, spasm in deficiency induced by malnutrition, alcoholism	Adults: 280-350 mg Pregnancy and Lactation: 320-355 mg Infants: 40-60 mg Children: 80-400 mg	Milk, cheese Meat, seafood Whole grains Legumes, nuts
Sodium (Na)	Readily absorbed Excretion chiefly by kidney, controlled by aldosterone	Major cation in extracellular fluid, water balance, acid-base balance Cell membrane permeability, absorption of glucose Normal muscle irritability	Losses in gastrointestinal disorders, diarrhea Fluid-electrolyte and acid-base balance problems Muscle action	Adults: 500 mg Infants: 120-200 mg Children: 225-500 mg	Salt (NaCl) Sodium compounds in baking and processing Milk, cheese Meat, egg Carrots, beets, spinach, celery
Potassium (K)	Readily absorbed Secreted and reabsorbed in gastrointestinal circulation Excretion chiefly by kidney, regulated by aldosterone	Major cation in intracellular fluid, water balance, acid-base balance Normal muscle irritability Glycogen formation Protein synthesis	Losses in gastrointestinal disorders, diarrhea Fluid-electrolyte, acid-base balance problems Muscle action, especially heart action Losses in tissue catabolism Treatment of diabetic acidosis: rapid glycogen production reduces serum potassium level Losses with diuretic therapy	Adults: 2000 mg Infants: 500-700 mg Children: 1000-2000 mg	Fruits Vegetables Legumes, nuts Whole grains Meat
Chlorine (Cl)	Readily absorbed Excretion controlled by kidney	Major anion in extracellular fluid, water balance, acid-base balance, chloride-bicarbonate shift Gastric hydrochloride—digestion	Losses in gastrointestinal disorders, vomiting, diarrhea, tube drainage Hypochloremic alkalosis	Adults: 750 mg Infants: 180-300 mg Children: 350-750 mg	Salt (NaCl)

Table 8-2

Summary of Major Minerals (required intake over 100 mg/day)—cont'd

Mineral	Metabolism	Physiologic functions	Clinical applications	Requirement	Food sources
Sulfur (S)	Elemental form absorbed as such; split from amino acid sources (methionine and cystine) in digestion and absorbed into portal circulation Excreted by kidney in relation to protein intake and tissue catabolism	Essential constituent of protein structure Enzyme activity and energy metabolism through free sulfhydryl group (−SH) Detoxification reactions	Cystine renal calculi Cystinuria	Diet adequate in protein contains adequate sulfur	Meat, egg Milk, cheese Legumes, nuts

The Study of Major Elements

By the simplest definition, an essential element is one required for existence; conversely, its absence brings death. For major elements that occur in relatively large amounts in the body, as we have seen, such determinations can be made easily because the quantity present is sufficiently available for study. However, for things that occur in very small amounts, this determination of essentiality is not easy to make. For example, of the 54 known chemical elements in the major part of the periodic table, 27 have been determined to be essential to human life and function. By far most living matter as we know it is made up of five fundamental elements: hydrogen (H), carbon (C), nitrogen (N), oxygen (O), and sulfur (S). We know these elements well because their concentrations are relatively large, hence more easily studied, and their requirements for human function can be stated in multiples of grams per gram of body weight. This is a recognizable quantity with which we can be comfortable. We have means for analysis of such quantities and can easily see that these are essential elements. Also, the major minerals you have just reviewed here occur in respectable amounts in the body, so their essentiality has been more easily studied and determined.

The Study of Microelements

A much larger number of elements—microelements or trace elements—occur in biologic matter in such very small amounts that measurement and analysis are exceedingly difficult. So in many cases we know little about them and understand even less. It is much harder to determine the essentiality of these trace elements because we apparently require so little of them.[10] In general, trace elements have been defined as those having a required intake of less than 100 mg/day. Yet some of them exist in fairly large amounts in our diet and our environment.

Trace Elements: The Concept of Essentiality

Essential Function

Despite difficulties in determining the essentiality of these very small amounts of trace elements in our bodies, studies have indicated that essentiality can be determined on the basis of function and effect of deficiency.

Basic functions of trace elements. An element is essential when a deficiency causes an impairment of function and supplementation with that substance, but not with others, prevents or cures this impairment. Studies in this field have identified the two basic functions of trace elements in terms of *catalytic* and *structural* components of larger molecules.

Deficiency and requirement. Because these small amounts of trace elements are not easily measured, specific needs have been stated only for the following: (1) iron (Fe), because it has a long history; (2) zinc (Zn), because it occurs in higher concentration than some of the others; and (3) iodine (I), because it has only one specific known function. Thus far the RDA standard only estimates requirements for the others as a general range of need.

Essential Trace Elements: Definite and Probable

On the basis of current knowledge, these small trace elements may be classed in two groups: those that are definitely essential and those that are probably essential.

Definitely Essential Elements

Ten trace elements have been assigned essential roles in human nutrition based on defined function and need determined from research. This group includes iron (Fe), iodine (I), zinc (Zn), copper (Cu), manganese (Mn), chromium (Cr), cobalt (Co), selenium (Se), molybdenum (Mo), and fluorine (Fl).

Probably Essential Elements

All the remaining eight trace elements are probably essential, but a more complete understanding awaits the development of better means of analysis and tests for function. These elements include silicon (Si), vanadium (V), nickel (Ni), tin (Sn), cadmium (Cd), arsenic (As), aluminum (Al), and boron (B).

We will look first at iron and iodine because of their long history and clearly defined specific function. Then in turn we will briefly review the remainder. These essential elements are summarized in Table 8-3.

Iron

Forms of Iron in the Body

The human body contains only about 45 mg iron/kg body weight. This iron is distributed in four forms that point to its basic metabolic function.

Transport Iron

A trace of iron, 0.05 to 0.18 mg/dL, is in plasma bound to its transport carrier protein *transferrin*.

Hemoglobin

Most of the body's iron, about 70%, is in red blood cells as a vital constituent of the heme portion of **hemoglobin.** Another 5% is a part of the muscle hemoglobin *myoglobin*.

Hemoglobin
Protein that gives the color to red blood cells. A conjugated protein composed of an iron-containing pigment called heme and a simple protein, globin. Carries oxygen in the blood; combines with oxygen to form oxyhemoglobin.

Table 8-3

Summary of Trace Elements (required intake less than 100 mg/day)

Element	Metabolism	Physiologic functions	Clinical applications	Requirement/day	Food sources
Iron (Fe)	Absorption controls bioavailability; favored by body need, acidity, and reduction agents such as vitamins; hindered by binding agents, reduced gastric HCl, infection, gastrointestinal losses Transported as transferrin, stored as ferritin or hemosiderin Excreted in sloughed cells, bleeding	Hemoglobin synthesis, oxygen transport Cell oxidation, heme enzymes	Anemia: hypochromic, microcytic Excess: hemosiderosis, hemochromatosis Growth and pregnancy needs	Adults: men, 10 mg; women, 15 mg Pregnancy and lactation: 30 to 15 mg supplement Infants: 6-10 mg Children: 10-15 mg	Liver, meats, egg Whole grains Enriched breads and cereals Dark green vegetables Legumes, nuts (iron cookware)
Iodine (I)	Absorbed as iodides, taken up by thyroid gland under control of thyroid-stimulating hormone (TSH) Excretion by kidney	Synthesis of thyroxine, which regulates cell metabolism, BMR	Endemic colloid goiter, cretinism Hypothyroidism and hyperthyroidism	Adults: 150 μg Infants: 40-50 μg Children: 70-150 μg	Iodized salt Seafood
Zinc (Zn)	Absorbed with zinc-binding ligand (ZBL) from pancreas Transported in blood by albumin; stored in many sites Excretion largely intestinal	Essential coenzyme constituent: carbonic anhydrase, carboxypeptidase, lactic dehydrogenase	Growth: hypogonadism Sensory impairment: taste and smell Wound healing Malabsorption disease	Adults: 15 mg Infants: 3-5 mg Children: 10-15 mg	Widely distributed: Seafood, oysters Liver, meat Milk, cheese, egg Whole grains
Copper (Cu)	Absorbed with copper-binding protein metallothionein Transported in blood by histidine and albumin Stored in many tissues	Associated with iron in enzyme systems, hemoglobin synthesis Metalloprotein enzymes constituent	Hypocupremia: nephrosis and malabsorption Wilson's disease, excess copper storage	Adults: 1.5-3.0 mg Infants: 0.4-0.7 mg Children: 1-5 mg	Widely distributed: Liver, meat Seafood Whole grains Legumes, nuts (Copper cookware)

Continued.

Table 8-3

Summary of Trace Elements (required intake less than 100 mg/day)—cont'd

Element	Metabolism	Physiologic functions	Clinical applications	Requirement/day	Food sources
Manganese (Mn)	Absorbed poorly Excretion mainly by intestine	Enzyme component in general metabolism	Low serum levels in diabetes, protein-energy malnutrition Inhalation toxicity	Adults: 2.0-5.0 mg Infants: 0.03-1.0 mg Children: 1-5 mg	Cereals, whole grains Legumes, soybeans Leafy vegetables
Chromium (Cr)	Absorbed in association with zinc Excretion mainly by kidney	Associated with glucose metabolism; improves faulty glucose uptake by tissues; glucose tolerance factor	Potentiates action of insulin in persons with diabetes Lowers serum cholesterol, LDL-cholesterol Increases HDL	Adults: 50-200 μg Infants: 10-60 μg Children: 20-200μg	Cereals Whole grains Brewer's yeast Animal proteins
Cobalt (Co)	Absorbed as component of food source, vitamin B_{12} Elemental form shares transport with iron Stored in liver	Constituent of vitamin B_{12}, functions with vitamin	Deficiency only associated with deficiency of B_{12}	Unknown; evidently minute	Vitamin B_{12} source
Selenium (Se)	Absorption depends on solubility of compound form Excreted mainly by kidney	Constituent of enzyme glutathione perioxidase Synergistic antioxidant with vitamin E Structural component of teeth	Marginal deficiency when soil content is low Deficiency secondary to parenteral nutrition (TPN), malnutrition Toxicity observed in livestock	Adults: 55-70 μg Infants: 10-15 μg Children: 20-50 μg	Varies with soil Seafood Legumes Whole grains Low-fat meats and dairy products Vegetables
Molybdenum (Mo)	Readily absorbed Excreted rapidly by kidney Small amount excreted in bile	Constituent of oxidase enzymes, xanthine oxidase	Deficiency unknown in humans	Adults: 75-250 μg Infants: 15-40 μg Children: 25-250 μg	Legumes Whole grains Milk Organ meats Leafy vegetables
Fluorine (Fl)	Absorption in small intestine; little known of bioavailability Excreted by kidney—80%	Accumulates in bones and teeth, increasing hardness	Dental caries inhibited Osteoporosis: may help control Excess: dental fluorosis	Adults: 1.5-4.0 mg Infants: 0.1-1.0 mg Children: 0.5-2.5 mg	Fish Fish products Tea Foods cooked in fluoridated water Drinking water

Storage Iron

About 20% of the body iron is stored as the protein-iron compound **ferritin,** mainly in liver, spleen, and bone marrow. Excess iron is stored in the body as *hemosiderin.*

Cellular Tissue Iron

The remaining 5% of body iron is distributed throughout all cells as a major component of oxidative enzyme systems for the production of energy.

Absorption-Transport-Storage-Excretion Balance

In the body, iron follows a unique system of interrelated absorption-transport-storage-excretion. Optimal levels of body iron are not maintained by urinary excretion as is the case with most plasma constituents. Rather, the mechanisms of iron control lie in the absorption-transport-storage complex.

Absorption

The main control of the body's iron balance is at the point of intestinal absorption. Dietary iron enters the body in two forms: **heme** and **nonheme** (Table 8-4). By far the larger portion is nonheme—all plant sources plus 60% of animal sources. But it is absorbed at a much slower rate than the smaller heme portion, because nonheme iron is tightly bound in its food sources to organic molecules in the form of ferric iron (Fe^{+++}). In the acidic medium of the stomach, it must be disassociated and reduced to the more soluble ferrous iron (Fe^{++}).[11] This is a source of nutritional concern because of nonheme's greater quantity in the diet. A protein receptor in the intestinal mucosal cells, **apoferritin,** then receives iron to form ferritin. The amount of ferritin already present in the intestinal mucosa determines the amount of ingested iron that is absorbed or rejected. When all available apoferritin has been bound to iron to form ferritin, any additional iron that arrives at the binding site is rejected, returned to the lumen of the intestine, and passed on for excretion in the feces. Only 10% to 30% of the ingested iron is absorbed, mostly in the duodenum. The remaining 70% to 90% is eliminated.

Factors Favoring Absorption

The following factors favor absorption:
1. **Body need.** In deficiency states or in periods of extra demand as in growth or pregnancy, mucosal ferritin is lower and more iron is absorbed. When tissue reserves are ample or saturated, iron is rejected and excreted.
2. **Acidity and reduction agents.** Vitamin C (ascorbic acid) aids iron ab-

Ferritin
Protein-iron compound in which iron is stored in the tissues; the storage form of iron in the body.

Heme
Iron-containing, nonprotein portion of hemoglobin.

Nonheme
Protein portion of hemoglobin that does not contain the heme.

Apoferritin
Protein base found in intestinal mucosa cells, which will bind with ion (from food) to form ferritin, the storage form of iron.

Table 8-4

Characteristics of Heme and Nonheme Portions of Dietary Iron

	Dietary iron	
	Heme smallest portion	Nonheme largest portion
Food sources	None in plant sources; 40% of iron in animal sources	All iron in plant sources; 60% of iron in animal sources
Absorption rate	Rapid; transported and absorbed intact	Slow; tightly bound in organic molecules

sorption by its reducing action and effect on acidity. Other agents have similar effects, as does the gastric hydrochloric acid, which provides the optimal acid medium for the preparation of iron for utilization.

3. **Calcium.** An adequate amount of calcium helps bind and remove agents such as phosphate and phytate, which would combine with iron and prevent its absorption.

Factors Hindering Absorption

The following factors hinder absorption:

1. **Binding agents.** Materials such as phosphate, phytate, and oxalate bind iron and remove it from the body. Tea and coffee inhibit nonheme iron absorption.
2. **Reduced gastric acid secretion.** Surgical removal of stomach tissue (gastrectomy) reduces the number of cells that secrete hydrochloric acid, thus reducing the necessary acid medium for iron reduction.
3. **Infection.** Severe infection hinders iron absorption.
4. **Gastrointestinal disease.** Malabsorption or any disturbance that causes diarrhea will hinder iron absorption.

Thus the bioavailability of iron essentially depends on its absorption, which in turn depends on a number of influencing factors in the body. This is both a unique and precarious arrangement.

Transport

In the mucosal cells of the duodenum and proximal jejunum, iron is oxidized and bound with the plasma *transferrin* for transport to body cells. Normally, only about 20% to 35% of the iron-binding capacity of transferrin is filled. The remaining capacity forms an unsaturated plasma reserve for handling variances in iron intake.

Storage

Hemosiderin
Insoluble iron oxide−protein compound in which iron is stored in the liver when the amount of iron in the blood exceeds the storage capacity of ferritin, e.g., during rapid destruction of red blood cells (malaria, hemolytic anemia).

Hemosiderosis
Condition in which large amounts of hemosiderin are deposited, especially in the liver and spleen. Occurs with the excessive breakdown of red blood cells, as in malaria and hemolytic anemia, or after multiple blood transfusions.

Bound to plasma transferrin, iron is delivered to its storage sites in bone marrow and to some extent in the liver. Here it is transferred to the storage form, ferritin, and drawn on as needed for hemoglobin in red blood cells and for general tissue metabolism. A secondary, less soluble storage compound, **hemosiderin,** is used as reserve storage in the liver; excess storage causes the condition **hemosiderosis.** From these storage compounds, iron is mobilized for hemoglobin synthesis as needed, from 20 to 25 mg/day in an adult. The body avidly conserves the iron in hemoglobin, recycling the iron when red cells are destroyed after their average life span of about 120 days. These interrelationships of body iron absorption-transport-storage mechanisms are diagrammed in Figure 8-3 for review.

Excretion

Since the main mechanism controlling iron levels in the body occurs at the point of absorption, only minute amounts are lost by renal excretion. Essentially none is in the urine, as is the case with other circulating minerals. Rather, the small amounts of iron excreted normally come from the sloughing off of skin tissue, gastrointestinal cells, and normal gastrointestinal and menstrual blood loss. Unusual blood loss such as that from heavy menstrual flow, childbirth, surgery, acute and chronic hemorrhage, gastrointestinal disease, or parasitic infestation may bring severe iron loss.[12]

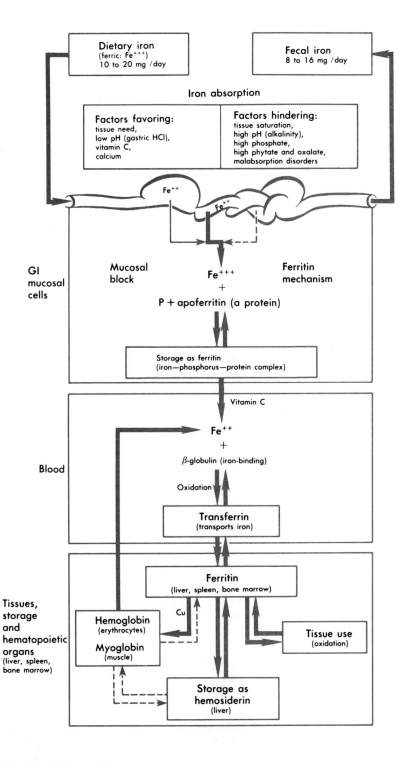

Figure 8-3
Summary of iron metabolism, showing its absorption, transport, main use in hemoglobin formation, and its storage forms (ferritin and hemosiderin).

Physiologic Functions of Iron
Oxygen Transport

Iron is the core of the *heme* molecule, the fundamental nonprotein part of hemoglobin in the red blood cells. As such, iron functions as a major transport of vital oxygen to the cells for respiration and metabolism.

Cellular Oxidation

Although iron exists in smaller amounts in cells, it also functions there as a vital component of enzyme systems for oxidation of glucose to produce energy.

Growth Needs and Clinical Problems
Normal Life Cycle

During rapid growth, positive iron balance is imperative. At birth, the infant has about a 4- to 6-month supply of iron stored in the liver during fetal development. Breast-fed infants obtain iron in breast milk. However, since cow's milk does not supply iron, it is added to commercial formulas. Supplementary iron-rich and fortified foods are added to the diet at about 4 to 6 months of age. Iron is also needed for continued growth and building of reserves for the physiologic stress of adolescence, especially the onset of menses in girls. The woman's need for iron is increased markedly during pregnancy, and normal blood loss during delivery reduces iron stores further.

Anemias

Iron deficiency occurs in both developed and underdeveloped countries. The small dietary supply may not be readily absorbed and there may be sources of potential loss. Iron deficiency results in a hypochromic microcytic **anemia.** This deficiency may result from several causes:

1. **Nutritional anemia.** An inadequate dietary supply of iron and other nutrients needed for hemoglobin and red blood cell production.
2. **Hemorrhagic anemia.** Excessive blood iron loss.
3. **Postgastrectomy anemia.** Lack of gastric hydrochloric acid necessary to liberate iron for absorption.
4. **Malabsorption anemia.** The presence of iron-binding agents that prevent its absorption or mucosal lesions that affect the absorbing surface.

Iron Requirement

The RDA standard is 10 mg/day for men, and a larger amount—15 mg/day—for women during the childbearing years. This larger amount is needed to cover menstrual losses. During pregnancy, an added 15 mg is needed. Individual iron needs vary with age and situation, and growth allowances for infants and children are designed to provide margins for safety.

Food Sources of Iron

By far the best sources of iron are organ meats, especially liver. Other food sources include meats, seafood, egg yolk, whole or enriched grains, legumes, green leafy vegetables, and nuts.

Iodine

Anemia
Blood condition characterized by decrease in number of circulating red blood cells, hemoglobin, or both.

The body of the average adult contains a small amount of the trace element iodine, from 20 to 50 mg. Approximately 50% of this is in the muscles, 20% in the thyroid glands, 10% in the skin, and 6% in the skeleton. The remaining 14% is scattered in other endocrine tissue, in the central nervous system, and in plasma transport. By far, the greatest iodine tissue concentration is in the thyroid glands, where its one function is to participate in the synthesis of the thyroid hormone *thyroxine*.

Absorption-Excretion Balance
Absorption

Dietary iodine is absorbed in the small intestine in the form of iodides. These are loosely bound with proteins and carried by the blood to the thyroid gland. About one third of this iodide is selectively absorbed by the thyroid cells and removed from circulation.

Excretion

The remaining two thirds of the iodide is usually excreted in the urine within 2 to 3 days after ingestion.

Hormonal Control

A pituitary hormone, *thyroid-stimulating hormone (TSH)*, stimulates the uptake of iodine by the thyroid cells in direct feedback response to the plasma levels of the hormone. This normal physiologic **feedback mechanism** maintains a healthy balance between supply and demand.

Physiologic Function of Iodine
Thyroid Hormone Synthesis

Iodine participates in the synthesis of thyroid hormone as its only known function in human metabolism. The hormone, thyroxine, in turn stimulates cell oxidation and regulates basal metabolic rate (BMR), apparently by increasing oxygen uptake and reaction rates of enzyme systems handling glucose. In this role iodine indirectly exerts a tremendous influence on the body's total metabolism.

Plasma Thyroxine

The free thyroxine is secreted into the blood stream and bound to plasma protein for transport to body cells as needed. After being used to stimulate oxidation in the cell, the hormone is degraded in the liver and the iodine is excreted in bile as inorganic iodine.

Clinical Needs
Abnormal Thyroid Function

Both hyperthyroidism and hypothyroidism affect the rate of iodine uptake and use, and subsequently influence the body's overall metabolic rate.

Goiter

Endemic colloid **goiter,** characterized by great enlargement of the thyroid gland, occurs in persons living where water and soil and thus locally grown foods contain little iodine. When iodine intake is insufficient, the gland cannot produce a normal quantity of thyroxine, and the blood level of the hormone remains low. As a result, the pituitary continues to put out TSH. The only response the iodine-starved thyroid gland can make is to increase the amount of colloid tissue of which it is composed, and the gland becomes increasingly engorged. It may attain a tremendous size, weighing 500 to 700 g (1 to 1.5 lb) or more (Figure 8-4). Unusual "goiter zones" have been reported in various parts of the world where, despite iodine supplementation, large numbers of persons have developed goiter as a result of contamination of the drinking water with goiter-producing chemicals such as resorcinol and phthalate esters, or from a water supply that carried an excessive amount of

Feedback mechanism
Mechanism that regulates production and secretion by an endocrine gland (A_g) of its hormone (A_h), which stimulates another endocrine gland (T_g— the *target gland*) to produce its hormone (T_h). As sufficient T_h is produced, blood levels of T_h signal A_g to stop secreting A_h.

Goiter
Enlargement of the thyroid gland caused by lack of sufficient available iodine to produce the thyroid hormone, thyroxine.

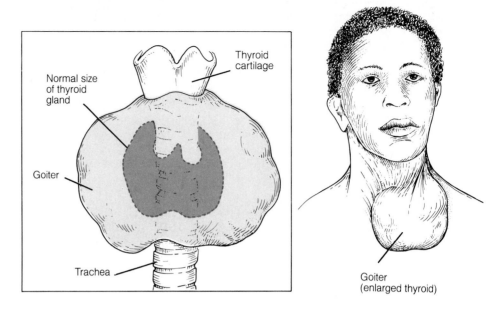

iodine. For example, endemic "iodine goiter" has been found on populations having excessive iodine in their drinking water in areas near oil fields or environmental iodine sources.

Iodine Overload

Increased incidental intake of iodine may also cause problems. Most of this excess comes through dairy products from such sources as iodized salt licks for the animals, and *iodophors,* iodine-containing chemicals used to sanitize udders, milking machines, and milk tanks. Other iodine-containing food additives are *iodates* used as dough conditioners in breads, *erythrosine* used as a coloring agent, and iodine supplements added to animal feeds. Various reports, including those of the FDA, indicate that levels of iodine in American diets usually exceed by many times the dietary recommendation. More is added by individual overuse of salt, iodized salt, both in seasoning and large use of processed foods. Excess iodine may result first in acne-like skin lesions or may worsen preexisting acne of adolescents or young adults. The "iodine goiter" from excessive iodine could be misdiagnosed as regular goiter caused by insufficient iodine.

Iodine Requirement

The RDA standard is 150 μg/day for adults. These needs normally increase during periods of accelerated growth such as adolescence and pregnancy and decrease in older adulthood.

Food Sources of Iodine

Seafood provides a considerable amount of iodine. The quantity in natural sources varies widely depending on the iodine content of the soil and the iodine compounds used in food processing. The commercial iodizing of table salt (1 mg to every 10 g salt) provides a main dietary source.

Other Essential Trace Elements

Zinc

Zinc has come to nutritional prominence as an essential trace element with wide clinical significance. But much is still to be learned about the details of its metabolism. Its wide tissue distribution reflects its broad metabolic activity as a component of key cell enzymes. It occurs in many tissues including pancreas, liver, kidney, lung, muscle, bone, eye (cornea, iris, retina, lens), endocrine glands, prostate secretions, and spermatozoa.

Clinical Problems

Because of its widespread metabolic use, a number of clinical problems caused by zinc deficiency (see the box on p. 178) can occur:

1. **Hypogonadism.** Diminished function of the gonads and dwarfism result from marked human zinc deficiency during critical growth periods.
2. **Taste and smell defects.** *Hypogeusia* (diminished taste) and *hyposmia* (diminished smell) in a number of clinical situations are improved with zinc supplementation.
3. **Wound healing.** Such defects occur in zinc-deficient persons, an effect common in long-term hospitalization. Patients in such situations may benefit from zinc supplementation.
4. **Chronic illness in aging.** Older patients with poor appetites who subsist on marginal diets in the face of unhealed wounds and debilitating illness may also need zinc supplementation.
5. **Malabsorption disease.** Zinc deficiency can occur with malabsorption diseases such as Crohn's disease.

Zinc Requirement and Food Sources

As with the trace element iron, an optimal intake of zinc in the U.S. population cannot be assumed. The adult standard is 12 to 15 mg/day with 10 to 15 mg for children and 5 mg for infants. The best sources of dietary zinc are seafood (especially oysters), meat, and eggs. Additional less rich sources are legumes and whole grains. Since animal food sources supply the major portion of dietary zinc, pure vegetarians, especially women, may be at risk for development of marginal zinc deficiency.

Copper

This trace element has frequently been called the "iron twin." The two elements are metabolized in much the same way and share functions as cell enzyme components. Both are related to energy production and hemoglobin synthesis. The average American diet, previously thought to provide about 2 to 4 mg of copper each day, is now known to contain only 1 to 2 mg, which is less than sufficient for adults. It is widely distributed in natural foods, so a serious dietary deficiency is rare. Its main food sources include meat, shellfish, nuts, seeds, legumes, and whole grains.

Manganese

The total adult body content of manganese is about 20 mg, occurring mainly in the liver, bones, pancreas, and pituitary. It functions like other trace elements as an essential part of cell enzymes that catalyze a number of important metabolic reactions. Manganese deficiency, evidenced by low serum levels, has been reported in diabetes and pancreatic insufficiency, as well as in protein-energy malnutrition states such as *kwashiorkor*. Toxicity occurs as an industrial disease syndrome, *inhalation toxicity,* in miners and other workers who have prolonged exposure to manganese dust. In such cases, excess manganese accumulates in the liver and central nervous system, producing se-

To Probe Further

Zinc Barriers

Are people eating more zinc but absorbing it less? Current trends toward a "heart-healthy" diet may be one of the reasons. Some Americans may be at risk for developing a zinc deficiency, not because they are avoiding zinc-rich foods, but because they are choosing foods and supplements that reduce its availability for absorption. For example:

- Animal foods, rich in readily available zinc, are consumed less by an increasingly cholesterol-conscious public.
- Fiber, being promoted by some persons as a cardiovascular panacea, may create a negative zinc balance.
- Phytate, a component of fiber-rich foods, is another zinc antagonist, although its effect on zinc absorption is controversial.
- Vitamin-mineral supplements may contain iron-to-zinc ratios greater than 3:1 and provide enough iron to inhibit zinc absorption.

Other factors that reduce zinc availability include such unusual cravings as pica, for example, *geophagia,* a clay- or earth-eating habit practiced primarily in the southeastern United States, especially among children and pregnant women. Also, such clinical conditions as cystic fibrosis, alcohol cirrhosis, celiac disease, and diarrhea limit zinc absorption.

The risk for deficiency is greatest among pregnant and breast-feeding women. Low levels can reduce the amount of protein available to carry iron and vitamin A to the target tissues and reduce the mother's appetite and taste for foods. As a result, the fetus is at even greater risk for inadequate growth and development.

All these conditions, plus milling processes that remove excessive amounts of zinc from grains, have resulted in an average per capita intake of 12.5 mg/day. This is less than the 15 mg/day recommended for most persons, and less than the 15 to 19 mg/day recommended for pregnant and lactating women.

To put more zinc in their diets, persons may:

- Include some form of animal food—meat, milk, eggs—in the diet each day to ensure a minimal intake of zinc.
- Avoid extensive use of alcohol.
- Avoid "crash" diets.

Signs of zinc deficiency are still fairly rare in the United States but becoming more apparent among at risk persons, such as older adults with long-term chronic illness and hospitalization. There is no need, though, for the general public to overprotect themselves with massive doses. These can lead to nausea, abdominal pain, and anemia. As with all other nutrients, too much of a good thing can sometimes be bad as too little—or even worse.

REFERENCES

Lawler MR and Klevay LM: Copper and zinc in selected foods, J Am Diet Assoc 84(9):1028, 1984.

Solomans NW: Biological availability of zinc in humans, Am J Clin Nutr 35(5):1048, 1982.

Solomans NW, Helitzer-Allen DL, and Villar J: Zinc needs during pregnancy, Clin Nutr 5(2):63, 1986.

vere neuromuscular symptoms that resemble those of Parkinson's disease. The RDA adult standard for manganese is 2.0 to 5.0 mg/day, with 1.0 to 5.0 mg for children. The best food sources of manganese are plants: cereal grains, legumes, seeds, nuts, leafy vegetables, tea, and coffee. Animal foods are poor sources.

Chromium

The precise amount of chromium present in body tissues is not well defined because of difficulties in analysis. Although large geographic variations occur, the total body content is low, less than 6 mg. Highest concentrations have been found in skin, adrenal glands, brain, muscle, and fat. Serum levels are extremely low, less than 10 mg/mL. Chromium functions as an essential component of the organic complex **glucose tolerance factor (GTF),** which stimulates the action of insulin. Insulin resistance manifested by impaired glucose tolerance has responded positively to chromium supplementation by restoring normal blood sugar. Also, significant reduction of elevated serum cholesterol has been observed in some studies, but not all, of persons treated with chromium supplementation. The RDA standard estimates an adequate intake of chromium for adults at a range of 50 to 200 μg/day. Brewer's yeast is a rich source. Most grain and cereal products contain significant amounts.

Glucose tolerance factor (GTF)
Chromium compound associated with glucose and lipid metabolism and insulin activity.

Cobalt

Cobalt occurs in only minute traces in body tissues and the main storage area is the liver. As an essential component of cobalamin (B_{12}), cobalt's only known function is associated with red blood cell formation. The normal cobalt blood level, representing the trace element in transit and in red blood cells, is exceedingly small, about 1 μg/dL. Cobalt is provided in the human diet only by vitamin B_{12}. The human requirement is unknown but is evidently minute. For example, as little as 0.045 to 0.09 μg/day maintains bone marrow function in patients with pernicious anemia. Cobalt is widely distributed in nature. However, for our needs cobalt is obtained in preformed vitamin B_{12}, synthesized in animals by intestinal bacterial flora.

Selenium

Selenium is deposited in all body tissues except fat. Highest concentrations occur in liver, kidney, heart, and spleen. Serum levels are about 0.22 μg/dL. Selenium functions as an integral component of an antioxidant enzyme that protects cells and lipid membranes against oxidative damage. In this role, selenium balances with tocopherol (vitamin E), each sparing the other. This protective function is widespread, since the enzyme is found in most body tissues. Selenium also acts as a structural component, incorporated into the protein matrix of the teeth. The new RDA standard for adult intake of selenium is 55 to 70 μg/day. Food sources vary with the selenium soil content. Usually good sources include seafood, legumes, whole grains, low-fat meats and dairy products, with additional amounts in vegetables.

Molybdenum

The precise occurrence of molybdenum in human tissues and its clear role is still under investigation. The amount in animal tissue is exceedingly small,

0.1 to 3.0 parts per million (ppm), based on dry tissue weight. The largest amounts are deposited in liver, kidney, bone, and skin. Molybdenum is required as a catalytic component of the metalloenzymes: xanthine oxidase, aldehyde oxidase, and sulfite oxidase. As such, it is essential for a number of metabolic reactions. The RDA standard estimates an adequate adult intake of molybdenum of 75 to 250 µg/day. Food sources include legumes, whole grains, milk, leafy vegetables, and organ meats.

Fluorine

The trace element fluorine, or fluoride, accumulates in all body tissues showing calcification, mostly in bones and teeth. In human nutrition fluoride functions mainly to inhibit *dental caries.* The principal cause of caries is acid dissolution of tooth enamel. This acid is produced by microorganisms feeding on fermentable carbohydrates, especially sucrose, adhering to the teeth after a meal or snack. Fluoride therapy enhances the ability of the tooth structure to withstand the erosive effect of the bacterial acid. Establishment of a fluoride requirement is difficult because it appears to be retained in the bones regardless of the intake level. The RDA adult standard estimates a need in the range of 2.0 to 5.0 mg/day. Fish, fish products, and tea contain the highest concentration of fluoride. Cooking in fluoridated water raises the level in many foods. The public health measure of artificial *fluoridation* of community water supply to 1 ppm provides adequate amounts and has largely been responsible for the remarkable decline in dental caries. Less well defined, but promising, is fluoride's possible role in helping to control the development of *osteoporosis.* It may provide protection from the demineralizing of bone that characterizes this condition.

Probably Essential Trace Elements

The remaining trace elements that have been found in human tissue have less well-defined metabolic functions. But they have been found to be essential in animal nutrition and are probably essential in human nutrition in a similar manner as well, both as cofactors for cell enzymes in key metabolic reactions and as structural components in special tissues, for example, the role of boron with calcium in bone building.[13] These eight trace elements are silicon (Si), vanadium (V), nickel (Ni), tin (Sn), cadmium (Cd), arsenic (As), aluminum (Al), and boron (B). Apparently, most of these trace elements are needed in such minute amounts that primary dietary deficiency is highly unlikely. However, with increased use of long-term total parenteral nutrition (TPN) therapy, induced deficiencies may be of increasing clinical concern.

Water Balance

A number of the major minerals described above in the first section of this chapter have basic functions as electrolytes in controlling the body's vital water balance. This collective function is fundamental to health and often a vital part of patient care. Thus, in brief summary here, we will look at the three basic interdependent factors that control this balance: (1) the water itself, the solvent base for solutions; (2) the various particles (solutes) in solution in the water; and (3) the separating membranes that control the flow.

Water-Electrolyte Balance
Body Water Distribution

If you are a woman, your body is about 50% to 55% water. If you are a man, your body is about 55% to 60% water. The higher water content in most men is a result of their greater muscle mass. *Striated* muscle contains more water than any body tissue other than blood. The remaining 40% of a man's weight is about 18% protein and related substances, 15% fat, and 7% minerals. A woman's remaining body composition is about the same except for a somewhat smaller muscle mass and a larger fat deposit.

Water Functions

Body water performs three essential functions: (1) helps give structure and form to the body through the turgor it provides for tissues, (2) creates the water-based environment necessary for the vast array of chemical actions and reactions that comprise the body's metabolism and sustain life, and (3) provides the means for maintaining a stable body temperature.

Water Compartments

Consider the water in your body in two **compartments,** as shown in Figure 8-5: (1) the total water outside of cells—the *extracellular fluid compartment (ECF)*—and (2) the total water inside of cells—the *intracellular fluid compartment (ICF)*.

1. **ECF.** Water outside of cells makes up about 20% of the total body weight. It consists of four parts: (a) *blood plasma,* which accounts for about 25% of the ECF and 5% of body weight; (b) **interstitial** *fluid,* the water surrounding the cells; (c) *secretory fluid,* the water circulating in transit; and (d) *dense tissue fluid,* water in dense connective tissue, cartilage, bone.
2. **ICF.** Water inside cells makes up about 40% to 45% of total body weight. As the body cells handle our vast metabolic activity, it is no surprise that the total water inside cells is about twice the amount outside.

Overall Water Balance: Intake and Output

The average adult metabolizes from 2.5 to 3 L of water/day in a constant turnover balanced between intake and output. This water enters and leaves the body by various routes, controlled by basic mechanisms such as thirst and hormonal activity.

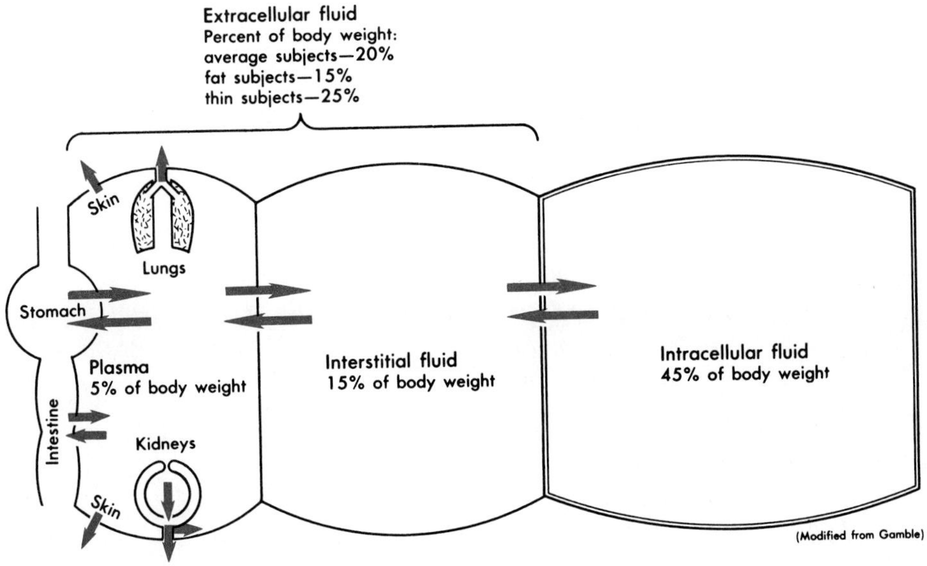

Compartment
Collective quantity of material in a given type of tissue space in the body.

Interstitial
Refers to spaces or interstices between the essential parts of an organ that comprise its tissue.

Figure 8-5
Body fluid compartments. Note the relative total quantities of water in the intracellular compartment and in the extracellular compartment.

Extracellular fluid
Percent of body weight:
average subjects—20%
fat subjects—15%
thin subjects—25%

Skin

Lungs

Stomach

Plasma
5% of body weight

Interstitial fluid
15% of body weight

Intracellular fluid
45% of body weight

Intestine

Kidneys

Skin

(Modified from Gamble)

Intake

Water enters the body in three main forms: (1) preformed water as such and in other beverages that are consumed, (2) preformed water in foods that are eaten, and (3) metabolic water, a product of cell oxidation.

Output

Water leaves the body through the kidneys, skin, lungs, and fecal elimination through the large intestine.

These routes of intake and output must be in constant balance. This balance is summarized in Table 8-5. Abnormal conditions, such as diarrhea or dysentery, produce much greater losses, causing serious clinical problems if prolonged. Extensive loss of body fluids can be especially dangerous in infants and children. Their bodies contain a greater percentage of the total body water, and much more of the water is outside of cells and easily available for loss.

Forces Controlling Water Distribution

Forces that influence and control the distribution of body water revolve around two factors: (1) the **solutes,** particles in solution in body water, and (2) the *separating membranes* between water compartments.

Solutes

A variety of particles with varying concentrations occur in the body. Two main types, electrolytes and plasma protein, control water balance:

1. **Electrolytes.** Several minerals provide major electrolytes for the body. In this role, these small inorganic elements are called **electrolytes** because they are free in solution and carry an electrical charge. These free, charged forms are *ions,* atoms or elements or groups of atoms that, in solution, carry either a positive or negative electrical charge. An ion carrying a positive charge is called a *cation;* examples are sodium (Na^+)—major cation of water outside cells, potassium (K^+)—major cation of water inside cells, calcium (Ca^{++}), and magnesium (Mg^{++}). Conversely, an ion carrying a negative charge is called an *anion;* examples are chloride (Cl^-), carbonate (HCO_3^-),

Solute
Dissolved substance; particles in solution.

Electrolyte
Chemical element or compound, which in solution dissociates by releasing ions. The process of dissociating into ions is termed ionization.

Table 8-5

Approximate Daily Adult Intake and Output of Water

	Intake (replacement) mL/day		Ouput (loss)	
			Obligatory (insensible) mL/day	Additional (according to need) mL/day
Preformed		Lungs	350	
Liquids	1200-1500	Skin		
In foods	700-1000	Diffusion	350	
Metabolism (oxidation of food)	200-300	Sweat	100	±250
		Kidneys	900	±500
		Feces	150	
TOTAL	2100-2800	TOTAL	1850	750
	(approx. 2600 mL/day)		(approx. 2600 mL/day)	

phosphate (HPO_4^{--}), and sulfate (SO_4^{--}). Because of their small size, these ions or electrolytes can diffuse freely across body membranes. Thus they produce a major force controlling movement of water within the body.

2. **Plasma proteins.** Organic substances of large molecular size, mainly albumin and globulin of the plasma proteins, influence the shift of water in and out of capillaries in balance with their surrounding water. In this function, these plasma proteins are called *colloids* (Gr. *kolla,* glue) and form *colloidal solutions.* Because of their large size, these particles or molecules do not pass readily through separating capillary membranes. Therefore they normally remain in the blood vessels, where they exert **colloidal osmotic pressure (COP)** to maintain the integrity of the blood volume.

3. **Organic compounds of small molecular size.** Other organic compounds of small size, such as glucose, urea, and amino acids, diffuse freely but do not influence shifts of water unless they occur in abnormally large concentrations. For example, the large amount of glucose in the urine of a patient with uncontrolled diabetes mellitus causes an abnormal osmotic diuresis or excess water output.

Water and solutes move across the body's separating membranes by the basic physiologic mechanisms that operate fluid balances according to body need. These mechanisms include osmosis, diffusion, filtration, active transport, and pinocytosis.

Influence of Electrolytes on Water Balance
Measurement of Electrolytes

The concentration of electrolytes in a given solution determines the chemical activity of that solution. It is the *number* of particles in a solution that is the important factor in determining chemical combining power. Thus electrolytes are measured according to the total number of particles in solution, each one of which contributes chemical combining power according to its **valence,** rather than their total weight. The unit of measure commonly used is an *equivalent.* Since small amounts are usually in question, most physiologic measurements are expressed in terms of *milliequivalents.* The term refers to the *number* of ions—cations and anions—in solution, as determined by their concentration in a given volume. This measure is expressed as the number of *milliequivalents per liter (mEq/L).*

Electrolyte Balance

Electrolytes are distributed in the body water compartments in a definite pattern, which has physiologic significance. This distribution pattern maintains stable *electrochemical neutrality* in body fluid solutions. According to biochemical and electrochemical laws, a stable solution must have equal numbers of positive and negative particles. It must be electrically neutral. When shifts and losses occur, compensating shifts and gains follow to maintain this dynamic balance, essential *electroneutrality.*

Electrolyte Control of Body Hydration

As indicated, ionized sodium is the chief cation of ECF, and ionized potassium is the chief cation of ICF. These two electrolytes control the amount of water retained in any given compartment. The usual bases for these shifts in water from one compartment to the other are ECF changes in concentration of these electrolytes. The terms *hypertonic* and *hypotonic* dehydration refer to

Colloidal osmotic pressure (COP)
Pressure produced by the protein molecules in the plasma and in the cell.

Valence
Power of an element or a radical to combine with (or to replace) other elements or radicals. Atoms of various elements combine in definite proportions. The valence number of an element is the number of atoms of hydrogen with which one atom of the element can combine.

the electrolyte concentration of the water *outside* the cell, which in turn causes a shift of water into or out of the cell to maintain balance.

Influence of Plasma Protein on Water Balance

Capillary Fluid Shift Mechanism

Water is constantly circulated throughout the body by the blood vessels. However, it must get out of the vessels to service the tissues and then be drawn back into circulation to maintain the normal transporting flow. Two main opposing pressures—*colloidal osmotic pressure (COP)* from plasma protein (mainly albumin) and *hydrostatic pressure* (blood pressure) of the capillary blood flow—provide balanced control of water and solute movement across capillary membranes. The body maintains this constant flow of water and the materials it is carrying to and from the cell by means of a shifting balance of these two pressures. It is a filtration process operating according to the differences in osmotic pressure on either side of the capillary membrane.

When blood first enters the capillary system, the greater blood pressure forces water and small solutes (glucose, for example) out into the tissues to bathe and nourish the cells. The plasma protein particles, however, are too large to go through the pores of capillary membranes. Hence the protein remains in the vessel and exerts the now greater colloidal osmotic pressure that draws the returning fluid and its materials back into circulation from the cells. This process is called the **capillary fluid shift mechanism.** It provides one of the most important and widespread *homeostatic* mechanisms in the body to maintain water balance, without which cells would die.

Cell Fluid Control

Much as plasma protein provides colloidal osmotic pressure to maintain the integrity of extracellular fluid, cell protein helps to provide the osmotic pressure that maintains the integrity of fluid inside the cell. Also, ionized potassium within the cell guards cell water in balance with ionized sodium guarding water outside the cell. This balance supports the flow of water, nutrients, and metabolites in and out of cells to sustain life.

Influence of Hormones on Water Balance

ADH mechanism

The **antidiuretic hormone (ADH),** also called **vasopressin,** is secreted by the posterior lobe of the pituitary gland. Its causes reabsorption of water by the kidney according to body need. Thus it is a water-conserving mechanism. In any stress situation with threatened or real loss of body water, this hormone is triggered to hold on to precious body water.

Capillary fluid shift mechanism
Process that controls the movement of water and small molecules in solution (electrolytes, nutrients) between the blood in the capillaries and the surrounding interstitial area.

Antidiuretic hormone (ADH) or vasopressin
Hormone secreted by the posterior pituitary gland in response to body stress. It acts on the renal tubules (chiefly the distal tubule) to cause reabsorption of water.

Aldosterone Mechanism

Aldosterone is primarily a sodium-conserving hormone, related in its operation to the renin-angiotensin system, but in doing this job it also exerts a secondary control over water loss. This mechanism's full name is the *renin-angiotensin-aldosterone mechanism,* because **renin,** an enzyme from the kidney, and **angiotensin,** the active product of its substrate (angiotensinogen) from the liver, are the intermediate substances used to trigger the adrenal glands to produce in turn the aldosterone hormone. Both aldosterone and ADH are activated by stress situations such as injury or surgery.

Angiotensin
Pressor substance produced in the body by interaction of the enzyme, *renin,* produced by the renal cortex and a serum globulin fraction, angiotensinogen, produced by the liver.

To Sum Up

Minerals are inorganic substances that are widely distributed in nature. They build body tissues; activate, regulate, and control metabolic processes; and transmit neurologic messages.

Minerals are classified as (1) *major minerals,* required in relatively large quantities, which make up 60% to 80% of all the inorganic material in the body, and (2) *trace elements,* required in quantities as small as a microgram, which make up less than 1% of the body's inorganic material. Seven major and ten trace minerals are known to be essential in human nutrition, with another eight trace elements probably essential, and still others constantly being examined for possible essentiality.

Overall water balance in the body is controlled by fluid intake and output. The distribution of body fluids is mainly controlled by two types of solutes: (1) *electrolytes,* charged mineral elements and other particles derived from inorganic compounds, and (2) *plasma protein,* mainly albumin, consisting of particles too large to pass through capillary membranes but capable of influencing the flow of fluid from one compartment to another. These solute particles influence the distribution of fluid passing across cell or capillary membranes, separating body fluid into its two compartments.

Questions for Review

1. List the 7 major minerals, describing physiologic function and problems created by dietary deficiency or excess.
2. List the 10 trace elements with proven essentiality for humans. Which have established RDA standards? Which have "safe and adequate intake" limits established? Why is it difficult to establish RDAs for everyone?
3. What accounts for the edema of starvation?
4. Why does potassium depletion occur in prolonged diarrhea?

References

1. Solomans NW: Calcium intake and availability from the human diet, Clin Nutr 5(4):167, 1986.
2. Spencer H: Factors contributing to osteoporosis, J Nutr 116:316, Feb 1986.
3. Horowitz M and others: Lactose and calcium absorption in postmenopausal osteoporosis, Arch Intern Med 147:534, March 1987.
4. Allen LH: Calcium and age-related bone loss, Clin Nutr 5(4):147, 1986.
5. Lindsay R: Managing osteoporosis: current trends, future possibilities, Geriatrics 42:35, March 1987.
6. Francis RM and Peacock M: Local action of oral 1,25-dihydroxycholecalciferol on calcium absorption in osteoporosis, Am J Clin Nutr 46:315, Aug 1987.
7. Allen LH: Calcium and osteoporosis, Am Fam Physician 36:178, Dec 1987.
8. American Council on Science and Health: Osteoporosis, Summit, NJ, 1986.
9. Avioli LV: Calcium and phosphorus. In Shils ME and Young VR, editors: Modern nutrition in health and disease, ed 7, Philadelphia, 1988, Lea & Febiger.
10. Iyengar V: Dietary intake studies of nutrients and selected toxic elements in human studies: analytical approaches, Clin Nutr 6(3):105, 1987.
11. Fairbanks VF and Beutler E: Iron. In Shils ME and Young VR, editors: Modern nutrition in health and disease, ed 7, Philadelphia, 1988, Lea & Febiger.
12. Monsen ER and Balintfy JL: Calculating dietary iron bioavailability: refinement and computerization, J Am Diet Assoc 80(4):307, 1982.
13. Nielsen FH: Boron—an overlooked element of potential nutritional importance, Nutr Today 23(1):4, 1988.

Applegate E: Just a trace, Health 20(6):59, 1988.

This nutritionist's brief updated review of trace minerals in a popular journal, complete with a large summary table, makes an excellent tool for review or resource for clients.

Beard JL: Iron fortification—rationale and effects, Nutr Today 21(4):17, 1986.

Crosby WH: Yin, yang, and iron, Nutr Today 21(4):14, 1986.

This pair of articles presents the two views of iron fortification: the first gives a defense for a moderate controlled program; the second, the conservative charge that the "viciously partisan FDA bureaucrats" have once again foiled the public.

Mertz W: Our most unique nutrients, Nutr Today 18(2):6, 1983.

This little classic gem is worth going back to for a rich account that relates these important trace elements in human nutrition to our geologic environment over the ages.

Nielsen FH: Boron—an overlooked element of potential nutritional importance, Nutr Today 23(1):4, 1988.

This nutrition researcher tells us about his current studies on boron, a lesser known trace element, and his evidence that it has a potential role important to metabolism of major minerals and to osteoporosis.

Swartz MW: Potassium imbalances, Am J Nurs 87:1292, 1987.

This article provides a good review of potassium imbalances—causes, symptoms, treatment—complete with many illustrations, making it an excellent teaching and learning tool.

Further Readings

Do We Need More? Guidelines for Trace Element Supplementation

Currently in the consumer marketplace, trace elements have become popular in both sales and discussions of supplementation. Are there any reasonable guidelines for supplementation based on reliable and current research?

Ten trace elements have generally been identified as essential for optimum health. These elements are chromium, cobalt, copper, fluorine, iodine, iron, manganese, molybdenum, selenium, and zinc. Nutritionists are concerned about toxicity, in terms of dietary and supplemental contributions leading to excess intake, as well as deficiency, in terms of eliminating factors interfering with bioavailability and evaluating the possible need for supplements.

The following list may serve as a basic guide for examining the need for supplementing the U.S. diet with trace minerals.

Iron is provided by organ meats, dried fruits, whole grains, fortified breakfast cereals, legumes, and dark green leafy vegetables. Men require 10 mg/day, women 15 mg. The need for supplements has long been established for pregnant and breast-feeding women, who require *daily supplements of 15 mg*. Other high-risk groups may also need to supplement their diets: adolescent girls, low-income adolescent boys, athletes, and elderly Blacks. Before recommending a supplement to these individuals, however, you should evaluate their intake of iron antagonists such as fiber and caffeine.

Iodine is provided by foods grown in iodine-rich soil, seafood, and iodized salt. Daily requirements are 75 to 150 μg/day, although the average intake is several times that amount because of the widespread use of iodine-containing compounds in the dairy and baking industries. Since greater levels can result in thyrotoxicosis, *supplementation is not recommended*.

Zinc is supplied by oysters, whole grains, legumes, nuts, and meats. The recommended intake is 12 to 15 mg/day. Pregnancy and lactation increase the need to 15 to 19 mg, respectively, to avoid deficiency signs of slow growth, impaired taste and smell, poor wound healing, and skin problems. Others at risk include alcoholics and individuals on long-term, low-calorie diets. It takes 3 to 24 weeks for symptoms to appear but *supplementation relieves deficiency symptoms* in a matter of days. To avoid an overdose, characterized by gastrointestinal upset, nausea, and bleeding, check the client's eating habits for zinc antagonists, for example, an excessive intake of fiber or iron.

Copper is widely available in liver, oysters, shellfish, nuts, whole grains, and legumes. The average diet was previously believed to provide 2 to 5 mg/day, easily meeting the minimum RDA recommendation of 1.5 to 3 mg/day. Intake levels are now believed to range from less than 1 mg to no more than 2 mg/day, based on new analysis methods, thus placing a larger segment of the population at risk for developing a mild deficiency. Before recommending supplementation, however, examine factors that reduce copper bioavailability, such as a low protein intake, or high levels of zinc, cadmium, fiber, or ascorbic acid.

Chromium is provided by brewer's yeast, animal products, and whole grains. Daily adult requirements have been estimated between 50 to 200 μg. Deficiency signs include resistance to insulin and other signs of diabetes. Supplementation not only reduces insulin resistance but also increases HDL cholesterol, thereby offering some protection against coronary heart disease. While reliable diagnostic tests have not been developed yet, it is estimated that current intakes fall below recommended levels. However, because it has only shown effectiveness in small, controlled studies, *supplementation recommendations have not been made yet for any population groups*.

Selenium is provided by fish, whole wheat, and plants grown in selenium-rich soil. Intakes of the new RDA standards for adults is 55 to 70 µg/day, with the average diet providing 50 to 150 µg/day. Selenium is believed to offer protection against breast cancer. One group of researchers believes that "optimal cancer protection" is provided at levels of 150 to 300 µg/day, although the connection between blood levels and cancer patients and cancer-free individuals has not been established. In addition to cancer, selenium is believed to protect against heart disease, arthritis, heavy metal poisoning, sexual dysfunction, and aging. As there is no current evidence of selenium deficiency in the general population, *supplementation is not recommended.*

Manganese is provided by whole grains, green vegetables, and dried beans. Safe intakes are estimated in the range of 2.0 to 5.0 mg/day. Deficiency signs in humans have not been reported, but signs of toxicity have. These signs include weakness and psychologic problems. Toxicity is associated mainly with industrial exposure. However, the possibility of an excess suggests that *supplementation is not recommended.*

Silicon requirements for humans are not known, nor are reliable food sources. Deficiency has been associated with poor bone growth in chicks and statistically correlated with cardiovascular disease in humans. However, *the need for supplementation has not been established.*

Nickel is provided by legumes, cocoa, wheat, shellfish, milk, meats, and a variety of vegetables and fresh fruits. Requirements are estimated at about 75 µg/day, though U.S. intakes have been estimated between 300 to 600 µg/day. In light of this excessive intake, plus the existence of at least one sign of toxicity, a nickel-sensitive dermatitis, *supplementation is not recommended.*

Vanadium requirements are unknown, as are reliable food sources. However, it is estimated that the average American diet provides 1 to 2 mg/day. Some individuals are apparently sensitive to this amount, exhibiting severe depression. They improve when given megadoses of vitamin C, which blocks vanadium activity. *The need for supplementation is not indicated* because of its potential for toxicity in at least this one sensitive population group.

REFERENCES

Allen LH: Trace minerals and outcome of human pregnancy, Clin Nutr 5(2):72, 1986.

Beard JL: Iron fortification—rationale and effects, Nutr Today 21(4):17, 1986.

Helman AD and Darnton-Hill I: Vitamin and iron status in new vegetarians, Am J Clin Nutr 45:785, April 1987.

Krishnamachari KAVR and Krishnamachari R: Trace elements and human health, Clin Nutr 6(3):126, 1987.

Pennington JAT and Jones JW: Molybdenum, nickel, cobalt, vanadium, and strontium in total diets, J Am Diet Assoc 87(6):744, 1987.

Turnlund JR: Copper nutriture, bioavailability, and the influence of dietary factors, J Am Diet Assoc 88(3):302, 1988.

Part II

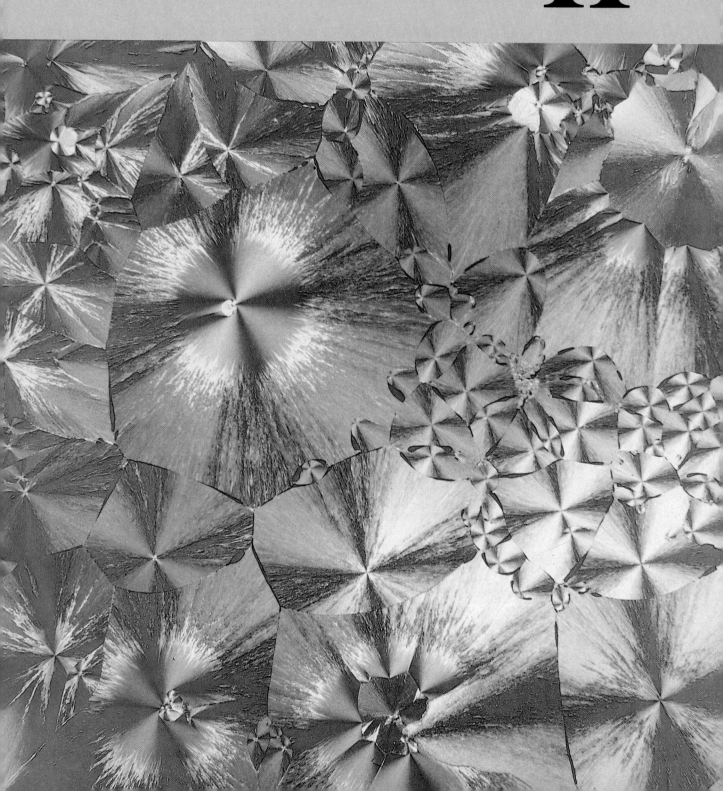

Community Nutrition: The Life Cycle

9 The Food Environment and Food Habits

Chapter Objectives

After studying this chapter, the student should be able to:

1. Identify personal and environmental forces that determine food choices and nutritional status.
2. Relate social, psychologic, and cultural factors to the development of personal food habits.
3. Examine personal food beliefs and habits of clients and patients in helping them plan nutritional food patterns.
4. Identify ways public food safety and quality are protected in the United States.
5. Describe changing food pattern trends in the United States today and account for their development.

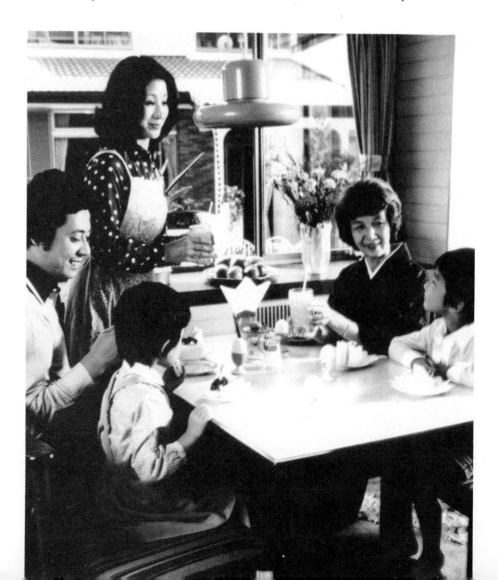

PREVIEW

We live in a rapidly changing environment. As a result, health care is changing and the needs of people it seeks to serve are changing. It is inevitable in the face of such change that the *real* needs of persons must be learned and met, if good health care is to be provided. Nutrition is basic to such health care.

Thus far, in the first part of your study, you have reviewed some basic principles of the science of human nutrition. But these principles can only come alive in terms of *personal need.* Knowledge alone is not enough to meet these health care needs. Human compassion and concern are necessary, as well as practical guides and skills, to apply knowledge in a useful and helpful manner.

The chapters in this second section of your study on community nutrition and the life cycle will provide a background on which you can build as you help to fulfill some of these human needs in your own practice. We begin here with a look at our changing food environment and the web of influences that determines personal food choices and habits.

The Food Environment and Malnutrition

Out of necessity, our food habits are inevitably linked to our environment. As a result, our rapidly changing human environment, with its problems of imbalance such as pollution and malnutrition, often threatens health. The word **ecology** comes from a Greek word, *oikos,* meaning "house." Just as many factors and forces within a family interact to influence its members, so even greater forces in our physical environment and social system interact to produce disease.

The public health significance of **malnutrition,** local to worldwide in scope, continues to grow.[1,2] Observation and experience have brought deepened awareness of two important interrelated facts: (1) having adequate food *alone* is not the complete answer, although it fulfills a fundamental need for all persons, and (2) a national high standard of living does not necessarily eliminate the problem of malnutrition. Even in the midst of plenty here in America, malnutrition exists.[3,4] It is found among vulnerable groups such as elderly and hospitalized persons. It is found among persons suffering from alcoholism and drug addition. It is associated with poverty and homelessness. It is partner to a distorted obsession with thinness. Human misery and human waste of life from malnutrition, more stark in some regions of our country and the world than in others, occurs nonetheless in both world hemispheres. The extent of this human suffering is impossible to quantify.

At its fundamental biologic level, malnutrition results from an inadequate supply of nutrients to the cell. However, this lack of essential nutrients at the cell level is by no means a simple problem. It is caused by a complex web of factors: psychologic, personal, social, cultural, economic, political, and educational. Each of these factors is more or less important at a given time and place for a given individual. If these factors are only temporarily adverse, the malnutrition may be short term, alleviated rapidly, and cause no long-

The Ecology of Human Nutrition

Ecology
Relations between organisms and their environment.

Malnutrition
Faulty nutrition resulting from poor diet, malassimilation, or overeating.

Epidemiology
Branch of medicine dealing with the study of various factors that determine the frequency and distribution of disease in given populations.

standing results or harm to life. But if they continue unrelieved, malnutrition becomes chronic. Irreparable harm to life follows (see the box on p. 197) and eventually death ensues. For the **epidemiologist** a triad of variables influences disease: (1) agent, (2) host, and (3) environment. These three factors describe malnutrition.

Agent

The fundamental agent in malnutrition is *lack of food*. Because of this lack, certain nutrients in food that are essential to maintaining cell activity are missing. As indicated, many factors may interact to cause or modify this lack of food: inadequate quantity and quality of food, insufficient amounts for children during critical growth periods, loss of supply through famine or poverty or maldistribution or war, or unwise choices made from foods available.

Host

The host is the person—infant, child, or adult—who suffers from malnutrition. Various personal characteristics may influence the disease: presence of other diseases, increased need for food during times of growth, pregnancy, or heavy labor, congenital defects or prematurity, and personal factors such as emotional problems and poverty.

Environment

Many environmental factors influence malnutrition. These include sanitation, social problems, culture, economic and political structure, and agriculture.

The interactive, tangled web of some of these factors leading to malnutrition is shown in Figure 9-1.

Economic and Political Environment
Food Availability and Use

In any society, at both governmental and personal levels, food availability and use involve both money and politics. It is plainly evident that money is a basic necessity for getting an adequate food supply. Sometimes, however, the role of politics and government structure and policies are not always as evident. Nonetheless, both are always intertwined in securing human nutrition.[5]

Government Food and Agriculture Programs

In any country, food and agricultural programs at any level of government influence food availability and distribution. A number of factors may be involved, such as land management practices and erosion, water distribution and its consequent pollution from long-term use of questionable pesticides, food production and distribution policies, and food assistance programs for individual persons in need.

Problem of Poverty

We are all made increasingly aware through the daily news that malnutrition, even famine and death, exists in countries such as India, parts of Africa, and mid-Eastern nations. Closer to home, peoples of Central and South America are hard-pressed by social conditions such as revolution, inequity,

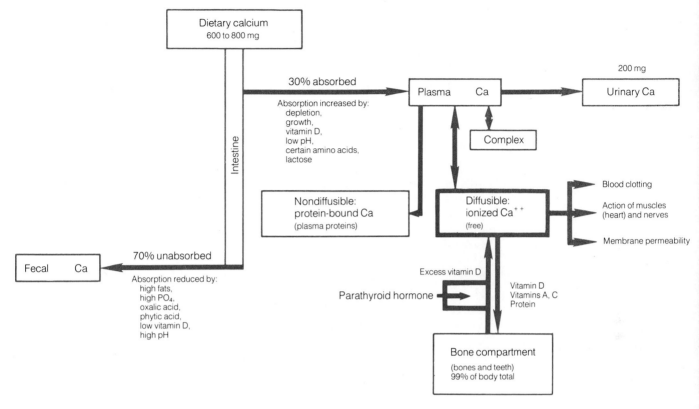

Figure 9-1
Multiple etiology of malnutrition.
(Modified from Williams CD:
Malnutrition, Lancet 2:342, 1962.)

and desperate poverty. But even here in the United States, one of the wealthiest nations on earth, many studies document widespread hunger and malnutrition among the poor, especially among minority groups, with increasing numbers of infants and young children involved.[4] For example, Black infants in the United States still have twice the chance of dying in their first year than white infants do.

Tremendous problems exist among the poor, and at times they seem almost insurmountable. Often a "culture of poverty" develops and is reinforced and perpetuated by society's values and attitudes, which wall off such persons more completely than do physical barriers. As a result of extreme pressures caused by living conditions, poverty-stricken persons become victims of negative attitudes and characteristics, feeling isolated and powerless and insecure, feelings that influence their use of community health services.

The national infant mortality rate for Blacks is about 22/ 1000 live births. For whites the rate is about 11.5/1000.

Isolation

Strong feelings of alienation from mainstream society are common among the poor. In many communities few if any channels of communications are open between the lowest income groups and the rest of society. In most instances a poor person responds to such feelings of alienation by further withdrawal. Each person feels isolated and alone and concludes that no one is really concerned. Hazards to health are inherent in poor housing and poor nutrition and are often compounded by distance from the sources of health care.

Powerlessness

It is ironic that often those persons most exposed to risks and emergencies have the fewest coping resources. Extreme frustration is inevitable and persons become overwhelmed. Why try, they conclude, if they have no control over the situation? Why plan, if there is no future different from today? In such a day-to-day struggle to exist, the poor person often sees little value in long-range preventive health measures.

Insecurity

Subjected to forces outside their control, poor individuals and families have little or no security. Insecurity and anxiety often incapacitate them. In such a setting, where hunger may be a constant companion, food—which has for poor people the same deep psychologic and emotional meaning that it has for all people—assumes even greater meaning than it has for persons who rarely know hunger.

Role of the Health Worker

How can concerned health workers help individuals and families conditioned by years of poverty or crushed by new poverty? In the face of such overpowering feelings of isolation, helplessness, and insecurity, what attitudes are necessary to be of real help? What methods and approaches are most likely to reach our clients and patients and supply their needs? Some basic principles can help.

Self-Awareness

First, we must explore our own feelings about the poor. We must be aware of our own distorted vision, our own class values and attitudes. If we are to be agents of constructive change, true "helping vehicles," we must first have some understanding of the person's situation and its broad social setting. We must also understand ourselves better and confront our own cultural conditioning and biases.

Rapport

Genuine rapport between persons is born of mutual respect and trust.

Genuine warmth, interest, friendliness, and kindness grow from within. **Rapport** is that feeling of relationship between persons that is born of mutual respect, regard, and trust. This sense of relationship gives both helper and helped a deep feeling of working *together*. Its most basic ingredient is a concern for people and persons, a positive orientation toward human beings in general and concern for individuals in particular. It is born of a deep knowledge of what it means to be human.

Acceptance

This term is another way of stating the principle that one must begin where the client or patient is. Each person's own concerns should be the primary consideration. Often we work with other team specialists to cut through the maze of factors involved in a given situation before the client or patient is ready to accept or even to consider the health practice or diet counsel that is needed or desired. Much time may have to be spent, for example, in coming to understand the meaning of food to this person, before practical dietary matters can begin to be explored.

Clinical Application

Functional Consequences of Malnutrition

In addition to specific disorders associated with deficiencies of particular nutrients, other human factors are related to malnutrition. These factors include immunocompetence, reproductive competence, work output, mental ability, and social or behavioral traits. The impact of inadequate nutrition on these aspects of human health and life is currently the subject of intense multilateral investigation.

We have long assumed a linear relationship between intake and well-being, at least up to the point of adequacy. We have relied on anthropometric measures, especially those measuring growth rates in children, to tell us how badly undernourished an individual or a population is. Measurements such as weight-for-age or height-for-age are compared with those of reference populations that are well nourished. The definitions of malnutrition, then, are as follows:

Degree of malnutrition	Weight for age
First degree: mild	75% to 90% of standard
Second degree: moderate	60% to 75% of standard
Third degree: severe	Less than 60% of standard

Scientists are now exploring the possibility that a *threshold of tolerance* exists, that a person may be able to adapt successfully to lowered intakes of kilocalories up to a point, or threshold. If the kilocalorie intake is chronically below this threshold, the individual is then likely to suffer functional disabilities, but if the kilocalories consumed fall chronically between what is recommended and this lower threshold point, the individual lives a marginal life barely free of impairment.

Studies have validated that long-term severe malnutrition leads to stunting of mental and emotional, as well as physical, development. However, the effects of chronic malnutrition, even in the early years of life, may be reversible by improved diet and social-emotional care later in the child's development. Of course, serious deficits of food are often accompanied by poverty in other areas of life, and a family may not be capable of "making up" for the early years of hardship.

REFERENCES
Beardslee WR and others: The effects of infantile malnutrition on behavioral development: a follow-up study, Am J Clin Nutr 35(6):1437, 1982.
Calloway DH: Functional consequences of malnutrition, Rev Infect Dis 4(4):736, 1982.
Grantham-McGregor S, Schofield W, and Powell C: Development of severely malnourished children who received psychosocial stimulation: six-year follow-up, Pediatrics 79:247, Feb 1987.
Scrimshaw NS: Consequences of hunger for individuals and societies, Fed Proc 45:2421, Sept 1986.

Listening

Here, more than elsewhere, the art of listening—positive, active, creative listening—is vital. Clients must tell their story in their own way, with no interruption by distracting statements or questions and no deflecting of the conversation to another's problems. This listening must also be observant. Sequence of statements, subjects introduced, areas of intense feeling, and areas ignored give clues to needs. Throughout we must proceed with sensitivity and create a relaxed, nonthreatening atmosphere, in which persons feel free to talk—*and we must listen.* The reason that some frustrated persons finally take their problems to the streets may well be that *no one listens to them unless they do.*

Worldwide Factors in Malnutrition

The world's affluent countries consume 70% of the world's grain. But only about 7% of that amount is consumed directly as human fare in the form of grains or flour. Most of it is used to feed livestock, and a sizeable portion is used to make alcoholic beverages.

On a broader level, international problems of population increase and export-import policies compound problems of malnutrition for two reasons: (1) the world population is rising at an alarming rate—a matter of grave concern; (2) regarding who feeds whom, it is a common conception that the rich world feeds the poor world. But this is not always the case. In fact, our grain exports go predominantly to other industrialized nations. Only about one fifth of the exports go to developing nations. Developed countries export nearly four times as much food to other developed countries as they do to the developing world. Less developed countries also export about three times as much to the industrialized countries as they do to other less developed nations.

Development of Food Habits

In addition to these factors of poverty and politics, other aspects of our lives influence our food patterns. Food habits, like other forms of human behavior, do not develop in a vacuum. They result from many personal, cultural, social, and psychologic influences. For each of us these factors are interwoven to develop a whole individual. To study these basic influences on food habits, we will look at each one of them separately.

Cultural Influences
Strength of Personal Culture

Culture
System of customs, habits, and values developed over time by a people, usually resulting from adaptation to environment, interpretation of life experiences, and religious beliefs.

Often the most significant thing about a society's **culture** is what it takes for granted in daily life. Culture involves not only the more obvious and historical aspects of a person's communal life—that is, language, religion, politics, technology, and so on—but also all the little habits of everyday living, such as preparing and serving food and caring for children, feeding them, and lulling them to sleep. These facets of a person's culture are *learned* gradually as a child grows up in a given society. Through a slow process of conscious and unconscious learning, we take on our culture's values, attitudes, habits, and practices through the influence of our parents, teachers, and others. Whatever is invented, transmitted, and perpetuated—socially acquired knowledge and habits—we learn as part of our culture. These elements become internalized and entrenched.

Food in a Culture

Food habits are among the oldest and most deeply rooted aspects of many cultures and exert deep influence on the behavior of the people. The cultural and subcultural background determines what shall be eaten, as well as when and how it shall be eaten. There is, of course, considerable variation. But rational or irrational, beneficial and injurious customs are found in every part of the world. Nevertheless, food habits are primarily based on food availability, economics, and personal food meanings and beliefs. Included among these influential factors are the geography of the land, the agriculture practiced by the people, their economic and marketing practices, their view about healthy or safe food, and their history and traditions. Within every culture there are certain foods that are deeply infused with symbolic meaning. These symbolic foods are related to major life experiences from birth through death, to religion, to politics, and to general social organization. From early times ceremonies and religious rites have surrounded certain events and seasons. Food gathering, preparing, and serving have followed specific customs and commemorated special events of religious and national significance and heritage. Many of these customs remain today.

Since America is a unique nation of many different ethnic heritages, a large number of different cultural food patterns are represented here in community life. Many have contributed characteristic dishes or modes of cooking to American eating habits, and in turn many food habits of subcultures have been Americanized. Traditional foods tend to be used more consistently by the older members of the family, whereas younger members may use such foods only on special occasions or holidays. Nevertheless, these traditional food patterns have strong meanings and serve to bind families and cultural communities in close fellowship. However, among persons of different cultures, individual tastes and geographic patterns vary. Economic factors cause wide differences, as does educational level. In various food patterns the type of food may be unique with special dishes and methods of preparation that represent certain ethnic or regional groups and use foods that are readily available. Other food patterns develop in relation to religious beliefs and festivals. Whatever the origin, such food practices are usually deeply ingrained in the lives of the people. A few of these representative cultural food patterns are briefly outlined here.

Traditional Cultural Food Patterns

Jewish Food Patterns
Dietary Food Laws

Jewish dietary food laws are different for the three basic groups within Judaism: (1) Orthodox—strict observance, (2) Conservative—nominal observance, and (3) Reform—less ceremonial emphasis and minimal observance. The Jewish body of dietary laws is called the *Rules of Kashruth* and foods selected and prepared accordingly are called *kosher* foods. The basis of these traditional laws is primarily self-purification and a means of service to God, although they probably also had some hygienic or ethical foundation in the beginning. Most of these rules relate to ordinances given to the ancient Hebrews, as recorded in the Old Testament books of the Law (Leviticus and Deuteronomy), and to the Jewish traditions accumulated over the centuries. These traditions were collected and interpreted in the Talmud, a body of laws set down in the fourth to the sixth centuries BC. Since the original Hebrew religion was centered in practices of animal sacrifice and the blood had special ritual significance, the present Jewish dietary laws apply specifically to the slaughter, preparation, and service of meat, to the combining of meat and milk, to fish, and to eggs.

Both words come from the Hebrew word *kashar*, meaning "right" or "fit."

Food Restrictions

As a result, traditional food restrictions include the following:
1. **Meat.** Only meat from cloven-hoofed quadrupeds that chew a cud

(cattle, sheep, goats, and deer) is used, and only the forequarters of these animals are allowed. The hindquarters may be eaten only if the sinew of Jacob (hind sinew of the thigh) is removed (Leviticus 11:1-8). Chickens, turkeys, geese, pheasants, and ducks may also be eaten (Leviticus 11:13-19).

2. **Blood.** Ritual slaughter follows rigid rules based on minimum pain to the animal and maximum blood drainage. It involves several steps. First, the meat is water-soaked in a special vessel, then rinsed, and thoroughly salted with coarse salt. Then it is placed on a perforated board and left to stand for an hour. Finally, after draining thoroughly, it is washed three times before being cooked. No blood may be eaten as food in any form. Blood is considered synonymous with life (Genesis 9:4; Leviticus 3:17).

3. **Meat and milk.** No combining of meat and milk is allowed (Exodus 23:19). Milk or food made from milk, such as cheese and ice cream, may be eaten just before a meal, but not for 6 hours after eating a meal that contains meat. In the Orthodox Jewish household, the custom is to maintain two sets of dishes, one for serving meat meals and the other for serving dairy meals.

4. **Fish.** Only those fish with fins and scales are allowed. No shellfish or eels may be eaten (Leviticus 11:9-12). Fish of the type permitted may be eaten with either dairy or meat meals.

5. **Eggs.** No egg that contains a blood spot may be eaten. Eggs may be taken with either dairy or meat meals.

Foods for Special Occasions

Many of the traditional Jewish foods are related to festivals of the Jewish calendar. These holidays commemorate events in Jewish history (Table 9-1). Often special Sabbath dishes are used. In Orthodox Jewish homes, no food is prepared on the Sabbath, which begins at sundown on Friday and ends when the first star becomes visible Saturday evening. Foods are prepared on Friday and held for use on the Sabbath. A long-honored custom is that of inviting a guest to share the Sabbath meal as a remembrance of the biblical statement, "For you were once strangers in the land of Egypt" (Exodus 22:20). A few representative Jewish foods include these:

1. **Challah.** A special Sabbath loaf of white bread, shaped as a twist or beehive coil, used at the beginning of the meal after kiddush (the blessing over wine).
2. **Gefüllte (gefilte) fish.** From a German word meaning "stuffed fish," usually the first course of the Sabbath evening meal and made of fish filet, chopped, seasoned, and stuffed back into the skin or minced and rolled into balls.
3. **Bagels.** Doughnut-shaped, hard yeast rolls.
4. **Blintzes.** Thin, filled, and rolled pancakes.
5. **Borscht (borsch).** Soup of meat stock and beaten egg or sour cream made with beets, cabbage, or spinach, served hot or cold.
6. **Kasha.** Buckwheat groats (hulled kernels), used as a cooked cereal or as a potato substitute with gravy.
7. **Knishes.** Pastry filled with ground meat or cheese.
8. **Lox.** Smoked, salted salmon.
9. **Matzo.** Flat unleavened bread.
10. **Strudel.** Thin pastry, filled with fruit and nuts, rolled, and baked.

Table 9-1

Jewish Holidays and Associated Foods

Holiday	Month	Event	Traditional foods
Rosh Hashanah (New Year)	September or October	Beginning of Jewish New Year (Tishri 1)	Honey, honey cake, carrot tzimmes
Yom Kippur	September or October	Day of Atonement	Fast day (total)
Sukkoth	October	Feast of Booths, Harvest festival; symbolizes booths in which Israelites lived on flight from Egypt and Wilderness wanderings	Kreplach or holishkes (chopped meat wrapped in cabbage leaves), strudel
Chanukah	December	Feast of Lights; celebrates heroic battle of the Maccabees for Jewish independence (165 BC); Home festival with candles	Grated potato latkes, potato kugel
Chamise Oser b'Sh'vat	January	Festival of the Trees (Arbor Day); blossoming time of trees in Palestine	Bokser (St. John's Bread), fruits, nuts, raisins, cakes
Purim	March	Feast of Esther, celebrates downfall of Haman and deliverance of Hebrews by influence of Queen Esther to King Xerxes of Persia	Hamantaschen (three-cornered pastry), apples, nuts, raisins
Passover (Pesach)	April	Festival of Freedom, celebrates escape of Israelites from Egyptian slavery	Seder meal, matzoth and matzoth dishes, wine, nuts
Shevuoth	May	Feast of Weeks (Pentecost); celebrates the day Moses received Ten Commandments on Mt. Sinai	Cheese blintzes, cheese kreplach, dairy foods

Mexican Food Patterns
Basis of Present Food Patterns

A blending of the food habits of Spanish settlers and native Indian tribes forms the basic of traditional food patterns of persons of Mexican heritage who now live in the United States, chiefly in the Southwest. Three foods are basic to this pattern—dried beans, chili peppers, and corn. Variations and additions may be found in different localities or among those of different income levels.

Traditional Use of Food

In general, food use habits include these:

1. **Milk.** Little milk is used. A small amount of evaporated milk may be purchased for babies.

2. **Meat.** Because of its cost, little meat is taken. Beef or chicken may be eaten two or three times a week. Eggs are also used occasionally, but fish is rarely eaten.

3. **Vegetables.** Corn, fresh or canned, and chili peppers are the main vegetables. *Chicos* is steamed green corn dried on the cob. *Pasole* is similar to whole-grain hominy (lime-treated, hulled whole kernels). Chili peppers provide a good source of vitamin C; they are usually dried and ground into a powder. Pinto or chalice beans are used daily. They may be reheated by frying (refried beans) or cooked with beef, garlic, and chili peppers (chili con carne).

4. **Fruits.** Depending on availability and cost, oranges, apples, bananas, and canned peaches are used.

5. **Bread and cereals.** For centuries corn has been the basic grain used as bread and cereal by the Mexican people. *Masa* (dough) is made from dry corn that has been heated, soaked in lime water, washed, and ground wet to form a mass with the consistency of putty. This dough is then formed into thin, unleavened cakes and baked on a hot griddle to make the typical *tortilla.* Wheat is now replacing corn for making some tortillas. Unless the wheat flour is enriched, however, the calcium in the previously used lime-treated corn is lost. Cornmeal gruel, or *atole,* is served with hot milk. Rice cooked in milk may be used as a dessert. Oatmeal is a popular breakfast cereal.

6. **Beverages.** Large amounts of coffee are generally used. In some families coffee is also given to young children.

7. **Seasonings.** Chili pepper, onions, and garlic are used most frequently. Occasionally other herbs may be added. Lard is the basic cooking fat.

Puerto Rican Food Patterns
Basis of Traditional Food Patterns

The Puerto Rican people share a common Spanish heritage with the Mexicans. A large part of their food pattern is similar. However, the use of tropical fruits and vegetables that grow on their homeland island have formed a base for the Puerto Rican food pattern. Some of these habits are carried over to Puerto Ricans living in America when the foods are available in the neighborhood markets. Almost everyone eats the main food, *viandas,* which are starchy vegetables and fruits such as plantain and green bananas. The two other diet staples are rice and beans. Milk, meat, yellow and green vegetables, and other fruits are used in limited quantities.

General Food Use Habits

Patterns of general food use include these:

1. **Viandas.** The many kinds of viandas eaten daily include green bananas, green and ripe plantains, white and yellow sweet potatoes, white yams, breadfruit, and cassava. These foods are cooked in many ways. Usually codfish and onion are added. If income permits, some avocados and hard-boiled eggs are also added. This dish is called *serenata.* A soup containing viandas and meat is called *sancocho.*

2. **Rice.** A large portion of daily kilocalories is obtained from rice. Most Puerto Ricans eat about 7 oz daily, usually cooked in salted water and seasoned with lard. Other rice dishes include a rice stewed with beans and *sofrito*—a sauce of tomatoes, green pepper, onion, garlic, salt pork, lard, and herbs; rice with chicken, seasoned with olives, red pepper, and sofrito; a dessert made with rice, sugar, and spices; and a thick soup of chicken and rice.

3. **Other cereal grains.** Some wheat is used in the form of bread, noodles, and spaghetti. Oatmeal and cornmeal mush may be added if income permits.

4. **Beans.** Legumes used include chickpeas (garbanzos), navy beans, red kidney beans (preferred), and dried peas. Usually they are boiled until tender and cooked with sofrito.

5. **Meat.** Most families cannot afford much meat, although pork and chicken are used when income allows. The only animal protein that the majority can buy is dried codfish.

6. **Milk.** Low-income groups can afford little milk. Most of what is taken is boiled and used with coffee; some cocoa and chocolate are used in the same way.

7. **Vegetables and fruits.** Small amounts of other vegetables are used by the Puerto Rican people. Many tropical fruits are available on the island. Puerto Rico is the home of the *acerola,* the tiny, sour, West Indian cherry, which looks like a miniature apple and has the highest quantity of ascorbic acid known to be contained in any food—about 1000 mg/100 g. Other fruits include oranges, pineapples, grapefruits, papayas, and mangoes.

General Meal Pattern

In most Puerto Rican households a typical day's food pattern would include coffee with milk for breakfast; a large plate of viandas with codfish for lunch; and rice, beans, and viandas for dinner. If income permits, egg or oatmeal may be added to breakfast, some meat to dinner, and fruit between meals. This simple daily diet contrasts with a holiday meal such as that enjoyed at Christmas time. This feast would include whole pig roasted on a spit, blood sausage, green bananas or plantain cooked in the ashes, rice, *pasteles* (plantain dough filled with chopped pork, sofrito, olives, raisins, and boiled peas), rice pudding, and wine, beer, or brandy.

Chinese Food Patterns
Basis of Traditional Food Habits

Traditional Chinese cooking is based on three principles: (1) natural flavor must be developed, (2) texture and color must be maintained, (3) any undesirable qualities of foods must be masked or modified. Like the French, Chinese cooks believe that refrigeration diminishes natural flavors. So they select the freshest possible foods, hold them the shortest possible time, and then cook them quickly at a high temperature in small amounts of liquid or fat. This is called *stir-frying,* commonly done in a wok. By these means natural flavor, color, and texture are preserved. Vegetables are cooked just before serving, so that they are still crisp and flavorful when eaten. The only sauce that may be served with them is a thin translucent one lightly thickened with cornstarch. A thick gravy is never used. Foods that have been dried, salted, pickled, spiced, candied, or canned may be added as garnishes or relishes to mask some flavors or textures or to enhance others.

General Food Use Habits

Basic food use habits include these:

1. **Milk.** Little milk and limited amounts of cheese are used.

2. **Meat.** Pork, lamb, chicken, duck, fish, and shellfish are used in many ways. Usually they are cooked in combinations with vegetables, thus extending the small amount of meat. Eggs and soybeans in the form of soybean curd and milk add to the protein content of the diet. Some characteristic dishes include *egg roll,* a thin dough spread with meat and vegetable filling,

rolled, and fried in deep fat; *egg foo yung,* an omelet of egg, chopped chicken, mushrooms, scallions, celery, and bean sprouts; and *sweet and sour pork,* pork cubes fried and then simmered in a sweet-sour sauce of brown sugar, vinegar, and other seasonings. Chow mein, or chop suey, is purely an American invention. It is a mixture of meat, celery, and bean sprouts, served over rice or noodles, with added soy sauce.

3. **Vegetables.** Cooked by the characteristic method described, stir-frying, vegetables such as cabbage, cucumbers, snow peas, melons, squashes, greens, mushrooms, bean sprouts, and sweet potatoes are made into many fine dishes.

4. **Fruits.** Usually fruits are eaten fresh. Pineapple and a few others are sometimes used in combination dishes.

5. **Bread and cereals.** Rice is the staple grain used at most meals.

6. **Seasonings.** Soy sauce is a basic seasoning. Ginger, sesame seed, and almonds are also used. Most often used cooking fats are lard and peanut oil.

7. **Beverage.** The traditional beverage is unsweetened green tea.

Japanese Food Patterns
Basis of Traditional Food Patterns

Japanese food patterns are in some ways similar to Chinese. Rice is a basic grain of the diet, soy sauce is used for seasoning, and tea is the main beverage. However, some characteristic differences occur. The Japanese diet contains more seafood, especially raw fish. A number of taboos prohibit certain food combinations or the use of certain foods in specific localities or at specific times. Some of these taboos are associated with religious practices such as ancestor veneration.

General Food Use Habits

Traditional food use habits include these:

1. **Milk.** Little milk or cheese is used. Some evaporated or dried milk may be added in cooking or given to babies.

2. **Meat.** The main animal protein source is seafood. Many varieties of fish and shellfish such as raw squid or octopus are served. Other unusual salt water fare are eels, abalone, and globe fish (puffer fish—deadly if the chef's knife slips in cutting out a certain poisonous gland). More familiar to the Westerner are crab, shrimp, mackerel, carp, and salmon. Families living inland especially may also eat rabbits, chicken, and occasionally beef or lamb. Eggs are a source of additional protein.

3. **Vegetables.** Menus include many vegetables, usually steamed and served with soy sauce. Pickled vegetables are also well liked.

4. **Fruits.** Fresh fruits are eaten in season. A tray of fruit is a regular course of the main meal.

5. **Bread and cereals.** Although rice is the staple grain, some corn, barley, and oats are served, and white wheat bread is increasingly used.

Meal Pattern

A specific sequence of courses is usually followed at most traditional Japanese dinners: green tea, unsweetened; some appetizer, such as soy cake or red bean cake, a raw fish (sashimi) or radish (komono) relish; broiled fish or omelet; vegetables with soy sauce; plain steamed rice; herb relish; fruits in season; a broth-based soup; and perhaps more unsweetened gree tea. Typical dishes include tempura (batter-fried shrimp) and *aborakge* (fried soybean curd). *Sukiyaka,* a mixture of sautéed beef and vegetables served with soy sauce, is as American as chow mein. Soybean oil is the main cooking fat.

Italian Food Patterns
Basis of Traditional Food Patterns

The sharing of food and companionship is an important part of Italian life. Meals are associated with much warmth and fellowship, and special occasions are marked by the sharing of food with families and friends. Leisurely meals are customary, with a light breakfast, dinner in the middle of the day, and a small evening meal. Bread and pasta are basic Italian foods. On religious fast days, such as Fridays, Lent, and the period of Advent before Christmas, pasta is prepared with meatless sauces or with fish.

General Food Use Habits

Traditional food use habits include these:

1. **Milk.** Although milk is seldom used alone as a beverage, it is frequently consumed with coffee in a half and half mixture. Cheese, however, is a favorite food. Parmesan and Romano are hard, grating cheeses used in cooking; ricotta and mozzarella are two soft cheeses used in cooking or with bread.

2. **Meat.** Chicken baked with oil or in tomato sauce is often used. Beef and veal are eaten as meatballs, meat loaf, cutlets, chops, stews, and roasts. Roasted or fried Italian pork sausage is common. A number of Italian cold cuts are famous: *salami, mortadella* (bologna-type), *coppa* (peppered), and *prosciutto* (Italian cured ham). Many kinds of fish are used. Fresh fish are preferred, but some canned fish such as tuna, sardines, anchovies, and special salted codfish are also used. Some characteristic dishes are chicken browned in olive oil, then simmered in a sauce flavored with wine and herbs. Italian meatballs are served with spaghetti, and dry, salted codfish, soaked several days and browned in olive oil, is simmered with tomato sauce and herbs.

3. **Vegetables.** Favorite vegetables include zucchini and other types of squash, broccoli, spinach, eggplant, salad greens, green beans, peppers, and tomatoes. The latter are used in many ways—in sauces, either whole or as paste, or pureed. Vegetables are usually cooked in water, drained, and seasoned with olive oil or with oil and vinegar. A combination of salad greens, with simple dressing of olive oil, vinegar, garlic, salt, and pepper, is called *insalata.*

4. **Fruits.** Fresh fruit in season is eaten for dessert.

5. **Bread and cereals.** Bread is present at every Italian meal as a highly regarded principal food. It is made into loaves of many shapes, each one characteristic of a different Italian province. All breads are made of wheat flour and are white, crusty, and substantial. Some rice and cornmeal are used in special dishes. For example, *polenta* is a thick, yellow cornmeal mush, sometimes made into a casserole with sausage, tomato sauce, and cheese. *Pasta* in many forms and shapes is a basic food item. This term is used for a variety of wheat products in forms such as spaghetti, macaroni, and noodles. Pasta is served in many ways. Spaghetti is commonly used with a characteristic tomato sauce and cheese or with meatballs or fish. Special dishes of pasta filled with meat mixtures—ravioli, lasagna, manicotti, tortellini, cannelloni—are served on holidays. A dry red or white wine is usually served also.

6. **Soups.** Thick soups often serve as a main food for lighter meals. *Mine-strone* is made with vegetables, chickpeas, and pasta. Often a substantial bean soup is used.

7. **Seasonings and cooking method.** Herbs and spices characteristically used in Italian dishes include oregano, rosemary, basil, saffron, parsley, and nutmeg. Garlic is used often, as are wine, olive oil, tomato puree, salt pork, and cheese. The basic cooking process for main dishes is the initial browning of the vegetables and seasonings in olive oil, adding meat or fish for browning also, then covering with liquid such as wine, tomato sauce, or broth, and simmering slowly on low heat for several hours.

Greek Food Patterns
Basis of Traditional Food Patterns

In the close-knit, traditionally organized life of the Greek family, food and ceremonial aspects of meals are primary values. In many homes the meal is a family ritual. A blessing is said or sung, and hospitality is extended to guests. Everyday meals are simple, but holidays are occasions for serving a great variety of delicacies. Bread is always the center of every meal—indeed it *is* the meal—with other foods considered accompaniments to it, bread being eaten between bites of other food. During religious observances such as Lent, there are fast days of meatless meals with large use of vegetables.

General Food Use Habits

Traditional food use habits include these:

1. **Milk.** A relatively small amount of milk is used as a beverage by adults, who usually take this food in the form of yogurt. Children drink hot boiled milk sweetened with sugar. Cheese is a favorite food, however. Varieties include *feta*, a special white cheese made from goat's milk and preserved in brine, and two hard salty cheeses, *caceri* and *cephalotyri.*

2. **Meat.** Lamb is the favorite meat. Little beef and some pork and chicken are eaten. Frequent use is made of organ meats and fresh fish. Eggs are sometimes used as a main dish, but not at breakfast.

3. **Vegetables.** A variety of vegetables are eaten, usually cooked until soft and seasoned with meat broth or tomato with onions, olive oil, and parsley. They are often the main dish. Large amounts are consumed, with fresh ones preferred. Combination salad of thinly cut raw vegetables with a simple dressing of olive oil and vinegar or lemon juice is a frequent choice. Many legumes (beans, peas, lentils, and chickpeas) are eaten. Often a meal consists of cooked dried beans served with olives and pickles. A characteristic dish is *dolmathes,* a meat and rice mixture rolled in cabbage or grapevine leaves, steamed, and served with egg sauce.

4. **Fruits.** Large amounts of fruit are eaten fresh in season. Peeled raw fruit is an everyday dessert.

5. **Bread and cereals.** Bread is made of plain wheat flour, water, salt, and yeast. An indispensable part of every meal, it is preferred plain without butter, jam, or jelly. Dark breads are used by some families. Wheat products such as noodles, macaroni, and spaghetti may be used plain or with meat and tomato sauce. Rice is commonly served. A characteristic rice dish is *pilaf,* which is rice, first browned in butter, then covered with broth or water, and simmered until the liquid is absorbed.

6. **Desserts.** Other than raw fruit, special desserts are used in holiday meals. Such a characteristic dessert is *baklava*, made with many layers of paper-thin pastry, brushed with butter, sprinkled with nuts, sugar, and spices, cut in diamond shapes, baked, and served with honey.

Social Organization

The study of human group behavior reveals numerous activities, processes, and structures by which social life goes on. Human behavior can be understood in terms of social phenomena and problems—social change, urbanism, rural life, the family, the community, race relations, delinquency, drugs and crime. These social problems carry nutritional implications. Two aspects of social organization concern health professionals: class structure and value systems.

Class Structure

The structure of a society is largely formed by groupings according to such factors as economic status, education, residence, occupation, or family. Within a given society many of these groups exist, and their values and habits vary widely. Subgroups develop on the basis of region, religion, age, sex, social class, health concerns, occupation, or political affiliation. Within these subgroups there may be still smaller groupings with distinct attitudes, values, habits. A person may be a member of several subcultural groups, each of which influences values, attitudes, and habits. Our democratic philosophy, as well as the humanitarian ideals on which the health professions have been nurtured, combine to make the reality of class differences difficult for us to accept. Yet differences do exist, and they probably influence our approach to clients and patients, relationships with them, and the outcome of these encounters more than we may be aware of or care to admit.

Value Systems

A society's value systems develop as a result of its history and heritage. Traditionally four basic premises have influenced American value systems and have affected attitudes toward health care and food habits:

1. **Equality.** A high value on equality leads health workers to establish quality health care standards for all people, although in reality this does not always work out.

2. **Sociality.** The high respect accorded to a social nature builds peer group pressures and status seeking within social groups. Foods may be accepted because they are high status foods or rejected because they are low-prestige foods. Even the use of dietary supplements has been associated with the desire for prestige, along with health concerns.[6]

3. **Success.** The esteem in which success is held often leads persons to measure life in terms of competitive superlatives. They want to set the best table, provide the most abundant supply of food for the family, or have the biggest eater and the fattest baby of any in the neighborhood.

4. **Change.** The value placed on change leads families and individuals to seek constant variety in their diets, to be geared for action, to be a mobile society, and to seek quick-cooking, conveniently prepared foods. In response to such marketing demands, food technologists continually produce an array of new food products.

Social Influences on Food Habits

Food and Social Factors

Food habits in any setting are highly socialized. These habits perform significant social functions, some of which may not always be evident.

Social Relationships

Food is a symbol of social acceptance, warmth, and friendliness. People tend to accept food more readily from those persons they view as friends or allies. They accept advice about food from persons they consider to be authorities or with whom they can feel warm relationships. Persons tend to distrust food given them by strangers and outsiders. Emotional feelings about persons are transferred to their food. The more alien the authority figure, the more such persons are considered to be unconcerned, and their food suggestions will be considered outlandish or perhaps even harmful.

Food in Family Relationships

Food habits that are most closely associated with family sentiments are the most tenacious throughout life. Long into adulthood, certain foods trigger a flood of childhood memories and are valued for reasons totally apart from any nutritional value. Strong religious factors associated with food tend to have their origin and reinforcement within the family meal circle. Also, family income, community sources of food, and market conditions influence food habits and ultimately food choices. Persons eat foods that are readily available to them and that they have the money to buy.

Psychologic Influences on Food Habits

Social Psychology: Understanding Dietary Patterns

Social psychology is concerned with (1) social interaction in terms of its effect on individual behavior and (2) the social influences of individual perception, motivation, and action. How does a particular individual perceive a given situation? What basic needs motivate action and response? What social factors surround a particular action? Issues of particular concern include the effect of culture on personality, the socialization of the child, differences in individuals in groups, group dynamics, group attitudes and opinions, and leadership. The methods of social psychology have made important contributions to nutrition, medicine, nursing, and allied health care, especially to problems of human behavior under stress.

Food and Psychologic Factors

Individual behavior patterns, including those related to eating, result from many interrelated psychosocial influences. Factors that are particularly pertinent to the shaping of food habits are motivation and perception.

Motivation

People are not the same the world over. Those of differing cultures are not motivated by the same needs and goals. Even primary biologic drives such as hunger and sex are modified in their interpretation, expression, and fulfillment by many cultural, social, and personal influences. The kinds of food sought, prized, or accepted by one individual at one time and place are rejected by another living in different circumstances. For persons existing in a state of basic hunger or semistarvation, food is the whole perception and motivation. Such a person thinks, talks, and dreams about food. Under less severe circumstances, however, the concern for food may be on a relatively abstract level and may involve symbolism that is associated with other needs. For example, Maslow's classic hierarchy of human needs illustrates these human strivings.[7] He described five levels of need that operate in turn, each building on the prior ones:

1. **Basic physiologic needs.** Hunger, thirst.
2. **Safety needs.** Physical comfort, security, protection.
3. **"Belongingness" needs.** Love, giving and receiving affection.
4. **Recognition needs.** Self-esteem, status, sense of self-worth, strength, self-confidence, capability, adequacy.
5. **Self-actualization needs.** Self-fulfillment, creative growth.

Of course, these levels of need overlap and vary with time and circumstance. But we can use them to help us understand the needs of our clients and plan care accordingly.

Perception

To make sense out of an otherwise chaotic assortment of impressions, we perceive our environment in different ways. These perceptions enable us to live in an environment that feels relatively stable. However, perception also limits understanding. Every phenomenon that the outer world offers is filtered through our own social and personal lenses. In every experience of our lives, we perceive a blend of three facets: (1) the *external reality,* (2) the *message* of the stimulus that is conveyed by the nervous system to the integrative centers of the brain where thinking and evaluation go on, and (3) the *interpretation* that we put on every part of our personal experience. A host of subjective elements—hunger, thirst, hate, fear, love, self-interest, values, temperament—influence our response to the outer world's phenomena.

Personal Learning

On the basis, then, of personal motivation and perception, personal learning takes place. In the final analysis, all persons must learn in their own way according to their own needs. It is this very personal human dimension that makes a health professional's work profound. We cannot impose on our clients and patients mechanical routines of sanitation, hygiene, and nutrition born of our own antiseptic cultural values. Patients will not carry them out if they are presented in this way. Glib answers fail. Persons learn because they have an urgent need to know. They learn because their curiosity is aroused. They learn because they want to make meaning out of their lives. They learn by exploring, making mistakes and correcting them, testing, verifying. *All of these things individuals must do for themselves.* This is true of everyone's learning. It is true of the learning we desire for our patients. It is true of our own learning. The process cannot be changed or shortened or avoided.

Food Misinformation

Unscientific statements about food and nutrition often mislead the public and contribute to poor food habits. Persons have often surrounded their cultural eating habits with myths of various sorts.[8] But other more damaging false information may come from folklore, or it may be built on half-truths, innuendos, and outright deception. In contrast, nutritional science is a growing body of knowledge built on vigorously examined scientific evidence. Concern for food safety and wholesomeness clearly existed long before the scientific method was known. Nonetheless, in this rapidly changing world, it

Current Confusions Influencing Food Habits

is only on the sound basis of scientific knowledge that we may make wise food choices and recognize misinformation as such.

Types of Food Faddist Claims

Food faddists make exaggerated claims for certain types of food. These claims fall into four basic groups: (1) certain foods will cure specific conditions, (2) certain foods are harmful and should be avoided, (3) special food combinations are very effective as reducing diets or have special therapeutic effects, and (4) only **"natural" foods** can meet body needs and prevent disease. But these claims contain basic error and inherent dangers to health.

"Natural" food
Popular term for food said to be "as grown" without any food additives.

Basic error. Examine these claims carefully. You will notice that each one focuses on foods per se, not on their specific chemical components, the *nutrients,* which are the actual physiologic agents of life and health. Certain individuals may be allergic or intolerant to particular foods and should obviously avoid them. Also, certain foods may have particularly high concentrations of certain nutrients and therefore are good sources of such nutrients. But it is the *nutrients,* not any specific foods, that have specific functions in the body. Each of these nutrients may be found in a number of different foods. Remember, persons require specific nutrients, never specific foods.

Dangers of food fads. Why should the health worker be concerned about food faddism and its effect on food habits? What harm may it do? Essentially food fads involve four basic dangers:

1. **Dangers to health.** Responsibility for one's health is fundamental. However, self-diagnosis and self-treatment can be dangerous, especially where health problems are concerned. When such action is based on questionable sources, the dangers are multiplied. By following such a course, a person with a real illness may fail to seek appropriate medical care. Many ill and anxious patients have been misled by fraudulent claims of cures and postponed effective therapy.

2. **Money spent needlessly.** Some of these foods and supplements used by faddists are harmless, but most are expensive. In one recent year alone, the health food industry claimed $2.6 billion spent by consumers on nutrition supplements.[9] Money spent for needless food and supplements is wasted. When dollars are scarce, the family may neglect to buy foods that will fill its basic needs just to purchase a "guaranteed cure."

3. **Lack of knowledge of scientific progress.** Misinformation hinders the development of society along lines opened up by scientific progress. Superstitions that are perpetuated can counteract sound health teaching.

4. **Distrust of food market.** Our food environment is rapidly changing. We need intelligent concern and rational approaches to meet nutritional needs. A wise course is to select a variety of primary foods "closer to the source"—having minimal processing—and adding a few carefully selected processed items for specific uses. Blanket erroneous teaching concerning food and health breeds public suspicion and distrust of the common food products that are responsible for the many varied standard quality food items. Each food product must be evaluated on its own merits in terms of individual needs—nutrient contribution, aesthetic values, and cost.

Vulnerable Groups

Food fads appeal especially to certain groups of people with particular needs and concerns:

1. **Older persons.** Fear of changes that come with aging leads many middle-aged persons to grasp at exaggerated claims that some product will restore vigor. Older persons in pain and discomfort, perhaps facing chronic illness, reach out for the "special supplement" that promises a sure cure. Desperately ill and lonely individuals are easy prey for a cruel hoax.

2. **Young people.** Figure-conscious girls and muscle-minded boys frequently respond to advertisements that offer a crash program to attain the perfect body. Young people, those who are lonely or have exaggerated ideas of glamour, hope to achieve peer-group acceptance by these means.

3. **Obese persons.** One of the most disturbing personal concerns and frustrating health problems in America is obesity. Obese persons, faced with a bewildering barrage of propaganda advocating diets, pills, candies, wafers, and devices, are likely to succumb to fads.

4. **Athletes and coaches.** This group is a prime target for those who push miracle supplements. Always looking for the added something to give them the "competitive edge," athletes tend to fall prey to nutrition myths and hoaxes.

5. **Entertainers.** Persons in the public eye, such as entertainers, are often prey to those who make false claims that certain foods, drugs, or dietary combinations will enable them to attain the physical appearance and strength on which their careers depend.

These various groups are vulnerable for obvious reasons. But there seems to be no segment of the population that is completely free from food faddism's appeal. Particularly in metropolitan areas, large groups of persons present a constant array of misinformation that hinders the efforts of members of the legitimate health professions to raise the community's standards in nutrition.

What is the answer?

What can be done to counter food habits built on food faddism, misinformation, or outright deception? What can workers in the health professions do? What *should* they do? Several actions merit consideration:

1. **Assess your own attitudes and habits.** We cannot counsel or teach other persons until we have first examined our own position. Instruction based on personal conviction, practice, and enthusiasm will achieve far more than teaching that says, in effect, "Do as I say, not as I do."

2. **Use reliable sources.** Two types of background knowledge are vital: (1) knowledge of the product and the persons behind it, and (2) knowledge of human nutritional physiology and the scientific method of problem solving.

3. **Recognize human needs.** Consider the emotional needs that are symbolically fulfilled by the eating of foods and by the rituals surrounding the process. Respect these needs. Everyone has them. They are a part of life. Welcome the positive power that food and eating rituals possess in fulfilling these needs. Use this knowledge wisely and work it into the nutrition program. Food should not be disparaged as a mere "crutch." Even when there is reason to believe that the client is using food as a crutch for emotional adjustment, the value of such an adjustment must be considered. A wise

teacher of mine once put it well: "We must avoid 'breaking crutches' without providing alternative support."

4. **Be alert to community opportunities.** Grasp any opportunity that arises to present sound health information to groups or individuals, formally or informally. Learn about available community resources, such as local and state university agricultural extension services; volunteer agencies; clinic and hospital facilities; federal, state, county, and city public health departments; and professional health organizations. Develop communication skills. Avoid monotony. Use a well-disciplined imagination. Without these things, the message will not convince.

5. **Think scientifically.** We can teach even very young children to use the problem-solving approach to everyday situations. Children are naturally curious. With their eternal *why,* they often seek evidence to support statements they hear. Far too often our system of education fails to develop this natural spirit of inquiry. We need to teach them, and ourselves, the value of asking three simple but significant questions: "What do you mean?" "How do you know?" and "What is your evidence?"

6. **Know responsible authorities.** The Food and Drug Administration (FDA) has the legal responsibility of controlling the quality and safety of food and drug products marketed in the United States. But this is a monumental task and needs the help of vigilant consumers. Other governmental, professional, and private organizations can provide additional resources.

Influence of Food Safety Concerns on Food Habits

A number of chemicals have been developed by the agricultural and food processing industries to increase and preserve our food supply. They have also influenced consumers' beliefs about food chemicals and their subsequent food choices.[10] They have rapidly changed the character of America's present food market and its environment into a complex "feeding web," which has increasingly raised issues about nutritional ecology. Critics voice concerns about the effects these rapid changes have brought to our overall food environment and food habits.

Intentional Food Additives

In the past few decades chemicals intentionally added to foods have increased in our food supply, with both positive and negative results. True, our present variety of marketed food items would be impossible without them.[11] But they have also raised many health concerns and problems. They have been a major factor in the rapid evolution of the corner grocery store into the giant, fiercely competitive supermarket chains. These changes that have swept the food-marketing system during the last 30 years are rooted in a deeper social revolution and scientific advance.

Reasons for this development and use of food additives include:

1. **Population growth** requires increased food production.

2. **Publicized scientific discoveries** have increased consumers' awareness of nutritional needs and the values of a well-balanced diet. We have all benefitted from basic specific foods that have been **enriched** or **fortified** to help supply these needs.

3. **Desire for variety** in foods and creativity in cooking has increased. Foods from local and distant places, both fresh and processed, provide great variety and choice.

Enriched
Food with added nutrients, usually to replace some of those lost in processing, such as addition of several B vitamins and iron to white flour.

Fortified
Food with added nutrients to make it a comparable substitute for a similar regular food, such as vitamin A fortified margarine used for butter; or food having a needed nutrient added, such as vitamin D fortified milk.

4. **Complexity of family life** and the increasing number of working women, now about half of the total work force, have created a need for convenience foods that require little or no preparation.

5. **Safe, quality food** is a public desire. Americans are more health-conscious and aware that their health depends on an adequate supply of fresh and properly preserved foods. Consumer efforts to buy quality foods are backed by laws governing food production, processing, and sale. However, the rapidly changing food environment requires constant reevaluation of these regulations to ensure their adequacy to meet needs.

Food additives serve a variety of purposes in modern food products. They (1) add specific nutrients to enrich products; (2) produce uniform properties such as color, flavor, aroma, texture, and general appearance; (3) standardize many functional properties, such as thickening or stabilization; (4) preserve foods by preventing oxidation; and (5) control acidity or alkalinity to improve flavor, texture, and the cooked product. Some examples of intentional food additives and their functions in certain food products are given in Table 9-2.

Problems with Food Additives

However, despite their useful purposes, food additives have created problems. These problems are of increasing concern to consumers and producers. They have accrued over time, based on the history of food additive development and use.

Food Additives Amendment and Delany Clause. The Food Additives Amendment of the Federal Food, Drug, and Cosmetic Act of 1938 was passed by Congress on September 7, 1958. This admendment, which took effect on March 6, 1960, completely altered the U.S. government's method of regulating the use of additives in food. For the first time, the law provided that no additive could be used in food unless the FDA, after careful review of all the test data, agreed that the compound was safe at the intended levels of use. An exception was made for all additives in use at the time, which, because of years of use without bad effects reported, were "generally recognized as safe" (GRAS) by experts in the field. This approach was a compromise between giving blanket approval to all additives then in use or banning all untested additives until several years of laboratory safety studies could be conducted. The now famous Delany Clause was attached in the final hours of congressional debate on the legislation. This clause to the amendment states that "no additive shall be deemed safe if it is found to induce cancer when ingested by man or animal, or it is found, after tests which are appropriate for the evaluation of the safety of food additives, to induce cancer in man or animal."

GRAS list. The result of this amendment was to establish what is now known as the GRAS list, large numbers of food additives "generally recognized as safe" but not having undergone rigid testing requirements. This list included thousands of common food additives, with such diverse items as salt, sugar, baking powder, spices, flavorings, vitamins, minerals, preservatives, emulsifiers, and nonnutritive sweeteners. Some of these items were restricted to uses in certain foods and at certain levels, but most were limited

Table 9-2
Some Examples of
Intentional Food
Additives

Function	Chemical compound	Common food uses
Acids, alkalis, buffers	Sodium bicarbonate Tartaric acid	Baking powder Fruit sherbets Cheese spreads
Antibiotics	Chlortetracycline	Dip for dressed poultry
Anticaking agents	Aluminum calcium silicate	Table salt
Antimycotics	Calcium propionate Sodium propionate Sorbic acid	Bread Bread Cheese
Antioxidants	Butylated hydroxyanisole (BHA) Butylated hydroxytoluene (BHT)	Fats Fats
Bleaching agents	Benzoyl peroxide Chlorine dioxide Oxides of nitrogen	Wheat flour
Color preservative	Sodium benzoate	Green peas Maraschino cherries
Coloring agents	Annatto Carotene	Butter, margarine
Emulsifiers	Lecithin Monoglycerides and diglycerides Propylene glycol alginate	Bakery goods Dairy products Confections
Flavoring agents	Amyl acetate Benzaldehyde Methyl salicylate Essential oils; natural extractives Monosodium glutamate	Soft drinks Bakery goods Candy; ice cream Canned meats
Nonnutritive sweeteners	Saccharin Aspartame	Diet packed canned fruit Low-calorie soft drinks
Nutrient supplements	Potassium iodide Vitamin C Vitamin D Vitamin A B vitamins, iron	Iodized salt Fruit juices Milk Margarine Bread and cereal
Sequestrants	Sodium citrate Calcium pyrophosphoric acid	Dairy products
Stabilizers and thickeners	Pectin Vegetable gums (carob bean, carrageenan, guar) Gelatin Agar-agar	Jellies Dairy desserts and chocolate milk Confections "Low-calorie" salad dressings
Yeast foods and dough conditioners	Ammonium chloride Calcium sulfate Calcium phosphate	Bread, rolls

only to their "intended use" and to "good manufacturing practice"—a vague regulation at best.

Problems, however, have existed with the GRAS list. First, from the beginning of food additive use, there has been uncertainty about how many GRAS items there are, and only with computer aid was this large list finally tabulated.[12] Second, in the years since the GRAS list was formulated, two developments have had direct bearing on the soundness of the original GRAS concept: (1) we know much more now about toxicity testing, so relying merely on a lack of reported human adverse effect as the sole measure of safety is inadequate; and (2) we see the demands of modern technology increase the uses of certain GRAS items well beyond our original exposure patterns. In short, the total food environment has changed radically, creating new problems.

Need for Review

As a result, in 1977 the U.S. government directed the FDA to reevaluate all the items on the GRAS list for safety and this large task continues. Also, the Delany Clause is again being debated. Many scientists and government officials now consider it to be too rigid. It is seen as an example of congressional understanding during the 1950s that there was no way to tell safe levels for carcinogens. Now the FDA is moving toward a policy of *risk assessment*.[13] The options being considered by the FDA include what is called *constituent policy*, which proposes two requirements for an additive to trigger the Delany Clause: (1) the additive *as such* would have to be carcinogenic in tests, not just the particular constituents of it; and (2) if the constituent *is* carcinogenic, it would have to be judged a significant risk by a quantified risk assessment test. Under such an agreement, the FDA could reinstate some substances now banned, such as yellow food dye No. 1 and red food colors Nos. 10, 11, 12, and 13. But how do we assess a degree of risk? This is particularly perplexing in the area of human health, where errors of judgment can result in tragedy. This risk-benefit debate goes on.

Incidental Food Additives: Pesticides

Modern American agriculture uses a number of chemicals to control a wide variety of insects, kill weeds, control plant disease, control maturation of fruit and stop fruit from dropping prematurely, make leaves drop so that harvesting will be easier, make seeds sprout, keep seeds from rotting before they sprout, increase yield, and improve marketing qualities. Concerns and confusion continue about pesticide *residues* in food.[14] Farm workers, consumers, and the general public have increasing questions about the accumulating effects of current levels of agricultural chemicals used to increase needed food production. These practices have led to our present "pesticide dilemma," because agricultural chemicals bring hazards and gains. Today the FDA directs a pesticide control program in two phases: (1) requirement for initial approval and (2) continued surveillance.

Control Agencies

Numerous government and private agencies and professional organizations are charged with the responsibility of ensuring the safety and high quality of our food supply. Concerned groups in the U.S. Department of Health and Human Services (HHS) are the FDA and the Public Health Service (PHS). In the U.S. Department of Agriculture are the Agricultural Research Service and the Consumer Marketing Service. Also protecting the consumer are the Federal Trade Commission and the National Bureau of Standards.

FDA. The broad work of the FDA serves as an example of the U.S. government's effort to protect and control our food supply. In essence, the FDA is a law enforcement agency charged by Congress to ensure, among other things, that the food supply is safe, pure, and wholesome. The agency enforces federal regulations through a number of basic projects related to food safety. This work includes activities such as food sanitation and quality control, control of chemical contaminants and pesticides, control of food additives, regulating movement of food across state lines, nutrition and nutrition labeling of foods, safety of food service, meat, and milk. Methods of enforcement available to FDA are recalls, seizure, injunction, and prosecution. The use of recalls is the most common method, with seizures of contaminated foods second.

Food labeling. Nutritional labeling is currently a controversial area, and the legislative debate is increasing.[15] This is especially true concerning FDA proposals for health claims on product labels (see Issues and Answers on p. 224). Although the FDA passed basic "Truth-in-Packaging" regulations in the mid-1960s, many persons are concerned that nutritional labeling is inadequate. Sodium leads the list of labeling topics, closely followed by macronutrients, cholesterol, saturated fat, and additives such as sulfiting agents, to which some persons are dangerously allergic. The FDA is reviewing different approaches to labeling to develop a system that adequately describes the food but is not overwhelming or incomprehensible to the consumer.

Food standards. Section 401 of the Federal Food, Drug, and Cosmetic Act was designed to "promote honesty and fair dealing in the interest of consumers." The FDA has the responsibility for establishing and enforcing uniform national food standards. The label must indicate these standards and tell what is in the package. It must not be false or misleading in any particular.

1. **Standards of identity.** Reference standards have been set for a number of common foods. On such identified foods, there is no requirement to list the ingredients, since they are named in the standard. For many less common ones with no established standard of identity, the label must list the ingredients in the order of their predominance in the food product.
2. **Standards of quality.** For a number of canned fruits and vegetables, minimum standards have been set concerning such properties as tenderness, color, and freedom of defects. If the food is safe to eat but does not meet these standards, it must specifically indicate this on the label.
3. **Standards of fill of container.** For many foods, standards have been set to protect the consumer against slack fillings. These are specially necessary for products that settle after filling, such as cereals, or products that consist of a number of pieces packed in liquid, such as fruit cocktail.
4. **Standards for enriched products.** Standards are set for enrichment of flour, cereals, margarine, and other foods with specific quantities of vi-

tamins and minerals. Any product labeled "enriched" or "fortified" must contain precisely the specified amount of added nutrients.

Consumer education. The FDA Division of Consumer Education conducts an active program of consumer protection through education and public information. Special attention is given to nutrition misinformation. Sound materials are prepared and distributed to individuals and students and community groups. Consumer specialists work through all FDA district offices.

Food contamination in disasters. In cooperation with local and state officials, the FDA inspects food that has been damaged by flood, hurricane, fire, or other disasters and removes contaminated items from the market. USDA commodities are made available in such disasters for community use.[16]

Scientific research. As a basis for all its activities in a world of burgeoning technology, FDA scientists continually provide background evaluation through their own research (Figure 9-2). Precise policies have varied with different administrators, and bureaucratic entanglements sometimes occur. Nevertheless, the declared intent of persons in charge of FDA is that food safety must be interpreted not only in the traditional sense that food must be free from danger, but also in the more positive sense that its nutritional value must be clear. It is reasonable for consumers to insist that additives introducing possible hazard without adding any benefits to the food must be avoided. An attempt is being made to develop nutritional guidelines for a variety of food products, including formulated main dishes, new foods such as meat analogs, foods having high malnutrition risks, fruit juices and fruit drinks, and snack foods. This is a broad jump from the former attitude of a purely regulatory function and should go far in meeting changing needs in these changing times.

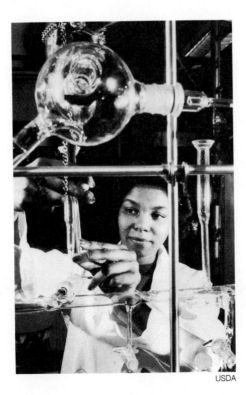

USDA

Figure 9-2
Research in food chemistry. A chemist in the U.S. Department of Agriculture's Agricultural Research Service makes an adjustment on a molecular still used in a project to aid in the manufacture of dry milk.

Changes in American Food Habits

Determinants of Food Choice
Basic Influences

Clearly some of the basic and universal determinants of food choice focus on physical, social, and physiologic factors (Table 9-3). We have discussed the broad areas of culture, sociology, and psychology in terms of their influence on food habits. Attempting to change our own eating patterns or helping our clients to make needed changes is difficult. It requires a sensitive, flexible understanding of the complex factors that influence choices persons make when they eat what they do.

Conservative and Dynamic Influences

Two sets of factors—conservative and dynamic—influence our eating habits in opposite directions. The group processes of ethnic patterns and regional and cultural habits precondition our food choices and exert a conservative influence to resist change. On the other hand, new dynamic factors arise when we no longer have to spend most of our time getting food. We are thrust in the direction of diversity and change and also into dissatisfaction with our current situation. These new factors include the following:

1. **Wealth.** A sufficient income affords us increasing amounts of both choice and time and a desire to try the unusual.
2. **Technology.** Our expanding technology has vastly increased what is available to us from our food supply.
3. **Environment.** We are reassessing our relationship with our world, realizing that we cannot afford to endlessly exploit it.
4. **Vision.** Mass media, especially television, and greatly improved communications have made us aware of multiple options, changed our expectations, and developed a new sense of perspective.

Changing American Food Patterns

The stereotype of the all-American family with parents and two children eating three meals a day with a ban on snacking is no longer the common pattern. In the past two decades we have undergone far-reaching changes in our way of living and subsequently in our food patterns.

Table 9-3

Factors Determining Food Choices

Physical factors	Social factors	Physiologic factors
Food supply available	Advertising	Allergy
Food technology	Culture	Disability
Geography, agriculture, distribution	Education, nutrition and general	Health-disease status
Personal economics, income	Political and economic policies	Heredity
Sanitation housing	Religion and social custom	Personal food acceptance
Season, climate		Needs, energy, or nutrients
Storage and cooking facilities	Social class, role	Therapeutic diets
	Social problems, poverty, or alcoholism	

Households

Changes evident in the turbulent 1970s and continuing through the 1980s have had far-reaching effects on our daily lives. For example, between 1970 and 1980 there was a 25% increase (or 15.7 million) in the number of American households. Most of these are groups of unrelated persons or persons living alone, an increase of 73%, whereas family households have climbed only 13%. The average size of the American household is now 2.75 persons instead of the 3.17 in 1970.[17] These trends indicate a very significant change in the American social picture, sometimes lamented as the "deterioration" of the family but more appropriately seen as one facet of a dynamic and rapidly changing society.

Working Women

The number of women in the work force continues to increase rapidly, a trend that is not likely to reverse. This increase reflects the increased educational opportunities for women: 51% of college undergraduates are now women. Women account for 30% of the enrollment in law schools, 25% in medical schools, 30% in business schools, and 12% in technical graduate schools. This phenomenon of working women is not restricted to one social, economic, or ethnic group. It is a widespread societal change, bringing with it changes in the functioning of the family. Working mothers rely on food items and cooking methods that save time, space, and labor.

There has been a 50% increase in single-person households in the last 5 years.

Meal Times

There has been a dramatic increase in flexibility about when we eat and whether it is with our families or not. Midmorning snacks are commonplace, a midafternoon snack similar to a European "tea" is popular, with snacks over television and a midnight refrigerator raid at the day's end. Nutrition hardliners from the old school decry this snacking behavior, but Americans are moving toward a concept of "balanced days" rather than "balanced meals." Studies indicate that frequent, small meals are better for the body than three larger meals a day, depending on what snacks are included (see the box on p. 221).

Americans are increasing the number of times a day they eat, sometimes having as many as 11 "eating occasions" a day, a pattern recently termed "grazing."

Health and Fitness

Americans' interest in physical fitness continues. This has taken primarily two forms. First, there is a more general nutrition awareness. Americans are becoming increasingly aware of the nutritional content of their foods and are demanding a wholesome, safe, nutritious food supply. This is reflected in the interest in **"natural"** or **"organic"** foods and many similar items. Second, there is more attention to "weight watching." More than half of the American population at any given time is on a weight-reducing diet. Our weight consciousness has affected the foods we choose to eat, and foods perceived as lower in calories, including the new lines of "light" foods, are popular.

"Organic" food
Popular term for food said to be grown without pesticides.

Economy

More and more Americans are economizing on food. Many supermarket shoppers are changing their diets primarily to save money. Consumers are stocking up on bargains and cutting back on expensive "convenience" foods. They are buying items in larger packages and in bulk and doing much less "store hopping" for bargains, staying with the store they consider to have the lowest overall prices. There has been a decline in brand loyalty and an upsurge in the purchase of generic products. Shoppers are using labels for both unit pricing and calorie-counting.

Gourmet Cooking

The demand for gourmet foods has risen, and food specialty shops have sprung up in every shopping center. Gourmet cooking has become a popular hobby, and entertaining guests at home over a gourmet meal has been called a "new elitism." This phenomenon parallels the general trend toward meals that are easy to fix, take little time, and fulfill the consumers' nutritional needs. As a result, two new food industry markets have developed: (1) nutritional products and (2) entertainment products or fun foods.

Fast Foods

Over the past decade, sales of fast food products rose 300%, from $6.5 billion to $23 billion per year, and are still rising. Some 90% of all Americans eat in a fast-food restaurant at least once a year, and about 10% eat fast foods more than five times a week.[18] As family income rises, so does the consumption of fast foods, especially among the upper middle class. This trend is continuing.

> Over the last decade sales of fast-food products rose 300%, from $6.5 billion to $23 billion per year.

Report from Industry

Profits in the food industry are rising. Cereal products are selling better, as more people see it as a nutritious item. Sales of frozen vegetables, low-fat and nonfat milk, cheese, yogurt, and coffee, especially decaffeinated varieties, are rising. Sales of whole milk and canned goods have dropped, and sales of white bread have dropped about 45% in the last 20 years. There has been a spectacular rise in ethnic packaged foods and in fast food outlets. The fitness movement has spawned a new line of "light" foods, from beer to pizza. There are more pure fruit juices, yogurts, and decaffeinated products, including soft drinks. There are many new spreads, sauces, processed meats, and snack foods; leading the list of popular snack foods is tortilla chips. Nuts and dried fruit are popular. Also, we are seeing a variety of new breads and brands of bottled water. And more and more new foods are being developed specifically for preparing in microwave ovens.

To Probe Further

Snacking: The All-American Food Habit

The United States market for snacks continues to grow at a rate of more than 10% a year. People are buying more chips, crackers, and cookies. College students show preferences for soft drinks, candies, gum, and fresh fruit as snacks, followed by bakery items, milk, and both corn and potato chips.

The old adage is that snacking "ruins your appetite." And we certainly consume far too many soft drinks. But is snacking all bad?

Reports indicate that adolescents get more complete nutrition with increases in snacks—those who snack more show higher percentages in the "adequate" range of the recommended daily allowances of nutritional needs. Surveys also show that many persons snack on foods that aren't "empty extras," but essential contributions to nutritional adequacy. These snack items include cheese, poultry, eggs, bread, crackers, and fruit.

Snacking is clearly a significant component of food behavior. In fact, studies have indicated that adolescent snacks contribute as much nutrition as do their meals, and that snacking frequency may range upward to as many as seven eating occasions per day. Health workers need to remain aware of this food behavior. Rather than rule against the practice of snacking, we need to actively promote snack foods that enhance nutritional well-being.

REFERENCES

Bigler-Doughten S and Jenkins RM: Adolescent snacks: nutrient density and nutritional contribution to total intake, J Am Diet Assoc 87(12):1678, 1987.

McCoy H and others: Snacking patterns and nutrient density of snacks consumed by Southern girls, J Nutr Educ 18(2):61, 1986.

Story M and Resnick MD: Adolescents' views on food and nutrition, J Nutr Educ 18(4):188, 1986.

To Sum Up

We all grow up and live our lives in a social context. We each inherit at least one cultural background and live in our particular society's social structure, complete with food habits and attitudes about eating. It is from a social perspective that we can best examine changes in food habits. We need to understand the effects on health that are associated with major social and economic shifts. We also need to understand current social forces to best help persons make new dietary changes that will benefit their health. We must meet concerns about food misinformation and food safety.

America is changing a number of its food patterns. We increasingly rely on food technology in our fast, complex life. More women are working, households are getting smaller, more and more persons are living alone, and our meal patterns are different. We search for less fancy, lower-cost food items, and also creative gourmet cooking. In general, we are more nutrition and health conscious. Fast food outlets and snacking are social habits here to stay.

Questions for Review

1. What is the meaning of culture? How does it affect our food patterns?
2. What are social and psychologic factors that influence our food habits? Give examples of personal meanings related to food.
3. Why does the public tend to accept nutrition misinformation so easily? What groups of people are more susceptible? Select one such group and give some effective approaches you might use in reaching them with sound nutrition.
4. What is the basis of concern about food additives and pesticide residues?
5. Name seven trends in the American mainstream of food patterns and discuss their implications for nutrition and health.

References

1. World hunger: grim accounting, Nutr Week 13(22):4, 1983.
2. Bloom BR: A new threat to world health, Science 239:9, Jan 1, 1988.
3. American Dietetic Association: Hunger—a worldwide problem, J Am Diet Assoc 86(10):1414, 1986.
4. Foerster S and Hinton A: Hunger in America: an American Dietetic Association perspective, J Am Diet Assoc 87(11):1571, 1987.
5. Cross AT: Politics, poverty, and nutrition, J Am Diet Assoc 87(8):1007, 1987.
6. Greger JL: Food, supplements, and fortified foods: scientific evaluations in regard to toxicology and nutrient bioavailability, J Am Diet Assoc 87(10):1369, 1987.
7. Maslow AH: Motivation and personality, New York, 1954, Harper & Row.
8. Harper AE: Nutrition: from myth and magic to science, Nutr Today 23(1):8, 1988.
9. Cordaro JB and Dickinson A: The nutritional supplement industry: realities and opportunities, J Nutr Educ 18(3):128, 1986.
10. Betterly CJ, Hathcock JN, and Fanslow AM: Cooperative Extension Service clientele's beliefs about food chemicals, J Nutr Educ 18(5):221, 1986.
11. Hannigan KJ and Przybyla AE: Market battle for the market basket, Food Engineering 58:53, Oct 1986.
12. Smith MV and Rulis AM: FDA's GRAS review and priority-based assessment of food additives, Food Technol 35:71, Dec 1981.
13. Labuza TP: Food research, Cereal Foods World 32:830, Nov 1987.
14. Lecos C: Pesticides and food: public worry no. 1, FDA Consumer 18:12, 1984.
15. Leonard R: Nutrition legislation: the year ahead, Food Management 23:20, Jan 1988.
16. Gerem Y: When disaster strikes, Food Nutr 17:20, April 1987.
17. Report: Will there be more households and fewer families in the 1980s? J Am Diet Assoc 81(6):738, 1982.
18. "Fast foods" and the American consumer, J Am Diet Assoc 81(5):579, 1982.

Further Readings

Bell LS and Fairchild M: Evaluation of commercial multivitamin supplements, J Am Diet Assoc 87(3):431, 1987.

Cordaro JB and Dickinson A: The nutritional supplement industry—realities and opportunities, J Nutr Educ 18(3):128, 1986.

Guthrie HA: Supplementation: a nutritionist's view, J Nutr Educ 18(3):130, 1986.

These three articles provide good background for some hard thinking about the use and misuse of food supplements, balancing the industry's marketing view against the view of nutritionists from scientific research and personal concern.

Chery A, Sabry JH, and Woolcott DM: Nutrition knowledge and misconceptions of university students: 1971 vs 1984, J Nutr Educ 19(5):237, 1987.

This interesting report compares nutrition beliefs over time and finds misconceptions persisting, despite increased general public knowledge.

Harper AE: Nutrition: from myth and magic to science, Nutr Today 23(1):8, 1988.

This excellent article traces the development of nutrition as a biologic science with important application to human health, addresses the dichotomy today between scientific nutrition and popular pseudonutrition, and gives some thoughts about why such divergent views exist.

Does Nutrition-Health Labeling Really Affect Food Choices?

In the midst of an increasing health-consciousness among consumers in the highly competitive modern American food marketplace, this is a very serious question. Should health claims be allowed on food labels? Do they really affect food choices? But further, do they actually border on health fraud? An intense debate about these issues is currently going on and the answers are by no means all in.

Nutrition labeling for processed food has been with us since the FDA's initial proposal became effective in 1975 and established a standardized label format. Over the time since then, nutrition labeling has grown to involve a sales volume of more than half of all the processed foods regulated by the FDA in American supermarkets. Driven by market competition, about two thirds of this volume comes voluntarily from the food industry. The remaining amount results from food enrichment regulations or the use of nutrition claims on labels or in advertising.

But nutrition labeling is expensive, as both industry and FDA officials can testify. It requires constant new food assays, increases mislabeling risks, and requires new labeling with new findings—all of which require money, for which the consumer must pay in higher prices. It even reaches into the taxpayer's pocket as more tax monies must cover increased FDA surveillance and control. So we must ask the question, "Is it worth it?" From a marketing standpoint, the answer seems to be "yes." In consumer surveys conducted by large supermarket chains in collaboration with the FDA, shoppers' food choices have been influenced both by the product label and by shelf information at the site of purchase. So straightforward label information about basic nutrient content seems to have positive value for consumers.

But from straight nutrition information to health claims on food product labels is a giant leap, and the waters at that point get murkier. Seeking to control emerging product statements that capitalize on health concerns involving unresolved issues in nutritional and medical science, the FDA has made a proposal entitled "Food Labeling: Public Health Messages on Food Labels and Labeling." This proposal requires that health-related statements on labels be (1) truthful and not misleading, (2) based on valid, reliable scientific data, (3) consistent with a sound total diet, and (4) accompanied by full nutritional labeling.

On the face of it, this proposal may sound simple. But that is far from the case. First, as opponents have stated, "telling the truth" on food product labels may actually be deceptive and misleading when it is not the *whole* truth. And just what is the "whole truth?" The fact is that there is no scientific consensus as yet on the three most-debated issues—the value of high-fiber diets in preventing colorectal cancer and the role of high-fat diets and of elevated serum cholesterol levels in atherosclerosis or in breast cancer. The scientific base for decision making is inadequate owing to individual dietary and biochemical variability, as well as the differing bioavailability of food nutrients. Effects of individual nutrients do not occur alone, but in conjunction with the entire diet. Indeed, good nutrition cannot come from a certain food product—it is a function of the person's *total* diet.

Advertising and food labeling do have an impact on the public. And there are certainly high stakes involved in the food industry. Because of the politics involved, it may be up to Congress to mandate some type of health claim labeling scheme. But it won't be easy. And the results are certain not to satisfy everyone involved.

REFERENCES

Carr CJ: The scientific base for decision-making, Am J Clin Nutr 44:571, Oct 1986.
Herbert V: Health claims in food labeling and advertising, Nutr Today 22(3):25, 1987.
Labuza TP: A perspective on health claims in food labeling, Cereal Foods World 32:256, March 1987.

Schucker RE: Does nutrition labeling really affect food choices? Nutr Today 20(6):24, 1985.
Stone MB: Health claims for food—where are we now? Cereal Foods World 32:875, Dec 1987.

10 Family Nutrition Counseling: Food Needs and Costs

After studying this chapter, the student should be able to:

1. Describe the role of the nutrition counselor-educator in health care settings.
2. Identify the primary focus and components of the counseling or teaching-learning process and apply these components to the nutrition interview.
3. Identify available community food assistance resources for families with economic problems and assist them with wise buying approaches.

Chapter Objectives

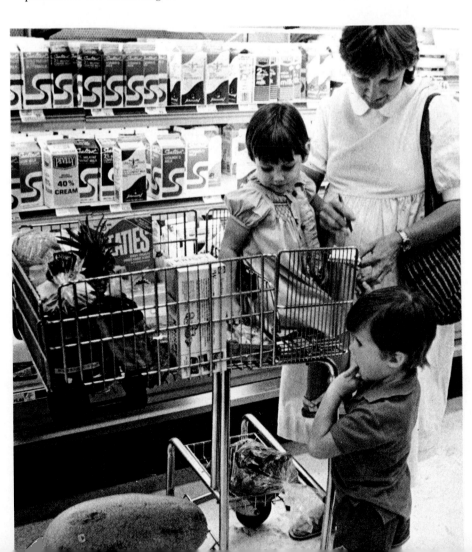

PREVIEW

Health care that is helpful to the client or patient must always be based on the individual's particular health needs. Therefore our first task in providing that care is to discover what those needs are. Then we can plan *with the client* the best way of meeting these needs. This is the necessary beginning and continuing part of all health care and education.

Health counseling in its broad sense centers on this basic type of activity—helping the client to meet personal health needs and develop habits of good ongoing self-care. Good health depends on sound nutrition. Thus a basic part of meeting health needs always involves attention to nutritional needs.

In a variety of situations, health care providers will be closely involved with the health care team. This may be the general primary health care team, the nursing care team, or the nutritional care team. In each case, under the guidance of the team's nutrition expert (the clinical nutritionist or registered dietitian), the goal is to help meet each patient's nutritional care and education needs.

Family Nutrition Counseling

Person-Centered Goals

Realistic family diet counseling must be *person-centered*. It involves close attention to personal and family needs, nutrition and health problems, and food choices and costs. In our work we have three main goals: (1) to obtain basic information about the client(s) and the living situation that relates to nutrition and health needs; (2) to provide basic health teaching to help meet these needs; and (3) to support the client and family in all personal efforts to meet needs through encouragement, reinforcement, general caring and concern, and practical resources. A basic skill that all health workers must learn, therefore, is the skill of talking with clients in a helpful manner. Skills in *interviewing* are essential in health care.

Interviewing

Interviewing does not necessarily mean only the more formal or structured diet history or other history-taking activity. Frequently it means a purposeful "planned conversation" either in the hospital or clinic or home. It may be a simple telephone call to the home to determine ongoing needs or progress. General principles of interviewing should guide these activities, including the purpose or focus, means used to achieve the purpose, and measuring results.

Focus and Purpose

As indicated, the focus of all health care is the individual client and personal health needs. It may be a small intermediate goal relating to some aspect of the overall care, or it may be a long-term goal. Our ultimate purpose is to provide whatever help the individual or family may need to determine personal health needs and goals and to work with the person or family in finding ways of meeting these needs and goals.

Means Used to Achieve Purpose

Relationship. Counseling is a **dynamic** person-centered process built upon a helping relationship. This is reflected in the common use of the word *services* for all health care related activities. The most important means of helping a person is establishing a relationship of mutual trust and respect. The most significant tool we ever have for helping others is *ourselves*. Our role is that of a "helping vehicle." Within this kind of relationship, true healing can take place.

Climate. The kind of climate we create involves both the physical setting and the psychologic feelings involved. The physical setting should be as comfortable as possible in relation to space, ventilation, heating, lighting, and sitting or lying down. Other important factors include providing sufficient time for the interview, in a quiet setting free from interruptions and with sufficient privacy to assure confidentiality. If it is in an office setting, the desk should be to the side, not between the therapist and client.

Attitudes. The word *attitude* refers to that aspect of personality that accounts for a consistent behavior toward persons, situations, or objects. Our attitudes are *learned*. Hence they develop from life experiences and influences. Because they are learned, they can be examined. We can become more aware of them. We can try to strengthen those attitudes that are desirable and constructive and at the same time seek to change or modify those attitudes that are less desirable and more destructive. If a health worker is to be able to help meet clients' needs, certain attitudes are necessary components of behavior:

1. **Warmth.** A genuine concern for the client or patient is displayed by interest, friendliness, and kindness. We convey warmth by being human and thoughtful.

2. **Acceptance.** We must meet the client "as he is, where he is." To accept the client does not necessarily mean approval of behavior. It does mean a realization that clients or patients usually regard their behavior as purposeful and meaningful. It may well be for them a means of handling stress. An attitude of acceptance conveys that a person's thoughts, ideas, and actions are important and worth attention simply because a person—a human being—has the right to be treated as having worth and dignity.

3. **Objectivity.** To be objective is to be free of bias. It is having a nonjudgmental attitude. Of course, complete objectivity is impossible, but reasonable objectivity is certainly a goal that can be attained. We must be aware of our own feelings and biases and we should attempt to control them. The evaluation of a situation must be based on what is actually happening, the facts as we perceive them, not on mere opinions, assumptions, or inferences.

4. **Compassion.** This attitude enables us to feel with and for another person or oneself. It means accepting the impact of an emotion, holding it long enough to absorb its meaning, and entering into a kind of "fellowship of feeling" with the person who is moved by the emotion. There is nothing soft or easy in developing the attitude of compassion. It requires emotional maturity.

Dynamic
Pertaining to change. A dynamic process is one that is constantly changing.

Measuring Results

Continuous and terminal evaluation of our interviews is an ongoing part of our activity. Evaluation is measuring how behavioral changes in the client and in ourselves are related to the needs and goals that have been identified. In summary, therefore, health workers will always be dealing with the following sequence of questions in interviewing:

1. **Need.** What is wrong? What is the health problem or *need* of the client or patient?
2. **Goal.** What does the client want to do about it? What is the client's immediate *goal*? What is the long-range goal?
3. **Information.** What *information* do I need to know to help the client? What does the client need to know to help take care of personal needs? What knowledge and skills are necessary to solve the health problem?
4. **Action.** What has to be done to help meet the need? What *plan of action* is best for solving the health problem and meeting the client's personal needs?
5. **Result.** What happened? What was the *result* of the action planned and carried out? Did it solve the problem or meet the need? If not, why not? What change in plan is indicated?

Important Actions of the Interview

Five important actions of an interview can be identified: observing, listening, responding, terminating, and recording. Each of these requires study, practice, and development of skills.

Observing

Ordinarily we do not deliberately and minutely look at all the persons we meet. However, in the care of persons with health needs the helping role requires such behavior. Our purpose is to gather information that will guide us in understanding clients or patients and their environment. Valid observation is a skill that is developed through concentration, study, and practice. Areas of such needed observation include the following:

1. **Physiologic functioning and features.** Refer to Table 1-1 in the first chapter and review the clinical signs of nutritional status. Such features as these may be used as a basis for making detailed observations of physical features. Learning to take an organized look at the person may help develop greater accuracy and objectivity. We tend to see what we have the mind-set, sensitivity, or awareness to see. Therefore we need to develop certain sensitivities that can detect pertinent details that can provide important clues to real needs.

2. **Behavior patterns.** Observe closely not only the physical features but also the immediate behavior of the client or patient in the health care situation. Attempt to look at the behavior in terms of its meaning to the person in relation to self-concept and the illness. From these observations, certain assumptions or "educated guesses" about immediate and long-term needs and goals can be made. But realize all the while that these are only assumptions and hence need to be validated and clarified with the client to determine whether they are indeed factual. This action helps us to understand our own feelings and rule out our own biases, prejudices, or distortions of the situation.

3. **Environment.** Observing the client's immediate environment in an organized manner is also helpful. This may be the home and community environment on a visit, or it may be the immediate environment in a clinic or hospital setting.

Listening

Hearing and listening are not the same thing. Hearing is purely a physiologic function, only the first phase of the listening process. The function of the listening is to hear, to identify the sound, to understand its meaning, and to learn by it.

Although the senses have amazing powers of perception, they are limited. The nervous system must constantly select and discriminate among the millions of bits of information it confronts. Listening is also limited. A large part of communication time is spent in listening, but the average person without special training has only about 25% listening efficiency. In other words, one "hears" only a small percent of the total surrounding communication.

The task of the health worker is to learn the art of "creative listening." First of all, we must learn to be comfortable as a listener. Usually our lives are so filled with activity and *noise* that to sit and listen quietly is often difficult. Actually, when you think about it, most of us have had little experience during our own development of being listened to, so that listening to others must be learned. We practice listening by staying close by, assuming a comfortable position, and giving our full attention to the person who is speaking. We show genuine interest by indicating agreement or understanding with a nod of the head or making such sounds as "uh-huh," "I see," or "And then?" at the appropriate moments in the conversation. We must learn to remain silent when the other person's comment jogs some personal memory or parallel experience of our own. We learn to listen not only for words the patient uses but also the repetition of key words, to the rise and fall of the tone of voice, to hesitant or aggressive expression of words and ideas, and to the softness or harshness of tone. We listen to the overall content of what is being said, to the main ideas being expressed, and to the topics chosen for discussion. We listen for the feelings, needs, and goals that are being stated. We learn to listen to the silences and to be comfortable with them, giving the person time to frame thoughts and express them.

Responding

The responses we give to the client or patient may be verbal or nonverbal. Nonverbal responses include signs and actions, such as gestures and movements, silences, facial expressions, and touch. Verbal responses make use of language—words and meanings (Table 10-1). But we must remember that we give our own meanings to the words we use. A word is only a symbol, not the thing itself. Thus we must give attention to our choice of words—we must "begin where the person is." And all the while we must provide a supportive environment for responses (see the box on p. 231). Also, we must watch the level and pace of our speaking. Questions should be clear, concise, free from bias, and always nonthreatening. Sometimes a verbal response may be a simple restatement of what the client has said. This enables the person to hear the statement again, think about it and thus reinforce, expand, or correct it. At other times the response may be a reflection of what the ex-

The eye can handle about 5 million bits of information per second, but the resolving power of the brain is only about 500 bits per second.

Creative listening—listening with a sincere effort to see matters from the patient's point of view.

Table 10-1

Verbal Responses Used
by the Helping
Professions

Purpose of response	Type of response	Description
Clarification	Content	Counselor summarizes content of conversation up to that point
	Affective	Counselor paraphrases or defines concern that client has implied but not actually stated
Leading	Closed question	Question that can be responded to with "yes" or "no," or with very few words
	Open question	Question that cannot be answered briefly; often triggers discussion or a flow of information
	Advice	Provision of an alternative type of behavior by counselor for client; may be an activity or thought
	Teaching	Information presented by counselor with intention of helping client acquire knowledge, skills, and so on to perform appropriate nutrition-related behaviors
Self-revealing	Self-involving	Response made to client's statements that reflects the personal feelings of counselor
	Self-disclosing	Response made to client's statements that reflects factual information about counselor
	Aside	Statement counselor makes to self

pressed feelings seem to be. This enables the client to respond, to verify or to deny that this was indeed the feeling. We must never act on our assumptions about the client's feelings without verifying them first.

Terminating the Interview

The close of the interview should meet several needs. It may be used to summarize the main points covered or to reinforce learning. If contact with the client is to continue, it can include plans for the follow-up visits or activities. It should always leave the person with the sense that the health worker's concern has been sincere and that the door is always open for further communication, should the person so desire.

Recording

Some means of recording the important points of the interview should be arranged. This should be as unobtrusive as possible, with little note-taking, if any, during the interview itself and completion of the record immediately afterward. If some recording device is used, the client's permission must always be obtained. Give full assurance that identity will be erased and that the recording will only be used for a specific purpose, such as to help the health worker improve interviewing skills or to learn the health needs of a particular group of people, as in gathering research data.

To Probe Further

**Creating a
Supportive Nutrition
Counseling
Environment**

Over 50 years ago a sensitive physician expressed truths about the client-patient interview in a healing environment that are human verities today as much as then—perhaps even more so in our more complex world. He reminds us anew that we must *listen*—really listen—to our clients if we are to help them.

Listening

"Now hear this," he seems to be imploring us still. "We must listen," he is saying, "for what the client wants to tell us, what he does not want to tell us, and for what he cannot tell us. He does not want to tell us things that are shameful or painful. And he cannot tell us his implicit assumptions that even he does not know." Sounds like *creative listening,* as a more modern philosopher and counselor, Carl Rogers, used to call it. This is no mere passive thing. It is a very active counseling skill. Only thus can we really hear and respond wisely.

Also, nutrition counselors may inadvertently close communication channels by failing to ask questions or otherwise verbally discouraging the client from expressing real concerns and expectations or by using "body language" that is distracting, inappropriate, or misinterpreted by the client because of cultural differences.

Questions and reflections

Questions or statements that reflect what the client says or feels and encourage further expression are usually *open-ended,* making a simple yes-or-no response inadequate, or *affective,* reflecting feelings that the client may have implied but not expressed directly. Closed questions and self-directed statements do little to encourage the person to "open up." (See Table 10-1.)

Body language

Body language can be distracting or intimidating, or it can make the client feel "comfortable." The key here is to understand the client's concept of the following:

Personal space. Americans like lots of room. Try sitting next to the only passenger on a city bus and note the amount of anxiety created! In other cultures, such as the Middle East, closeness, even to the point of pushing and shoving, is considered acceptable behavior. Thus we must understand that our *distance* from our clients may affect their sense of comfort.

Eye contact. Americans show respect by looking at each other straight in the eye. Asians do the same thing by looking downward. Attempts to interchange these behaviors can be interpreted as rude.

Speech inflection. The tone of voice and its loudness and inflection may be interpreted as threatening or comforting, depending on the region or country of origin of the listener.

Continued.

To Probe Further

**Creating a
Supportive Nutrition
Counseling
Environment—cont'd**

You cannot always be aware of your clients' attitudes toward body language ahead of time. However, you can take note of any signs of uneasiness and at least invite them to discuss anything about the interview that may be causing concern.

Yes, Dr. Henderson, we still hear you. We can—and must—listen.

REFERENCES

Henderson L: Physician and patient as a social system, N Engl J Med 212:819, 1935.
Heppner PP, Rogers ME, and Lee LA: Carl Rogers: reflections on his life, J Counsel Dev 63:14, 1984.
Spenser H: The hidden meaning of body language, Am Pharm NS21(7):416, 1981.
Vickery CE and Hodges PAM: Counseling strategies for dietary management: expanded possibilities for effecting behavior change, J Am Diet Assoc 86(7):924, 1986.

Various members of the health team contribute information about the client or patient and the health problem in a system of written reports. This is the patient's chart, a legal document which in case of litigation could be used in court. There is an obligation to the client or patient to respect confidentiality and to determine what and how much information is shared and with whom. At the same time health workers have a responsibility for relaying to other health team members pertinent information to aid in the total planning of care.

What aspects, then, of the interview should be recorded? Data from two basic areas of communication are needed: (1) a description of the client or patient's general physical and emotional status and concerns, followed in some instances by judgment of the immediate and ongoing care needs; and (2) description of whatever care and teaching were given and results observed. In addition, we may sometimes include follow-up plans made with the client or patient and the family or notes concerning needs that were passed on to other health team members or to other agencies. Similar information is often communicated through oral team reports and various case conferences.

Nutrition History and Analysis
Personal Life Situation and Food Patterns

First, working closely with the nutritionist on the health care team, learn the family's situation and values and identify health and nutrition needs through a general nutrition history and its analysis. Several methods for such interviewing may be used:

1. **24-hour recall.** Ask the person to recall all food and drink consumed during the previous day, noting the nature and amount of each item. This method has disadvantages with some persons, such as elderly people or young children, whose memory may be limited, and it does not reveal long-term food habits.

2. **Food records.** Persons are asked to record their food intake for a brief period of time, usually about 3 days, or on certain days periodically. Each

person is taught how to describe the food items used singly or in combination, and how to measure amounts consumed. Often a 3-day record is used following an initial diet history as a periodic monitoring tool.

3. **Food frequency.** Use a structured questionnaire that lists common food items or food groups to obtain information about quantity and frequency of use. This tool may be helpful in relation to a particular disease risk or incidence by helping to determine use of specific groups of foods over an extended period of time.

4. **Diet history.** At the initial individual or family contact, a nutrition interview provides needed information for planning continuing care. Professional nutritionists and dietitians use a comprehensive form of this approach in a variety of clinical and community settings, usually evaluating their findings by detailed computer analysis. Other health team members working with the dietitian may contribute helpful nutrition information through use of a simplified version, such as the *activity-associated general day's food pattern* given here in Tool A (see the box on p. 234). Most people eat in relation to activity or work throughout the day, where they were, what they were doing, and whom they were with at the time. So using such an activity-associated guide through the day gives both interviewer and client a structure, a beginning, middle, and end, and provides a series of "memory jogs" to flesh out the information in greater detail to permit constructive counseling. With respect to each item, questions are asked in terms of general habits—nature of food items, form, frequency, preparation, portion, seasoning—not in terms of a specific day's intake. All through such an interview important clues to food attitudes and values can be communicated. Note these for later thought and exploration. If your manner is interested and accepting, the information should be valid and straightforward. Conversely, if you are judgmental and authoritarian, persons will probably only tell you what they think you want to hear.

Changing American Eating Behavior

A basic reason for using an activity-associated general day's food intake as the structure for a diet history is the fact that America's eating behavior is changing from traditional patterns. Recent surveys indicate that current eating behavior has become much more fragmented into frequent light feedings—called "grazing" by many observers—than the traditional family meals. Actually, one study that compared American eating patterns over the past 15 years found that the smallest and fastest shrinking population segment is that group called "Happy Cookers" who still cook "three square meals" a day.[1] These investigators found that this traditional group now accounts for only 15% of the American population and that their numbers have declined 35% from the previous 15-year period. On the other hand, the largest and fastest growing segment, whom the researchers called the "Chase and Grabbits," is composed of those eating easily portable items that don't take much time to cook or consume. This group now accounts for 26% of the population and its numbers have swelled 136% over the past 15 years.

Plan of Care

On the basis of the diet history and review of any health problems requiring diet modification, a realistic personal food plan can be developed with the

Clinical Application: Tool A

Nutrition History: Activity-Associated General Day's Food Pattern

Name _____ Date _____

   Height _____ Weight (lb) _____ (kg) _____ Age _____

   Ideal weight _____

Referral

Diagnosis

Diet order

Members of household

Occupation

Recreation, physical activity

Present food intake			Frequency, form, and amount
	Place	Hour	checklist
Breakfast			Milk
			Cheese
			Meat
			Fish
Noon meal			Poultry
			Eggs
			Cream
			Butter, margarine
Evening meal			Other fats
			Vegetables, green
Extra meals			Vegetables, other
			Fruits (citrus)
			Legumes
Summary			Potato
			Bread—kind
			Sugar
			Desserts
			Beverages
			Alcohol
			Vitamins
			Candy

individual and family. Then any related follow-up care can be developed as needed. This may take the form of return visits to the clinic, home visits, consultation and referral with other members of the health care team, or use of community resources. Follow-up work requires patience and a steady focus on the goal, knowing that there are options, no one way, of reaching it. Imagination and good humor are invaluable. Take one step at a time. Guide the client and family in applied nutrition principles, give support as needed,

Clinical Application: Tool B

I. Assess nutrition needs

   A. Define the person

      1. Who the person is: age, sex, family, occupational role, cultural background, socioeconomic status, personal characteristics, limitations, strengths

      2. Where the person is: physical setting—place of care, its possibilities and limitations; and personal setting—mental, psychologic, emotional, and physical, in relation to health or disease, adaptation

      3. Nutritional status: food habits and general nutritional analysis; clinical observations and signs (Table 10-1)

   B. Determine the disease or normal physiologic stress (such as pregnancy and growth)

      1. The general disease or physiologic process: anatomy and physiology, signs and symptoms, general treatment or management, pathology, course, prognosis

      2. Patient's unique experience with the disease or physiologic stress: duration, intensity, medical management, prior diet therapy, adaptation, problems and solutions, knowledge of disease and its care—source, form, attitude, behavior response

II. Identify and define problems and develop plan of care

   A. Explore present needs

      1. Day-to-day nutritional support: maintenance, optimum intake, basic nutritional requirements

      2. Nutritional therapy: treatment by modified diet

      3. Teaching: basic nutrition knowledge or principles of special diet modification

   B. Explore future needs

      1. Continuity of care: home, responsible significant others, extended-care facility

      2. Plan for medical management: health team conferences, nursing team conferences

      3. Plan for nutritional care: diet modification, practical food management (family situation, living alone, degree of disability), follow-up diet counseling and nutrition education, community resources

III. Carry out plan of care

   A. Physical, psychosocial responses: diet and its meaning

   B. Teaching plan: materials needed, content, sequence, methods, approaches, plan for evaluation

   C. Records of action for study

IV. Check results

   A. Follow-up care: planned with patient, family, and health team

   B. Reinforcement to strengthen learning

   C. Revision: as needed

Guide for Assessment and Care of Nutrition Needs

Clinical Application: Tool C

Stages of a Nutrition Interview

I. The patient as a person
  A. Introduction
    1. Developing a relationship: establishing rapport; putting the patient at ease; gaining the patient's confidence and trust; mutual trust
    2. Defining roles: selling health worker's role as helper, health counselor, teacher; determining patient's role as learner and active participant in taking increasing responsibility for own learning and care according to individual capacity
    3. Determining the patient's health need or problem and related personal goals: discovering whether the patient's goals are different from what was expected; deciding whether underlying objectives exist other than those concerning the immediate dietary problem
    4. Redefining objectives in light of patient's goals: Seeing couseling goals in terms of those of patient
  B. Patient profile: Who and what kind of person is the patient?
    1. Gathering physical data: How do these data affect the dietary problem? How long has the problem existed? Has the patient known anyone with a similar problem?
      a. Age
      b. Height
      c. Weight—present and past history
      d. Experience with disease or weight problem
    2. Understanding the patient's setting: the patient's environment: social and economic factors involved
      a. Family: identity of family (ethnic); number in family; who cooks, markets
      b. Work: hours, extent of activity; effect on eating habits; education
      c. Social activity: recreation; physical exercise
    3. Interpreting the patient's attitudes toward disease or weight problem: How has the patient's experience with the problem influenced personal belief about it? Have family members or friends influenced the patient? Has the patient expressed fears, misconceptions, misunderstanding?
II. The patient's food habits
  A. Nutrition history
    1. Determining present food intake: What does the patient usually eat? (flavorings, seasonings, condiments, beverages, other relevant additions)
    2. Learning place and time: Where and when does the patient eat? How do these affect what is eaten? Can any times or places be changed or eliminated?
    3. Referring to checklist of various food groups and some individual foods: keeping some form of reminder for the counselor to make sure that relevant foods have been covered

4. Determining who prepares the food and how: possible consulta-
      tion with wife or mother
   B. Physical exercise and reaction: activities associated with the patient's
      food habits (work, school, social gatherings, travel)
   C. Food reactions: patient's likes, dislikes, intolerances, allergies: Could
      food be accepted in a different form or by using another method of
      preparation? Possible substitutes?
III. Diet counseling
   A. Choosing the diet: What is the diet ordered by the physician or the
      nutritionist? What form will be best understood by the patient?
   B. Explaining the reasons for the diet: Why the increases in certain
      foods or restrictions on other; the effect of food on the disease
   C. Planning a daily food pattern with the patient: considering the
      patient's likes and dislikes, usual habits, and restrictions because of
      dietary problem; developing a dietary plan that fits into daily
      activity
   D. Reviewing the diet and answering questions: answering inquiries
      throughout interview but asking specifically for questions or
      feedback toward the end
      Does the patient understand?
IV. Termination of the interview
   A. Planning for follow-up: When will the patient be seen again?
      Encouraging recording of questions or problems that may develop
      to discuss next time
      Should the patient keep food records of any kind?
   B. Recording the interview: completing any needed charting of the
      interview; keeping any needed notes in records

---

help with adjustments of the plan, provide reinforcement of prior learning, and continue to add new learning opportunities as the family's needs develop. Tool B and Tool C (see boxes) provide general guides for reviewing nutritional needs of individuals and helping to plan their ongoing care.

Learning and Changed Behavior

There is far more to teaching and learning than merely dispensing information. But the myth still prevails in much of health education that if enough information is provided, harmful health practices will be changed. This is not the case. A vast difference exists between a person who has learned and a person who has only been informed. Learning must ultimately be measured in terms of *changed behavior*. As with counseling, valid education focuses not on the practitioner-teacher or the content, but on the *personal learner*. The health teacher's major task is to create situations in which clients and their families can learn, succeed, and develop self-direction, self-motivation, and self-care. These learning goals are especially important in dealing with adult patients and clients (see Issues and Answers on p. 250).

The Teaching-Learning Process

Aspects of Human Personality Involved in Learning

The teaching-learning experience involves three fundamental aspects of the human personality—thinking, feeling, and the will to act.

Thinking

We grasp information through our personal thinking process. We take in information selectively, then process and shape it according to our needs. The total thought process provides the background knowledge that is the basis for reasoning and analysis. The learner senses the contribution of this thinking to the learning process as "I know how to do it."

Feeling

In each of us specific feelings and responses are associated with given items of knowledge and given situations. These emotions reflect desires and needs that are aroused. Emotions provide impetus, creating the tensions that spur us to act. The learner senses the contribution of emotion to the learning process as "I want to do it."

Will to Act

The will to act arises from the conviction that the knowledge discovered can fulfill the felt need and relieve the symptoms of tension. The will focuses the decision to act on the knowledge received so that attitude, value, thought, or pattern of behavior can be changed. The learner senses the contribution of the will to the learning process as "I will do it."

Principles of Learning

Learning follows three basic laws: (1) learning is *personal,* occurring in relation to perceived personal needs; (2) learning is *developmental,* building on prior knowledge and experience; and (3) learning means change, resulting in some form of *changed behavior.*

Individuality

Learning can only be individual. In the final analysis we must all learn for ourselves, according to our own needs, in our own way and time, and for our own purpose. The teacher must discover who the learner is by asking questions that clarify the learner's relationship to the problem. New approaches to realistic nutrition education can help teachers vary teaching-learning strategies to meet the differing needs of learners and learning situations.[2]

Need Fulfillment

Motivation
Providing something that prompts an individual to act in a certain way.

An important initial force in learning is personal **motivation.** Persons learn only what they believe will be useful to them, and they retain only what they think they need or shall need. The sooner persons can put new learning to use, the more readily they grasp it. The more it satisfies their immediate goals, the more effective the learning will be.

Contact

Learning starts from a point of contact between prior experience and knowledge, an overlap of the new with the familiar. Find out what the individual already knows and to what past experiences the present situation can be related. Start the process of learning at this point. Search for the areas of association that are present, then relate your teaching to that point of contact.

Active Participation

Since learning is an active process through which behavior can change, learners must become personally involved. They must participate actively. Indeed, effective teaching strategies *require* active participation of learners to bring about desired changes in attitudes and behaviors.[3] One means of securing participation is through *planned feedback*. Feedback may take several forms: (1) Ask questions that require more than a "yes" or "no" answer and that reveal a degree of understanding and motivation, such as those in Table 10-1. (2) Use guided return demonstrations, which are brief periods in which procedures are practiced and skills discussed. Such guided practice develops ability, self-confidence, and security. It enables the learner to clarify the principles involved as a basis for decision making about particular situations and actions. (3) Have the learner try out the new learning in personal experiences outside the teacher-directed situation. Alternate such trials with return visits to review these experiences. Answer, or help the person to answer, any questions raised and provide continued support and reinforcement.

Appraisal

At appropriate intervals take stock of the changes that your clients or patients have made in outlook, attitude, and actions toward their specific goals in health and nutrition care and education. Careful, sympathetic questioning may reveal any blocks to learning. In addition to speeding the learning process, such concern will show you whether you are communicating successfully, making contact, or making the best choices of method. It may help you to recall principles that you may have glossed over. In the final analysis, the measure of success in teaching lies not in the number of facts transferred, but in the change for the better that has been initiated in your client.

In all, the nutrition educator who builds on clients' needs and goals, imparts a strong knowledge and interest in the subject, shows respect and concern for each individual in the program, and projects self-confidence has the greatest chance for success. In the long run, clients following a personal goal-setting approach in their nutrition counseling and education will have more opportunity to develop self-care responsibility and personal choice than those following a purely diet-prescription approach.[4] Initially the personal goal-setting approach may take longer, but it achieves far greater long-term results.

In your counseling you will discover economic stress among many clients and their families. Some may need financial help. In such situations you will need to discuss available food assistance programs and make appropriate referrals through your team nutritionist and social worker or directly to community agencies and programs involved.

Family Economic Needs: Food Assistance Programs

Commodity Distribution Program

In the post-Depression years, legislation was initiated to stabilize agricultural prices. This legislation provided for the federal government to purchase market surpluses of perishable goods. Later the resulting accumulation of food stocks led to the creation of distribution programs as a means of disposing of the stored products (Figure 10-1). Such surplus has been defined as ei-

Figure 10-1
Warehouse for food surplus goods used in Commodities Distribution Program.

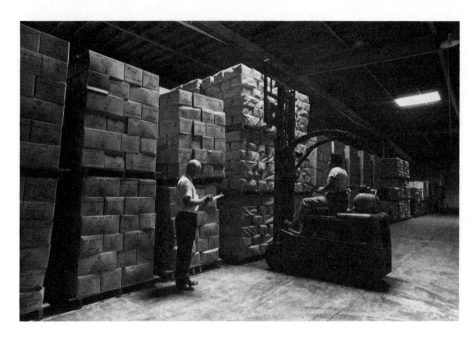

ther physical (exceeding requirements) or economic (prices below desired levels). Foods coming under these regulations include meat and poultry, fruits and vegetables, eggs, dried beans and peas. Most of these items purchased under this program have been donated by the Food and Nutrition Service of the U.S. Department of Agriculture (USDA) to schools through the National School Lunch and School Breakfast Programs. Foods accumulated through other aspects of the legislation are price-supported basic and nonperishable items. These foods have been donated to child-feeding programs, summer camps, Indian reservations, trust territories, nutrition programs for the elderly, charities, disaster-feeding programs, and the Commodities Supplemental Food Program (Figure 10-2).

Food Stamp Program

Also growing out of the post-Depression years, the Food Stamp Program was founded to help low-income families purchase needed food. The program became part of permanent legislation by the Food Stamp Act of 1964, which made the program available to all counties wishing to participate. The program has developed from a $13 million program in 1961 to one of nearly $12 billion in 1985.[5] Although it has suffered federal administration budget cuts through the 1980s, it remains the largest U.S. food assistance program.

Under this program the participant is issued coupons, or food stamps. The coupons are distributed to participating "households," defined by the program as a group of people living in the same house who buy, store, and eat food together. These coupons are supposed to be sufficient to cover the household's food needs for 1 month. These households must have a net monthly income below the program's eligibility limit to qualify. This limit is quite low, and usually families who qualify simply aren't making enough money to buy food. Eligibility is based on gross, not actual net, income. For example, the Poverty Index Ratio (PIR) used, as that with the U.S. Department of Health and Human Services for its National Health and Nutrition

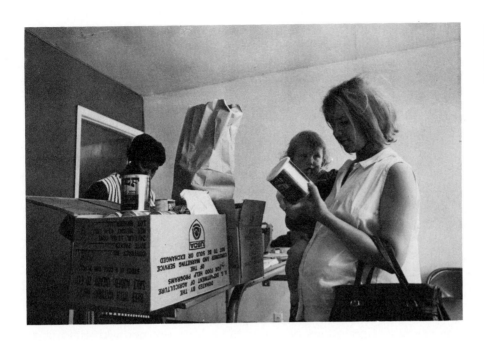

Figure 10-2
Pregnant mother and her child participating in the supplemental Commodities Distribution Program.

Examination Survey (NHANES), is calculated on gross family income.[6] This PIR compares household income to three times the cost of the lowest USDA Thrifty Food plan. Households with a PIR of less than 1 are below the official poverty line.

Child Nutrition Programs

After the Surplus Commodities Program was started, the government faced a glut of accumulated food items and needed a means of disposing of them. Then during World War II the military discovered a distressing rate of nutrition-related disorders that prevented a number of its draftees from serving in the army. Out of these two situations the National School Lunch Program of 1946 was born. From this initial program came all of today's child nutrition programs.

National School Lunch and Breakfast Program

These programs provide financial assistance to schools to enable them to provide nutritious lunches and breakfasts to all their students. The program allows poor children to eat free meals or meals at reduced prices, whereas other students pay somewhat less than the full cost of the meal. Commodity foods, as described above, are available to participating schools, and the programs usually entail minimal costs to the school district. All public and private nonprofit schools are eligible to participate in the program if their average tuition per student does not exceed $1500. Children's residential institutions, preschools, and Head Start programs run as part of a school system are also eligible. Lunches served must fulfill approximately one third of the child's Recommended Dietary Allowance (RDA) for nutrients.

Child Care Food Program

This program provides USDA food commodities, cash equivalents, and meal reimbursements for most or all of the meal and administrative costs of feeding children up to 12 years of age who are enrolled in organized child care programs. These settings include day care centers, recreation centers, settlement houses, and some Head Start programs. The children's eligibility for free and reduced-price meals is the same as for the school lunch and breakfast programs.

WIC

The Special Supplemental Food Program for Women, Infants, and Children, commonly called by its basic initials *WIC*, provides nutritious foods to low-income women who are pregnant or breast-feeding and to their infants and children under age 5. The food is either distributed free or purchased by free vouchers (Figure 10-3). It is designed to supplement the diet with rich sources of iron, protein, and certain vitamins. The vouchers are good for such foods as milk, eggs, cheese, juice, fortified cereals, and infant formulas. The program includes funding to cover clinic visits for medical checkups and for nutrition education and counseling by public health nutritionists. It is administered by the USDA through state health departments and native American tribes, bands, or groups and run locally by public health facilities or organizations. Participants must be pregnant or postpartum mothers (up to 6 months), lactating mothers (up to 12 months), or women with children under age 5. They must be at nutritional risk and must have an income under the reduced-price guidelines for the school lunch program. Factors indicating nutritional risk include evidence of an inadequate diet, poor growth patterns, a lack of nutrition understanding, or a medical history of nutrition-related problems, such as low birth weight or premature infants, pregnancy-induced hypertension (toxemia), spontaneous abortions (miscarriages), and anemia. Current reports indicate that the prevalence of anemia among infants and children in low-income families has steadily declined over the past decade, largely owing to the positive impact of public health programs such as WIC.[7] Also, WIC prenatal supplementation has helped reduce the incidence of low birth weight, though it remains a problem, and raise the mean birth weight.[8] By the early 1980s the WIC program served the needs of about 2 million persons who received benefits at just over 1000 clinics across the United States. Unlike the food stamp or school lunch programs, however, WIC is not an "entitlement" program. This means that eligibility does not automatically entitle one to benefits. There is an absolute ceiling each year on funding and therefore on participation.

For a family of two to participate in the WIC program, the family income must be less than $10,530 annually.

By the early 1980s the WIC program served the needs of about 2 million persons who received benefits at just over 1000 clinics across the United States.

Nutrition Program for Elderly Persons

Congress has provided two types of food programs to benefit the growing numbers of elderly citizens in the United States. Regardless of their income level, all persons over 60 years of age are eligible to receive meals from the Congregate Meals Program or the Home-Delivered Meals Program. Elderly persons often face many social, physical, and economic difficulties and do not eat adequately to fulfill their nutritional needs. Many of them suffer from isolation and social deprivation. The main difference in these two programs is their setting and social aspect: (1) the *Congregate Meals Program* provides ambulatory elderly persons with a hot nourishing noon meal at a community center where they can share food once a day, 5 days a week, with a group of their peers at no charge. Free transportation is often provided. Social events and nutrition information accompany the meals. (2) In compari-

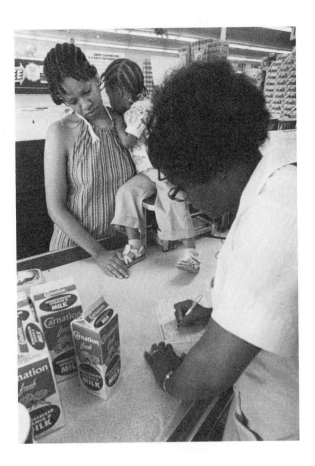

Figure 10-3
Mother in WIC program using program vouchers at a super-market to buy groceries.

son, the *Home-Delivered Meals Program,* sometimes called Meals-on-Wheels, provides homebound elderly persons who have difficulty preparing their own meals with at least one nutritious meal delivered to them in their home Monday through Friday. Both programs are allowed to accept voluntary contributions for meals.

General family nutrition counseling may also involve guidance in planning for control of family food costs.

Food Buying Guides

USDA Food Plans

The USDA periodically issues low-cost food plans to serve as guides for food assistance programs. These plans are called liberal, moderate, low, and thrifty or very low-cost food plans, but in comparison to modern consumer food costs in general they are all low-cost plans. These very low-cost food plans are developed by nutritionists, economists, and computer experts at USDA on the basis of a predetermined level of spending appropriate to the prevailing policy identifying the **poverty** threshold. The lowest of these plans is used to determine allotments of food stamp coupons to poor households.

Family Food Costs

A number of factors influence the way a family divides its food dollar. Some of these factors as listed here can help your client's family work out their their household food plan.

Poverty
Having little or no money, goods, or means of support; scantiness, insufficiency; meagerness. The 1981 federal government definition of the poverty level was an annual income of less than $9,287 for a family of four.

1. Family income
2. Number, sex, ages, and general activities of family members
3. Any family food produced or preserved at home
4. Likes and dislikes of family members and special family dishes
5. Special dietary needs of any family member
6. Time, transportation, and energy for food shopping and preparation
7. Skill and experience in food management: planning, buying, cooking
8. Storing and cooking facilities in the home
9. Amount and kind of entertaining, if any
10. Meals eaten away from home
11. Value family places on food and eating

Good Shopping and Food Handling Practices

Today's American family spends more time shopping for food than cooking it. Food marketing is big business, and buying food for a family may seem to be a more complex affair than the preparation of food at home. A large American supermarket may stock some 8000 or more different food items and add more daily. A single food item may be marketed in a dozen different ways at as many different prices. Frequently client families ask for more help with food buying than with any other aspect of fulfilling their diet needs. The following four food handling practices will help control costs.

Plan Ahead

Completely unplanned purchases account for more than half of the items usually bought in supermarkets.

Use market guides in newspapers, plan general menus, keep a kitchen supply checklist, and make out a market list ahead according to location of items in a regularly visited market. Such planning helps avoid impulse buying and extra trips.

Buy Wisely

Know the market, market items, packaging, grades, brands, portion yields, measures, and food value in a market unit. Watch for sale items and buy in quantity if it results in savings and the food can be adequately stored or used. Be cautious in selecting convenience foods. The time saved may not be worth the added cost.

Store Food Safely

The kitchen waste that results from food spoilage and misuse can be controlled. Conserve food by storing items according to their nature and use and by using dry storage, covered containers, and refrigeration as needed. Keep opened and partly used food packages at the front of the shelf for early use. Avoid plate waste by preparing only the amount needed by the family and use leftovers intelligently and creatively.

Cook Food Well

Retain maximum food value in cooking processes and prepare food with imagination and good sense. Give zest and appeal to dishes by using a variety of seasonings and combinations.

In all family nutrition counseling, however, we must remember that as much as the family may have learned about nutrition, this is not always a primary factor. Family members usually eat because they are hungry or because the food looks and tastes good, not necessarily because it is nutritious.

The Best Food Buys
Vegetables and Fruits

In addition to minerals, these foods supply vitamins A and C, two nutrients found in surveys to be most often lacking in the average American diet. Give your clients the following guidelines:

1. Buy fresh items in season to save on out-of-season foods transported in from warmer, distant places.

2. Select fresh produce that is firm, crisp, and heavy for size. Medium size items are usually better buys than large, most of which may need to be discarded in preparation.

3. Distinguish between types of fresh produce defects. Small surface defects do not affect quality or food value and may cost less. Many or deep defects cause more waste, as does decay that is even slightly evident.

4. Compare cost of fresh produce sold by weight or count. The resulting price per item can be computed by each method of sale to make the best choice.

5. Avoid fancy grades in canned vegetables and fruits. Grading is based on shape, size, and perfection of pieces. Lower grades contain small, broken, or imperfect pieces but are equal in taste and food value and thus are good buys.

6. Buy vegetables and fruits in large cans, if family size warrants it.

7. Select low-cost dried foods. Dehydrated foods vary in price. Dried beans, peas, and lentils are excellent food buys. But specialty dried foods, such as potatoes or dried fruits, are usually more expensive than fresh ones.

8. Compare cost of frozen, canned, and fresh vegetable and fruit items. Frozen items are usually more expensive. However, specials and family-sized packages can be compared weight for weight with canned or fresh items in season.

9. Cook vegetables with care. Excess cooking water and time destroy or eliminate vitamins and minerals and rob the vegetable of color, texture, and taste. Such unappetizing food often goes uneaten and causes costly waste.

Breads and Cereals

Most bread and cereal products are well liked, inexpensive, and fit easily into meal plans. This group of foods, along with potatoes and other vegetables, provides complex carbohydrate, which nutritionists advise should be the staple food of most persons' diets. Whole-grain foods are good sources of dietary fiber and are high in important vitamins and minerals. They are also important sources of amino acids and, in combination with other grains and legumes, form complete or "complementary" proteins. Many foods in this group can be excellent bargains:

1. Whole-grain or enriched products are much more nutritious than refined grains and products and are usually no more expensive.

2. Enriched specialty breads, such as French or Italian, cost up to three times more than whole-grain bread with similar or better nutritive value.

3. Precooked rice is much more expensive than unprocessed and often lacks many of the nutrients lost in processing.

4. Many cereals have nutrients added. Cereals that advertise 100% of the RDA for vitamins and minerals are usually more expensive. If the diet is adequate, such levels of supplementation are unnecessary.

5. Ready-to-eat cereals and instant hot cereals and those packaged for individual servings are usually much more expensive. Buy grains in bulk if adequate storage can be provided.

6. Baked goods made at home, from scratch or even from some mixes, are usually much cheaper than bakery goods.

7. A large loaf of bread may not weigh more than a small loaf. Compare prices of equal weights of bread to find the better buy.

8. Try unusual forms of grains. For example, bulgur, buckwheat groats (hulled kernels), barley, and millet are excellent grains and can be used in many meals. Bulgur, which is cooked like rice, has a toast-like color, is rich in wheat flavor, and is equal in food value to whole wheat.

Protein Foods
Plant Proteins

Dried beans and peas, grains, nuts, and seeds are inexpensive sources of complementary proteins. Legumes and grains contribute different ratios of needed amino acids and in various mixes complement one another to provide food sources of complete protein (see Chapter 6). These foods store well, are versatile in preparation, low in fat, and free of cholesterol, which is purely an animal product. They are also good sources of vitamins and minerals, including iron, zinc, and the B vitamins. For example, tofu, a curd made from soybean milk, has been the low-cost protein backbone of the East Asian diet for more than 2000 years.

A quarter pound of tofu has about 85 kcal, 8 to 10 g of protein, and 5 g of fat, most of which is unsaturated.

Eggs

Eggs provide high-quality complete protein and are sold according to grade and size, neither of which is related to food value. Egg grades are based on qualities such as firmness of egg white, appearance, and delicacy of flavor, not on food value or quality. Shell color varies with species and has no effect on quality.

Milk and Cheese

Dairy products are good sources of high-quality complete protein. However, whole milk products carry saturated fat, so distinguish among them those that are lower in fat, as well as lower in price:

1. Fluid nonfat milk, buttermilk, and canned evaporated milk cost less than whole, fluid milk. So-called low-fat milks consist of 2% butterfat; whole milk is 4%. To produce these lower fat milks, part of the butterfat is removed and and dry milk solids are added. Low-fat milk contains 135 kcal per cup (8 oz). Whole milk contains 170 kcal per cup; nonfat milk contains 80 kcal per cup.

2. Nonfat dried milk is the best bargain of all forms. Reconstituted with water it provides a fluid nonfat milk at less than half the cost of fresh form. It can also be used many ways in cooking to add valuable nutrition and the base for making yogurt.

3. If family size warrants it, buy milk in large bulk containers.

4. If cheese is used often, buy it in bulk. It costs less per unit of weight and keeps better. Cheese standards set by the FDA are based on percentage of fat and moisture. The most commonly used, cheddar cheese (American, Daisy, Longhorn), is 50% fat and 30% moisture. Spread cheeses and imported cheeses are much more expensive.

5. Cottage cheese is an unripened, soft curd (80% moisture) and hence a rapidly perishable item. Buy it only as used to avoid waste from spoilage.

Poultry

Buy poultry by the whole bird. Usually the larger, more mature birds cost less than the young broilers and fryers, and they can be made equally tender with longer, moist cooking methods, such as braising, stewing, or pressure cooking.

Organ Meats

Liver, kidney, and heart carry many nutrients, especially iron, although liver is high in cholesterol. However, in some areas they may actually be more expensive than some other boneless cuts of meat. A good cookbook will have appetizing ways of cooking them for family acceptance.

Fish

This is sometimes a fairly expensive food in many areas, depending on the season and the kind. Shellfish is more costly. Less expensive packed styles of canned fish may be available. For example, tuna is packed according to sizes of pieces, with fancy or solid pack (large pieces) being most expensive.

Red Meats

Since meat is commonly one of the most costly food items, learn how it is graded, cut, processed, and marketed. Excellent learning material is available through the local county home advisor, USDA Extension Service. Avoid cuts with large amounts of gristle, bone, and fat. The lower grades provide good quality and less fat at a lower cost. A new, leaner form of beef, developed by genetic engineering and animal feeding changes, is beginning to enter our markets.[9]

Additional Resources

Farmers' Markets

In community farmers' markets local produce is made available directly to consumers. This outlet has the advantage of fresh produce at prices lower than those found in the supermarket. It also offers opportunities for socializing experiences between growers and consumers and gives a sense of community cohesion.

Consumer Cooperatives

Consumer cooperatives focus on the economics of food marketing, as well as on the issues of nutrition and ecology. The newer food cooperatives usually deal in bulk sales of whole or minimally processed foods. Belonging to a food cooperative increases personal responsibility and individual choice and brings food issues into the hands of the consumer.[10] Many of these food cooperatives stress the purchase of locally grown foods, thus strengthening local farmers while providing very fresh foods for consumers.

Home Gardens

With a little effort any extra yard space may be turned into a home garden. Many persons are now turning to their backyards, interspacing vegetable plants among flowers and shrubbery in frontyards, using alloted community spaces, window boxes, planter boxes on porches, and even indoor pots to grow at least a portion of their own produce.

To Sum Up

A major role of health care professionals is to translate the large amount of nutrition information available so that it can meet the needs of clients and families. They must present it in such a way that it is easily understood, is retained and applied by the learner, and can be evaluated to improve its effectiveness and ability to meet continuing care needs. Valid health and nutrition education must focus on the needs of the learner. Goals for planning counseling and educational activities and the methods for meeting these goals must be based on identifiable client and family needs.

Families and individuals under economic stress need counseling concerning financial assistance. Various U.S. food assistance programs operate to help families in need. Referrals to appropriate agencies may be made. The nutrition counselor may also need to assist the family in planning the most economic and nutritious meals possible within their limited circumstances. The family may need help in learning good shopping and food handling practices—planning ahead, buying wisely, storing safely, and cooking appropriately to preserve nutritional values and make food appetizing.

Questions for Review

1. Identify and describe the skills necessary for an effective nutrition counseling session.
2. Identify the basic principles of learning and describe how they may be used in planning nutrition education for one of your clients and family.
3. What government food assistance programs are available to help low-income families? What other local food resources are available in your community?
4. List and discuss the "best food buys" described in this chapter. How many of the recommended practices do you follow in selecting, storing, and preparing foods?

Physical factors affecting the counseling session—limited or no vision, limited hearing ability, and so on—may require more time, patience, or specially designed audiovisuals to facilitate learning. Involving a "significant other," such as family member, in the session might help to reinforce behavior changes at home.

Economic factors can influence the outcome of counseling if the client believes that new food choices will be expensive. Explaining wise buying practices and the benefits of dietary changes vs the cost of continued health care in a nonintimidating way may help overcome this anxiety. If cost is a barrier, the counselor may refer the client to any social service organization that could provide assistance.

Above all, counselors and teachers of adult clients must treat them as the adults they are. Such wise practitioners will develop approaches and methods that help their adult learners enhance their own creative thinking and problem-solving skills. At the beginning of every counseling or teaching session, they will strive to establish the empathy and good rapport that are essential for effective communication. Only in this way can sufficient information be obtained about the client's concerns and expectations and learning needs to develop an effective strategy for solving nutrition-related problems.

REFERENCES

Brown HW: Lateral thinking and androgyny: improving problem solving in adulthood, Lifelong Learning 8(7):22, 1985.

Gorham J: Differences between teaching adults and pre-adults: a closer look, Adult Ed Quarterly 35(4):194, 1985.

Holt GA: Patient characteristics: how adults learn, Am Pharm NS21(7):414, 1981.

Long HB: Adult learning—research and practice, Chicago, 1983, Follett Publishing Co.

11 Nutrition During Pregnancy and Lactation

Chapter Objectives

After studying this chapter, the student should be able to:

1. Relate the mother's specific increased maternal nutrition demands to her changed physiology during pregnancy.
2. Plan realistic food patterns to meet these increased maternal nutrition needs.

3. Identify functional problems some times encountered during pregnancy and make general dietary suggestions for their management.
4. Identify possible complications of pregnancy and related dietary management.
5. Develop food plans to meet the nutritional needs of breast-feeding mothers.

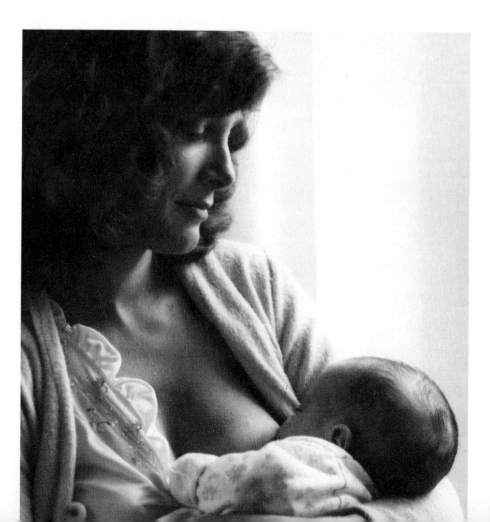

PREVIEW

Human reproduction involves complex processes of rapid, specialized growth. Given a positive environment, including sufficient nutritional support, both mother and child possess tremendous powers of adaptation that enable them to meet these demands.

We have seen in the previous chapters of our study that healthy body tissues depend directly on certain essential nutrients in food. Here we see that the infant's development relates directly to the diet of the mother.

In this chapter we start our journey through human needs during the life cycle. Here we look first at the beginnings of life. We will explore the nutritional needs of pregnancy and the vital role this basic support plays in its successful outcome.

Early Medical Practice

For centuries, in all cultures, a great body of folklore has surrounded pregnancy. Various traditional practices and diets have been followed, many of which have had little basis in fact, and much clinical advice has been based only on supposition. For example, early obstetricians even held the notion that semistarvation of the mother was really a blessing in disguise because it produced a small baby of light weight who would be easier to deliver. To this end they used diets restricted in kilocalories and protein, water, and salt. Despite the lack of any scientific evidence to support such ideas, two erroneous assumptions, now known to be false, governed practice: (1) the *parasite theory*: whatever the fetus needs it will draw from the stores of the mother despite the maternal diet; and (2) the *maternal instinct theory*: whatever the fetus needs, the mother will instinctively crave and consume.

The Healthy Pregnancy

It is clear now that until recently much of the counsel given to pregnant women over the past few decades has been based more on tradition than on scientific fact. Increasing evidence indicates that positive nutritional support of pregnancy, rather than past negative restrictions born of limited knowledge and false assumptions, promotes a positive successful outcome with increased health and vigor of mothers and infants alike. This struggle over the past four decades, particularly to define the positive "healthy pregnancy," has not been easy. Jacobson describes such a healthy pregnancy in broader terms of mother and infant and family.[1] We are beginning to understand more now just what this really means, especially as we see around us the current fetal damages from malnutrition and drug abuse. We know that we must assess and support more fully the fundamental nutritional needs and the quality of life of each mother and her family, if we are to approach the healthy pregnancy we desire for all mothers and have a healthier society.

Directions for Current Practice

Clinical observations and developing science in both nutrition and medicine have provided directions for healthier pregnancies. They have refuted previous false ideas and laid a sound base for our current practice. A benchmark

Maternal Nutrition and the Outcome of Pregnancy

Figure 11-1
A healthy child and mother—happy participants in the WIC program.

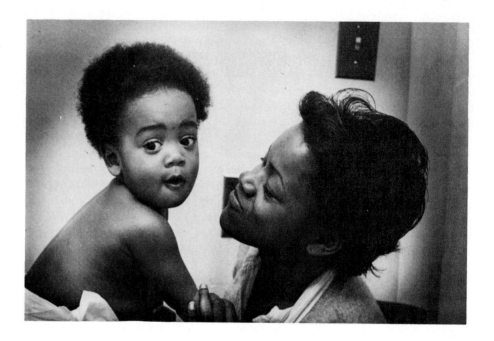

report of the National Research Council (NRC) first reflected this applied scientific base and led the way. This report, *Maternal Nutrition and the Course of Human Pregnancy*, was a clear turning point and provided undeniable direction for a new positive approach to the management of pregnancy.[2] Indeed, continuing research has reinforced this positive direction. On the basis of the significant NRC findings, guidelines for nutritional care of pregnant women were then issued by the American College of Obstetrics and Gynecology and the American Dietetic Association.[3,4] These reports have continued to provide guidelines for physicians, nutritionists, dietitians, and nurses in their prenatal care. We are reminded by these guides that a child is nutritionally 9 months old at birth, even older when we consider the significance of the mother's preconception status. Ancient Chinese wisdom has indeed embodied this truth in its counting of age at birth as 1 year.

Factors Determining Nutritional Needs

It is now evident from increased knowledge and the wide experience of many clinicians that maternal nutrition is critically important to both the mother and the child. It lays the fundamental foundation for the successful outcome of pregnancy—a healthy and happy mother and child (Figure 11-1). Several vital considerations emerge as factors that determine the nutritional requirements of the mother during her pregnancy.

Age and Parity

The teenage mother adds her own immaturity and growth needs to those imposed on her by her pregnancy.[5] At the other end of the reproductive cycle, hazards increase with age. Also, the number of pregnancies, **parity,** and the time intervals between them greatly influence the mother's nutrient reserves, her increased nutritional needs, and the outcome of the pregnancy.

Parity
The number of children born alive.

Preconception Nutrition

The mother brings to each pregnancy all of her previous life experiences, including her diet and food habits. Her general health and fitness and her state of nutrition at the time of conception are products of her lifelong dietary habits and her genetic heritage.

Complex Metabolic Interactions of Gestation

Three distinct biologic entities are involved in pregnancy: the mother, the fetus, and the **placenta.** Together they form a unique biologic whole. Constant metabolic interactions go on among them. Their functions, while unique, are at the same time interdependent.

Basic Concepts Involved

As a result of our increased knowledge of pregnancy and nutrition, we can provide better nutritional guidance. Three basic concepts form a fundamental framework for assessing maternal nutrition needs and for planning supportive prenatal care for both parents.

Perinatal Concept

The prefix *peri-* comes from the Greek root meaning "around, about, or surrounding." Thus the word *perinatal* refers more broadly to the scope of factors that surround a birth than merely to the 9 months of the physical gestation. Certainly, as nutrition knowledge and understanding have increased, health professionals realize that all of a woman's life experiences surrounding her pregnancy need to be considered. Her nutritional status and food patterns, which have developed over a number of years, and the degree to which she has established and maintained nutritional reserves are all important factors. Cultural and social influences have shaped beliefs and values of both parents about pregnancy. All of these influences come to bear upon any pregnancy.

Synergism Concept

The word *synergism* is a term used to describe biologic systems in which the cooperative action of two or more factors produces a total effect greater than and different from the mere sum of the parts. In short, a new whole is created by the unified, joint effort of blending the parts in which each part makes more powerful the action of the others. Of the many biologic and physiologic examples of synergism, pregnancy is a prime case in point. Maternal organism, fetus, and placenta combine to produce a new whole, a system not existing before and producing a total effect greater than and different from the sum of the parts, all for the sole purpose of sustaining and nurturing the pregnancy and its offspring. Physiologic measures change. Blood volume increases, cardiac output increases, ventilation rate and tidal volume of breathing increase, and basal metabolic rate increases. The physiologic norms of the nonpregnant woman do not apply. The normal physiologic adjustments of pregnancy cannot be viewed as pathologic with application of treatment procedures for that same type of response in the nonpregnant state. For example, a normal physiologic generalized edema of pregnancy is a protective response. It reflects the normal increase in total body water necessary to support the increased metabolic work of pregnancy and is associated with enhanced reproductive performance.

Placenta
Tissue that becomes active during pregnancy, providing a selective exchange of soluble particles in the blood to and from the fetus.

Synergism
The joint action of agents, which, when they act together, are more productive than when they act separately.

Life Continuum Concept

In a real sense, throughout her life a woman is providing for the ongoing continuum of life through the food that she eats. Each child obviously becomes a part of this continuing process during the pregnancy when the mother's diet directly sustains growth. But in the broader sense both parents carry over their nutritional heritage, practices, and beliefs in the teaching of their growing children, who in the next generation pass on this heritage both genetically and culturally.

Positive Nutritional Demands of Pregnancy

Basic Nutrient Allowances and Individual Variation

The period of **gestation** is an exceedingly rapid growth period. During this brief 9-month period, the human life grows from a single fertilized egg cell (ovum) to a fully developed infant weighing about 3 kg (7 lb). On the basis of this intense physiologic growth and development of the fetus, what nutrients must the mother supply? What must her diet provide to meet the nutritional demands of the fetus and of her own changing body during this critical period of human growth? Throughout the pregnancy there is an increased need for all the basic nutrients (Table 11-1). But it is important to remember that these are guidelines and individual variances in need must be examined

Gestation
The period of embryonic and fetal development from fertilization to birth; pregnancy.

Table 11-1

Recommended Daily Dietary Allowances of Some Selected Nutrients for Pregnancy and Lactation (National Research Council, 1989 revision)

Nutrients	Nonpregnant girl 12-14 yr 47 kg (103 lb)	Nonpregnant girl 14-18 yr 55 kg (120 lb)	Nonpregnant women 25 yr 58 kg (128 lb)	Pregnancy Added need	Pregnancy Girl 12-14 yr	Pregnancy Girl 14-18 yr	Pregnancy Woman 25 yr	Lactation (850 ml daily) Added need	Lactation Girl 12-14 yr	Lactation Girl 14-18 yr	Lactation Woman 25 yr
Kilocalories	2200	2200	2200	300	2500	2500	2500	500	2700	2700	2700
Protein (g)	46	46	50	10-15	60	60	60	15	65	68	65
Calcium (g)	1.2	1.2	0.8	0.4	1.6	1.6	1.2	0.4	1.6	1.6	1.2
Iron (mg)	15	15	15	15	30	30	30	0	15	15	15
Vitamin A (RE)*	800	800	800	0	800	800	800	500	1300	1300	1300
Thiamin (mg)	1.1	1.1	1.1	0.4	1.5	1.5	1.5	0.5	1.6	1.6	1.6
Riboflavin (mg)	1.3	1.3	1.3	0.3	1.6	1.6	1.6	0.5	1.8	1.8	1.8
Niacin equivalent and tryptophan (mg)	15	15	15	2	17	17	17	5	20	20	20
Ascorbic acid (mg)	50	60	60	10	60	70	70	35	95	95	95
Vitamin D (μg)†	10	10	5	5	15	15	10	5	15	15	10

*Retinol equivalents.

†Cholecalciferol; 10 μg equals 400 IU vitamin D.

for each pregnancy. Individual variations such as body size, activity, and multiple pregnancy would need to be considered. Also, quantitative need for nourishment of pregnant adolescents must be noted.[5] The need for individual counseling and for correct use of the Recommended Dietary Allowances (RDAs) of the NRC as guidelines is clearly stated by the NRC: "They are not called 'requirements,' because they are not intended to represent merely literal (minimal) requirements of average individuals, but to cover substantially the individual variations in the requirements of healthy people."[6] In considering the needs of the healthy pregnant woman, we will review the nutrient elements in terms of general amounts of increased intake indicated, why this increase is recommended, and how it may be obtained in basic foods.

Energy Needs

Kilocalories must be sufficient to (1) supply the increased energy demanded by the increased metabolic workload and (2) spare protein for tissue building. A minimum of about 36 kcal/kg is required for efficient use of protein during pregnancy. The RDA standard recommends an additional amount of energy, 300 kcal, representing about a 10% to 15% increase over the previous prepregnant standard, or about 2500 kcal. This amount may be insufficient for active, large, or nutritionally deficient women, who may need as much as 2500 to 3000 kcal. Remember that a minimum of 1800 kcal is required just to avoid negative nitrogen balance, to say nothing of the added pregnancy and activity needs. This primary positive emphasis on sufficient kilocalories is critical to the support of the pregnancy and necessary to ensure nutrient and energy needs. Appropriate weight gain during the pregnancy will indicate whether sufficient kilocalories are being provided.

Protein Needs

An additional daily allowance of 10 g of protein is indicated throughout the pregnancy, raising the 50 g recommended for the healthy nonpregnant woman to at least 60 g daily. This represents about a 20% increase.

Protein, with its essential nitrogen, is the nutrient basic to growth. Nitrogen balance studies give some indication of the large amounts of nitrogen used by the mother and child during pregnancy and emphasize the importance of maternal reserves to meet initial needs even before the pregnancy is confirmed. More protein is necessary to meet tissue demands posed by (1) rapid growth of the fetus; (2) enlargement of the uterus, mammary glands, and placenta; (3) increase in maternal circulating blood volume and subsequent demand for increased plasma proteins to maintain colloidal osmotic pressure and circulation of tissue fluids to nourish cells; and (4) formation of amniotic fluid and storage reserves for labor, delivery, and lactation.

Milk, egg, cheese, and meat are complete protein foods of high biologic value. Protein-rich foods also contribute other nutrients such as calcium, iron, and B vitamins. Additional protein may be obtained from legumes and whole grains, with lesser amounts in other plant sources such as nuts, seeds, and vegetables.

Mineral Needs

All of the major and trace minerals play roles in maternal health. Two that have special functions in relation to pregnancy—calcium and iron—deserve particular attention.

Calcium

The pregnant woman needs to increase her daily calcium intake by 400 mg. The suggested intake for the nonpregnant woman is about 800 mg, so the total daily intake during pregnancy should be 1200 mg, about a 50% increase.

The size of the recommended increase indicates the importance of calcium to the mother and fetus. Calcium is the essential element for the construction and maintenance of bones and teeth. It is also an important factor in the blood-clotting mechanism and is used in normal muscle action and other essential metabolic activities. The rapid fetal mineralization of skeletal tissue during the final period of rapid growth demands more calcium.

Dairy products are a primary source of calcium. Some increase in milk or equivalent in milk foods (cheese, ice cream, nonfat milk powder used in cooking) is recommended. Additional calcium is obtained in whole or enriched grains and in green leafy vegetables.

Iron

A woman needs to maintain a daily intake of 15 mg of iron throughout her childbearing years. This amount would replenish menstrual losses and restore tissue and liver reserves after each pregnancy, but surveys generally show that the iron stores of most women are only marginal. To meet the increased demands of pregnancy, iron supplements are usually recommended in addition to dietary sources because the "iron cost" of a pregnancy is high. With the increased demands for iron, often inadequate maternal stores, and insufficient provision through the usual diet, a daily increase of 15 mg of iron is the RDA standard. If the woman is anemic at conception, a larger therapeutic amount, usually 120 to 200 mg of iron, is recommended.

To obtain the needed amount of iron, check the percentage of elemental iron in the iron preparation being used. For example, the commonly used compound *ferrous sulfate* is a hydrated salt [$(FeSO_4) \cdot 7\ H_2O$], which contains 20% iron. It is usually dispensed in tablets containing 195, 300, or 325 mg of the ferrous sulfate compound. Each tablet, then, would contain 39, 60, or 65 mg of iron, respectively. Thus to supply a regular daily supplement of 60 mg of iron, one 300 mg tablet of ferrous sulfate would be used, and for a therapeutic dose of 120 mg iron, two tablets.

However, there are problems with routine iron supplementation for all pregnant women, such as unpleasant gastrointestinal side effects that interfere with maintaining a good diet. Also, there may be imbalances with other trace elements, such as zinc, which must compete with iron for absorption.[7] Actually, excess iron intake when not needed may potentially mask inadequate pregnancy-induced hemodilution, a normal pregnancy adaptation that puts less strain on the maternal heart, minimizes hemoglobin loss with blood loss at delivery, and may increase nutrient flow to the fetus. Thus some prenatal clinics are currently following revised protocols that prescribe regular prenatal vitamins with iron at the first clinic visit, then individual additional iron supplementation only if hemoglobin falls to 10.5 g/dL or less at any time during the pregnancy.[8]

During pregnancy the maternal circulating blood volume normally increases from 40% to 50% and more with multiple births. An individual mother's iron supplement need will have to be assessed accordingly. Maternal iron is also needed to supply iron stores for the developing fetal liver.

And adequate maternal iron stores help fortify the mother against serum iron losses at delivery.

It is no surprise then that our major food source of iron by far is liver. Its use can be encouraged by preparing it in many appetizing ways. Other food sources include meat, legumes, dried fruit, green vegetables, eggs, and enriched bread and cereals.

Vitamin Needs

Increased amounts of vitamins A, B-complex, C, and D are needed during pregnancy. If these needs are met, sufficient amounts of vitamins E and K will be available.

Vitamin A

According to the new RDAs, most healthy American women do not need a daily increase of vitamin A during pregnancy. However, malnourished women will need more. Vitamin A is an essential factor in cell development, maintenance of epithelial tissue, tooth formation, and normal bone growth. Liver, egg yolk, butter and fortified margarine, dark green and yellow vegetables, and fruits are good food sources.

B Vitamins

A special need exists for the various B vitamins during pregnancy. These are usually supplied by a well-balanced diet that is increased in quantity and quality to supply needed energy and nutrients. The B vitamins are important as coenzyme factors in a number of metabolic activities related to energy production, tissue protein synthesis, and function of muscle and nerve tissue. Therefore they play key roles in the increased metabolic work of pregnancy.

There is a particular increased metabolic demand for the B vitamin folic acid during pregnancy. Folic acid deficiency usually occurs in conjunction with general malnutrition, making the pregnant woman in high-risk, low socioeconomic conditions especially vulnerable. A specific megaloblastic anemia caused by maternal folate deficiency sometimes occurs and warrants supplementation of the diet with folic acid. This added amount is particularly needed where such demands are greater, as in a multiple pregnancy. The RDA standard recommends a daily intake of 400 μg of folic acid to prevent such potential deficiency.

Vitamin C

Special emphasis must be given to the pregnant woman's need for ascorbic acid. It is essential to the formation of intercellular cement substance in developing connective tissues and vascular systems. It also increases the absorption of iron that is needed for synthesis of increased quantities of hemoglobin. A daily increase of 10 mg is recommended. Added to the adult recommendation of 60 mg, this makes a total daily need of 70 mg during pregnancy. Additional food sources such as citrus fruit and other vegetables and fruits should be included in the mother's diet.

Vitamin D

Adults that lead active lives entailing adequate exposure to sunlight probably need little additional source of vitamin D. However, during pregnancy the increased need for calcium and phosphorus presented by the developing fetal skeletal tissue requires additional vitamin D to promote the absorption and utilization of these minerals. The recommended amount for pregnancy is 400 IU (15 μg calciferol) daily. Food sources include fortified milk, liver, egg yolk, and fortified margarine.

Dietary Patterns: General and Alternative
General Daily Food Pattern

A variety of familiar foods can usually supply the mother's need for added nutrients and make eating a pleasure. The increased quantities of essential nutrients needed during pregnancy may be met in many ways by planning around a daily food pattern and using key types of suggested foods. A general daily food pattern, which meets basic nutrient needs but not necessarily sufficient kilocalories, is suggested in Table 11-2. It may be used as a guide, with additional foods added according to energy and nutrient needs, as well as personal desires. This pattern represents the "orthodox middle-class American diet." It has been labeled the "biomedically recommended prenatal diet," which is generally used in some form by most health professionals in industrialized affluent countries worldwide.

Alternative Food Patterns

But there are alternative food patterns and it is always important to use the mother's own personal, cultural, and social food patterns in diet counseling. Sometimes we rigidly adhere to the "orthodox medical" pattern above as the *only* pattern for all pregnant women. However, it is but one alternative pattern among many others from different cultures, belief systems, and lifestyles. An extremist, unquestioning pursuit of "science as magic" may well lead us to label in turn *any* alternative practice as unscientific and unreasonable and to close our minds to some possibly fruitful avenues of scientific exploration. Remember, *specific nutrients,* not specific foods, are required for a successful pregnancy, and these nutrients are found in a wide variety of food choices. If we are wise, we will encourage our clients to use foods that serve their nutritional needs, *whatever* those foods might be. A number of resources have been developed to serve as guides for a variety of alternative food patterns, ethnic and vegetarian.

In essence then, two important principles govern the diet: (1) the pregnant woman must eat a sufficient quantity of food, and (2) she must eat regularly, avoiding any habit of fasting or skipping meals, especially breakfast following the night's fast of sleep.

General Dietary Problems

Functional Gastrointestinal Problems
Nausea and Vomiting

These symptoms are usually mild and short-term, the so-called morning sickness of early pregnancy because it occurs more often on arising than later in the day. At least 50% of all pregnant women, most of them in their first pregnancy, have this condition, beginning during the fifth or sixth week of the pregnancy and usually ending about the fourteenth to sixteenth week. A number of factors may contribute to the situation. Some are physiologic, based on hormonal changes that occur early in pregnancy. Others may be psychologic, based on situational tensions or anxieties about the pregnancy itself. Still others may be dietary problems, based on poor food habits. Sim-

Table 11-2
Core Food Plan for Daily Intake During Pregnancy and Lactation*

Food	Nonpregnant woman	Pregnancy	Lactation
Milk, cheese, ice cream, skimmed or buttermilk (food made with milk can supply part of requirement)	2 cups	3-4 cups	4-5 cups
Meat (lean meat, fish, poultry, cheese, occasional dried beans or peas)	1 serving (3-4 oz)	2 servings (6-8 oz); include liver frequently	2½ servings (8 oz)
Eggs	1	1-2	1-2
Vegetable† (dark green or deep yellow)	1 serving	1 serving	1-2 servings
Vitamin C–rich food† Good source: citrus fruit, berries, cantaloupe Fair source: tomatoes, cabbage, greens, potatoes in skin	1 good source or 2 fair sources	1 good source and 1 fair source or 2 good sources	1 good source and 1 fair source or 2 good sources
Other vegetables, fruits, juices	2 servings	4-6 servings	4-6 servings
Bread‡ and cereals (enriched or whole grain)	6 servings	10 servings	10 servings
Butter or fortified margarine	Moderate amount	Moderate amount	Moderate amount

*Meets nutrient needs; add additional foods as needed for energy (kilocalorie) demands.
†Use some raw daily.
‡One slice of bread or ½ cup starch (grains or vegetables) equals 1 serving.

ple treatment generally improves food toleration. Small frequent meals and snacks, fairly dry and consisting chiefly of easily digested energy-yielding foods, such as carbohydrates, mainly starches, are usually more readily tolerated. Also, it sometimes helps to avoid cooking odors as much as possible. Liquids are best taken between meals instead of with meals. In about 2% of pregnant women, the nausea may continue and develop into severe and prolonged vomiting that can be life-threating, a condition called **hyperemesis gravidarum.** In such cases, the mother is usually hospitalized and receives peripheral parenteral nutrition (see Chapter 23), followed by careful oral refeeding. Continued personal support and reassurance are important.

Hyperemesis gravidarum
Severe vomiting that is potentially fatal.

Constipation

This complaint is seldom more than minor. Placental hormones relax the gastrointestinal muscles, and the pressure of the enlarging uterus on the lower portion of the intestine may make elimination somewhat difficult. Increased fluid intake, use of naturally laxative foods containing dietary fiber, such as whole grains, fruits and vegetables, dried fruits (especially prunes and figs), and other fruits and juices help induce regularity. Laxatives should be avoided.

Weight Gain During Pregnancy
General amount of weight gain

Healthy women produce healthy babies over a wide range of total weight gain. It is the individual assessment of need and the quality of the weight gain that are of paramount importance. Optimal weight gain of the mother during pregnancy is a significant reflection of good nutritional status and contributes to a successful course and outcome. It should not be a problem or a source of contention. An average weight gain during pregnancy is about 25 to 30 lb (11 to 14 kg). Around this average many individual variations occur. There is no specific rigid norm or restriction to which all women should be held regardless of individual needs. Such a course is obviously unwise and unscientific. Current recommendations, therefore, are usually stated in terms of ranges to accommodate variances in needs. An initial base for evaluation, however, may be the average weight of the products of pregnancy as shown in Table 11-3. In addition to the components of growth and development usually attributed to a pregnancy, an important part is maternal stores, which vary according to preconception nutritional status. This laying down of extra adipose fat tissue is necessary for maternal energy reserves to sustain rapid fetal growth during the latter half of pregnancy, as well as energy for labor and delivery and maintaining lactation after birth. About 4 to 8 lb (1.8 to 3.6 kg) or more of adipose tissue is commonly deposited for these needs. So although a relatively wide range of weight gains can support healthy pregnancies and healthy babies, some approximate ranges based on prepregnant weight may be recommended and can serve as general guidelines[9]:

1. *Normal weight women*: 24 to 32 lb (10 to 14.5 kg)
2. *Underweight women*: 28 to 36 lb (13 to 16.5 kg)
3. *Overweight women*: 16 to 24 lb (7.3 to 11 kg)

Quality of Weight Gain

The important consideration, as indicated, lies in the *nutritional quality* of the gain. The foods consumed should be nutritious foods to meet the nutrient requirements, not foods contributing only "empty" kilocalories. Also, there has been failure in some cases to distinguish between weight gained as a result of edema and that owing to deposition of fat, maternal stores for energy to sustain the latter rapid fetal growth, and needs for labor, delivery, and early lactation. Analysis of the total tissue gained in an average pregnancy shows that the largest component, 62%, is water. Fat accounts for 31% and protein for 7%. Water is also the most variable component of the tissue gained, accounting for a range of 8 kg (18 lb) to as much as 11 kg (24 lb). Of the 8 kg of water usually gained, about 5.5 kg (12 lb) is associated with fetal tissue and other tissues gained in pregnancy. The remaining 2.5 kg (6 lb) accumulates in the maternal interstitial tissues.[10] Gravity causes the maternal tissue fluids to pool more in the lower extremities, leading to general swelling of the ankles, which is seen routinely in pregnant women. This fluid retention is a normal adaptive phenomenon designed to support the pregnancy and exert a positive effect on fetal growth. The connective tissue becomes more **hygroscopic** because of the estrogen-induced changes in the ground substance. The connective tissue thus becomes softer and more easily distended to facilitate delivery through the cervix and the vaginal canal. Also, the increased tissue fluid provides a means for handling the increased

Hygroscopic
Taking up and retaining moisture readily.

Products	Weight
Fetus	3400 g (7.5 lb)
Placenta	450 g (1 lb)
Amniotic fluid	900 g (2 lb)
Uterus (weight increase)	1100 g (2.5 lb)
Breast tissue (weight increase)	1400 g (3 lb)
Blood volume (weight increase)	1800 g (4 lb) (1500 ml)
Maternal stores	1800-3600 g (4-8 lb)
TOTAL	11000-13000 g (11-13 kg; 24 to 28 lb)

Table 11-3

Approximate Weight of Products of a Normal Pregnancy

metabolic work and circulation of numerous nutrients and metabolites necessary for fetal growth.

Clearly, severe caloric restriction in pregnancy is unphysiologic and potentially dangerous to the developing fetus and to the mother. It is inevitably accompanied by restriction of the vitally needed nutrients essential to the growth process. Thus *weight reduction should never be undertaken during pregnancy.* To the contrary, sufficient weight gain should be encouraged with the use of a nourishing diet as outlined.

Rate of Weight Gain

On the whole, about 1.0 to 2.3 kg (2 to 5 lb) is an average weight gain during the first trimester. Thereafter, about 0.5 kg (1 lb) per week, more or less, during the remainder of the pregnancy is usual. There is no scientific justification for routinely limiting weight gain to lesser amounts. Moreover, an individual woman who needs to gain more should not have unrealistic "grid patterns" imposed upon her. It is only unusual patterns of gain, such as a sudden sharp increase in weight after the twentieth week of pregnancy, which may indicate excessive, abnormal water retention, that should be watched.

Despite efforts of practitioners over the past few years to dispel former myths and practices, many women still have misconceptions about how much weight they should gain during pregnancy. In a recent study there was evidence that some of these misconceptions may stem from inappropriate advice about weight gain given to pregnant women by their physicians.[11] The majority of the mothers were given no weight gain advice or were being advised to gain less than is currently deemed advisable, a particular concern among many high-risk mothers. The investigators concluded that appropriate weight gain advice, especially for high-risk groups, could have a positive effect on birth outcomes.

Sodium

Sometimes in relation to weight gain, questions are raised about the use of salt during pregnancy. A regular moderate amount of dietary sodium is needed, because it is the major mineral required for guarding the extracellular fluid compartment, which is increased during pregnancy to support its successful outcome. Current practice usually follows a regular diet with moderate sodium intake, 2 to 3 g/day, including light salt use to taste. Limiting sodium beyond this general use is contrary to physiologic need in pregnancy and is unfounded. A recent study, measuring general sodium intake as desired by pregnant women during their second and third trimesters, found their daily sodium intake in the two trimesters to be 2.57 g (112 mmol) and 2.34 g (102 mmol), respectively.[12] Both the NRC and professional obstetric guidelines have labeled routine salt-free diets and diuretics as dangerous practices that should *not* be used.[2-4] Maintaining the needed increase in circulating blood volume during pregnancy requires adequate amounts of both sodium and protein.

High-Risk Mothers and Infants

Identify Risk Factors Involved

To avoid the consequences of poor nutrition during pregnancy, mothers at risk must be identified as soon as possible. Risk factors that identify women with special nutritional needs during pregnancy are given in Table 11-4. These nutrition-related factors are based on clinical evidence of inadequate nutrition. However, rather than waiting for clinical symptoms of poor nutrition to appear, a better approach would be to identify poor food patterns that will bring on nutritional problems and prevent these problems from developing. Look for three types of dietary patterns that will not support optimal maternal and fetal nutrition: (1) insufficient food intake, (2) poor food selection, and (3) poor food distribution throughout the day.[10] These patterns, added to the list of risk factors in Table 11-4, would provide a much more sensitive measure of nutritional risk.

Plan Personal Care

On the basis of such early assessment, practitioners can then give more careful attention to women identified as having higher risks in their pregnancies. By working closely with each woman and her own patterns of food intake and living situation, a personal food plan can be developed with her to ensure an optimal intake of all the nutrient increases demanded for support of the pregnancy and its successful outcome.

Recognize Special Counseling Needs

In addition to avoiding dangerous practices, such as diet fads, macrobiotics or fruitarianism, and **pica,** several special needs require sensitive counseling.

Age and Parity

Pregnancies at either age extreme of the reproductive cycle pose special problems. The adolescent pregnancy carries many social and nutrition-related risks. Imposed on a still immature teenaged body are the additional demands of the pregnancy. **Nulligravidas** 15 years old and younger are especially at risk, since their own growth is incomplete. Sensitive counseling provides both information and emotional support. It should involve family or other persons significant to the young mother. On the other hand, the older **primigravida** (over 35 years of age) also requires special attention. She may be more at risk for hypertension, either preexisting or pregnancy-induced, and may need more attention to rate of weight gain and excessive

Pica
Perverted appetite or craving for unnatural foods, such as chalk or clay, sometimes seen in pregnancy or in malnourished children.

Nulligravida
A woman who has never been pregnant.

Primigravida
A woman pregnant for the first time.

Table 11-4

Nutritional Risk Factors
in Pregnancy

Risk factors presented at the onset of pregnancy	Risk factors occurring during pregnancy

Age
  15 years or younger
  35 years or older
	Low hemoglobin and/or hematocrit
	  Hemoglobin less than 12.0 g
	  Hematocrit less than 35.0 mg/dL

Frequent pregnancies: three or more during a 2-year period	Inadequate weight gain
	  Any weight loss
	  Weight gain of less than 2 lb per month after the first trimester

Poor obstetric history or poor fetal performance	Excessive weight gain: greater than kg (2 lb) per week after the first trimester
Poverty	
Bizarre or faddist food habits	
Abuse of nicotine, alcohol, or drugs	
Therapeutic diet required for a chronic disorder	

Inadequate weight
  Less than 85% of standard weight
  More than 120% of standard weight	

use of sodium. In addition, several pregnancies within a limited number of years leave a mother drained of nutritional resources and entering each successive pregnancy at a higher risk. Counseling may well include discussions of acceptable means of contraception and nutrition information and support.

Social Habits: Alcohol, Cigarettes, and Drugs

These three personal habits cause fetal damage and are contraindicated during pregnancy. Extensive or habitual alcohol use leads to the well-described and documented *fetal alcohol syndrome,* which is currently a leading cause of mental retardation.[13-15] Cigarette smoking during pregnancy poses special problems of placental abnormalities and fetal damage, including prematurity and low birth weight (see the box on p. 266), largely because of impaired oxygen transport.[16] Counseling with mothers who smoke should certainly stress the importance of quitting.

Drug use, both recreational and medicinal, also poses numerous problems. Self-medication with over-the-counter drugs carries potential adverse effects. The use of "street drugs" is especially hazardous to the developing fetus, causing the baby to be born addicted or with AIDS from the mother's use of contaminated needles in her drug injections. Dangers come not only from the drug itself or contaminated needles but also from the impurities such street drugs contain.[17]

In addition, drug abuse from megadosing with basic nutrients such as vitamin A during pregnancy may also bring fetal damage. Especially dangerous are drugs made from vitamin A compounds, retinoids such as Accutane or etretinate, prescribed for severe acne, which have caused spontaneous abortion of malformed infants by women who conceived during such acne

Clinical Application

Who Will Have the Low-Birth-Weight Baby?

The number of babies weighing less than 2500 g (5 lb) at birth is still a problem. Perinatal nutritionists are well aware of the dietary factors that may influence this increase, especially poor weight gain during pregnancy. The prevalence of that turn-of-the-century adage to "grow the baby to fit the pelvis" continues to influence some physicians, nurses, and expectant mothers alike to limit prenatal weight gain to 9 kg (20 lb) or less to avoid obstetric problems, especially at delivery. This practice is harmful and is refuted by recent evidence that a gain of 11 to 15 kg (25 to 25 lb) is correlated with birth weights of greater than 2500 g (5 lb).

The obsession with weight control during pregnancy can lead to harmful restrictions of vital energy and nutrients. Weight reduction should *never* be attempted during pregnancy. Such regimens are extremely dangerous to the fetus. Even the common practice of skipping breakfast, especially late in pregnancy, may potentially impair intellectual development (as seen in studies with rats) by inducing a ketotic, pseudostarvation state very quickly. Increased ketoacidosis from fat breakdown can cause neurologic damage to the fetus.

Nondietary factors influencing this growing trend toward more low-birth-weight (LBW) babies were identified in a Baltimore study:

- Rise in number of older primigravidas (that is, over 35 years of age)
- Rise in number of teenage pregnancies
- Previous induced abortions
- Single marital status (often an indicator of low economic status)
- Technologic advances in neonatal care, which keeps premature infants alive longer
- Race: nonwhites have higher rates of LBW infants than whites do

To reduce the risk of LBW infants in populations being served by your facility, you may want to:

- Explain the rationale for gaining around 11 to 15 kg (25 to 30 lb)
- Discourage the use of cigarettes and alcohol
- Monitor excessive weight gain and sodium intake in older primigravidas, who are at risk for prenatal essential hypertension and obesity
- Explore eating habits of adolescents in the local community, working with the girl and her "significant others" to incorporate nutrient-dense foods into her meal and snack selections
- Keep abreast of federal, state, and local supplemental food progams (for example, WIC) available to low-income women to ensure an adequate intake of nutrients and kilocalories
- Encourage regular eating patterns throughout pregnancy

REFERENCES

Behrman RE: Premature births among black women, N Engl J Med 317:763, September 17, 1987.

Brown JE and others: Prenatal weight gains related to the birth of healthy-sized infants to low-income women, J Am Diet Assoc 86(12):1679, 1986.

Endres J and others: Older pregnant women and adolescents: nutrition data after enrollment in WIC, J Am Diet Assoc 87(8):1011, Aug 1987.

Paige DM and Davis LR: Fetal growth, maternal nutrition, and dietary supplementation, Clin Nutr 5(5):191, 1986.

Villar J and Cassio TG: Nutritional factors associated with low birth weight and short gestational age, Clin Nutr 5(2):78, 1986.

treatment.[18,19] Thus the use of these drugs without contraception is definitely contraindicated.

Caffeine

Although milder in its effect, depending on extent of use, than agents discussed above, caffeine is still a widely used drug that can cross the placenta and enter fetal circulation. Its use at pharmacologic levels has been associated with low birth weight.[20] A pharmacologic dose of caffeine—250 mg—is contained in 2 cups of coffee, 3.5 cups of tea, or 5 12-oz colas, so such use is not recommended.[21] Most responsible health agencies have recommended that pregnant women avoid caffeine-containing beverages, and that products containing caffeine be plainly labeled to inform consumers.

Socioeconomic Problems

Special counseling is required for women and young girls living in low-income situations or extreme poverty. Numerous studies and clinical observations indicate that lack of prenatal care, often associated with racial prejudices and fears, as well as poverty, places the expectant mother in grave difficulty. Special counseling, sensitive to personal needs, is needed to help plan resources for care and financial assistance. Resources include programs such as WIC (Figure 11-1) and the Commodity Distribution Program, both of which are described in the previous chapter.

Anemia

Anemia is common during pregnancy. About 10% of all women in large prenatal clinics in the United States have hemoglobin concentrations of less than 10 g/dL and a hematocrit reading below 32%. Anemia is far more prevalent among the poor, many of whom live on diets barely adequate for subsistence. However, anemia is by no means restricted to lower economic groups.

Iron-Deficiency Anemia

A deficiency of iron is by far the most common cause of anemia in pregnancy. The total cost of a single normal pregnancy in iron stores is large—about 500 to 800 mg. Of this amount nearly 300 mg is used by the fetus. The remainder is used in the expanded maternal blood volume and its increased red blood cells and hemoglobin mass. This iron requirement exceeds the available reserves in the average woman. Thus, in addition to including iron-rich foods in the diet, a daily supplement of may be needed. Treatment of highly deficient states requires more, a daily therapeutic dose of 120 to 200 mg, which is usually continued for 3 to 6 months after the anemia has been corrected to replenish the depleted stores.

Folate-Deficiency Anemia

A less common **megaloblastic anemia** of pregnancy results from folic acid deficiency. During pregnancy the fetus is sensitive to folic acid inhibitors and therefore has increased metabolic requirements for folic acid and its derivatives. To prevent this anemia, the RDA standard recommends a preventive intake for pregnant women of 400 μg of folic acid daily.

Complications of Pregnancy

Megaloblastic anemia
Reduction in the number of red blood cells associated with the presence of large, premature cells in the bone marrow. Caused by a folic acid deficiency.

Hemorrhagic Anemia

Anemia caused by blood loss is more likely to occur during labor and delivery than during pregnancy. Blood loss may occur earlier, as a result of abortion or ruptured tubular pregnancy. Most patients undergoing these physiologic problems receive blood by transfusion, and iron therapy may be indicated for adequate replacement hemoglobin formation.

Pregnancy-Induced Hypertension (PIH)

Relation to Nutrition

A number of clinicians have presented clinical and laboratory evidence that pregnancy-induced hypertension, formerly labeled **toxemia,** is a disease of malnutrition, especially related to diets poor in protein, kilocalories, calcium, and salt. Such malnutrition affects the liver and its many metabolic activities. Classically, it is associated with poverty and found most often in women subsisting on inadequate diets and having little or no prenatal care, which inherently includes attention to sound nutrition. A woman's fitness during pregnancy is a direct function of her past good state of nutrition and her optimal nutrition throughout pregnancy.

Clinical Symptoms

PIH is defined according to its manifestations, which generally occur in the third trimester toward term. These symptoms are hypertension, abnormal and excessive edema, albuminuria, and in severe cases, convulsions or coma, a state called **eclampsia.**

Treatment

Specific treatment varies according to the individual patient's symptoms and needs. Optimal nutrition is a fundamental aspect of therapy in any case.[22] Emphasis is placed on adequate dietary protein. Correction of plasma protein deficits stimulates the capillary fluid shift mechanism and increases circulation of tissue fluids, with subsequent correction of the **hypovolemia** (see Chapter 8). In addition, adequate salt and sources of vitamins and minerals are needed for correction and maintenance of metabolic balance.

Maternal Disease Conditions

Preexisting clinical conditions in the mother further complicate pregnancy. In each case, management of these conditions is based on general principles of care related both to pregnancy and to the particular disease involved. Examples of three such maternal disease complications are given here.

Hypertension

Preexisting hypertension in the pregnant woman can cause considerable maternal and fetal consequences. Many of these problems can be prevented by initial screening and continued monitoring by the prenatal nurse, with referral to the clinical nutritionist for plan of care. The hypertensive disease process begins long before signs and symptoms appear and later symptoms are inconsistent. Risk factors for hypertension before and during pregnancy are compared in Table 11-5. Nutritional therapy will center on (1) prevention of weight extremes, underweight or obesity, (2) correction of any dietary defi-

Toxemia
Formerly used term (current official term of American College of Obstetricians and Gynecologists is *pregnancy-induced hypertension—PIH*); a metabolic disturbance that usually manifests itself in the third trimester with symptoms of hypertension, abnormal edema, and albuminemia. If uncontrolled, it can lead to coma or convulsions.

Eclampsia
Advanced pregnancy-induced hypertension (PIH) manifested by convulsions.

Hypovolemia
Abnormal reduction in volume of circulatory plasma.

Before pregnancy	During pregnancy
Nulligravida	Primigravida
Diabetes mellitus	Large fetus
Preexisting condition (hypertension, renal or vascular disease)	Glomerulonephritis
Family history of hypertension or vascular disease	**Fetal hydrops**
Diagnosis of pregnancy-induced hypertension in a previous pregnancy	**Hydramnios**
Dietary deficiencies	Multiple gestation
Age extremes 20 years or younger 35 years or older	**Hydatidiform mole**

Table 11-5

Risk Factors in Pregnancy-Induced Hypertension

Fetal hydrops
Extensive edema of the entire fetus associated with severe anemia.

Hydramnios
An excess of amniotic fluid.

Hydatidiform mole
An abnormal pregnancy resulting in a cystic mass resembling a bunch of grapes, formed by a pathologic ovum in the uterus; a molar pregnancy.

ciencies and maintenance of optimal nutritional status during pregnancy, and (3) management of any related preexisting disease such as diabetes mellitus. Sodium intake may be moderate but should not be unduly restricted, because of its relation to fluid and electrolyte balances during pregnancy and its controversial therapy in hypertension in general. Initial and continuing client education and a close relationship with the nurse-nutritionist care team contribute to successful management of the hypertension and prevent problems that may occur.

Diabetes Mellitus

The management of preexisting insulin-dependent diabetes mellitus (IDDM) in pregnancy presents special problems. Today, however, improved expectations for the diabetic mother's pregnancy constitute one of the success stories of modern medicine.[23] Contributing factors to this improved outlook include advances in technology for monitoring fetal development, increased knowledge of nutrition and diabetes, and especially management refinements in "tight" blood glucose control through self-monitoring.[24] Routine screening is necessary to detect gestational diabetes, and team management is required for IDDM. Refer to Chapter 21 for a detailed discussion of diabetes care.

Maternal Phenylketonuria (MPKU)

Successful detection and management of PKU babies through U.S. newborn screening programs in all states has ensured their normal growth and development to adulthood. PKU is a genetic metabolic disease caused by a missing enzyme for the metabolism of the essential amino acid phenylalanine. It is controlled by a special low-phenylalanine diet initiated at birth. Now a new generation of young women with PKU since birth are beginning to have children of their own. However, maternal PKU presents potential fetal hazards. Experience has shown how crucial it is for the mother to follow a strict low-phenylalanine diet before conception, whenever possible, to minimize risks of fetal damage in the early cell differentiation weeks of pregnancy.[25]

Currently, to study these effects of maternal PKU on pregnancy outcome, the U.S. National Institute of Child Health and Human Development of the National Institutes of Health (NIH) is conducting a 7-year collaborative project, begun in 1984.[26] This large Maternal PKU Collaborative Study involves all 50 states and the District of Columbia, as well as all the provinces of Canada. The diet protocol is planned around a specially formulated phenylalanine-free supplemented medical food of amino acids and carbohydrate—a powder to be mixed with free liquids and used at meals as a beverage. Foods are selected from special lists of low-phenylalanine vegetables, fruits, and grains, and numerous free foods. Early reports of pregnancy outcomes among the women in the study are encouraging.

Nutrition During Lactation

Current Breast-Feeding Trends

An increasing number of mothers in America and other developed countries are choosing breast-feeding for their infants (see Issues and Answers on p. 274). Several factors have contributed to this choice: (1) more mothers are informed about the benefits of breast-feeding; (2) practitioners recognize the ability of human milk to meet infant needs (Table 11-6); (3) maternity wards and alternative birth centers are being modified to facilitate successful lactation; and (4) community support is more available, even in work places. Exclusive breast-feeding by well-nourished mothers can be adequate for periods ranging from 2 to 15 months. Solid foods are usually added to the baby's diet at about 6 months of age.

Nutritional Needs

The basic nutritional needs for lactation include the following additions to the mother's prepregnant allowances.

Protein

An increase of 20 g of protein over the amount recommended for the nonpregnant woman is needed during lactation. This makes a total protein allowance of about 65 g/day.

Energy

The recommended caloric increase is 500 kcal more than the usual adult allowance. This makes a daily total of about 2700 kcal. This additional energy need for the overall total lactation process is based on three factors as follows

1. **Milk content.** An average daily milk production for lactating women is 850 ml (30 oz). Human milk has a kcal range of 20 to 70 kcal/oz or an average of 24 kcal/oz. Thus 30 oz of milk has an energy value of about 700 kcal.
2. **Milk production.** The metabolic work involved in producing this amount of milk requires from 400 to 450 kcal.
3. **Maternal adipose tissue storage.** The additional energy need for lactation is drawn from maternal adipose tissue stores deposited during pregnancy in normal preparation for lactation to follow in the maternal cycle. Depending on the adequacy of these stores, additional energy input may be needed in the lactating woman's daily diet.

Milk component	Colostrum	Transitional	Mature	Cow's milk
Kilocalories	57.0	63.0	65.0	65.0
Vitamins, fat-soluble:				
A (μg)	151.0	88.0	75.0	41.0
D (IU)	—	—	5.0	2.5
E (mg)	1.5	0.9	0.25	0.07
K (μg)	—	—	1.5	6.0
Vitamins, water-soluble:				
Thiamin (μg)	1.9	5.9	14.0	43.0
Riboflavin (μg)	30.0	37.0	40.0	145.0
Niacin (μg)	75.0	175.0	160.0	82.0
Pantothenic acid (μg)	183.0	288.0	246.0	340.0
Biotin (μg)	0.06	0.35	0.6	2.8
Vitamin B_{12} (μg)	0.05	0.04	0.1	0.6
Vitamin C (mg)	5.9	7.1	5.0	1.1

Table 11-6

Nutritional Components of Human Milk (per 100 ml)

Minerals

The quantities of calcium and iron required by the lactating mother are not greater than those needed during the pregnancy. The increased amount of calcium that was required during gestation for mineralization of the fetal skeleton is now diverted into the mother's milk production. Iron, because it is not a principal mineral component of milk, need not be increased for milk production.

Vitamins

An increased quantity of vitamin C above that needed by the pregnant woman is recommended for the lactating mother. An increase of 35 mg is indicated, making her total ascorbic acid requirement 95 mg/day. Increases over the mother's prenatal intake are recommended also for vitamin A and the B-complex vitamins involved as coenzyme factors in energy metabolism. The quantities needed therefore invariably increase as kilocalorie intake increases.

Fluids

Adequate fluid intake is needed, but contrary to common beliefs, additional fluid beyond this need will not increase the mother's milk supply further.[27] The more critical factor necessary for successful milk production is the increased energy intake. The basis for this increased caloric need is described above. Additional beverages such as juices and milk contribute both fluid and kilocalories.

Rest and Relaxation

In addition to the increased diet, the nursing mother requires rest, moderate exercise, and relaxation. Both parents may benefit from counseling focused on reducing the stresses of their new family situation, as well as meeting their own personal needs.

To Sum Up

Pregnancy involves synergistic interactions among three distinct biologic entities: the fetus, the placenta, and the mother. Maternal needs reflect the increasing nutritional needs of the fetus and the placenta, as well as the need to meet maternal needs and to prepare for lactation. An optimal weight gain of about 11 kg (25 lb), or more as needed, is recommended during pregnancy to accommodate the rapid growth taking place. Even more significant than the actual weight gain, though it must be sufficient, is the quality of the diet.

Common problems occurring during pregnancy include nausea and vomiting, heartburn, or constipation. In most cases they are easily relieved without medication by simple, often temporary changes in the diet. Unusual or erratic eating habits, age, parity, prepartum weight status, and low income are among the many related conditions that also place the woman at risk for complications.

The ultimate goal of prenatal care is a healthy infant and a mother physically capable of breast-feeding her child, should she choose to do so. Human milk provides essential nutrients in quantities required for optimal infant growth and development.

Questions for Review

1. List and discuss five factors that influence the nutritional needs of the woman during pregnancy. Which factors would place a woman in a high-risk category? Why?
2. List six nutrients that are required in larger amounts during pregnancy. Describe their special role and identify four food sources of each.
3. Identify two common problems associated with pregnancy and describe the dietary management of each.
4. List and discuss five major nutritional factors of lactation.

References

1. Jacobson HN: A healthy pregnancy: the struggle to define it, Nutr Today 23(1):30, 1988.
2. Food and Nutrition Board, Committee on Maternal Nutrition, National Research Council: Maternal nutrition and the course of human pregnancy, Washington, DC, 1970, National Academy of Sciences.
3. American College of Obstetricians and Gynecologists, Committee on Nutrition: Nutrition in maternal health care, Chicago, 1974.
4. American College of Obstetricians and Gynecologists and American Dietetic Association, Task Force on Nutrition: Assessment of maternal nutrition, Chicago, 1978.
5. Rees JM and Mahan K: Nutrition in adolescence. In Williams SR and Worthington-Roberts BS, editors: Nutrition throughout the life cycle, St Louis, 1988, The CV Mosby Co.
6. National Research Council: Recommended dietary allowances, ed 9, Washington, DC, 1980, National Academy of Sciences.
7. Solomans NW, Helizer-Allen DL, and Villar J: Zinc needs during pregnancy, Clin Nutr 5(2):63, 1986.
8. Reece J, Donovan PP, and Pellet AY: Iron supplementation in pregnancy: testing a new clinic protocol, J Am Diet Assoc 87(12):1682, 1987.
9. Brown JE: Nutrition services for pregnant women, infants, children, and adolescents, Clin Nutr 3(3):100, 1984.
10. King JC: Dietary risk patterns during pregnancy, Nutr Update 1:206, 1983.
11. Taffel SM and Keppel KG: Advice about weight gain in pregnancy and actual weight gain, Am J Pub Health 76:1396, Dec 1986.

12. Brown MA and others: Comparing methods to assess dietary sodium intake in pregnancy, J Am Diet Assoc 87(8):1058, 1987.

13. Weiner L and Rosett HL: Pregnancy and alcohol, Clin Nutr 4(1):10, 1985.

14. Abel EL and Sokol RJ: Fetal alcohol syndrome is now leading cause of mental retardation, Lancet 2:1222, Nov 22, 1986.

15. Raymond CA: Birth defects linked with specific level of maternal alcohol use, but abstinence is still the best policy, JAMA 258:177, July 10, 1987.

16. Bureau MA and others: Maternal cigarette smoking and fetal oxygen transport, Pediatrics 72:22, 1983.

17. Enig MG: Pharmacologic basis of drug-nutrient interaction related to drug abuse during pregnancy, Clin Nutr 6(6):235, 1987.

18. Watson RR: Vitamin A and teratogenesis: recommendations for pregnancy, J Am Diet Assoc 88(3):364, 1988.

19. Ellis CN and Voorhees JJ: Etretinate therapy, J Am Acad Dermatol 16:267, 1987.

20. Leonard TK, Watson RR, and Mohs ME: The effects of caffeine on various body systems: a review, J Am Diet Assoc 87(8):1048, 1987.

21. Leonard-Green TK and Watson RR: Caffeine and health risk, J Am Diet Assoc 88(3):370, 1988.

22. Williams SR: Management of pregnancy complications and special disease conditions of the mother. In Worthington-Roberts BS and Williams SR: Nutrition in pregnancy and lactation, ed 4, St Louis, 1989, The CV Mosby Co.

23. Freinkel N, Dooley SL, and Metzger BE: Care of the pregnant woman with insulin-dependent diabetes mellitus, N Engl J Med 313:96, 1985.

24. Beebe CA: Self blood glucose monitoring: management of the patient with diabetes, J Am Diet Assoc 87(1):61, 1987.

25. Rohr FJ and others: The New England Maternal PKU Project: prospective study of untreated and treated pregnancies and their outcomes, J Pediatr 110:391, 1986.

26. Rohr FJ, Friedman EG, and Koch R: Maternal PKU: report from the Maternal PKU Collaborative Study, Metabolic Currents 1(1):1, 1988.

27. Stumbo PJ and others: Water intakes of lactating women, Am J Clin Nutr 42:870, Nov 1985.

Further Readings

Berenbaum S: How to build a better baby, J Nutr Ed 17:100D, Aug 1985.

Canada's National Guidelines on Prenatal Nutrition, Nutr Today 22(4):34, 1987.

These two Canadian resources provide helpful guides for nutrition in pregnancy and a practical teaching tool for pregnant women for helping them meet these excellent goals.

Endres J and others: Older pregnant women and adolescents: nutrition data after enrollment in WIC, J Am Diet Assoc 87(8):1011, 1987.

This study focuses on the age risk in pregnancy, as well as on the low income factor, and the effect of WIC participation in meeting needs.

Jacobson HN: A healthy pregnancy: the struggle to define it, Nutr Today 23(1):30, 1988.

This article traces the struggle of the past four decades to define positive guidelines for a healthy pregnancy and describes where we are now and how far we still have to go.

Worthington-Roberts BS: Nutritional support of successful reproduction: an update, J Nutr Ed 19(1):1, 1987.

The Dynamic Nature of Human Milk

Mother Nature is determined to give every breast-fed infant all the nutrients he or she needs, no matter *when* the child is born or *how*.

Mothers and physicians alike have been reluctant to consider breast-feeding for babies born prematurely or delivered by cesarean section, for fear that there may be some negative effect on the quantity or quality of human milk. Uncertainty about the nutritional quality of mother's milk has also led them to encourage adding formula and/or solid foods to the diet to make sure the baby is "well fed." These practices are usually unnecessary. They may contribute to obesity, allergies, and digestive problems because of the extra stress placed on an immature gut.

Breast milk for the preterm infant

Levels of nutrients in mother's milk shift according to the gestational age of the infant at birth. The preterm infant is often "spared" its mother's milk by some hospital workers because they think of it as "mature" milk having too little protein and too much lactose to meet the child's needs. An analysis of the nutritional quality of preterm milk, however, revealed energy and fat concentrations that were 20% to 30% *higher,* protein levels 15% to 20% *higher,* and lactose levels 10% *lower* than those found in mature milk. Premature milk *can* meet the preterm infant's needs.

Breast milk during weaning

Nutrient levels continue to change with time to match changing growth patterns and developing digestive abilities. Mother's milk *does* provide sufficient kilocalories and nutrients to keep babies well fed without supplemental formula and food. Even when the infant is being weaned, Mother Nature ensures adequate nutrients, just in case the new, solid-food diet can't meet the child's needs. In a study in which human milk was collected during gradual weaning, it was found that the milk had higher concentrations of protein, sodium, and iron. Lactose levels fell, possibly so that higher amounts of kilocalories could be supplied by fats, a more concentrated source.

Breast milk and the cesarean-section infant

The quality of human milk is not influenced by the way in which babies come into the world either. Many women fear that a baby born by cesarean section cannot be nursed, because this method delays or prevents the production of "mature" milk. Milk production is stimulated by the release of the placenta, which occurs whether the delivery is vaginal or not. A recent study of 19 women confirmed *no* significant difference in the length of time it took mature milk to "come in" after vaginal versus cesarean deliveries.

Thus premature or cesarean deliveries shouldn't discourage women from breast-feeding. Mothers should not underestimate the nutritive quality of their milk simply because it does not appear as rich and thick as cow's milk. In nutritional and immunologic terms, breast milk remains the *best* milk for baby.

REFERENCES

Cunningham AS: Breast-feeding and health, J Pediatr 110:658, April 1987.

Ferris AM and others: Macronutrients in human milk at 2, 12, and 16 weeks postpartum, J Am Diet Assoc 88(6):694, 1988.

Garza C and others: Changes in the nutrient composition of human milk during gradual weaning, Am J Clin Nutr 37(1):61, 1983.

Jensen RG and Neville MC, editors: Human lactation: milk components and methodologies, New York, 1985, Plenum Press.

Karra MV and others: Changes in specific nutrients in breast milk during extended lactation, Am J Clin Nutr 43:495, April 1986.

Lonnerdal B: Effects of maternal dietary intake of human milk composition, J Nutr 116:499, April 1986.

12 Nutrition for Growth and Development

After studying this chapter, the student should be able to:

1. Describe the normal physical growth pattern during the life cycle.
2. Identify ways of measuring childhood growth.
3. Relate basic nutrients to the growth process and identify nutritional needs for normal growth and development of children at each age level.
4. Relate food choices and feeding practices to basic physical and psychosocial development at each age period.

Chapter Objectives

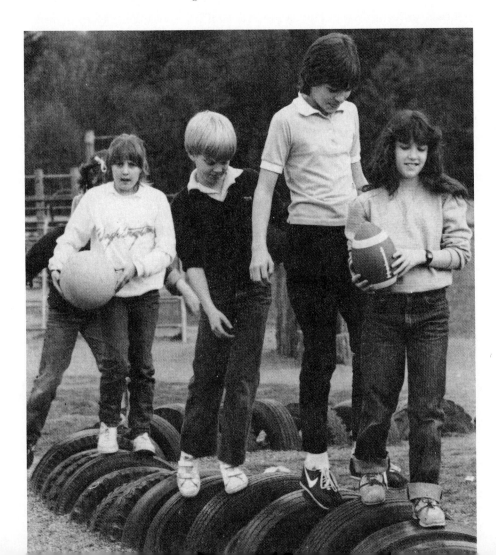

PREVIEW

Human growth and development involves far more than physical processes alone. It encompasses social and psychologic influences and relationships. Indeed, it enfolds the entire environment and culture that nurtures individual growth potential.

Food and feeding practices are highly significant during the childhood years. They do not and cannot exist apart from the broader overall human growth and development process. The *whole* process produces the *whole* person.

In this chapter, therefore, we will consider food and feeding as an integral part of the whole development of the child. We will relate age-group nutritional needs and food habits to individual psychosocial development, as well as to physical maturation normally achieved at each age level.

Human Growth and Development

Individual Needs of Children

Growth may be defined as an increase in size. Biologic growth of an organism occurs through cell multiplication. Development is the associated process in which growing tissues and organs take on increased complexity of function. Both of these processes are part of one whole, forming a unified inseparable concept of growth and development. Through these changes a small dependent newborn is transformed into a fully functioning independent adult. However, each child is a unique individual with individual needs. This is a paramount principle in working with children. Thus we must always seek to discover these individual human needs if we are to help each child reach his or her greatest growth-and-development potential.

Normal Life Cycle Growth Pattern

The normal human life cycle follows four general stages of overall growth and development.

Infancy

The infant grows rapidly during the first year of life, with the rate tapering off in the latter half of the year. At age 6 months an infant will probably have doubled the birth weight and at 1 year may have tripled it.[1]

Childhood

The latent period of childhood between infancy and adolescence reflects a slowed and erratic growth rate. At some periods there are plateaus. At others small spurts of growth occur. The overall variable rate affects appetite accordingly. At times children will have little or no appetite, and at other times they will eat voraciously. Parents who know that this is a normal pattern will relax and not make eating a battleground with their children.

Adolescence

With the beginning of puberty the second rapid growth period occurs. Because of the hormonal influences involved, multiple body changes develop. These changes include the growth of long bones, development of sex characteristics, and the growth of fat and muscle mass.

Adulthood

In the final stage of a normal life cycle, growth levels off on the adult plateau. Then it gradually declines during old age.

Measuring Childhood Physical Growth
Growth Charts

Children grow at widely varying individual rates. In practice a child's pattern of growth is compared with percentile growth curves derived from the measurement of numbers of children throughout the growth years. Contemporary growth charts, developed by the National Center for Health Statistics (NCHS), reflect a broad base for growth patterns in children today.[2] These charts are based on data from large numbers of a nationally representative sample of children. Two age intervals are used: birth to 36 months and 2 to 18 years, with separate curves for boys and for girls.

Anthropometric Measures

Practitioners use *anthropometry* to monitor a child's growth, with the growth charts and other clinical standards as reference. A number of methods and measures may be employed:

1. **Weight and height.** These are common general measures of physical growth. They provide a basic measure but give only a crude index of growth without giving finer details of individual variations. They are used mainly to look for patterns of growth over time, as the individual child's pattern is plotted on the related age group chart (Figure 12-1). The *recumbent length* of infants and small children is measured initially, then standing height as they grow older.

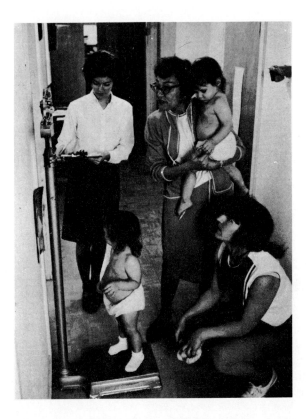

Figure 12-1
Growth and development study being conducted at the University of California in Berkeley. Here weight of twins in the study is being recorded. Many other measurements are taken, some by use of calipers.

2. **Body circumferences and skinfolds.** The head circumference is a valuable measure in infants but is seldom taken routinely after 3 years of age. Measures of abdomen, chest, and the leg at its maximal girth of the calf are usually included at periodic intervals. Other measures for monitoring muscle mass growth and body composition include the *midarm circumference* and the *triceps skinfold* at the same point. From these two measures the *midarm muscle circumference* can be calculated from a special formula. Skinfold measures, including a number of body sites, are done with special calipers and require skill and practice for accuracy. Longitudinal growth studies in research centers employ many measures of development in addition to these basic monitoring ones used in general practice.

Clinical Signs

Various clinical signs of optimal growth may be observed as measures of a child's nutritional status. These include such factors as general vitality; a sense of well-being; good posture; healthy gums, teeth, skin, hair, and eyes; muscle development; and nervous control. Refer back to Table 1-1 (Chapter 1) for a review of these general signs and observations.

Laboratory Tests

In addition, other measures of growth can be obtained by various laboratory tests. These may include studies of blood and urine to determine levels of hemoglobin, vitamins, and similar substances. X-ray films of the hand and wrist may be used to measure degree of bone development.

Nutritional Analysis

A nutritional analysis of general eating habits (see Chapter 10) provides helpful information for assessing growth needs. The nutritionist uses results of such an analysis, usually done by computer, as a basis for diet counseling with the parents.

Mental and Psychosocial Development
Mental Growth

Measures of mental growth usually involve abilities in speech and other forms of communications, as well as the ability to handle abstract and symbolic material in thinking. Young children originally think in very literal terms. As mental capacity develops, they can increasingly handle more than single ideas and develop constructive concepts.

Emotional Growth

Measures of emotional growth reflect the capacity for love and affection, as well as the ability to handle frustration and its anxieties. It also involves the child's ability to control aggressive impulses and to channel hostility from destructive to constructive activities.

Social and Cultural Growth

Social development of a child is measured in terms of the ability to relate to others and to participate in group living in a cultural setting. These social and cultural behaviors are first learned through relationships with parents and family, all of which have much influence on food habits and feeding patterns. As horizons broaden, the child develops relationships with others outside the family, with friends and persons in the community, at school, at church, or at other social gatherings. For this reason a child's play during the early years is a highly purposeful activity.

Energy Needs

During childhood the demand for kilocalories is relatively great. However, there is much variation in need with age and condition. For example, the total daily caloric intake of a 5-year-old child is spent in the following way: (1) about 50% supplies *basal metabolic requirements;* (2) 5% is involved in the *specific dynamic action* of food ingestion in general stimulation of metabolism; (3) various *physical activities* require about 25%; (4) 12% is needed for *tissue growth;* and (5) about 8% is represented in *fecal loss.* Of these kilocalories, carbohydrate is the primary energy source and is also important to spare protein for its essential growth needs rather than having it spent for energy. Fat kilocalories are important as backup energy sources, but particularly as sources of essential fatty acids such as linoleic acid needed for growth. However, an excess of fat, especially from animal sources, should be avoided.

Protein Needs

Protein provides the essential building materials for tissue growth—amino acids. As a child grows, the requirements per unit of body weight gradually decrease. For example, during the first 6 months of life an infant requires 2.2 g/kg. This amount gradually decreases until adulthood, when protein needs are only 0.8 g/kg. Usually the healthy, active, growing child will consume the necessary amount of kilocalories and protein in the variety of foods provided.

Water Requirements

Water is essential to life. The infant's relative need for water is greater than that of the adult. The infant's body content of water is from 70% to 75% of the total body weight, whereas in the adult water constitutes only about 60% to 65% of the total body weight. Also, a large amount of the infant's total body water is *outside* the cell and more easily lost. The child's water need is related to the caloric intake and the urine concentration. Generally an infant drinks daily an amount of water equivalent to 10% to 15% of body weight. A summary of approximate daily fluid needs during the growth years is given in Table 12-1.

Mineral and Vitamin Needs

In your previous study of minerals (Chapter 8) and vitamins (Chapter 7), you learned of their essential roles in tissue growth and maintenance and in overall energy metabolism. Positive childhood growth and development depend on an adequate amount of these essential substances. For example, rapidly growing young bones require calcium and phosphorus. An x-ray film of a newborn's body would reveal a skeleton appearing as a collection of disconnected, separate bones requiring mineralization. Calcium is also needed for developing teeth, muscle contraction, nerve irritability, blood coagulation, and heart muscle action. Another mineral of concern is iron, essential for hemoglobin formation. The infant's fetal store is diminished in 4 to 6 months. Thus solid foods added then need to supply iron. Such initial foods as enriched cereal and egg yolk and later meat accomplish this. The use of

Nutritional Requirements for Growth

iron-fortified formulas and foods, especially by high-risk children enrolled in the WIC program, has greatly reduced the incidence of iron-deficiency anemia among children.[3]

Hypervitaminosis

Excess amounts of two vitamins, A and D, are of concern in feeding children. Excess intake of these vitamins may occur over prolonged periods because of misunderstanding, ignorance, or carelessness. Parents must be carefully instructed to use only the amount directed and no more. These excesses bring clear toxic symptoms:

1. **Vitamin A.** Symptoms of toxicity from excess vitamin A include lack of appetite, slow growth, drying and cracking of the skin, enlargement of the liver and spleen, swelling and pain of long bones, and bone fragility.

Table 12-1

Approximate Daily Fluid Needs During Growth Years

Age	ml/kg
0-3 months	120
3-6 months	115
6-12 months	100
1-4 years	100
4-7 years	95
7-11 years	90
11-19 years	50
> 19 years	30

Table 12-2

Recommended Daily Dietary Allowances for Growth (National Research Council 1989 version)

	Age (yr)	Weight		Height		Energy (kcal)	Protein (g)	Vitamin A (µg RE)	Vitamin D (µg*)	Vitamin E (mg α TE)	Vitamin K (µg)
		kg	lb	cm	In						
Infants	Birth-0.5	6	13	60	24	kg × 108	kg × 2.2	420	75	3	5
	0.5-1	9	20	71	28	kg × 98	kg × 1.5	500	10	4	10
Children	1-3	13	29	90	35	1300	16	400	10	6	15
	4-6	20	44	112	44	1800	24	500	10	7	20
	7-10	28	62	132	52	2000	28	700	10	7	30
Males	11-14	45	99	157	62	2500	46	1000	10	10	45
	15-18	66	145	176	69	3000	59	1000	10	10	65
Females	11-14	46	101	157	62	2200	46	800	10	8	45
	15-18	55	120	163	64	2200	44	800	10	8	55

*As cholecalciferol; 10 µg cholecalciferol equals 400 IU vitamin D

2. **Vitamin D.** Symptoms of toxicity from excess vitamin D include nausea, diarrhea, weight loss, excess urination especially at night, and eventual calcification of soft tissues, including those of renal tubules, blood vessels, bronchi, stomach, and heart.

A summary of the overall nutritional needs for growth, as recommended by the National Research Council, is given in Table 12-2.

The Stages of Human Life

Age Group Needs

Throughout the human life cycle food and feeding must not only serve to meet nutritional requirements for physical growth but also relate intimately to personal psychosocial development. The nutritional age group needs of children cannot be understood apart from the child's overall maturation as a *person*. Over the past 30 years Erikson's theory of human development has come to play a significant role in our view for the human life cycle.[4]

Psychosocial Development

Erikson has identified eight stages in human growth and a basic psychosocial developmental problem with which persons struggle at each age. The developmental problem at each stage has a positive ego value and a conflicting negative counterpart:

1. **Infancy:** Trust vs distrust
2. **Toddler:** Autonomy vs shame and doubt
3. **Preschooler:** Initiative vs guilt
4. **School-age child:** Industry vs inferiority
5. **Adolescent:** Identity vs role confusion
6. **Young adult:** Intimacy vs isolation
7. **Adult:** Generativity vs stagnation
8. **Older adult:** Ego integrity vs despair

Given favorable circumstances, a growing child develops positive ego strength at each life stage and therefore builds increasing inner resources and strengths to meet the next life crisis. The struggle at any age, however, is not forever won at that point. A residue of the negative remains, and in pe-

Water-soluble vitamins							Minerals						
Vit. C (mg)	Fola-cin (μg)	Nia-cin (mg)	Ribo-flavin (mg)	Thia-min (mg)	Vit. B$_6$ (mg)	Vit. B$_{12}$ (μg)	Cal-cium (mg)	Phos-phorus (mg)	Iodine (μg)	Iron (mg)	Mag-nesium (mg)	Zinc (mg)	Selenium (μg)
30	25	5	0.4	0.3	0.3	0.5	400	300	40	6	40	5	10
35	35	6	0.5	0.4	0.6	1.5	600	300	50	10	60	5	15
40	50	9	0.8	0.7	1.0	2.0	800	800	70	10	80	10	20
45	75	12	1.1	0.9	1.1	2.5	800	800	90	10	120	10	20
45	100	13	1.2	1.0	1.4	3.0	800	800	120	10	170	10	30
50	150	17	1.5	1.3	1.7	3.0	1200	1200	150	12	270	15	40
60	200	20	1.8	1.5	2.0	3.0	1200	1200	150	12	400	15	50
50	150	15	1.3	1.1	1.4	3.0	1200	1200	150	15	280	12	45
60	180	15	1.3	1.1	1.5	3.0	1200	1200	150	15	300	12	50

riods of stress, such as an illness, regression in some degree usually occurs. But as the child gains mastery at each stage of development, assisted by significant positive relationships of support, integration of self-control takes place. Various related developmental tasks surround each of these stages. These are skills that, when accomplished, contribute to successful resolution of the core problem.

Physical Growth

These psychosocial developmental tasks are integrated and associated with normal physical maturation at each point of growth. Various neuromuscular motor skills enable the child to accomplish related physical activities.

Food and Feeding Practices

In each of these stages of childhood, food choices and feeding practices are intimately related. Food habits do not develop in a vacuum. They are an integral part of both physical and psychosocial development. Here we will relate these two influences to the general age-group developmental characteristics at each stage.

Infancy (Birth to 1 Year)

The Premature Infant
Physical Characteristics

Special care is crucial for these tiny, immature babies, who vary in weight and development. But they are usually considered premature if they are born at fewer than 270 days of gestation or weigh less than 2500 g (5.5 lb). However, modern neonatology research and technology have currently pushed the edge of viability for premature babies to about 24 weeks (168 days) of gestation and weight of almost 600 g (1.25 lb). But such extremely underdeveloped babies have only about a 20% chance for survival.[5] The term *small for gestational age (SGA)* describes infants who, although full term, have suffered some degree of intrauterine growth failure and also have low birth weights and general growth retardation. The results of the National Infant Mortality Surveillance project indicate that the most important predictor for infant survival is birth weight.[6] All of these underdeveloped infants have problems catching up in growth and nutrition. Their body composition differs from that of full-term infants: (1) they have much more water and less protein and minerals per kilogram of body weight; (2) there is little subcutaneous fat to help maintain body temperature; (3) bones are poorly calcified; (4) the neuromuscular system is incompletely developed, making normal sucking reflexes weak; (5) digestive-absorptive ability and renal function are limited; and (6) the immature liver lacks developed enzyme systems or adequate iron stores.

Food and Feeding

If these tiniest babies are to survive, they require special feeding. Consideration has to be given to the type of milk used and methods of feeding.

Type of milk. Controversy continues regarding the relative merits of breast milk and special formulas for premature infants. Nonetheless, premature infants have done well on both forms of feeding. Indications are that the milk produced by mothers of premature infants may be especially suited to the

Table 12-3

Nutritional Value of Special Formulas and Human Milk for the Preterm Infant

Nutritional Component	Advisable intake Birth weight		Human milk content		Standard formulas	Special premature formulas		
	1.0 kg (2.2 lb)	1.5 kg (3.3 lb)	Preterm	Mature	Enfamil* Similac† SMA‡	Enfamil Premature with Whey*	Similac Special Care†	"Preemie" SMA‡
Kilocalories/deciliter			73	73	67	81	81	81
Protein (g/100 kcal)	3.1	2.7	2.3§	1.5	2.2	3.0	2.7	2.5
Vitamins, fat-soluble								
D (IU/120 kcal/kg/day)	600	600	—	4.0	70-75	75	180	76
E (IU/120 kcal/kg/day)	30	30	—	0.3	2-3	2	4	2
Vitamins, water-soluble								
Folic acid (μg/120 kcal/kg/day)	60	60	—	8.0	9-19	336	45	14
Vitamin C (mg/120 kcal/kg/day)	60	60	—	7.0	10	10	45	10
Minerals								
Calcium (mg/100 kcal)	160	140	40.0	43.0	66-78	117	178	92
Phosphorus (mg/100 kcal)	108	95	18.0	20.0	49-66	58	89	49
Sodium (mEq/100 kcal)	2.7	2.3	1.5‖	0.8	1.0-1.8	1.7	1.9	1.7

*Mead Johnson Nutritional Division, Evansville, Inc.
†Ross Laboratories, Columbus, Ohio.
‡Wyeth Laboratories, Philadelphia.
§Range: 1.9-2.8 g/100 kcal.
‖Range: 0.9-2.3 mEq/100 kcal.

needs of the preterm infant; in comparison to milk from mothers of full-term infants it has a higher protein and mineral content and its fat is more digestible. For a number of reasons, however, the majority of preterm babies are fed special formulas at some stage. Several newer commercial preterm formulas have been developed. Table 12-3 shows a comparison of these special formulas with standard full-term infant formulas and with human milk.

Methods of feeding. Tube feeding has been used for premature infants, but it is hazardous and usually avoided. Long-term peripheral vein feeding is difficult in tiny infants and may become complicated by infection and jaundice. For most of these infants, bottle-feeding can be instituted successfully with care and support, using one of these newer special formulas.

Physical Characteristics

The Full-Term Infant

The growth rate during infancy is rapid. Consequently energy requirements are high. The full-term infant has the ability to digest and absorb protein, a moderate amount of fat, and simple carbohydrate. There is some difficulty with starch, since amylase, the starch-splitting enzyme, is not being produced at first. However, as starch is introduced, this enzyme begins to function. The renal system functions well, but more water relative to size is needed than in an adult to manage urinary excretion. Since teeth do not erupt until about the fourth month, the initial food must be liquid or semiliquid. The infant has limited nutritional stores remaining from fetal development, especially in iron, so that supplements of vitamins and minerals are needed. These are first given in concentrated drops and later in **beikost**—solid or semisolid food additions to milk. The newborn's *rooting reflex* and somewhat recessed lower jaw are natural adaptations for feeding at the breast.

Beikost
Solid and semisolid baby foods.

Psychosocial Development

The core psychosocial problem during infancy is the development of *trust vs distrust*. Feeding is the infant's main means of establishing human relationships. The close mother-infant relationship in the feeding process fills the basic need to build trust. The need for sucking and the development of the oral organs, lips and mouth, as sensory organs represent adaptations to ensure an adequate early food intake for survival. As a result, food becomes the infant's general means of exploring the environment and is one of the early means of communication. As muscular coordination involving the tongue and the swallowing reflex develops, the infant will accept solid foods when such foods are started at about 6 months of age. As physical and motor maturation develop, the infant will want to help in the feeding process. When these stages of development occur, the exploration of new powers should be encouraged. If the needs for food and love are fulfilled in this early relationship with the mother, father, and other feeding adults, and in broadening relationships with other family members, trust is developed. The infant shows this trust by an increasing capacity to wait for feedings while they are being prepared.

Food and Feeding

Breast-Feeding

The ideal food for the human infant is human milk. It has specific characteristics that match the infant's nutritional requirements during the first year of life. The process of breast-feeding today, as in the past, is successfully initiated and maintained by most women who try. However, sometimes there are problems, as well as a high degree of variability among nursing mothers about frequency of feedings and intake and growth indexes.[7] Thus, in providing support for mothers who want to breast-feed their babies, experienced nutritionists and nurses, many of whom are certified professional lactation counselors, advise flexibility rather than a rigid approach.

The female's breasts, or mammary glands, are highly specialized secretory organs (Figure 12-2). They are composed of glandular tissue, fat, and connective tissue. The secreting glandular tissue has 15 to 20 lobes, each containing many smaller units called *lobules*. In the lobules secretory cells called *alveoli* or *ancini* form milk from the nutrient material supplied to them by a rich capillary system in the connective tissue. During pregnancy the breasts are prepared for lactation. The alveoli enlarge and multiply and toward the end of the prenatal period secrete a thin, yellowish fluid called *colostrum*. As the infant grows, the breast milk develops, adapting in composition to meet the needs of the developing child.

Breast milk is produced under the stimulating influence of the hormone *prolactin* from the anterior pituitary gland. After the milk is formed in the mammary lobules by the clusters of secretory cells (alveoli or ancini), it is carried through converging branches of the *lactiferous ducts* to reservoir spaces under the *areola,* the pigmented area of skin surrounding the nipple. Two other pituitary hormones, principally *oxytocin* and to a lesser extent *vasopressin,* stimulate the ejection of the milk from the alveoli to the ducts, releasing it to the baby. This is commonly called the *let down reflex.* It causes a tingling sensation in the breast and the flow of milk. The initial sucking of the baby stimulates this reflex. The newborn rooting reflex, oral needs for sucking, and the basic hunger drive usually induce and maintain normal relaxed breast-feeding for the healthy mother (Figure 12-3). A nutritionally adequate diet will support ample milk production.

Bottle-Feeding

Formula feeding by bottle may be preferred by some mothers. If the mother does not choose breast-feeding or stops early, bottle feeding of an appropriate formula is an acceptable alternative. About 90% of these mothers use a commercial formula. A variety of these formulas that approximate human milk composition are available. A description of the major types of standard commercial formulas for full-term infants is given in Table 12-4. The standards for levels of nutrients required in these formulas are set by the Infant Formula Act of 1980, P.L. 97-359, which is based on recommendations from

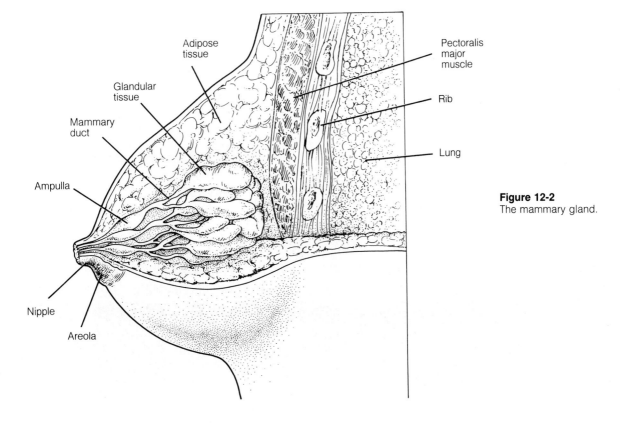

Figure 12-2
The mammary gland.

Table 12-4

A Comparison of Types of Formulas Manufactured for Full-Term Infants

Type of formula used		Protein content	Fat content	Carbohydrate content
Milk-based routine	Source:	Nonfat cow's milk	Vegetable oils	Lactose
	G/100 kcal:	2.2-2.3	5.4-5.5	10.4-10.8
	% Kcal:	9	48-50	41-43
Whey-adjusted routine	Source:	Nonfat cow's milk plus demineralized whey	Vegetable and oleo oils	Lactose
	G/100 kcal:	2.2	5.4	10.8
	% Kcal:	9	48	43
Soy isolate/cow's milk sensitivity	Source:	Soy isolate	Vegetable oils	Corn syrup solids and/or sucrose
	G/100 kcal:	2.7-3.2	5.1-5.6	9.9-10.2
	% Kcal:	12-13	45-51	39-40
Casein hydrolysate/ protein sensitivity, ga-lactosemia	Source:	Casein hydrolysate	Corn oil or corn oil and MCT*	Tapioca starch and glucose, sucrose, or corn syrup solids
	G/100 kcal:	2.8-3.3	3.9-4.0	13.1-13.6
	% Kcal:	11-13	35	52-54
Meat-based cow's milk sensitivity, galactosemia	Source:	Beef hearts	Sesame oil and beef heart fat	Tapioca starch and sucrose
	G/100 kcal:	4.0	4.8	9
	% Kcal:	16	47	37

*Medium-chain triglycerides.

Figure 12-3
Breast-feeding the newborn infant. Note that the nurse, in assisting the mother, avoids touching the infant's outer cheek so as not to counteract the natural rooting reflex at the touch of the breast.

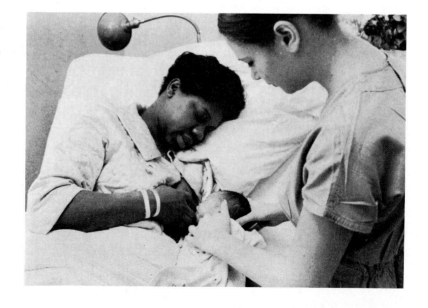

Nutrient	RDA (1980) (up to age 6 months)	Nutrient requirements of the Infant Formula Act of 1980	
		Minimum	Maximum
Energy (kcal)	570-870	670	
Protein (g)	13.2	12.1	30.2
Essential fatty acids			
Linoleate, % kcal	3.0	2.7	
Vitamins, fat-soluble			
A (IU)	1400 (420 µg)	1675 (503 µg)	5025 (1508 µg)
D (IU)	400 (10 µg)	268	670
E (IU)	4.5	4.7	
K (µg)	12.0*	27.0	
Vitamins, water-soluble			
C (mg)	35.0	54.0	
B$_1$ (thiamin) (µg)	300.0	268.0	
B$_2$ (riboflavin) (µg)	400.0	402.0	
B$_6$ (pyridoxine) (µg)	300.0	235.0	
B$_{12}$ (µg)	0.5	1.0	
Niacin	6.0 mEq	1.68 mg	
Folacin (µg)	30.0	27.0	
Pantothenic acid (mg)	2.0*	2.0	
Biotin (µg)	35.0	10.0	
Choline (mg)		47.0	
Inositol (mg)		27.0	
Minerals			
Calcium (mg)	360.0	335.0	
Phosphorus (mg)	240.0	168.0	
Magnesium (mg)	50.0	40.0	
Iron (mg)	10.0	1.0†	
Iodine (µg)	40.0	34.0	
Zinc (mg)	3.0	3.4	
Copper (µg)	500-700*	402.0	
Manganese (µg)	500-700*	34.0	
Sodium (mg)	115-350*	134.0	402.0
Potassium (mg)	350-925*	536.0	1340.0
Chloride (mg)	275-700*	369	1005.0
Fluoride (µg)	100-500*		
Chromium (µg)	10-40*		
Selenium (µg)	10-40*		
Molybdenum (µg)	30-60*		

Table 12-5
Nutrient Standards for Formulas Manufactured for Healthy, Full-Term Infants

*Based on estimated safe and adequate daily dietary intakes. Some figures are given in ranges because of a lack of information on which to base allowances.

†Based on iron content of nonfortified infant formula (0.15 mg/100 kcal). The Committee on Nutrition recommends that infants receive 1.0 mg/100 kcal formula.

the American Academy of Pediatrics.[8] These standards are given in Table 12-5 and can be compared to the RDA standards of the National Research Council for infants from birth to 6 months.

When formula is given, the baby should be cradled by the arm, as in breast-feeding. The close human touch and warmth are important. When the infant is obviously satisfied, extra milk should not be forced, regardless of the amount remaining in the bottle. Any remaining formula should be thrown away and not refrigerated for reuse. Infants usually take the amount of formula they need. Today most infants are fed on a so-called "demand schedule," which works out to about every 3 to 4 hours. A healthy infant will soon establish an individual pattern according to growth requirements.

Cow's Milk

Regular unmodified cow's milk is not suitable for infants. It may cause gastrointestinal bleeding; also its solute load is too heavy for the infant's renal system to handle. In addition, infants should *not* use reduced fat milks, such as nonfat or 2% fat, for two reasons: (1) *insufficient energy* is provided to support requirements, causing body fat to be used to make up the deficit, and (2) *linoleic acid* in the fat portion of milk is the essential fatty acid needed for growth and development of body tissues. A specific form of exzema has been observed in infants deficient in linoleic acid. To meet the special needs of infants, the American Academy of Pediatrics recommends breast milk or formulas up to 1 year of age, with a gradual addition of appropriate foods beginning at 6 months.

Beikost: Solid Food Additions

No nutritional need exists for introducing solid foods to infants earlier than 4 to 6 months of age. Earlier use may contribute to allergies. Nutritional and medical authorities agree that for the first 6 months of life the optimal single food for the infant is human milk, or alternative feeding of appropriate formula. Until that time the infant does not need any additional food and is not able to fully handle them. There is no one sequence of food additions that must be followed. A general guide is given in Table 12-6. Individual responses and needs may be a basis for choices. Single foods are given first, one at a time in small amounts, so that adverse reactions can be identified. The traditional initial transition food is fortified infant cereal mixed with a little milk or formula, then fruits, vegetables, egg, potato, and finally meat. Small amounts are given at first, usually offered before the milk feeding. Over time the child will learn to eat and enjoy a wide variety of foods, which is the basic goal. Many commercial baby foods are available, prepared today without the formerly used ingredients of sugar, salt, or monosodium glutamate. Some mothers prefer preparing their own baby food. This can easily be done by cooking and straining vegetables and fruits in a clean environment, freezing a batch at a time in ice cube trays, then storing the cubes in plastic bags in the freezer. Then a single cube can be reheated conveniently for use at a feeding.

Two basic principles should guide the feeding process: (1) *necessary nutrients* are needed, not any specific food, and (2) food is a main basis of early *learning*. Food not only serves for physical sustenance but also supplies other personal development and cultural needs. Good food habits begin early in

Table 12-6
Guideline for Adding of Solid Foods to Infant's Diet During the First Year*

When to start	Foods added	Feeding
Sixth month	Cereal and strained cooked fruit	10 AM and 6 PM
	Egg yolk (at first, hard boiled and sieved, soft boiled or poached later)	
	Strained cooked vegetable and strained meat	2 PM
	Zweiback or hard toast	At any feeding
Seventh to ninth month	Meat: beef, lamb, or liver (broiled or baked and finely chopped)	10 AM to 6 PM
	Potato: baked or boiled and mashed or sieved	

Suggested meal plan for age 8 months to 1 year or older

7 AM	Milk	240 ml (8 oz)
	Cereal	2-3 tbsp
	Strained fruit	2-3 tbsp
	Zweiback or dry toast	
12 NOON	Milk	240 ml (8 oz)
	Vegetables	2-3 tbsp
	Chopped meat or one whole egg	
	Puddings or cooked fruit	2-3 tbsp
3 PM	Milk	120 ml (4 oz)
	Toast, zweiback, or crackers	
6 PM	Milk	240 ml (8 oz)
	Whole egg or chopped meat	2 tbsp
	Potato: baked or mashed	2-3 tbsp
	Pudding or cooked fruit	
	Zweiback or toast	

*Semisolid foods should be given immediately before milk feeding. One or two teaspoons should be given at first. If food is accepted and tolerated well, the amount should be increased to 1 to 2 tbsp per feeding.
NOTE: Banana or cottage cheese may be used as substitution for any meal.

life and continue as a child grows older. By the time infants are approximately 8 or 9 months old, they should be able to eat family foods—chopped, cooked foods, simply seasoned—without needing special infant foods. Throughout the first year of life the infant's needs for physical growth and psychosocial development will be met by breast milk or formula, a variety of solid food additions, and a loving, trusting relationship between parents and child (Figure 12-4).

Toddler (1 to 3 years)
Physical Characteristics and Growth

After the rapid growth of the first year the growth rate of children slows. But although the rate of gain is less, the pattern of growth produces significant

Childhood (1 to 12 years)

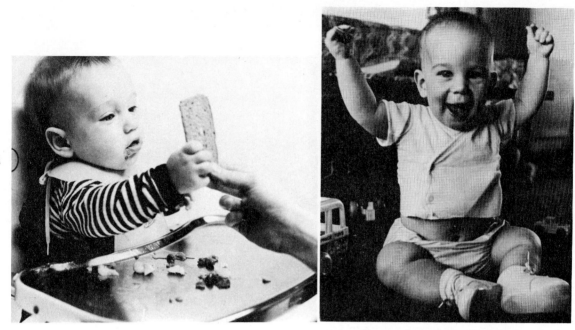

Figure 12-4
A, This 6-month-old boy is taking a variety of solid food additions and is developing wide tastes. Here feeding has become a bond of relationship between mother and child and is serving as a source not only of physical growth but also of psychosocial development. **B,** Optimum physical development and security are evident, the result of sound nutrition and loving care.

changes in body form. The legs become longer, and the child begins losing baby fat. There is less body water and more water inside the cells. The young child begins to look and feel less like a baby and more like a child. Energy demands are fewer because of the slackened growth rate. However, important muscle development is taking place. In fact, muscle mass development accounts for about one half the total gain during this period. As the child begins to walk and stand erect, more muscle is needed to strengthen the body. A special need exists, for example, for big muscles in the back, the buttocks, and the thighs. The overall rate of skeletal growth slows, but there is more deposit of mineral rather than lengthening of the bones. The increased mineralization strengthens the bones to support the increasing weight. The child has 6 to 8 teeth at the beginning of the toddler period. By 3 years of age the remainder of the deciduous teeth, "baby teeth," have erupted.

Psychosocial Development

The psychosocial development of toddlers is pronounced. The core developmental problem they struggle with is the conflict between *autonomy vs shame*. Each child has a profound increasing sense of self, of "I"—of being a distinct and individual person apart from the mother, not just an extension of her. As physical mobility increases, the sense of independence increases. A growing curiosity leads to much exploration of the environment, and increasingly the mouth is used as a means of exploring. Touch is important, providing

child's growing need for independence and ritual. Parents need to maintain a calm, relaxed attitude of sympathetic interest, to understand the child's struggle, and to give help where needed. But they must be careful to avoid both overprotection and excessive rigidity.

Preschooler (3 to 6 years)
Physical Characteristics and Growth

Physical growth continues in spurts. On occasion the child bounds with energy. Play is hard play—running, jumping, and testing new physical resources. At other times the child will sit for increasing periods of time engrossed in passive types of activities. Mental capacities are developing, and more thinking and exploring of the environment are done. Specific nutrients need emphasis. Protein requirements continue to be relatively high. Preschool children need about 24 g/day of high quality protein, such as found in milk, egg, meat, and cheese. They continue to need calcium and iron for storage. Since vitamins A and C may be lacking in the diets of preschool growing children, a variety of fruits and vegetables should be provided.

Psychosocial Development

Each age builds on the previous one. The core psychosocial developmental problem preschool children struggle with is essentially that of *initiative vs guilt*. They are beginning to develop the superego—the conscience. As powers of active movement increase, they have increasing imagination and curiosity. This very capacity often leads them into troubled feelings about their changing attitudes, especially toward parents. This a period of increasing imitation and of sex identification. The little boy imitates his father or other male role models. The little girl imitates the mother or other female role models. In their play much of this becomes evident in the use of grownup clothes and role-playing in domestic or job situations. Wise parents will avoid sex stereotyping responses, especially during this formative period. Eating assumes greater social aspects. The family mealtime is an important means of socialization and sex identification, as the children imitate their parents and others at the table.

Food and Feeding

The preschool child is beginning to form definite responses to various types of foods.

1. **Vegetables and fruits.** Of all the food groups, vegetables usually are less well liked by children, yet these foods contain many vitamins and minerals needed for growth. Parents need to consider ways these foods are prepared and served. Children usually dislike strong vegetables such as cabbage and onions. They have a keen sense of taste, so flavor and texture are important. They like pieces of crisp raw vegetables or fruits to eat as finger foods. Tough strings cause problems, and tough parts are hard to manage and therefore should be removed. Children also react to consistency of vegetables, disliking them overcooked.

2. **Milk, cheese, egg, and meat.** It is helpful if children can set their own goals in quantities of food. Portions need to be relatively small. Often children can pour their own milk from a small pitcher into a small glass and subsequently drink more. The quantity of milk needed usually declines during these years. The child will drink 2 or 3, rarely 4, cups of milk during the day.

Smaller children like their milk more at room temperature, not icy cold. Also, they prefer it in small glasses that hold about 4 to 6 oz rather than in large, adult-sized glasses. Cheese is liked as a good finger food or snack. Egg is usually well liked if cooked with sufficient body to pick up with the fingers, such as scrambled or boiled. Meat should be tender, easy to chew or cut; hence ground meat is popular.

3. **Grains.** The wide variety in which grains can be eaten adds to their appeal to children, who enjoy various breads, cereals, and crackers.

4. **Temperature.** Since children prefer their foods lukewarm, not hot, some foods may remain on their plates and become dry and gummy and so refused. Thus very small portions should be served at first.

5. **Single foods.** Children usually prefer single foods to combination dishes such as casseroles or stews. This a period of language learning for children. They like to learn names of foods and be able recognize and name them from their shape, color, texture, taste. So these identifiable characteristics need to be retained as much as possible.

6. **Finger foods.** Children like food they can eat with their fingers. Frequently when appetites lag, fruits can be substituted for vegetables. Often a variety of raw fruits or raw vegetables cut in finger-sized pieces and offered to children for their own selection provides a source of needed nutrition.

7. **Food jags.** Because of developing social and emotional needs, preschool children frequently follow "food jags," eating only a particular food. This may last for several days. But it is usually short-lived and is of no major consequence.

The preschool period is one of increasing growth for the young child. Lifetime food habits are forming. Food continues to play an important part in the developing personality, and group eating becomes significant as a means of socialization. The child learns food patterns at the family table or in group situations away from home. For example, if the family is vegetarian, they will need to give special attention to the child's energy and protein needs for growth. The child may be involved in a child care or preschool situation in which group eating occurs. Food habits of preschoolers are greatly affected by peer modeling, and food preferences grow according to what the group is eating. In such situations the child learns a widening variety of family food habits and forms new social relationships and food patterns.

The School-Age Child (6 to 12 years)
Physical Characteristics and Growth

The school-age period has been called the latent time of growth. The rate of growth slows, and body changes occur gradually. However, resources are being laid down for the rapid adolescent growth ahead. Sometimes this has been called the lull before the storm. By now the body type has been established, and growth rates vary widely. Girls usually outdistance boys in the latter part of this period.

Psychosocial Development

The core psychosocial developmental problem children struggle with during these early school years is the tension between *industry vs inferiority*. They have widening horizons, new school experiences, and challenging learning opportunities. They develop increased mental powers and ability to work out

"Food jags"
Colloquial expression referring to repeated use of single foods over a brief period of time.

problems and face competitive activities. They develop abilities to cooperate in group activities and begin to have a sense of adequacy and accomplishment and sometimes the frustration of not winning. The child begins moving from a dependence on parental standards to those of peers, first steps in preparing for coming maturity and self-growth. Pressures are generated for self-control of the growing body. These pressures produce changes in previously learned habits, and negative attitudes sometimes expressed are evidence of these struggles for growing independence. There is a temporary disorganization of previous learning and personality, a sort of loosening up of the pattern for the inevitable changes ahead in adolescence. It is a diffuse period of gangs, cliques, hero worship, pensive daydreaming, emotional stresses, and learning to get along with other children.

Food and Feeding

The slowed rate of growth during this period results in a gradual decline in the food requirement per unit of body weight. This decline continues up to the latter part of the period just before approaching adolescence. Likes and dislikes are a product of earlier years. Family food attitudes are imitated, but increasing outside activities often compete with family mealtimes and family conflicts arise. Research has firmly established the close relation of sound nutrition and childhood learning. Breakfast is particularly important for a school child. It breaks the fast of the sleep hours and prepares the child for problem solving and memory spans in the learning hours at school. The school breakfast and lunch programs provide nourishing school meals that many children would not otherwise have.[12] Here a child can observe many food attitudes and taste new foods that he or she may not normally know or accept. Some favorite foods of American children are listed in Table 12-7.

The school-age child has increasing exposure to influences on food habits. Television becomes a strong source of food selection. Positive learning opportunities exist in the classroom, particularly when parents provide support and reinforcement at home and nutrition education is integrated into other activities.

Table 12-7

Favorite Food Choices of American Children (listed in order of priority)*

Breakfast	Lunch or dinner	Vegetables	Fruit	Beverage	Desserts	Sandwiches
Cereal	Steak or roast beef	Corn	Apple	Cola or soda	Ice cream	Peanut butter and jelly
Pancakes or waffles	Pizza	Carrots	Orange	Milk	Cake	Meat or cold cuts
Eggs	Spaghetti	Beans	Peach	Fruit punch	Pie	Ham
French toast	Chicken	Tomatoes	Grape	Root beer	Pudding	Tuna fish
Toast	Hamburger	Peas	Banana	Juices (other than orange)	Gelatin dessert	Cheese
Sweet rolls	Fish	Greens, collards, or spinach	Watermelon	Orange juice	Banana split	Bacon, lettuce, and tomato
Doughnuts	Macaroni and cheese	Potatoes	Pear	Lemonade	Brownie	Roast beef

*Adapted from survey data of Lamme AJ, and Lamme LL: Children's food preferences, J Sch Health 50(7):397, 1980.

Adolescence (12 to 18 years)

Physical Characteristics and Growth

During the adolescent period, with the onset of puberty, the final growth spurt of childhood occurs. Maturation during this time varies so widely that chronologic age as a reference point for discussing growth ceases to be useful, if indeed it ever was. *Physiologic age* becomes more important in dealing with individual boys and girls. It accounts for wide fluctuations in metabolic rates, food needs, scholastic capacity, and even illness. These capacities can be more realistically viewed only in physiologic growth terms.

The profound body changes in the adolescent period result from hormonal effects regulating the development of the sex characteristics. The rate at which these changes occur varies widely and is particularly distinct in growth patterns that emerge between the sexes. In girls the amount of subcutaneous fat deposit increases, particularly in the abdominal area. The hip breadth increases, and the bony pelvis widens in preparation for reproduction. A pelvic girth of subcutaneous fat results. This is often a source of anxiety to many figure-conscious young girls. In boys physical growth is manifested more by an increased muscle mass and long-bone growth. His growth spurt is slower than that of the girl, but he soon passes her in weight and height.

Psychosocial Development

Adolescence is an ambivalent period full of stresses and strains. On the one hand teenagers look back to the securities of earlier childhood; on the other they reach for the maturity of adulthood. The core psychosocial developmental problem adolescents struggle with is that of *identity vs role diffusion*. The search for self begun in early childhood reaches its climax in the identity crisis of the teen years. The profound body changes associated with sexual development cause changes in body image and resulting tensions in maturing girls and boys. Individual variance is great in response to these tensions, depending on the resources that have been provided for them in earlier developmental years.

The identity crisis of the adolescent years, largely revolving around sexual development and preparation for an adult role in a complex industrialized and technologic society, produces many psychologic, emotional, and social tensions. The actual period of rapid physical growth is relatively short, only 2 or 3 years. However, the attendant psychosocial development continues over a much longer period. The pressure for peer-group acceptance is strong, and fads in dress and food habits are common. Also, in a technically developed society such as in the United States, where high values are placed on education and achievement, prolonged preparation for careers often delays marriage and family far beyond the initiation of the reproductive years. Social tensions and family conflicts are created. These conflicts may have nutritional consequences as teenagers eat away from home more often and develop a snacking pattern of personal and peer-group food choices.

Food and Feeding

With the rapid growth of adolescence come increased demands for energy, protein, vitamins, and minerals.

1. **Energy.** Caloric needs increase with the metabolic demands of growth and energy expenditure. Although individual needs vary, girls consume fewer kilocalories than boys—from 1800 to 2500 kcal/day; boys need 2500 to 3500 kcal/day. Sometimes the large appetite characteristic of this rapid growth period leads adolescents to satisfy their hunger with snack foods that are high in sugar and fat and low in essential protein.

2. **Protein.** Adolescent growth needs for protein are great, especially during the pubertal changes in both sexes and for the developing muscle mass in boys. From 45 to 55 g/day of protein sustains daily needs and maintains nitrogen reserves.

3. **Minerals.** Calcium and iron are particularly needed. Bone growth demands calcium. Menstrual iron losses in the adolescent girl predispose her to simple iron-deficiency anemia.

4. **Vitamins.** The B vitamins are needed in increased amounts, especially by boys, to meet the extra demands of energy metabolism and muscle tissue development. Intakes of needed vitamins C and A may be low because of erratic food intake, especially in vegetables and fruits.

Eating Habits

Physical and psychosocial pressures influence adolescent eating habits (see Issues and Answers on p. 300). By and large, boys fare better than girls. Their large appetites and the sheer volumes of food they consume usually ensure intake of adequate nutrients. But the adolescent girl may be less fortunate. Two factors combine to place her under pressures concerning body weight:

Physiologic Sex Differences

Because of the girl's physiologic sex differences associated with fat deposits during this growth period and her comparative lack of physical activity, she may gain excess weight easily.

Social and Personal Tensions

These pressures and tensions concerning figure control sometimes cause adolescent girls to follow unwise, self-imposed crash diets for weight loss. In some cases actual self-starvation regimens may result in complex and far-reaching eating disorders such as **anorexia nervosa** and **bulimia** (see Chapter 15). Usually these problems, which may assume severe proportions, involve a distorted self-image and a morbid, irrational pursuit of thinness.[13,14] Even in less clinical situations, constant "dieting" among teenage girls can bring varying degrees of poor nutrition at the very time in life when their bodies need to be building reserves for potential reproduction. The harmful effects that bad eating habits can have on the future course of a pregnancy are clearly indicated in many studies relating preconception nutritional status to the outcome of gestation (see Chapter 11).

Anorexia nervosa
Psychologic condition manifested by a refusal to eat to achieve a thin, usually abnormally thin, appearance.

Bulimia
Practice of binging on food, then inducing vomiting to prevent weight gain.

To Sum Up

Growth and development depend on nutrition to support heightened physiologic and metabolic processes. Nutrition, in turn, depends on a multitude of social, psychosocial, cultural, and environmental influences that affect individual growth potential throughout the life cycle. Four types of growth are usually measured during each phase of development: physical, mental, emotional, and sociocultural. Each type of growth is evaluated in assessing the child's nutritional status and planning an effective counseling approach.

Nutritional needs change with each growth period. *Infants* grow rapidly. Breast-feeding is preferred during the first 6 months of life. Solid foods are not needed, nor can they be handled, until about 4 to 6 months of age. *Toddlers, preschoolers,* and *school-age children* undergo a slowed and erratic latent growth of childhood. Their energy requirements per unit of body weight are not as great as the infant's. Their nutritional needs center on protein for growth with attendant minerals and vitamins. Social and cultural factors influence the development of food habits.

Adolescents undergo a second large growth spurt before reaching adulthood. This rapid growth is accompanied by sexual maturation and physical growth. Increased caloric and nutrient needs on the average are easier for boys to achieve than for girls, who frequently feel social and peer pressures to restrict food intake for weight control. This pressure may inhibit their ability to acquire the nutritional reserves necessary for later reproduction.

Questions for Review

1. How is physical growth measured? What signs are used to measure mental, emotional, and sociocultural growth?
2. What factors are responsible for the major differences in nutritional and feeding needs of the preterm and full-term infant?
3. Why is breast-feeding encouraged for feeding infants? Describe some types of commercial formulas that would provide appropriate alternative feeding.
4. Outline a general schedule for a new mother to use as a guide for adding solid foods to her infant's diet during the first year of life.
5. What changes in physical growth and psychosocial development influence eating habits in the the toddler, preschool child, and school-age child? How do these factors influence the nutritional needs of each age group?
6. What factors influence the changing nutritional needs of adolescents? Who is usually at greater nutritional risk during this phase—boys or girls? Why? What nutritional deficiencies may be associated with this more vulnerable age?

1. Picciano MF: Nutrient needs of infants, Nutr Today 22(1):8, 1987.

2. Hamill PV and others: Physical growth: National Center for Health Statistics percentiles, Am J Clin Nutr 32:607, 1979.

3. Yip R and others: Declining prevalence of anemia among low income children in the United States, JAMA 258:1619, 1987.

4. Erikson E: Childhood and society, New York, 1963, WW Norton Co.

5. Kantrowitz B, Wingert P, and Hager M: Preemies, Newsweek, p 62, May 16, 1988.

6. Hague CJ and others: Overview of the National Infant Mortality Surveillance (NIMS) project—design methods, results, Public Health Rep 102:126, March/April 1987.

7. Matheny R and Picciano MF: Feeding and growth characteristics of human milk-fed infants, J Am Diet Assoc 86(3):327, 1986.

8. US Congress, Infant Formula Act of 1980, Washington, DC, P.L. 96-359, Sept 26, 1980.

9. Anderson SA, Chinn HL, and Fisher KD: History and current status of infant formulas, Am J Clin Nutr 35:381, 1982.

10. Birch L and Marlin DW: I don't like it; I never tried it: effect of exposure on two-year-old children's food preferences, Appetite J Intake Res 3:353, 1982.

11. Pelchat ML and Pliner P: Antecedents and correlates of feeding problems in young children, J Nutr Ed 18:23, Feb 1986.

12. McConnel PE, Shaw JB, and Egan, M: Child nutrition services: ADA technical support paper, J Am Diet Assoc 87(2):218, 1987.

13. Kirkley BG: Bulimia: clinical characteristics, development, and etiology, J Am Diet Assoc 86(4):468, 1986.

14. Killen JD and others: Depressive symptoms and substance abuse among adolescent binge eaters and purgers: a defined population study, Am J Public Health 77(12):1539, 1987.

References

Bosma JF: Development of feeding, Clin Nutr 5(5):210, 1986.

This pediatrician-professor provides an excellent background for understanding the development process by which infants first learn to drink and then to eat, by suckling, sucking, swallowing, and transitional feeding to solids.

Farthing MC and Phillips MG: Nutrition standards in day-care programs for children: ADA technical support paper, J Am Diet Assoc 87(4):504, 1987.

McConnell PE, Shaw JB, and Egan M: Child nutrition services: ADA technical support paper, J Am Diet Assoc 87(2):218, Feb 1987.

These two articles provide statements of the American Dietetic Association about important child-care nutrition services, with support and recommendations.

Lifshitz F: Nutrition and growth, Clin Nutr 4(2):40, 1985.

This article provides a clear discussion of the growth process, with concerns of physicians and nutritionists about the effects of inappropriate dieting and social fads on normal growth of children.

Picciano MF: Nutritional needs of infants, Nutr Today 22(1):8, 1987.

This author describes current research knowledge of infant nutritional needs and how much more we need to learn with more sensitive and specific measures.

Satter EM: Child of mine: feeding with love and good sense, Palo Alto, CA 1986, Bull Publishing Co.

This skilled author and practitioner, both nutritionist (RD) and social worker (MSSW), provides a little gem of a book based on the title's premise that children thrive on good food fed with love and good sense. She provides much practical guidance for parents and practitioners alike.

Further Readings

Food Habits of Adolescents

Teenagers have gained the reputation of having the worst eating habits in the world. Is this justified? Here's a closer look at the actual eating habits of American adolescents during the last 15 years.

Skipping meals

A study of California teenagers revealed that lunch—not breakfast, as most people assume—was the meal most frequently skipped. Breakfast was skipped most frequently by obese children, however. In all cases the frequency of regular meals increased with income and social status.

Snacking

Another study indicated that 12- to 16-year-olds met or exceeded their RDA per 100 kcal for protein, riboflavin, and vitamin C through between-meal foods. Vitamin A, calcium, and iron levels fell considerably below the standard.

Fast foods

Having a limited range of items, fast-food restaurant menus are more likely to be lacking one or more essential nutrients. They are generally considered to be inadequate in calcium and vitamin A and too high in kilocalories, saturated fats, and sodium. Current marketing practices will continue to attract the young, who often consider fast-food restaurants as popular hangouts to escape the demands of an ever-encroaching adult world. Thus it is likely that these places will influence the nutritional quality of adolescent meals for some time.

Unusual food choices

Teenagers are likely to eat any type of food at any time of the day. Studies have shown that they are as likely to have barbecued chicken for breakfast as pancakes for dinner. These food choices are only unusual in terms of the time of day at which they are consumed, however, and usually present no threat to health or nutritional status.

Alcohol consumption

As adolescents approach the drinking age in their locale, alcohol begins to provide a more significant portion of their total caloric intake. As they begin to drink at younger and younger ages, even a mild form of abuse coupled with the elevated nutritional requirements of adolescence may compromise their nutritional status, especially in terms of folic acid, which is "destroyed" by excessive amounts of alcohol. Subclinical damage to the intestinal mucosa caused by chronic alcohol use could also influence the absorption of other nutrients.

In general the adolescent diet may be no worse than the average adult diet, although intakes of calcium, vitamin A, iron, and ascorbic acid are usually seriously inadequate during these years, especially among girls. In addition, eating habits and social pressures have made this age-group susceptible to at least two important nutritional problems: obesity and anorexia nervosa.

Obesity affects approximately 10% to 20% of the adolescent population. As in adults, an excessive intake of kilocalories is less often the cause than lack of exercise. Concern about personal appearance could make the adolescent more reluctant than an adult to participate in activities (team sports, dance classes) that are popular ways of controlling weight.

Anorexia nervosa is considered the flip side of the weight-management coin. It usually affects achievement-oriented, affluent girls, although the problem now crosses socioeconomic and sexual barriers. This self-induced starvation is often attributed to an obsession with attaining a slim figure—a desire that goes so far it results in self-starvation, emaciation, and serious health problems, including amenorrhea.

The food habits of adolescents reflect a reduced influence of parents on eating habits, increased peer pressure or desire to conform, extrasensitivity to appearance, and elevated needs for energy. The nutrition counselor must remember these influences when helping adolescents and their families plan food patterns that will enhance health and meet growth requirements during the teenage years.

REFERENCES

Bigler-Daughten S and Jenkins RM: Adolescent snacks: nutrient density and nutritional contribution to total intake, J Am Diet Assoc 87(12):1678, 1987.

Coctes TJ and others: Modifying the snack food consumption patterns of inner city high school students: The Great Sensations Study, Pre Med 14:234, March 1985.

Guenther PM: Beverages in the diets of American teenagers, J Am Diet Assoc 86(4):493, 1986.

13 Nutrition for Adults: Aging and the Aged

Chapter Objectives

After studying this chapter, the student should be able to:

1. Identify social and economic problems of adults as they grow older in American society today.
2. Define the role of nutrition in the general aging process and the changes it brings in specific nutrient needs.
3. Identify nutrition-related clinical problems of adults as they grow older.
4. Relate eating problems among older adults to practical daily living situations and identify community resources to help meet these needs.

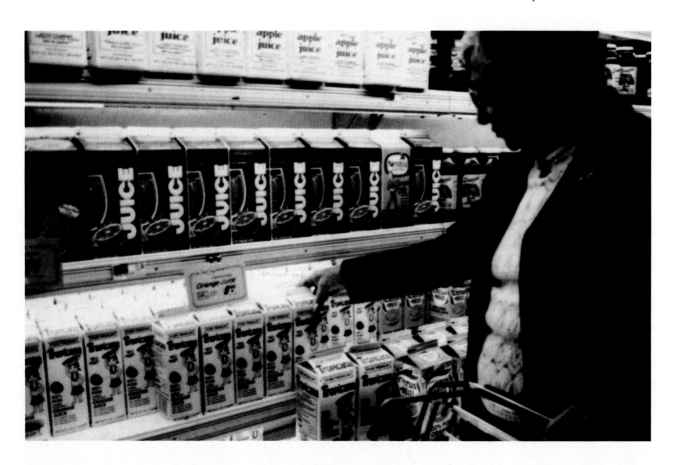

PREVIEW

Following the tumultuous adolescent years come the challenges, problems, and opportunities of maturity. The cycle of human growth and development continues throughout the adult years.

The American population has been changing. We have more adults now, and they are growing older. Thanks to the World War II "baby boom," the fastest growing group in America today is aged 35 to 44. This is an increase of almost 10% since the 1980 census, and this group now numbers about 28 million. Already there are about 26.3 million Americans aged 65 and over, and the second fastest growing group is aged 85 and over. During the 1980s the 65- to 74-year-old population has increased about 15%, and the 75-year-old and over population has increased some 33%.

Behind all these numbers are human beings, unique individual adults—young, middle, and older—experiencing the imprint of their personal life situation and facing problems, including health concerns. In our study here, two important concepts govern our approach: (1) aging throughout adulthood is a highly *individual* process, and (2) aging in adulthood is but part of the ongoing *total life* process from its beginning—biologic, nutritional, socioeconomic, psychosocial, and spiritual.

Aging Throughout the Life Cycle

Aging is a positive concept. It starts at conception and ends at death. It encompasses the whole of life, not merely its latter stages. Indeed, every stage has its unique potential and fulfillment and the periods of adulthood—young, middle, and older—are no exception. During adulthood both psychosocial and physical development continue, although in changing patterns, as persons mature and grow older. The three progressive adult stages of the human life span, as identified by Erikson (see Chapter 12), fulfill the whole of human development.

Psychosocial Development in Adulthood
Young Adulthood (18 to 40 years)

In the years of young adulthood, each person becomes launched in life as a mature individual. Now each person must resolve the core psychosocial developmental problem of *intimacy vs isolation*. The person who achieves the positive goal of intimacy is able to build close fulfilling relationships. Others who fail to do so become increasingly isolated. These are years of much stress but also of fulfillment. They are years of continuing education and career beginnings, of establishing one's own home, of parenthood, and of starting young children on their way through the same life stages. These are the years of early struggles to make one's way in the world, with their attendant joys and heartaches.

Middle Adulthood (40 to 60 years)

In the years of middle adulthood, the core psychosocial developmental task the individual faces is that of **generativity** *vs self-absorption*. Children are

Aging in America

Generativity
Pertaining to the reproduction or continuance of the species.

growing up and in the latter years of this period have grown to adulthood and gone on to make their own lives. For some middle adults these are the years of the "empty nest." For others it is an opportunity to expand personal growth—"it's my turn now." There is a coming-to-terms with what life is all about, together with opportunity for expressing stored learnings by passing on life's teachings to younger persons. It is a regeneration of one's life in the lives of young people following in the same way. To the degree that these inner struggles are not won, there is an increasing self-absorption, a turning on oneself, and a withering rather than a regenerating spirit of life.

Older Adulthood (60 to 80+ years)

In the last stage of life the final core psychosocial developmental problem is resolved between *integrity* vs *despair*. Depending on a person's resources at this point, there is either a predominant sense of wholeness and completeness or a sense of bitterness and revulsion and of wondering what life was all about. If the outcome of life's basic experiences has been positive, the individual arrives at old age a rich person—rich in the wisdom of the years. Building on each previous level, psychosocial growth reaches its personal positive human resolution. But some of our older patients will not have resolved each of the core developmental problems along the way. They still struggle with those same problems that they have wrestled with in previous stages of life. Thus they arrive at middle and older years poorly equipped to deal with the adjustments of aging and health problems that may face them. On the other hand, many will have been enriched by life's human experiences in their maturing process. In turn they will bring enrichment to our lives. The resulting relationship is mutually rewarding.

Socioeconomic and Psychologic Factors

Increasing industrialization and urbanization of American society, the complexity of the culture it is building, and the changes in age distribution in the population have all brought about changes in the lives of adults in the United States today.

Population Changes

Not only has the general population been increasing rapidly, but also significant shifts have occurred in the age distribution. Increasing longevity has resulted in a greater number of adults in the older age groups. One out of every 7 Americans is now over age 60, and the number of older Americans has increased 2.5 times as fast as the overall population. Now at age 65 the average life expectancy is 16 more years; at age 75, another 10. Although poverty exists in both inner cities and some isolated rural areas, recent surveys do indicate generally that many adults are not only living longer but are also living better.[1] These middle-aged and older adults are growing older but feeling and thinking younger. Many are active and able to take care of themselves for longer than the general American myths and stereotyping of **ageism** would picture them. But many persons are increasingly concerned about the *quality* of life, not merely its length.[2] They are concerned about changing biologic, social, and environmental factors and their combined effect on the quality of lengthened life. Today our increased longevity has in general been influenced by two factors: medical care and living standards.

Ageism
Discrimination on the basis of age, usually applying to older persons.

Medical Care

Although we still have not fully addressed our basic problem of a relatively high infant mortality rate (the United States ranks eighteenth among the developed nations of the world in infant mortality), progress has been made in controlling childhood diseases and improving pediatric care in general. The increased availability and quality of medical care during adult years is also a factor in health during maturing years. However, relatively little progress has been made in controlling chronic disease in older ages or in relating general medical care practices to the needs of the aged.[1]

Living Standards

General U.S. living standards are high, but many "new poor" persons and families have begun to suffer more hardships since we all now live in an interdependent volatile world economy and political realities are changing. In general, however, compared to past generations more people have a better education, better housing, and improved nutrition through growth and early adult years, although in older age problems in socioeconomic status increase for many. The very factors that have contributed to our longer lifespan and the resulting increased number of older persons in the American population have also contributed to our medical, social, and economic concerns.

Social and Economic Factors

America's shifting work force, with changing industrialization and high technology, has affected the position of the older person in American society. For many, economic insecurity is creating added pressures (Figure 13-1). A

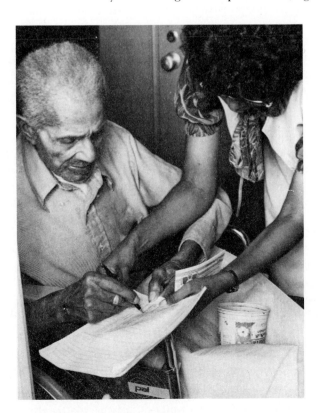

Figure 13-1
Elderly disabled man assisted by the Food Stamp Program to obtain needed food.

policy in industry of early retirement and employment difficulties with advancing age have created financial problems. However, corporate leaders are slowly beginning to recognize that changes in the workforce, the economic status of the federal Social Security system, and the value of older workers with much experience and skill are factors that will profoundly affect the composition of the workforce in the years ahead. In some instances changing social attitudes toward older adults and their capacities have increased institutional care and segregation in living situations. Many elderly persons, however, are able to live with extended families or in a variety of group or self-help situations. Actually, only 1 in 20 elderly persons lives in a health care facility, and only 10% of those over 65 are confined in any serious way (see the box on the facing page). Every effort needs to be made to provide the stimulus of involvement in the activities of society for as long as possible.

Psychologic Factors

Financial pressures and a decreasing sense of self-worth and accomplishment cause many older adults anxieties and loss of personal values. Many may feel inadequate. All persons need a sense of belonging, achievement, and self-esteem. Instead many older persons are often lonely, restless, unhappy, and uncertain. The greater part of the aging process in any area is primarily culturally determined. Unfortunately in many instances our culture imposes a set of negative roles on persons as they grow older. Basic needs common to older persons include economic security, personal effectiveness, suitable housing, constructive and enjoyable leisure-time activities, satisfying social relationships, and spiritual values. These needs we must seek to remember in our health care if our efforts are to be helpful.

General Physiologic Changes

The general biologic process of growth and gradual decline extends over the entire life span. It is conditioned by all previous life experiences and the imprint of these experiences on individual genetic heritage.

The Aging Process

Nature of Biologic Change

During middle and older adulthood, there is a gradual cell loss and reduced cell metabolism, with a related gradual reduction in the performance capacity of most organ systems. These changes, both physical and mental, may occur rapidly in one organ system and slowly in others, and individuals vary widely in the rate and order in which these changes occur.[3] But in general, lean body mass continues an age-related decline that accelerates in later life. For example, by age 70 the kidneys and the lungs lose about 10% of their weight in comparison with values in young adults, the liver loses 18% of its weight, and skeletal muscle diminishes by 40%. Also, an overall, gradual reduction in the body's reserve capacities takes place. An important cause is the gradual reduction in cellular units. For example, functioning units of the kidney—the nephrons—are lost as the "aging Western kidney," which evolved in prior ages of vastly different food intake needs, now responds to our modern high-protein diet (see Chapter 22).

Effect of Biologic Change on Food Patterns

Some physiologic factors may affect food patterns. For example, secretion of digestive juices is diminished, and motility of the gastrointestinal tract is de-

Clinical Application

The number of elderly Americans in nursing homes is increasing, and many suffer from malnutrition. Over the past three decades the number of nursing home beds has increased from about 880,000 to 1.5 million, and the need by the year 2000 is expected to exceed 3.5 million. Some 80% of these residents are 75 years old or older. Up to 50% cannot feed themselves. A reported 85% have moderate to severe protein-energy malnutrition, decreasing their response to rehabilitative efforts.

Food is a critical issue for older adults in long-term care facilities. These residents have a wide spectrum of needs. They place particular significance on food and daily meals, a fact that some facilities with otherwise excellent care in nursing and imaginative cultural programs sometimes fail to realize in their food service. The use of full-time nutritionists can change this situation.

Improvements in the nutritional status of residents when professional nutrition services by qualified nutrition specialists are provided has been documented many times over. These skilled and sensitive persons address various factors in quality care that must be present to ensure the optimal nutritional status of their clients.

Administrative activities

- Developing cyclic menus based on the nutritional requirements and food needs and desires of the population
- Training staff to ensure proper food preparation with appetizing seasoning, as well as appropriate storage and distribution
- Providing in-service education for all health professionals and kitchen staff regarding the nutritional needs of residents

Clinical activities

- Making regularly scheduled nutritional assessments—measures of weight and body composition, as well as laboratory tests and so on—upon admission and at intervals thereafter as needed
- Conducting a nutritional assessment of *every* resident at least once
- Making accurate calculations for diets, as needed, such as those for persons with insulin-dependent diabetes mellitus (IDDM)
- Discouraging abuse of alcohol, nicotine, drugs
- Developing resident education programs, such as appropriate exercise and weight management groups
- Encouraging eating by planning special events such as picnics, which may include family members; creating a home-like atmosphere in the dining hall; preparing meals in the residential area to "entice" residents with the aroma; encouraging residents to serve themselves; and so on.

Many of these same activities in modified form can be used in teaching and supervising caretakers in the emerging alternate setting of foster home care. We are learning from this new approach that residents tend to remain more mobile, develop the valuable skill of choice, and seem to have a better prognosis.

Continued.

Improving the Nutritional Status of the Elderly in Long-Term Care Facilities

Clinical Application

Improving the Nutritional Status of the Elderly in Long-Term Care Facilities—cont'd

REFERENCES
Ford AB: Looking after the old folks, Am J Pub Health 77(12):1499, 1987.
Kerschner PA: Breaking a long-term stereotype, Food Management 20:25, Dec 1985.
Gardner J and Kelley A: Long-term care facilities: the benefits of having a dietitian, J Can Diet Assoc 44(1):68, 1983.
Oktay JS and Vollard PJ: Foster home care for the frail elderly as an alternative to nursing home care: an experimental evaluation, Am J Pub Health 77(12):1505, 1987.
Sullivan D, Chernoff R, and Lipschitz D: Nutritional support in long-term care facilities, Nutr Clin Pract 2(1):6, 1987.

creased. This contributes to decreased absorption and the use of nutrients. Sensory perceptions of taste, smell, and vision also diminish.[4] These senses influence appetite and the amount of food consumed, so food for older adults needs more, not less, enhancement in seasoning. Also, along with these biologic changes often come an increased concern about body functions, increasing social stress, personal losses, and diminished social opportunities to maintain self-esteem. All of these responses can affect food intake.

Individuality of the Aging Process

The biologic changes in aging are general. But in reality persons in the advancing years of life will display a wide variety of individual reactions. We all simply get old at different rates. Every person bears the imprint of individual trauma and accumulation of disease experience, and we grow older at our own individual and unique gene-controlled nature and rate of the process of aging.[5] All of these factors directly affect individual aging. We can discuss aging and its nutritional needs in general terms, but individual situations and needs vary widely and must always be individually assessed. Actually, as we increasingly realize, the greatest influence of nutrition on the aging process takes place in earlier growth years when resources for later times are being built. Thus nutrition's most effective role is in growth and middle years, which prepare each one of us to meet the gradually declining metabolic processes of older age.

Nutritional Needs

Energy
Standard Allowances

Kilocalorie requirements vary according to degree of activity.

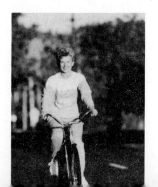

The reduced basal metabolic requirements caused by losses in functioning cells and reduced physical activity combine to create less energy demand as age advances. Some studies have indicated that the concept of a limited, less rich diet—"undernutrition without malnutrition"— may actually lengthen life.[6] The RDA standard is based on estimates of decreased metabolic activity of about 5% in middle and later years. The average estimate of adult energy need is an approximate caloric requirement of 2200 kcal for men and 1900 kcal for women.

Major gaps still exist in our knowledge of energy and nutrient needs of elderly adults. For example, nutrient uptake by cells may decline with aging, so that older persons may need higher plasma levels to maintain optimal tissue concentrations. Also, because living situations vary widely among older adults, much more information is needed on their daily life activities and the degree of energy they may be capable of expending. Kilocalorie requirements are highly individual, according to activity. Primary consideration must be given to the living situation of the person and the degree of activity in various phases of life. Perhaps the simplest criterion for judging adequacy of caloric intake is the maintenance of *normal* weight. However, there is rethinking of what is "normal" weight, a reexamination of traditional standards for ideal desired weight based on life insurance weight-for-height tables (see Chapter 15). Recent assessment of these and other data has raised the possibility that the greatest longevity is not associated with the conventional "desirable" weights but with levels 10% to 25% greater.[7] In other words, very thin persons have a reduced life expectancy rather than a better outlook. This view has obvious nutritional implications in terms of optimal energy intake for adults of all ages. To meet these energy needs, adults need ample carbohydrates but limited fats.

Carbohydrates. The optimal need for energy from carbohydrate is unknown, but it is usually recommended that at least 50% to 55% of daily kilocalories in the diet come from carbohydrate foods, mostly complex carbohydrates such as starches. Easily absorbable sugars may be used, and generally carbohydrate metabolism is not disturbed. The fasting blood sugar level is essentially normal in the aged. They can can choose freely among carbohydrate foods, according to individual needs, desires, and physical responses. Current findings indicate that much of the observed carbohydrate intolerance of older persons may be caused by factors other than biologic aging per se and that diet and exercise modifications can substantially curtail age-related glucose intolerance and insulin resistance.[2]

Fats. Generally, Americans eat too much fat. Fat intake is best limited to about 20% to 25% of the total kilocalories. Some fat is needed as a source of energy, important fat-soluble vitamins, and essential fatty acids. A reasonable goal is to avoid large quantities of fat, with more emphasis on the quality of the smaller amount of fat consumed, using mostly plant sources rather than animal fats. Digestion and absorption of fats may be somewhat delayed in elderly persons, but these functions are not greatly disturbed with age. There is no need to be unduly restrictive. Sufficient fat for food palatability aids appetite. Excessive fat, however, should be avoided because of the delayed absorption capacity of elderly persons.

Protein

There is a basic need for quality protein, though not in excessive amounts, to meet the needs of adults in our society.

Basic needs. The RDA standard recommends a continuation of the daily protein intake for the middle and older adult at the same allowance given for young adults—0.8 g/kg of body weight. Even this amount provides an allowance for wide variation in individual needs. Also, although the need for protein may be increased during illness or convalescence or during a wasting disease, the overall mass of actively metabolizing tissue decreases with age.

No adequate data exist on just what levels of dietary protein can best preserve the lean body mass and tissue function of the aging adult.[7] We need to know whether populations receiving 0.8 g/kg or less show any accelerated losses of lean body mass. It is possible that to maintain nitrogen balance, elderly persons need relatively more protein as their total caloric intake is reduced.

Protein quality. Protein needs are influenced by two basic factors: (1) the biologic value of the protein, or the quantity and ratio of its essential amino acids, and (2) adequate caloric value of the diet. It is estimated that about 25% to 50% of the protein intake should come from animal sources, the only foods that are "complete" proteins with all the essential amino acids, with the remainder coming from plant protein sources. In a vegetarian diet, careful supplementary mixtures of plant proteins, with additions of acceptable milk and egg protein, must be selected to assure adequate quality protein intake. Protein should supply from 15% to 20% of the day's total kilocalories. For healthy individuals there is usually no need for supplemental amino acid preparations. They are an expensive and inefficient source of available nitrogen.

Vitamins

Additional vitamin intake is usually not needed in the healthy adult. Tissue stores may gradually decrease with normal aging, but the requirement is no different from that for normal adults. Individual problems may stem from inadequate normal intake rather than from an increased need. A well-selected mixed diet with a variety of foods should supply vitamins in normally needed quantities. Increased therapeutic needs in illness should be evaluated on an individual basis.

Minerals

Osteoporosis
Bone weakened by a loss of mineral content, mainly calcium.

Usually increased minerals are not needed in normal aging. The same adult allowances are sufficient if provided on a continuing basis by a well-balanced diet. However, two essential minerals need emphasis: calcium and iron. The adult RDA standard for calcium intake is 800 mg/day. But some recent evidence indicates that negative calcium balance can be prevented by increasing the level to 1200 mg in women over age 50 and in men over age 60 to prevent calcium loss from bone tissue and **osteoporosis** (see Chapter 8).[8,9] Poor diets may also be deficient in iron, which is needed to prevent iron-deficiency anemia. Some individuals may need increased attention and encouragement to ensure adequate dietary sources of these minerals among their daily food choices.

Water

Xerostomia
Dry mouth caused by decreased salivary secretions.

Too often the vital need for water in older adults is overlooked. The normal thirst mechanism sometimes diminishes with age and dehydration can easily occur (see Chapter 8). Many elderly persons suffer from **xerostomia,** dry mouth caused by a severe reduction in the flow of saliva, which in turn affects their food intake.[10] This condition may be associated with the use of certain medications, autoimmune diseases, or radiation therapy to the head and neck. Conscious attention to adequate fluid intake, not dependent on normal thirst, is an important aspect of health maintenance and care.

The Question of Nutrient Supplementation

There is no evidence that *healthy* adults in middle and older years require additional nutrient supplementation. The nutrition board of the National Research Council has stated that it is "aware of no convincing evidence of unique health benefits accruing from consumption of a large excess of any one nutrient."[11] Nonetheless the use of such supplements is apparently widespread among older adults.[12-14] There is some indication, however, that certain specific nutrient supplementation might be a rational approach to improve cognitive function (see the box on p. 312) in disoriented older adults.[15] In illness or debilitated states supplementation may well be needed to help restore tissue integrity and health (see Issues and Answers on p. 317).

Malnutrition

Personal Food Habits

Generally poor dietary habits in young adulthood, as with any personal habit, tend to be set and accentuated in older age. Frequently evidence of inadequate distribution of needed kilocalories in food choices is present. For example, there may be fewer animal proteins, such as meat, egg, cheese, and milk. There may be inadequate use of whole grains, fewer vegetables and fruits, and more sweets and desserts, even to the extent of about 20% of the day's kilocalories. Also, older persons are frequently prey to claims of food faddists concerning restorative food products, tonics, or regulators.

Oral Problems

As indicated above, the constant problem of a dry mouth from limited salivary secretions often hinders the eating process in some older adults.[10] Poor teeth, **periodontal disease,** or poorly fitting dentures also may make chewing difficult. A denture can be only as successful as the health of the tissue on which it rests. An analysis of the three stages of eating food—biting, chewing, and swallowing—will provide a basis for helping the person with new dentures adjust to using them. Poor appetite and limited financial means for adequate dental care discourage efforts to seek improvement in the situation. Also, mucosal changes in the mouth, as well as a decrease or change in the quality of salivary secretions, cause further difficulty in eating.

Gastrointestinal Problems

Numerous gastrointestinal complaints vary from vague indigestion or "irritable colon" to specific diseases such as peptic ulcer or **diverticulitis** (see Chapter 19). Such problems generally reduce appetite and food intake so the needed nutrients are not taken in. A variety of other illnesses may limit food intake or utilization. Limited absorption of nutrients curtails nourishment still further.

Personal and Social Factors

Financial resources may be limited, and little money may be available to purchase needed food. Persons may lack knowledge of food needed for a well-balanced diet. Boredom, loneliness, anxiety, insecurity, and apathy compound the problem. Especially if an older person lives alone, the social value of eating is gone. They may also lack adequate cooking, refrigeration, or storage facilities. They may have no means of transportation to obtain food. A vicious cycle often ensues: funds are low, the person hesitates to spend,

Health Maintenance and Clinical Needs

Periodontal disease
Disease (inflammation) occurring in tissue surrounding the teeth; facilitates tooth loss.

Diverticulitis
Inflammation of "pockets" of tissue (diverticuli) in the lining of the mucous membrane in the colon.

To Probe Further

Food for Thought Among the Elderly

Among elderly persons, as well as others, it is a common observation that poor mental function and malnutrition go hand-in-hand. Although scientists haven't yet figured out the precise connections, they find a strong correlation between nutritional deficiencies and poor cognitive performance and memory among elderly persons. A study of 260 noninstitutionalized adults over the age of 60 reveals that those with poor nutritional food intakes scored poorly on special tests that measure nonverbal abstract thinking ability and memory. Protein, vitamin C, and various B vitamins—folate, niacin, pyridoxine, riboflavin, thiamin, and B_{12}—emerged as the nutrients of particular significance to the subjects' ability to think and remember.

Researchers are reluctant at this point to say, on the basis of such studies, that poor nutritional status causes poor thinking abilities and memory loss. A number of factors may intervene:

- Persons with poor memories may forget to take a vitamin pill. Those who don't recognize objects or shapes may have such difficulties preparing meals that they often fail to eat, leading to a poor nutritional status.
- Educated persons may be more inclined to take nutritional supplements and because of their experience in taking tests, score better than average.
- In a population of basically healthy elderly persons, there may be a subgroup with undetected clinical problems that contribute to poor mental performances.

There is no doubt that mental problems affect diet practices. Less clear is just how poor nutritional status may precipitate, aggravate, or prolong mental problems in elderly persons. Some more obvious nutrient candidates involved are precursors for neurotransmitters: the four amino acids tyrosine, tryptophan, threonine, and histidine, as well as the vitamin choline. Other candidates would be nutrients affecting the metabolism of neurotransmitters: pyridoxine, vitamin C, thiamin, copper, and iron. Then still other candidates would be nutrients with general effects on brain metabolism: glucose, folate, cobalamins, nicotinic acid, riboflavin, zinc, potassium, and magnesium.

Thus we can make a strong presumptive case for the potential importance of nutritional status in mental abilities of older adults. But what we lack is precise knowledge of the possible mechanisms involved, which probably act in concert with many other contributory factors.

REFERENCES

Goodwin JS, Goodwin JM, and Garry PJ: Association between nutritional status and cognitive functioning in a healthy elderly population, JAMA 249(21):2917, 1983.

Hodkinson HM: Diet and maintenance of mental health in the elderly, Nutr Rev 46:79, Feb 1988.

Raskind M: Nutrition and cognitive function in the elderly, JAMA 249(21):2938, 1983.

goes without, and suffers increasing weakness and **lethargy.** This state leads to still less interest and incentive. Finally, illness results.

Lethargy
Drowsiness; indifference.

Implications for Patient Care

Any malnourished adult—young, middle, or older—needs much personal care and support to build improved eating habits. Helpful attitudes and actions are based on an understanding and realistic approach.

1. **Analyze food habits carefully.** Learn the patient's personal attitudes, the precise living situation, and its limitations or available options. Nutritional needs can be met with a variety of foods, so suggestions can be adapted to fit particular needs and personal situations and desires. Offer suggestions in a practical, realistic, and supportive manner.

2. **Never moralize.** The statement, "Eat this because it's good for you," should be struck from everyone's vocabulary. It has little value for anyone, much less a person who is struggling to maintain personal integrity and self-esteem in a culture that tends to alienate its aged.

3. **Encourage food variety.** An unattractive bland diet is presumed by many to be necessary for all elderly persons. *It is not.* A variety of foods and adventures with new foods, tastes, and seasonings often prove to be the needed stimuli for poor appetite and lack of interest in eating. A decreased taste sensitivity in aging needs all the help it can get. Sometimes smaller amounts of foods and more frequent mini-meals are helpful.

Weight Management

In a different sense, overweight, or rather overfat, may be considered a form of malnutrition. In middle and older adults it can be a potential health hazard in relation to hypertension or coronary heart disease or diabetes. Avoiding excessive weight in earlier growth years is a major nutritional measure for preventing problems in adult years.

Causes of Overweight

Many of the same living situations and emotional factors that have been described here may also contribute to overweight from compensatory overeating and poor food habits. Also, physical activity is usually decreased, and the caloric requirements for maintenance are lessened, but the same food habits continue.

Individual Approach

Long-standing eating habits or excessive weight are difficult to change. Certainly a reasonable approach should be followed, avoiding drastic measures or diet and planning only for a slow gradual loss. Moderate physical activity should be encouraged whenever possible. Personal and realistic planning with each client is mandatory, because individual energy requirements vary widely and individual personalities and problems are unique. This initial approach should be followed by supportive guidance and encouragement (see Chapter 15). Such an individual program usually pays the greatest dividends.

Government Programs for Older Americans
Older Americans Act—Title VII

Community Resources

In 1972 the Nutrition Program for Older Americans, Title VII of the Older Americans Act, was authorized by P.L. 92-258. The program was developed to meet both nutritional and social needs of persons 60 years of age and older who (1) cannot afford adequate diets, (2) are unable to prepare adequate meals at home, (3) have limited mobility, or (4) are isolated and lack incentive to prepare and eat food alone. The original program provided services such as outreach, escort and transportation, health services, information and referral, health and welfare counseling, and nutrition and consumer education.

In 1978 amendments were authorized by P.L. 95-478, which coordinated nutrition services with other services for older people. Under this amended act, Title III, the services funded after 1980 included the provision of meals, both congregate and home-delivered, and related nutrition services and education.

1. **Congregate meals.** The program provides older Americans, particularly those with low incomes, with low-cost, nutritionally sound meals in senior centers and other public or private community facilities. In these settings older adults can gather for a hot meal and receive both food and social support.

2. **Home-delivered meals.** For those persons who are ill or disabled and, as a result, unable to attend the congregate meals, meals are delivered by couriers to the home. This service provides both nutritional needs and human contact and support. Often the courier is the only person the homebound individual may contact during the day.

U.S. Department of Agriculture (USDA) Research Centers

Human nutrition research centers on aging are being established by the USDA in collaboration with universities and are authorized by Congress to study nutrition's role in aging. Current investigations include such areas as protein needs in the aged, the nutritional status of older men and women, and the prevention and slowing of osteoporosis.

USDA Extension Services

The USDA operates agricultural extension services in state universities and county agencies. Through these agencies, county home advisors aid communities with much practical nutrition material and counsel for older adults and community workers.

Public Health Departments

Skilled health professionals work in the community through local and state public health departments. Health guidance for older adults is available through their resources. The public health nutritionist is a significant member of the health care team and provides counseling and nutrition education services, as well as community program planning. Counseling is also provided concerning the various food assistance programs available (see Chapter 10).

Professional Organizations and Resources
National Council on Aging

The National Council on Aging, established in 1950, is located in Washington, DC. It is an organization for professionals and volunteers that works on many fronts to improve the quality of life for older Americans. It maintains a nonprofit central national resource for research, planning, training, information, technical assistance, advocacy, program and standards development, and publications that relate to all aspects of aging, including nutrition.

American Geriatric Society

This professional organization of physicians engaged in medical care of elderly patients promotes research in **geriatrics** to advance scientific knowledge of the aging process and the treatment of its disease. A number of nurses and other health professionals are associate members. The society publishes the *American Journal of Geriatrics*.

Geriatrics
The study and treatment of diseases of old age; a branch of medicine concerned with medical problems associated with old age.

The Gerontological Society

This society's membership includes a wide number of interested health professionals. Its committee on aging has stimulated increased interest among other related organizations and community and government agencies in **gerontology** and the problems of aging persons in our society. This organization publishes the *Journal of Gerontology*.

Gerontology
The study of the aging process and its phenomena.

Community Groups

Local community groups representing health professions such as the medical society, nursing organizations, and dietetic associations sponsor a variety of programs to help meet the needs of older adults. In addition, there are qualified nutrition experts—professional nutritionists and registered dietitians—in private practice available in most communities for individual counseling and community program support. Senior citizens' centers in local communities also provide a broad range of services and available nutrition education and counseling.

Volunteer Health Organizations

Many activities of volunteer health organizations such as the American Heart Association and the American Diabetes Association relate to the health and nutrition needs of older persons. These organizations include both professional and public members. They operate at national and community levels to fund and conduct research and education.

The challenge of meeting the nutritional needs of the older population is compounded by the lack of needed research in this area, the interaction of current and past social, economic, and psychologic factors, and the wide range of individual differences in the biologic process of aging. Nutritional requirements should, at least in part, be on data available for younger adult populations, as well as requirements to counteract chronic disease processes prevalent in aging, such as cardiovascular disease.

To Sum Up

Major illnesses found in older adults are often associated with malnutrition and obesity. In counseling the older client, the nutritionist should analyze food habits carefully. Each person must be encouraged to make needed dietary changes at his or her own rate, with supportive guidance, encouragement, and patience.

1. Identify three major biologic changes that occur with aging and give an example of each.

Questions for Review

2. Identify and give examples of three major factors contributing to malnutrition in older adults. How do these factors influence the nutrition counseling process?

3. List and describe the purpose of several agencies providing nutrition-related services for older adults or for health professionals in geriatric practice.

References

1. Gibbs NR: Grays on the go, Time 13(8):66, Feb 22, 1988.
2. Rowe JW and Kahn RL: Human aging: usual and successful, Science 237:143, July 1987.
3. Chernoff R: Aging and nutrition, Nutr Today 22(2):4, 1987.
4. Cain WS: Flavoring foods for a grayer US, Food Engineering 56: 103, May 1984.
5. Begley S: Why do we grow old? Newsweek 107(24):61, 1986.
6. Limited intake and longevity, Nutr Rev 40(10):314, 1982.
7. Munro HN: Nutrient needs and nutritional status in relation to aging, Drug-Nutrient Interactions 4(1/2):55, 1985.
8. Allen L: Calcium and age-related bone loss, Clin Nutr 5(4):147, 1986.
9. Allen L: Calcium and osteoporosis, Nutr Today 21(3):6, 1986.
10. Streebny LM and Valdini A: Xerostomia: a neglected symptom, Archives Intern Med 147:1333, July 1987.
11. Food and Nutrition Board, National Research Council: Recommended dietary allowances, ed 9, Washington, DC, 1980, Academy Press.
12. Gray GE and others: Vitamin supplement use in a southern California retirement community, J Am Diet Assoc 86(3):800, 1986.
13. Hartz SC and Blumberg J: Use of vitamin and mineral supplements by the elderly, Clin Nutr 5(3):130, 1986.
14. Ranno BS, Wardlaw GM, and Geiger CJ: What characterizes women who overuse vitamin and mineral supplements, J Am Diet Assoc 88(3):347, 1988.
15. Raskind M: Nutrition and cognitive function in the elderly, JAMA 249(21):2939, 1983.

Further Readings

Akin JS and others: Cluster analysis of food consumption patterns of older Americans, J Am Diet Assoc 86(5): 615, 1986.

Posner BE, Smigelski CG, and Krachenfels MM: Dietary characteristics and nutrient intake in an urban homebound population, J Am Diet Assoc 87(4):452, 1987.

These two articles help answer the question, "What do older Americans eat?", and identify areas of major risk of nutritional problems.

Natow AB and Heslin J-A: Nutritional care of the older adult, New York, 1986, Macmillan Publishing Co.

This little book packs in its very readable pages a wealth of information and practical help for health professionals working with older adults.

Posner BM and others: Nutrition, aging, and the continuum of health care, ADA technical support paper, J Am Diet Assoc 87(3):345, 1987.

This article points to professional responsibilities in education and practice to meet the growing needs for continuing health care in our expanding population of older adults.

Can We Eat to Live Forever?

The world is getting older. Our lifespan has extended from age 45 at the turn of the century to 77 (74 in men) today. It is expected to climb even higher.

We owe today's longevity to the conquest of infectious disease, the provision of safer work environments, and the development of more effective medical technology. In short, we have largely conquered our external environment. The time has come to conquer our *inner* environment— through proper nutrition.

Scientists are beginning to consider the importance of nutrition in combating the physical deterioration that accompanies old age—a 10% loss of kidney and lung tissue, 18% of liver tissue, 40% of skeletal tissue, and as much as 25% (12% in men) of bone by the seventh decade of life. One would think that scientists could simply make biochemical calculations to find optimal blood levels for nutrients that could retard these losses and make recommendations for dietary intake. However, achieving an optimal diet among elderly persons is much more complex than that. Consider the following.

Sensory deprivation

Elderly persons tend to live alone. Such physical and emotional isolation tends to diminish the desire to eat. When this is combined with the progressive deterioration in sight, smell, touch, and hearing, attempts to prepare meals are no longer merely frustrating—they become dangerous.

Taste and smell

Oral infections, poor hygiene, and a reduced salivary flow rate contribute to the increased difficulty in taste and smell. To what extent does this affect the desire to eat? No one knows. Some scientists say very little, suspecting poor research techniques in studies of this problem. Others believe it is serious enough to warrant further research to arrest on-going losses.

Bone and tooth loss

Approximately one half of all adults have lost their teeth by age 65. The main culprit is **periodontal disease.** Researchers are beginning to look at this problem as a possible manifestation of osteoporosis. Therefore they are focusing study on calcium:

- **Calcium RDAs** Some suggest that 1000 to 1200 mg/day may be necessary to prevent calcium loss, rather than the current RDA of 800 mg.
- **Phosphate** Calcium and phosphorus maintain an inverse ratio in the blood (p. 233). Processed foods contribute heavily to phosphate levels in the American diet and are suspected of promoting calcium resorption from bone.
- **Megavitamins** One report associates excessive vitamin A levels with a greater loss of bone in elderly persons. Another study of 100 elderly subjects revealed that 60% took vitamin supplements, with most taking three or more times the recommended daily allowance for vitamin A. This warrants further study.
- **Protein** America's obsession with meat may harm aging bones, as a high protein intake results in increased loss of calcium in the urine.

Caloric needs

It has repeatedly been reported that elderly persons fail to consume recommended amounts of kilocalories. Recent animal research indicates that they might have the right idea. Restricted kilocalorie intake in rats has been associated with longevity and has retarded development of respiratory, cardiovascular, and renal disease, as well as cancer. This factor is still controversial. A recent reassessment of the effect of body weight suggests that we should all weigh 10% to 25% more than we do to live longer. As the reassessment does not associate body size with detrimental health habits, such as smoking, it, in turn, is itself controversial. *Continued.*

Can We Eat to Live Forever—cont'd

Gastrointestinal problems

Reduced production of digestive juices, less **peristalsis,** and reduced mucosal surface area all work to inhibit nutrient absorption and promote such digestive disorders as constipation.

Drugs

The high prevalence of chronic disease means a high prevalence of drug use, both prescription and over-the-counter use. Drugs, either individually or in combination, can alter taste, appetite, and other factors affecting nutritional status.

Poverty

Frequently many elderly persons either cannot work or are forced into retirement. For these reasons they tend to be among the poorest citizens. Even those individuals in good health often lack the money to shop, the transportation to reach shopping areas, or the means for adequate food preparation and/or storage equipment to maintain a reasonably healthful diet.

Based on the information available thus far, the most nutritionally supportive environment for elderly persons is one in which they

1. Have company for meals, congregate meal sites, family support, and friends
2. Have foods with pleasant but distinctive aromas and flavors
3. Consume meals that are lower in protein-rich and processed foods, higher in fiber-rich foods (complex carbohydrates and a variety of fresh fruits and vegetables) and calcium (from nonbovine as well as bovine sources, to avoid excessive protein levels), and meals that provide a moderate amount of kilocalories
4. Avoid excess supplements, especially of vitamin A
5. Avoid unnecessary drugs and are informed of the action of each drug they do take
6. Are subsidized financially or live in situations such as senior centers, private homes, or with roommates that provide some financial, emotional, and nutritional support

These seem like reasonable recommendations for any age group. But nutrition in elderly persons presents such a myriad of long-standing compounding factors that a wide variety of services and professional assistance may be needed to avoid nutritional deficits. Thus counselors who hope to promote a nutritionally supportive environment for elderly clients must themselves maintain a network of professionals available for referrals and work together as a team to meet the unique needs of older persons.

REFERENCES

Chernoff R: Aging and nutrition, Nutr Today 22(2):4, 1987.

Munro HN: Nutrient needs and nutritional status in relation to aging. Drug-Nutrient Interactions 4(1/2):55, 1985.

Munro HN: Nutritional requirements in the elderly, Hosp Pract 10:143, Aug 1982.

Rowe JW and Kahn RL: Human aging: usual and successful, Science 237(4811):143, 1987.

Suter PM and Russell RM: Vitamin requirements of the elderly, Am J Clin Nutr 45:501, March 1987.

14 Nutrition and Physical Fitness

Chapter Objectives

After studying this chapter, the student should be able to:

1. Define physical fitness and describe how it is measured.
2. Identify sources of body fuel for different levels of physical activity.
3. Describe the nutritional needs of an active person.
4. Relate the degree of physical exercise to modern health problems.
5. Help individual clients develop realistic physical activity programs.
6. Describe an "optimal basic diet" for athletes and a wise plan for making "carbohydrate loading" adjustments for endurance events.

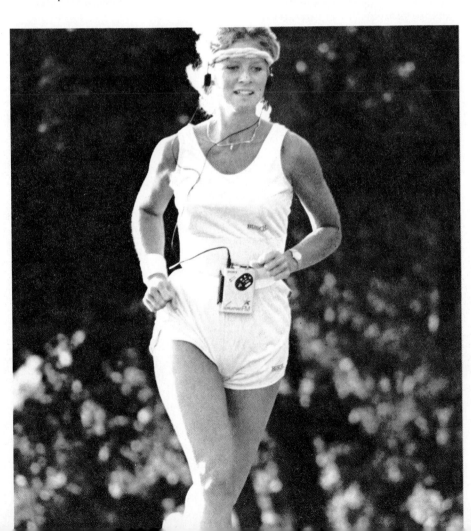

PREVIEW

During the human life cycle, three basic risk factors related to our changing lifestyles impinge on health maintenance. These factors are lack of exercise, excessive body fat (obesity), and stress. In the next three chapters we will look at each of these major risk factors in relation to health and nutrition. In this chapter we begin with physical fitness.

In recent years interest in physical fitness has been renewed. Presidents have exhorted us as a nation to improve our physical fitness level. And the surgeon general has issued reports relating physical fitness to health maintenance and chronic disease control in our aging society.

Judging from general public response, it seems that we are becoming more aware of the health toll of our inactivity. We search for ways to reverse our sedentary lifestyle born of society's technologic marvels. According to some estimates, 100 million Americans now practice some form of regular exercise, a twofold increase over the past 2 decades. Walking and swimming are our most popular activities, with bicycling and jogging close behind. And in the "big business" of athletics, the new specialty of sports medicine has developed.

For both recreational desires and health imperatives, we need to provide our clients and patients with sound physical fitness guidelines. We need to practice them ourselves.

Physical Activity and Energy Sources

Energy
The capacity for work; power to affect changes in self and surroundings.

Kinetic
Regarding or producing motion.

Substrate
The substance that enzymes act on.

The Nature of Energy

You will recall that you learned in Chapter 4 that the term **energy** refers to the body's ability, or power, to do work. The energy required to do body work takes several different forms: mechanical, chemical, electric, light, radiant, and heat. Energy, like matter, can neither be created nor destroyed. It can only be changed into another form and constantly cycled in the body and environment. We also speak of energy as being *potential* or **kinetic.** Potential energy is stored energy, ready to be used. Kinetic energy is active energy, being used to do work. Physical activity requires a base of sound nutrition to supply the **substrate** fuels, which along with oxygen and water meet widely varying levels of energy demand for body action.

Muscle Action: Fuels, Fluids, and Nutrients
Muscle Structures

The synchronized action of millions of specialized cells and structures that make up our skeletal muscle mass makes possible all forms of physical activity. A finely coordinated series of small bundles within the muscle fibers (Figure 14-1), triggered by nerve endings, produces a smooth symphony of action through simultaneous and alternating contraction and relaxation. These successively smaller muscle structures include the following:

1. **Skeletal muscle.** The largest bundle in the series is the complete muscle. Each particular muscle is composed of muscle fibers called *fasciculi.*
2. **Muscle fiber.** In turn each muscle fiber is composed of bundles of still smaller strands called myofibrils.

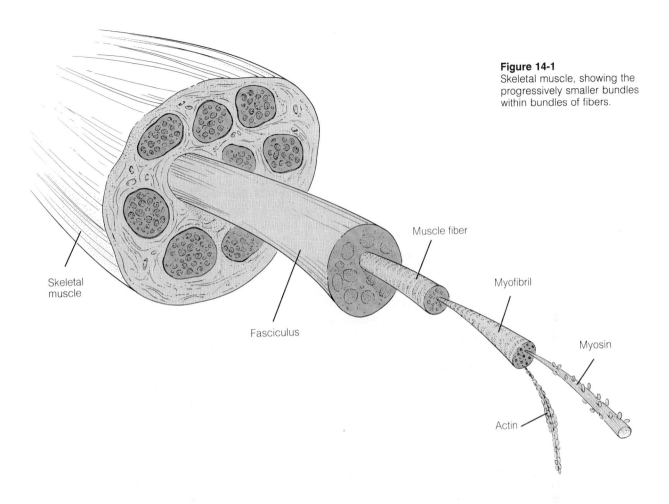

Figure 14-1
Skeletal muscle, showing the
progressively smaller bundles
within bundles of fibers.

Muscle fiber

Myofibril

Myosin

Skeletal
muscle

Fasciculus

Actin

3. **Myofibril.** Each single **myofibril** strand of the muscle fiber is made up
of the smallest of all the fiber bundles, called *myofilaments.* Contraction
occurs here.
4. **Myosin** and **actin.** Finally, within each myofilament are the contractile
proteins, **myosin** and **actin,** which are the smallest moving parts of every muscle.

Muscle Action

Inside the cell membrane these contractile proteins, myosin and actin, are arranged in long parallel rows. These parallel rows slide together and mesh
tightly when the muscle contracts and then pull apart when the muscle relaxes, allowing the muscle to shorten or lengthen as needed. When a specific
motor nerve impulse excites these molecules of myosin and actin in a myofilament, they mesh together and thereby shorten the muscle. This contraction
of the muscle bundles occurs instantly and simultaneously. Then periods of
relaxation occur between contractions. This alternating process continues
until muscle fatigue builds up and the muscle can no longer respond. Muscle
fatigue occurs for two reasons: (1) the supply of **glycogen,** the immediate
muscle fuel, is exhausted and thus insufficient to sustain the required chem-

Myofibril
Slender thread of muscle; runs
parallel to the muscle fiber's
long axis.

Myosin
A myofibril protein that acts in
conjunction with actin to cause
the contraction and relaxation of
muscle.

Actin
A myofibril protein that acts with
myosin to cause the contraction
and relaxation of muscle.

Glycogen
A polysaccharide, the main
storage form of carbohydrate,
largely stored in the liver and to
a lesser extent in muscle tissue.

Lactic acid
Produced by anaerobic glycolysis in muscles during exertion; can be converted to glucose by the liver.

ical reaction, and (2) **lactic acid,** the metabolic product of this chemical muscle reaction, accumulates during sustained high levels of exercise and cannot be removed fast enough.

Fuel Sources

Phosphate bonds form high-energy compounds in body metabolism (see Chapter 2). The main high-energy compound of the body cells is *adenosine triphosphate (ATP)*. It has rightly been called the "energy currency" of the cell. Various forms of energy are called on for successive energy needs.

1. **Immediate energy.** High-power or immediate energy demands over a short time depend on ATP being readily available within the muscle tissue. This amount is used up rapidly and a backup compound, *creatine phosphate (CP)*, is made available. These high-energy phosphate compounds, however, will sustain all-out exercise for only about 5 to 8 seconds.

2. **Short-term energy.** If an activity lasts longer than between 30 seconds and 2 minutes, *muscle glycogen* supplies the continuing need. Although the amount of available glycogen is small, it is an important rapid source of energy for brief muscular effort.

3. **Long-term energy.** Exercise continuing more than 2 minutes requires an oxygen-dependent, or **aerobic,** energy system. A constant supply of oxygen in the blood is necessary for continued exercise. Special cell organelles, the **mitochondria,** located within each cell, produce large amounts of ATP. The ATP is produced mainly from glucose and fatty acids and supplies continued energy needs of the body.

Aerobic
Requiring oxygen to proceed.

Mitochondrion
The cell's "powerhouse"; a small, spherical to rod-shaped organelle located in the cell cytoplasm; principal site of energy generation (ATP synthesis); contains enzymes of Krebs cycle and cell respiration, as well as RNA and DNA for synthesis of some proteins.

Fluids

An increased intake of water is essential in the course of exercise. A deficiency can be dangerous and limits capacity greatly. As exercise continues, the body temperature increases as part of the energy produced is released as heat. To control this temperature increase, the body shunts as much heat as possible to the skin, where it is released in sweat. Over time, and especially in hot weather, this excessive sweating can lead to **dehydration** (see Chapters 5 and 8). This is a serious complication.

Dehydration
Excessive water loss from body tissues.

Nutrients

The fuel nutrients also become depleted during continued exercise. As energy demands increase, the body burns blood glucose and muscle glycogen to provide energy. With prolonged exercise, levels of these nutrients fall too low to sustain the body's continued demands. Fatigue follows and exhaustion threatens.

Oxygen Use and Physical Capacity
Oxygen Consumption

The most profound limit to exercise is the person's ability to deliver oxygen to the tissues and use it for the production of energy. This vital ability depends on the fitness of the pulmonary and cardiovascular systems. In general, a person's *aerobic capacity* depends on the degree of fitness and body composition.

Body fitness. Physical fitness is defined in terms of aerobic capacity, which depends on the body's ability to deliver and use oxygen in sufficient quantities to meet the demands of increasing levels of exercise. Oxygen uptake increases with exercise intensity until either the demand is met or the ability to supply it is exceeded. This maximum oxygen (O_2) uptake, or aerobic capacity, is called the **VO$_2$ max,** maximum uptake volume of oxygen.[1] This capacity determines the intensity and duration of exercise that a person can perform. From the resting level, oxygen consumption rises steeply during the first 3 minutes of exercise. In about 6 minutes the rate levels off into a **steady state,** indicating an equilibrium between the energy required by the exercising muscles and the aerobic energy-producing system.[2] This aerobic capacity of an individual is measured in terms of milliliters of oxygen consumed per kilogram body weight per minute. Thus persons of differing sizes can be compared equally.

VO$_2$ max
Maximum uptake volume of oxygen.

Steady state
Equilibrium between energy required by exercising muscles and the aerobic energy-producing system.

Recovery period. During exercise, to accommodate the body's increased energy demands, the heart rate increases and breathing becomes deeper and more rapid. After exercise stops these functions do not immediately return to their preexercise levels, especially if the exercise has been strenuous. This recovery takes time because the body must replenish its "oxygen debt."

Body composition. Sex differences in aerobic capacity reflect the sex differences in body composition. In general, men have a higher aerobic capacity because of their larger **lean body mass,** the active metabolic body tissue. These highly metabolic tissues of the body thus use more oxygen than other tissues such as fat. When oxygen consumption is expressed only in terms of lean body mass instead of body weight, however, men and women have the same aerobic capacity. But women carry more body fat, a sex difference in body composition that serves critical biologic functions. Apart from stored adipose fat fuel, essential structural and functional body fat in women is about 12% of their body weight; in men it is only 3%. And since women must, of course, carry their entire body weight as part of their total workload, their performance will be affected accordingly.

Lean body mass
All component parts of the body, excluding neutral storage lipid; the entire fat-free mass.

Genetic influence. A person's aerobic capacity is mainly genetically determined. But the genetic heritage is influenced, as indicated, by body composition, which is associated with sex, and by aerobic training and age. Before puberty, lean body mass is about equal in boys and girls of comparable body size, but it increases rapidly in boys at puberty under the anabolic effect of testosterone. Maximal aerobic capacity then peaks at 18 to 20 years of age and declines gradually thereafter, largely because of age-related losses in lean body mass.[1,3]

Our diet must supply the necessary fuel substrate for meeting our energy needs. We require carbohydrate and fat as basic fuels but have very little need for protein. General needs apply to all individuals, but there are special needs for the young person, especially the growing child.

Diet and Exercise: Basic Nutrient Needs

Protein

Protein as a Fuel Substrate

Protein is usually discounted as a fuel substrate in energy production during exercise. Although some amino acids can feed into the cell's basic energy cycle, the extent of this input during exercise is minimal. There is evidence that some amino acid breakdown occurs during exercise, and there is some nitrogen loss in sweat. But authorities agree that under normal circumstances protein makes a relatively insignificant contribution to energy during exercise.[1,4]

Protein in the Diet

Most experts recommend 0.8 to 1.0 g protein/kg body weight to meet general needs of the active person. This amounts to the general RDA standard for adults, which contributes about 10% to 12% of the kilocalories in the diet. Most American eat about twice this amount of protein, putting a taxing load on the kidneys (see Chapter 22) and the liver. Nitrogen consumed in excess of need must be excreted. This requires an increased production of urea, which contributes to dehydration, a serious factor during strenuous exercise. High-protein diets can also increase calcium excretion in the urine.

Fat
Fat as Fuel Substrate

In the presence of oxygen, fatty acids are oxidized to provide energy. The rate at which this can occur is determined in part by the rate of mobilization of fatty acids from storage. But all stored fat is not alike. Actually, the body stores fat in two ways: (1) *depot fat* in adipose tissue, which is destined for transport back and forth to other tissues as needed for energy, and (2) *essential fat* in metabolically active tissue, such as bone marrow, heart, lungs, liver, spleen, kidneys, intestines, muscles, and nervous system, which is reserved in these places for necessary structural and functional use only.[5,6] Although storage depot fat in men and women is roughly comparable, essential fat reserves make the big difference—they are about four times greater in women.[7]

Free fatty acids, the fat fuel, are stored with glycerol as triglycerides in the body's adipose tissue. The enzyme *lipoprotein lipase* mobilizes these stores of fatty acids. This lipase is stimulated by exercise. Its activity is affected by levels of hormones also involved in exercise, especially growth hormone and epinephrine.

Fat in the Diet

It is important to recognize that fat as a fuel substrate is not drawn from the diet directly, but from the body's stored adipose fat. Dietary fat is not necessary to maintain these body fat stores, since excess kilocalories in the diet will be stored as fat regardless of their dietary source. We do not need to eat in excess of our dietary needs to burn fat, and there is no danger of depleting our fat stores before exercise has proceeded to exhaustion. Thus there is little basis for increased levels of fat in the diet. On the other hand, however, some fat in the diet is needed, especially as a source of the essential fatty acid, **linoleic acid.** In an apparent attempt to imitate the low-fat diet of the now-famous runners, the Tarahumara Indians of the mountains of Mexico, some compulsive runners in other countries have virtually eliminated fat from their diets, inducing a dangerous linoleic acid deficiency. Since the heart muscle prefers fatty acids, especially linoleic acid, as an energy source, deaths from cardiac arrest have been reported in some of these cases (see Issues and Answers on p. 338). Although some dietary fat is necessary, it should not exceed 25% to 30% of the total daily caloric intake.

Linoleic acid
Essential fatty acid; preferred fuel for the heart muscle.

Carbohydrate
Carbohydrate as Fuel Substrate

Although fat and protein have their special roles to play in maintaining general health, the major nutrient for energy support in exercise is carbohydrate. Carbohydrate fuels come from two sources, the circulating blood glucose and glycogen stored in muscle and liver.

Carbohydrate in the Diet

Carbohydrate should contribute about 55% or more of the daily caloric intake. Complex carbohydrates, starches, are preferable to simple ones, sugars. On the whole, the complex carbohydrates take longer to digest, provide a more sustained source of blood glucose, and are metabolized preferentially into glycogen. Simple sugars, on the other hand, are less efficient at maintaining the body's glycogen stores. They are mainly converted to fatty acids and stored as fat rather than glycogen. Simple sugars also provoke a sharper insulin response, contributing to the dangers of subsequent hypoglycemia. In addition, complex carbohydrates supply needed fiber, vitamins, and minerals.

In repeated bouts of intense exercise, diets low in carbohydrate have proved to be incapable of restoring tissue glycogen levels.[8] A low-carbohydrate diet decreases capacity for work, which intensifies over time. Conversely, a high-carbohydrate diet restores glycogen concentrations to their regular levels. Numerous studies have shown poor exercise performance on low-carbohydrate diets. Athletes especially experience fatigue, **ketoacidosis** (from excess **ketones**), dehydration, and hypoglycemia.[9-11] Sometimes athletes use a classic "glycogen-loading" regimen, as shown in Table 14-1, to build up glycogen reserves for endurance events, but this diet manipulation carries potential side effects and should not be used too often and certainly not without professional supervision. A more modern, less taxing approach,

Ketoacidosis
Abnormally high concentration of ketone bodies (ketones) in body tissues and fluids; a complication of low-carbohydrate diets, diabetes mellitus, and starvation.

Ketone
Intermediate fat metabolite; large class of organic compounds that contain the carbonyl group $C=O$, where the carbon atom is joined to two other carbon atoms.

Table 14-1

Stages of a Glycogen-Loading Program (2500 to 4000 kcal) Before an Endurance Athletic Event

Stage	Time period	Exercise	Diet	Nutrient ration (% total kcal)
Stage 1: muscle glycogen depletion	4-7 days before event	Exhausting exercise of same type in event first half of period; general training during diet change in second half of period	Second half: high protein, high fat, low carbohydrate	6% carbohydrate 54% protein 40% fat
Stage 2: muscle glycogen supersaturation	1-3 days before event	None	High carbohydrate, low fat, normal protein	80% carbohydrate 15% protein 5% fat
Stage 3: muscle glycogen use	Day of event	Endurance athletic event	Regular	50% carbohydrate 20% protein 30% fat

Adapted from Forgac MT: Carbohydrate loading—a review, J Am Diet Assoc 75(1)42, 1979.

Table 14-2

Modified Depletion-Taper
Precompetition Program
for Glycogen Loading

Day	Exercise	Diet
1	90-minute period at 70%-75% VO_2 max	Mixed diet 50% carbohydrate (350 g)
2-3	Gradual tapering of time and intensity	Diet above continued
4-5	Tapering of exercise time and intensity continues	Mixed diet 70% carbohydrate (550 g)
6	Complete rest	Diet above continued
7	Day of completion	High-carbohydrate pre-event diet

Adapted from Wright ED: Carbohydrate nutrition and exercise, Clin Nutr 7(1):18, 1988.

which consists of a depletion-tapering sequence,[8] as shown in Table 14-2, is in current use (see the box on p. 327).

Vitamins and Minerals
Vitamins and Minerals as Fuel Substrate

Vitamins and minerals cannot be used as fuel substrates. They are not oxidized or used up in the process of energy production. They are essential in the energy production process but only as catalytic cofactors in enzyme reactions.

Vitamins and Minerals in the Diet

Increased exercise levels are not correlated with increased dietary needs for vitamins or minerals, with the possible exception of riboflavin for very active women,[12] and of pyridoxine for active men.[13] A well-balanced diet will supply adequate amounts of vitamins and minerals, and exercise may well improve the body's efficient use of them. Because athletes, for example, have a dietary need for energy, their larger caloric intake from good food sources would automatically increase their general intake of vitamins and minerals. Studies indicate that multivitamin and mineral supplementation does not improve physical performance in healthy athletes eating a well-balanced diet.[14,15] And certainly the potential side effects from megavitamin supplements are well known (see Chapter 7). However, *therapeutic* iron supplements may be necessary for some athletes who have "sports anemia" (see the box on p. 329).

Exercise and Energy
Kilocalories

Physically active persons, especially athletes, need more fuel. Exercise raises the body's caloric need. Also, exercise has the benefit of helping to regulate appetite to meet these needs. At mild to moderate levels of exercise, persons have actually been shown to eat less than inactive persons do. This may relate to an internal "set point" regulating the amount of body fat the person will carry. According to this theory (see Chapter 15), the set point is raised—that is, more body fat is stored—when the individual becomes inactive. In any case, when exercise levels rise above mild or moderate amounts to strenuous levels, caloric needs also rise to supply needed fuel.

Carbohydrate Loading for Endurance

The marathon is the classic endurance sport. In this event the competitors run 42 km (26 mi)—if they can. To do this, they must have (1) sufficient glycogen stores to meet their needs throughout the race and (2) aerobic capacity large enough to enable them to "spare" glycogen by burning fatty acids at a high rate.

When the marathoner runs out of glycogen, exercise cannot continue. This is a classic phenomenon commonly known as "hitting the wall."

The effect of diet on glycogen stores has been known for a long time. In the mid-1960s Bergstrom and Hulman explored this relationship by subjecting their athletes to exhaustive exercise, feeding them for 3 days on a low-carbohydrate diet with continued exercise, feeding them for the next 3 days on a high-carbohydrate diet with little exercise, and then having them perform the exercise again. Needle biopsies documented the increase in muscle glycogen stores under this peculiar regimen. The athletes' subsequent performance was nearly twice the prior work load.

This became known as "carbohydrate loading," or glycogen supersaturation. The initial exhaustive exercise and 3 days of low-carbohydrate diet ensures a depletion of glycogen stores. In the absence of exercise but the presence of a high-carbohydrate diet the body is able to pack away more glycogen than it stored before depletion. However, there are dangers in this process, and if done too frequently, it takes a large toll. The phase of glycogen depletion through a low-carbohydrate diet is physically and psychologically taxing. The individual is nauseous, weak, irritable, and depressed. Exhaustive exercise at this point may be counterproductive to preparation for the event.

Some persons recommend a modified regimen that eliminates the depletion phase. By simply reducing the level of exercise to minimal, and eating a high-carbohydrate diet for 2 to 3 days before competition, the athlete's glycogen stores may be increased to levels comparable to the classic method of "loading" (see Table 14-2).

Each gram of glycogen is stored with 3 g of water. Glycogen loading thus leads to an increase in weight and sometimes to a sensation of muscle stiffness. However, added water is important in the prevention of dehydration during a long-distance effort.

Glycogen-loading will benefit performance only if the exercise is of extended duration, in excess of 1.5 to 2.0 hours. The procedure is specifically designated for endurance sports. The classic approach does carry dangers, and to prevent possible trauma to muscle tissues, most experts recommend that this more strenuous procedure not be practiced more than 2 or three times a year. However, the newer, more modified depletion-taper approach (Table 14-2) does not carry these dangers and may be used more often. And, in the long run, it is more productive.

REFERENCES
Katch FI and McArdle WD: Nutrition, weight control, and exercise, Philadelphia, 1986, Lea & Febiger.
Mirkin G and Shangold M: Sports medicine, JAMA 254:2340, 1985.
Wright ED: Carbohydrate nutrition and exercise, Clin Nutr 7(1):18, 1988.
Yoshida T: Effect of dietary modification on aerobic threshold, Sports Med 3(1):4, 1986.

Nutrition and Athletic Performance

Nutrient Fuels

Even for the athlete, the need for protein or fat is not significantly greater than for a nonactive person. Carbohydrate is the preferred fuel and critical foodstuff for the active person. These carbohydrates should mainly be complex in form, at an intake that will not only meet increased energy needs but also supply added vitamins and minerals. The following ratio is the approximate dietary composition recommended for support of physical activity:

Protein: 10% to 15% of total kilocalories (1.0 to 1.5 g/kg)

Fat: 30% of total kilocalories

Carbohydrate: 55% to 60% of total kilocalories (or remainder of kilocalories to meet energy needs)

Athletes and Coaches: A Vulnerable Group

Misinformation

Athletes and their coaches are particularly susceptible to myths and magic claims about foods and dietary supplements. They search relentlessly for the competitive edge (see Issues and Answers on p. 338). Knowing this, marketers unremittingly exploit this search, making this group particularly vulnerable. Manufacturers sometimes make distorted and false claims for products. For example, pangamic acid, trade-named "vitamin B_{15}" but not a vitamin at all, has carried claims about its ability to enhance oxygen transport during exercise. Naturally, if there were such a compound, it would be of interest to athletes and their trainers. However, scientific research has exposed these claims as unfounded.

Myths

In addition to specific fraud, the world of athletics is beset with superstitions and misconceptions. Some of these myths include the following:
- Athletes need protein for extra energy.
- Extra protein is needed to build bigger and stronger muscles.
- Muscle tissue is broken down during exercise, and protein supplements are needed to replace this breakdown.
- Vitamin supplements are needed to enable athletes to use more energy.
- Vitamins and minerals are burned up in workouts and training sessions.
- Electrolyte solutions are needed during exercise to replace sweat losses.
- A pregame meal of steak and eggs ensures maximal performance.
- Sugar is needed before and during performance to enhance energy levels.
- Drinking water during exercise will cause cramps.

Pregame Meal

Traditionally, steak and eggs have been the ritual foods for the precompetition meal. However, if such a meal is eaten less than 6 hours before the athletic event, it will still be in the stomach during the event. Protein and fat delay the emptying of the stomach and neither contributes to the glycogen stores needed during exercise (see the box on p. 327). On the contrary, the ideal pregame meal is a light, low-fat, low-protein meal high in complex carbohydrate (starches), eaten 3 to 4 hours before competition. This allows the body time to digest, absorb, and transform it into stored glycogen.

Clinical Application

Some athletes have periods of anemia with endurance exercise. Reduced hemoglobin in a runner's blood means reduced oxygen-carrying capacity, with obvious implications for aerobic capacity and ability to sustain an exercise workload.

The definition of anemia has been set at a hemoglobin (Hgb) value of less than 12 g% for women (normal 14) and less than 14 g% for men (normal 16). We know very little, however, about the relative influence on athletic performance of Hgb levels *within* the normal range. Some suggest that athletes' Hgb levels should be higher for optimal performance, although excessive concentrations of Hgb lead to increased blood viscosity and a decreased rate of flow. Maintenance of Hgb levels at least at the normal levels for women and men have been proposed.

Although frank anemia is rare among competitive athletes, low normal values are typical. Heavy exercise may induce transient anemia during the initial weeks of training, with Hgb stabilizing in the long run at the low end of normal. But strenuous continued exercise is also associated with low iron stores in athletes, which could pose long-term problems.

Possible causes of so-called sports anemia include (1) a diet inadequate in iron, (2) decreased iron absorption, and (3) increased iron losses. Few studies have revealed a diet low in iron; decreased absorption and increased loss are more probable causes. Women athletes have cyclic menstrual loss of iron, unless they have amenorrhea. Also, recent studies have shown significant amounts of iron lost in profuse sweating. Another possibility is occasional *intravascular hemolysis,* the rupture of red blood cells (RBC) as a result of the stresses of heavy exercise. This effect could be transient or chronic. It is manifested as free Hgb in the urine but is not reported often.

Another factor in athletes' low-normal Hgb levels may be *hemodilution.* Strenuous training leads to an increase in both plasma volume and absolute quantity of Hgb, but the increases may not be proportional—plasma volume increases more than Hgb. Hemodilution with increased iron loss and increased red blood cell turnover could account for the prevalence of low-normal values among athletes. Obviously, this situation is complicated if the diet is inadequate in bioavailable iron.

Sports Anemia

REFERENCES

Brotherhood JR: Nutrition and sports performance, Sports Med 1:350, 1984.
Clement DB and Sawchuk LL: Iron status and sports performance, Sports Med 1:65, 1984.
McDonald R and Keen CL: Iron, zinc, and magnesium nutrition and athletic perfomance, Sports Med 5(3):171, 1988.
Wardrop CAJ: Runners' anemia: a paper tiger, Br Med J 295:455, 1987.

Hydration: Water and Electrolytes

Water

Dehydration can be a serious problem for athletes. Its extent depends on the intensity and duration of the exercise, the surrounding temperature, the

Fluid replacement equivalent:
1 lb (2.2 kg) fluid weight = 500 ml.

level of fitness, and the preexercise or pregame state of hydration.[16,17] It is most severe in endurance events. For example, marathon runners sometimes collapse from dehydration. They may also have other problems such as cramps, delirium, vomiting, hypothermia, or hyperthermia—all caused by dehydration. With careful planning ahead of the event and providing fluid replacement along the way, many of these problems can be prevented.[18]

Cause. About 60% of the energy from the breakdown of glucose is released as heat. In minimal physical exercise this heat production maintains desirable body temperature. But during heavier exercise it exceeds the body's needs and sometimes its heat tolerance. Sweating is our main mechanism for dissipating body heat. The major source of fluid lost in sweat is plasma fluid. Endurance events can cause the loss of several liters of water as sweat, which is pulled from the plasma fluid to control body heat. Unless this amount is replaced, serious consequences can follow.

Prevention. The thirst mechanism fails to keep pace with the body's increased need for fluid during exercise. The dehydrated person, therefore, must push fluids. To prevent dehydration, athletes are advised to drink more water than they think is needed, without dependence on the normal thirst mechanism. Cold water, about the temperature inside a refrigerator, is absorbed more quickly from the stomach, so is the best "sports drink." It is important to speed rehydration and to minimize the discomfort that a full stomach can give the athlete. Small cups of cold water should be drunk every 15 minutes during athletic events of long duration. Until quite recently it was thought that drinking water immediately before or during an athletic event would cause cramps. This claim has no basis.

Electrolytes

Ergogenic
The tendency to increase work output.

There is much ado and money being made on electrolytes and special "sports drinks" (see the box on p. 331). The marketing of **ergogenic** aids claims that the electrolytes lost in sweat must be replaced. This is true, but how? Sweat is more dilute than our internal fluids, and thus we lose proportionately, not just absolutely, much more water than anything else. Adding electrolytes and sugar to water simply delays its emptying from the stomach.[19] Water is the rehydration of choice. Electrolytes will be replaced with the athlete's next meal.

Building a Personal Exercise Program

Health Benefits

In various other chapters we discuss physical activity in relation to different health problems. These chapters can be referred to for questions about particular conditions. Here we summarize health benefits of aerobic exercise for some of these conditions.

Coronary Heart Disease

Cardiac output
The volume of blood propelled from the heart with each contraction; also called *stroke volume.*

Aerobic exercise increases heart size and strength, improving its stroke volume and resulting blood circulation.[3] An increased **stroke volume** means that the heart puts out more blood with each beat so it needs to pump fewer times per minute to circulate the same amount of blood. This represents a long-term reduction in the heart's workload. This improved pulmonary and body circulation enhances the oxygen-carrying capacity of the blood and sus-

To Probe Further

Sort Out the Sports Drink Saga

A bevy of so-called sports drinks have been developed from the belief of some sports enthusiasts that water alone does not meet hydration needs during exercise. These beverages have now spawned a multimillion dollar industry. Their claims abound and sorting them out is not always easy for athletes and their coaches who forever seek that prize of the "competitive edge."

The current saga of the sports drinks began with a solution called Gatorade, a beverage its developers named for their university's football team. They reasoned that if they analyzed the sweat of their players they could replace the lost minerals and water, then add some flavoring, coloring, and sugars to make it acceptable, and it would do a better job than plain water. Although it has been highly profitable for the university and for the manufacturer, most athletes simply do not need it. Subsequent studies have shown that physically fit athletes engaged in regular nonendurance exercise do as well on plain water as on a solution such as this product, and they obtain their minerals from their regular diets.

However, what long-term endurance athletes do need, especially in hot weather, is water and fuel—carbohydrate. So much water is lost by a runner in a long distance marathon, for example, when the body sweats 2% to 6% of its weight, that it cannot keep cool enough and the overall system overheats, leading to heatstroke and collapse. Also, without adequate carbohydrate replacement, the muscles soon run out of glycogen stores and slow down. But simply adding sugar to water causes the water to be held in the stomach longer, where it does the body tissues no good for immediate needs. To meet this dual need for such marathon events, a second category of sports drinks using glucose polymers instead of so much sugar has been developed. These short chains of about five glucose molecules—maltodextrins—are produced in the breakdown of starch. They are not sweet and they leave the stomach rapidly, thus making them ideal as a continuing fuel source for the endurance athlete. Two such products in this category, marketed in powdered mix form, are Ross Laboratories' Exceed and Coca-Cola's Max. But don't look for them in supermarkets. They are provided mainly through pharmacies to professionals working with serious athletes.

Other sports drinks to enter the market have been Gatorade clones such as the product Recharge, which claims to add no sugar yet supplies an ample amount of it as fructose and glucose in its fruit juice base. And still another category has emerged in products such as Gear Up, which adds to its base of ten fruit juices ten vitamins in amounts yielding 137% of the RDA in a single 10-oz bottle, and contains no minerals. All of these extra vitamins won't help your performance at all, and on a hot day a sweating athlete could easily down a megadose in four or five bottles.

So sort out the claims of sports drinks. They are not for everyone. In the long run, special ones meet needs of the athlete in endurance events. But for nonendurance activities most persons don't need them. After all, water is the best solution for regular needs—and it costs far less. *Continued.*

To Probe Further

Sort Out the Sports Drink Saga—cont'd

REFERENCES

Flynn MG and others: Influence of selected carbohydrate drinks on cycling peformance and glycogen use.

Liebman BF: Sports drinks slug it out, Nutr Action Health Letter 13(7):10, 1986.

Murray R: The effects of consuming carbohydrate-electrolyte beverages on gastric emptying and fluid absorption during and following exercise, Sports Med 4:322, 1987.

Sports drinks, Am Family Physician 34:261, Nov 1986.

Wheeler KB and Banwell JG: Intestinal water and electrolyte flux of glucose-polymer electrolyte solutions, Med Sci Sports Exerc 18(4):436, 1986.

Wright ED: Fluid and electrolyte requirements during exercise, Clin Nutr 7(1):33, 1988.

tains the overall blood volume. Exercise also raises blood levels of high-density lipoproteins (HDL), creating a more favorable ratio of HDL to low-density lipoproteins (LDL), which carry cholesterol loads to cells.[20-23]

Diabetes Management

Exercise helps control diabetes by enhancing the action of insulin through an increased number of insulin receptor sites and by stimulating insulin-balancing hormones such as glucogon.[9,24] This effect is particularly useful in the management of non-insulin-dependent diabetes mellitus (NIDDM) in obese adults. However, in the management of insulin-dependent diabetes mellitus (IDDM) the nature and scheduling of physical activity must be balanced with food and insulin to prevent hypoglycemic reactions. But such management can be done and is a healthful tool of self-care.

Weight Management

Exercise is extremely beneficial in weight management because it helps to regulate appetite, increases the basal metabolic rate, and reduces the fat deposit "set point" level. Together with a well-planned diet, physical exercise corrects the energy balance in favor of increased energy output and decreased energy intake.[25]

Bone Disease

Exercise helps increase bone mineralization, thus reducing the risk of bone weakness and of potential osteoporosis.[26,27]

Mental Health

Exercise stimulates the production of brain opiates, associated with a decreased susceptibility to pain. These substances contribute to an improved mood, including a sense of exhiliration or kind of "high."

Assessment of Personal Health and Exercise Needs

There are many kinds of exercise. Choosing those kinds that are best depends on individual health and personal needs, the aerobic benefits involved, and personal enjoyment.

Health and Personal Needs

In planning an exercise program, it is important to assess individual health status, personal needs, present level of fitness, and resources required. What do you want to gain from your exercise? How much time can you commit to it? How much, if anything, does it cost? Perhaps it is even more important to ask yourself what you like to do. If the exercise you choose isn't fun, you will soon stop doing it, and it will benefit no one. Also, it is wise to start slowly and build gradually rather than risk injury and discouragement. Moderation and regularity are key guides in planning.

Beneficial Level of Exercise

To build aerobic capacity, the level of exercise must raise the pulse rate to within 70% of maximum heart rate. Unless you have had an exercise tolerance or stress test and know precisely what your maximum exercising heart rate is, a rule of thumb is to determine your **cardiac rate** by subtracting your age from 220 (Table 14-3). This calculation estimates your maximum heart rate, and 70% of this figure tells you the rate to which you want to raise your pulse in the course of exercise. This rate should then be maintained for an uninterrupted period of at least 20 minutes and be practiced at least 3 times a week to have aerobic benefits.[3] Check your resting pulse before starting the exercise period, then again during and immediately afterward to monitor your progress in developing your maximum exercising heart rate and aerobic capacity.

Cardiac rate
Number of heart beats per minute; pulse rate

Types of Physical Activity
General Exercise

There are many exercises from which you may choose. Many of them are enjoyable and healthful but do not reach aerobic levels. For example, golf is a passion for many, but it is far too slow and sporatic to be aerobic. Also, most sports in the hands of amateurs, rather than those with fast-paced extraordinary skill to provide sustained exercise, are too slow-paced to be aerobic. These include tennis, football, baseball, and basketball. Weight-lifting develops and strengthens muscles but is not an aerobic exercise.

Age	Maximal attainable heart rate (pulse: 220 minus age)	Target zone	
		70% Maximal rate	85% Maximal rate
20	200	140	170
25	195	136	166
30	190	133	161
35	185	129	157
40	180	126	153
45	175	122	149
50	170	119	144
55	165	115	140
60	160	112	136
65	155	108	132
70	150	105	127
75	145	101	124

Table 14-3

Target Zone Heart Rate According to Age to Achieve Aerobic Physical Effect of Exercise

Aerobic Exercise

Forms of exercise that can be sustained at a necessary level of intensity to provide aerobic benefits include such activities as swimming, running, jogging, bicycling, and the recently popular aerobic dancing routines and workouts (Table 14-4). Perhaps the simplest and most popular form of stimulating exercise is *walking*. If the pace is fast enough to elevate your pulse and it is maintained for the required 20 minutes at least, walking can be an excellent form of aerobic exercise. It is convenient and requires no equipment other than good walking shoes. It is also emotionally satisfying to many persons for whom running, swimming, cycling, and dancing may not be most appropriate.

Preparation for Exercise

Once a sport or exercise has been chosen, adequate preparation is essential. Safety precautions must be observed. Runners and joggers need quality, appropriate shoes; cyclists need good helmets. Before exercising, stretch the muscles to prevent stress and injury. Similarly take time after completing the exercise to cool down. Many exercise-related injuries, such as pulled muscles and stress fractures, are related to inadequate preparation. It is also possible to exercise beyond the limits of tolerance. Incidences of injuries in running, for example, start rising dramatically at the 25-miles-per-week marker. Some studies have compared the personality profiles of compulsive runners with those of anorexic persons (see Issues and Answers on p. 338). Certainly a level of compulsion that comes to dominate one's life is *unhealthy*. In short, listen to your own body. When you are tired, rest. When you hurt, stop. When the level of exercise is no longer a challenge and you want to increase it somewhat, do so—but only then.

Table 14-4

Aerobic Exercises for Physical Fitness (maintained at aerobic level for at least 30 minutes)

Type of exercise	Aerobic forms
Ballplaying	Handball
	Raquetball
	Squash
Bicycling	Stationary
	Touring
Dancing	Aerobic routines
	Ballet
	Disco
Jumping rope	Brisk pace
Running/jogging	Brisk pace
Skating	Ice skating
	Roller skating
Skiing	Cross country
Swimming	Steady pace
Walking	Brisk pace

The energy "currency" of the body is ATP. The cell's storehouse of energy is creatine phosphate (CP). These two high-energy phosphate compounds are in limited supply. They can provide energy for only a brief initial period and need to be replenished for exercise to continue. This added supply is made available by **anaerobic** glycolysis, with added energy made available for continued exercise by the body's aerobic system of energy production. The process of **glycolysis** metabolizes only carbohydrate substrate, furnished either by blood glucose or stored glycogen. Dietary carbohydrate is necessary to replenish these fuel sources. Protein contributes little to total energy production for exercise, whereas the body's ability to burn fat as fuel depends on the level of fitness. The higher the body's efficiency in using oxygen, the more fatty acids will contribute to the energy supply. Even in the best-trained athletes, fatty acid oxidation must be accompanied by glucose metabolism.

The protein needs of the diet are not increased by exercise, contrary to popular belief, and neither is the body's need for vitamins and minerals. Exercise does increase the body's need for kilocalories and water. Cold water taken in small, frequent amounts is the best way to prevent dehydration in endurance events. Electrolytes lost in sweat are replaced by a continuing diet of adequate quality and quantity. Adding electrolytes or sugar to water delays its emptying from the stomach and thus delays rehydration.

The optimal diet for the active person is 10% to 15% of the kilocalories from protein, 25% to 30% from fat, and 55% to 60% from carbohydrate. The pregame meal for athletes should be small, requiring little or no protein or fat and relying mainly on complex carbohydrate (starches).

The health benefits of general and aerobic exercise are many and increase with practice. A minimal level of aerobic exercise need for cardiovascular health is achieved by elevating the heart rate to 70% of maximum for a sustained period of at least 20 minutes at least 3 times a week. Excellent aerobic exercises include sustained fast walking, swimming, jogging, running, and aerobic dancing or workouts. Approach any exercise sensibly and choose those activities that are enjoyable.

To Sum Up

Anaerobic
Not requiring oxygen to function.

Glycolysis
Anaerobic enzymatic conversion of glucose to simpler compounds of lactate or pyruvate; results in stored energy in the form of ATP in muscles; differs from respiration in that organic substances, rather than oxygen, are used as electron receptors.

Questions for Review

1. What are the component muscle structures and how do they produce muscle action?
2. What type of substrate fuel does the body use for immediate energy needs? Short-term needs? Long-term needs?
3. Outline the nutrition and physical fitness principles you would discuss with a client who is an athlete. Plan a diet for this client that would meet nutrient and energy needs. How would you advise the athlete about "glycogen-loading" practices?
4. Why is fluid balance vital during exercise periods? How is water and electrolyte balance best achieved?
5. How would you conduct a counseling session for a patient with coronary heart disease about the role of exercise in cardiovascular health? With an overweight client with non-insulin-dependent diabetes mellitus (NIDDM)?

References

1. Wright ED and Paige DM: Physical exercise and energy requirements, Clin Nutr 7(1):9, 1988.
2. Astrand P-O and Rodahl K: Textbook of work physiology: physiological bases of exercise, New York, 1986, McGraw-Hill Book Co.
3. Katch FI and McArdle WD: Nutrition, weight control, and exercise, Philadelphia, 1986, Lea & Febiger.
4. Dohm CL and others: Protein metabolism during endurance exercise, Fed Proc 44:348, 1985.
5. Mc Ardle WD, Katch FI, and Katch VL: Exercise physiology: energy, nutrition, and human performance, Philadelphia, 1986, Lea & Febiger.
6. Arky RA and Perlman AJ: Hyperlipoproteinemia. In Rubinstein E and Federman DD, editors: Medicine, New York, 1986, Scientific American.
7. Wright ED and Paige DM: Lipid metabolism and exercise, Clin Nutr 7(1):28, 1988.
8. Costill DL: Carbohydrate before, during, and after exercise, Fed Proc 44:364, 1985.
9. Wright ED: Carbohydrate nutrition and exercise, Clin Nutr 7(1):18, 1988.
10. Coyle EF and Coggan AR: Effectiveness of carbohydrate feeding in delaying fatigue during prolonged exercise, Sports Med 1(6):446, 1984.
11. Kreider RB and Thompson WR: Ketone bodies and ketosis in exercise, Ann Sports Med 2(4):170, 1986.
12. Belko AZ and others: Effects of exercise on riboflavin requirements of young women, Am J Clin Nutr 37:509, 1983.
13. Dreon DM and Butterfield GE: Vitamin B_6 utilization in active and inactive young men, Am J Clin Nutr 43:816, 1986.
14. Weight LM, Myburgh KH, and Noakes TD: Vitamin and mineral supplementation: effect on the running performance of trained athletes, Am J Clin Nutr 47:192, 1988.
15. Van der Beek EJ: Vitamins and endurance training: food for running or faddish claims, Sports Med 2(3):175, 1985.
16. Wright ED: Fluid and electrolyte requirements during exercise, Clin Nutr 7(1):33, 1988.
17. Brotherhood JR: Nutrition and sports performance, Sports Med 1(5):350, 1984.
18. Moore M: Boston Marathon medical coverage: the road racer's safety net, Physician Sports Med 11(6):168, 1983.
19. Murray R: The effects of consuming carbohydrate-electrolyte beverages on gastric emptying and fluid absorption during and following exercise, Sports Med 4(5):322, 1987.
20. Haskell WL: Exercise-induced changes in plasma lipids and lipoproteins, Prev Med 13:23, 1984.
21. Hartung GH: Diet and exercise in the regulation of plasma lipids and lipoproteins in patients at risk of coronary disease, Sports Med 1(6):413, 1984.
22. Cook TC and others: Chronic low level physical activity as a determinant of high density lipoprotein cholesterol and subfractions, Med Sci Sports Exer 18(6):653, 1986.
23. Goldberg L and Elliot DL: The effect of exercise on lipid metabolism in men and women, Sports Med 4(5):307, 1987.
24. Holloway JF, Lewis SB, and Dohrmann ML: The role of exercise in the retardation of glucose intolerance and coronary risk factors in diabetics, Med Sci Sports Exer 15(2):91, 1983.
25. Pacy PJ, Webster J, and Garrow JS: Exercise and obesity, Sports Med 3(2):89, 1986.
26. Krolner B and others: Physical exercise as prophylaxis against involutional vertebral bone loss: a controlled trial, Clin Sci 64:541, 1983.
27. Allen LH: Calcium and age-related bone loss, Clin Nutr 5(4):147, 1986.

Grandjean AC: Nutrition for strength training, Sports Med Dig 10(3):1, 1988.

Coleman E: Nutritional supplements and weight training, Sports Med Dig 10(3):6, 1988.

Professional football players tackle lighter diets in training camp, J Am Diet Assoc 86(11):1528, 1986.

This collection of brief reports provides a sampling of sound directions for athletes and coaches, as well as their nutrition counselors. The first publication cited, *Sports Medicine Digest,* focuses on athletics and sports of all kinds with a wide variety of good reference material in each issue.

Grandjean AC: The vegetarian athlete, Physician Sports Med 15(5):191, 1987.

This nutritionist, chief nutrition consultant for the U.S. Olympic Committee, answers key questions about vegetarianism and athletics and indicates that vegetarians can be successful athletes, but only with a well-planned diet, which is true for any aspiring athlete.

Kris-Etherton PM: Nutrition and the exercising female, Nutr Today 21(2):6, 1986.

Manore MM and Leklem JE: Effect of carbohydrate and vitamin B_6 on fuel substrates during exercise in women, Med Sci Sports Exer 20(3):233, 1988.

Ouellette MG, MacVicar MG, and Harlan J: Relationship between percent body fat and menstrual patterns in athletes and nonathletes, Nurs Res 35:330, Nov/Dec 1986.

Risser WL and others: Iron deficiency in female athletes: its prevalence and impact on performance, Med Sci Sports Exer 20(2):116, 1988.

This group of articles provides background for exercising girls and women, whether they exercise for recreation or for competition, about special nutritional and energy needs, which vary throughout the life cycle.

Monmaney T and Robins K: The insanity of steroid abuse, Newsweek, p 75, May 23, 1988.

Yarrows SA: Weight loss through dehydration in amateur wrestling, J Am Diet Assoc 88(4):491, 1988.

These two reports focus sharply on two dangerous practices of body-builders and wrestlers—taking steroid hormones to gain weight and beef up muscles but becoming psychotic in the process, and inducing dehydration to lose weight and meet competition limits but becoming ill in the process.

Further Readings

The Winning Edge—or Over the Edge?

Athletes, their coaches, and indeed our entire culture have become increasingly aware that the percentage of body fat vs the percentage of lean body mass can be a major influence on athletic performance. Each extra pound of body fat an athlete carries into competition is extra, nonproductive weight. Muscles, the lean body mass, provide the strength, agility, and endurance required to win.

Athletes, therefore, strive to achieve as low a percentage of body fat as possible while still maintaining good health. In reaching for such a goal, however, many young athletes develop an abhorrence of body fat, resulting in food aversion and the undertaking of excessive weight loss regimens. These self-generated excesses are commonly reinforced by people surrounding the young athletes: coaches, teammates, and perhaps most demanding of all— parents. A fear of failure—failure to make the team, failure in competition, failure to live up to others' expectations—pushes the young person in his/her campaign to best this "opponent"—the level of body fat— and to win this particular contest by a large, decisive amount. Such an all-consuming focus can result in compulsive behavior that leads the young person to set unrealistic goals resulting in abusive weight loss. Fortunately, the reasons prompting such excessive voluntary weight loss in these young athletes are not the result of chronic emotional problems. Instead, they are superficial, resulting from an accumulation of immediate, short-term goals and concerns. These athletes usually respond to counseling in an excellent manner, reversing the excessive behavior, particularly with the support of concerned friends and teammates.

Yet for some individuals, excessive, compulsive fixation on lean body mass and the loss of body fat can become obsessive and enduring. For example, a compulsive runner's ideal of 5% body fat is found only in ballet dancers, gymnasts, models, and victims of anorexia nervosa. Our culture reinforces this "positive" attribute of beauty—slimness in women, physical prowess in men. But when a susceptible individual enters a time of stress or a search for a firm identity, he/she may see our cultural stereotypes as providing this self-concept. For women, this stress is usually encountered in adolescence, when physical attraction becomes important. For men, their sense of self is more closely tied to vocational and sexual effectiveness, both of which can be related to physical abilities. A man's abilities are tested more often in adulthood, resulting in a preoccupation with physical fitness as a way to deny any decline in strength or ability. This may be why the majority of compulsive runners—those who feel they must run despite everything, including injury or ill health—are men.

While our culture views compulsive dieting—anorexia nervosa—as a serious emotional disorder, compulsive training is seen as a positive personality trait showing dedication. In reality, both are symptomatic of an unstable self-concept and attempt to establish a firm sense of identity. They are perceptual disorders: whereas the anorexia victim sees herself as fat, the compulsive runner sees himself as out-of-shape. No goal, once attained, is sufficiently satisfying. If 5% body fat is achieved, 4% is strived for. Ignoring the physical indications against it, such striving has resulted in persons suffering permanent disabilities and even death, sometimes from cardiac arrest caused by linoleic acid deficiency. These driven individuals have a spartan attitude, unable to enjoy any of life's more passive, receptive pleasures.

While physical fitness and athletic accomplishments may be admirable goals, for a small percentage of participants the "thrill of victory" may be a hollow one if the victory is at the expense of their health and peace of mind. The ability to slow down, stop and "smell the roses," and enjoy life may mean more to the quality and quantity of a person's lifespan than the color of a coveted ribbon or medal.

REFERENCES

Evers CL: Dietary intake and symptoms of anorexia nervosa in female university dancers, J Am Diet Assoc 87(1):66, 1987

Herbert W: Runners and anorexics: an ascetic disorder? Sci News 123(7):102, 1983.

Scharf MB and Barr S: Craving carbohydrates: a possible sign of overtraining, Ann Sports Med 4(1):19, 1988.

Yates A, Leehy K, and Shisslak CM: Running—an analogue of anorexia? N Engl J Med 308:251, 1983.

15 Nutrition and Weight Management

Chapter Objectives

After studying this chapter, the student should be able to:

1. Identify social and physiologic costs of America's obsession with weight and thinness.

2. Identify causes of obesity and describe current related social trends.

3. Relate overweight to health.

4. Plan realistic weight management programs for clients based on a positive health model.

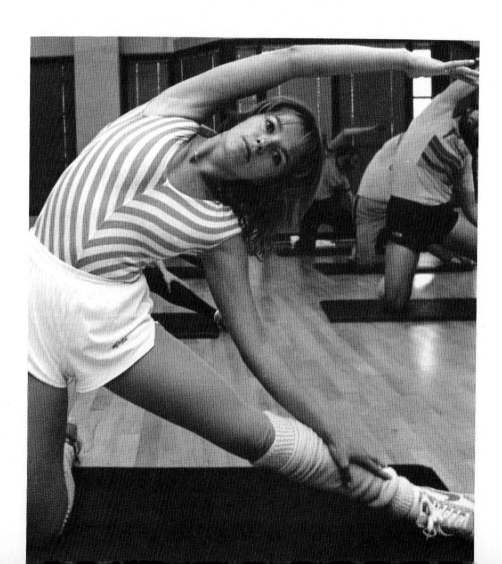

A second risk factor in health maintenance through the life cycle is overweight, or more correctly *overfat*, a source of great concern to many persons. Even as you read these lines, one out of every four Americans is on some kind of a weight-reduction diet. Use of these "diets" is increasing daily, with a bewildering array of them constantly appearing in the public press.

Even in the light of such an obsession with weight loss, however, we as a people are getting heavier. The average American has gained about 2.25 kg (5 lb) since the mid-1960s. A large part of the answer lies in our becoming less and less physically active since our growing technology is producing a sedentary society.

But the sad fact is that all of these reducing "diets" have one thing in common: the weight, once lost, is almost always put back on again. Only about 5% of these "dieters" manage to maintain their weight at the new lower level. Perhaps this result points to the failure of the traditional "medical (or illness) model" of obesity and the need for a more realistic "health model."

In this chapter we will move toward such a positive health model. In essence, we have two basic goals. First, we want to help individuals with weight problems feel better about themselves as persons, whatever their weight, and achieve a greater degree of physical fitness and sense of well-being. And second, we want to help those with related health problems such as diabetes or hypertension achieve positive health benefits through realistic weight control.

Body Weight vs Body Fat

Sometimes the common terms *obesity* and *overweight* are used without the necessary attention to *body composition*. It is helpful to consider first the distinct meanings and concepts embodied in each of these terms.

Obesity

As it is used in the traditional medical model, the word **obesity** is a clinical term for excess body weight, defining it in the sense of a disease. It is generally applied to a person who is 15% to 20% or more above the "ideal" weight. The problem, however, lies in defining the word *ideal*. It usually refers to an average weight according to height and frame. But an "average" person does not exist. Every person is individual, and *normal* values in healthy persons vary over a wide range. Also, until recently, *age* has been overlooked as an important variable in setting a reasonable or ideal body weight for a particular individual.[1] Investigators have indicated that no one best or ideal weight is associated with longevity in adults 25 to 60.[2,3] In terms of minimal mortality associated with coronary heart disease, for example, a desirable body weight is lower in young adults than in middle-aged adults.[4]

Overweight

We often use the term *overweight* as a synonym for obesity. But the two terms are not interchangeable, and the distinction is important. For example, a

Body Composition: Fatness and Leanness

Obesity
Excessive adipose fat tissue, more than is required for optimal body function.

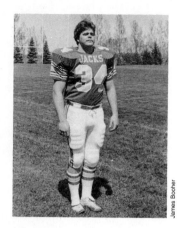

According to standard weight-height charts, a football player would be considered overweight. These charts should be used with discretion.

Body composition
A determination of how much of the body weight is fat and how much is lean body mass.

football player in peak condition can be markedly "overweight," according to standard weight-height charts. That is, he can weigh considerably more than the average man of the same height, but much of his greater weight is not fat at all. In clinical usage, the term *overweight* refers to persons with body weight in excess of the weight-height standard but below the 20% excess designated as obesity. In relation to health, however, the term *overfat* would be a more correct designation because it refers to the percentage of excess body fat in the overall total body composition. As a result of this understanding, experts in the field of nutrition now define *obesity* as "an excess of body *fat* frequently resulting in a significant impairment of health."[5]

Body Composition

What is critical in determining a reasonable body weight, then, is **body composition.**[4] For the most part, this refers to how much of the body weight comes from fat and how much is from *lean body mass* (see Chapter 5 and reread Issues and Answers on p. 145). On the basis of metabolic activity, hence energy (kilocalories) demand, and comparative size, the four components of body composition are as follows:

1. **Lean body mass (LBM).** This major body component of active fat-free cell mass largely determines the basal metabolic rate and energy and nutrient need. It changes through the life cycle and in adulthood accounts for some 30% to 65% of the total body weight. When persons gain or lose weight from diet changes, the loss reflects changes not only in body fat but also in LBM. But added exercise helps maintain or develop the relative LBM size.

2. **Body fat.** Gross body fat varies widely with individual degrees of fatness or leanness. These differences reflect the number and size of fat cells that make up the adipose tissue. In an adult man, for example, fat accounts for a range of 14% to 28% of total body weight. In a woman it is somewhat larger, about 15% to 29% of body weight. These amounts vary with age, climate, exercise, and fitness. About half the body fat is in the subcutaneous fat layers as insulation, thus providing a useful measure, the triceps skinfold, for estimating body fat in relation to LBM (see Chapter 17).

3. **Body water.** The body water content varies with relative leanness-fatness and with age, hydration, and health status. Generally it makes up about 20% of body weight. In fat persons it is about 15% of total body weight; in lean persons, about 25%. This results from the high water content of lean muscle tissue, which contains more water than any other body tissue except blood.

4. **Bone.** The remaining mineral mass, largely in the skeletal structure, accounts for only about 6% of the total body weight. The major mineral component is calcium, as you would expect, which makes up about 2% of the body weight.

Various indirect methods of measuring body composition have been developed. These include such classic means as water displacement (weighing under water) and measuring radioactive body emissions. Newer methods include ultrasonics, light absorption and reflection, electrical conductivity and resistance, radioactive absorption, and related estimates from various measurements of body circumferences and skinfold thicknesses.[6]

Body Mass Index (BMI)

Health professionals generally use the body mass index as a measure of relative body fatness in their evaluation of risk factors associated with obesity.[7,8] The BMI can be calculated easily by this simplified formula:

$$BMI = \frac{\text{weight (kg)}}{\text{height (meters)}^2}$$

The metric conversion factors involved are 1 kg = 2.2 lb; 1 m = 39.37 in. The desired health maintenance BMI range for adults is 20 to 25 kg/m^2. Health risks associated with obesity begin in the range of 25 to 30 kg/m^2. Values above 40 kg/m^2 indicate severe or "morbid" obesity.

Standard Weight-for-Height Measures

Two basic approaches have been used to evaluate body weight—a general guide and standard weight tables.

General Guide

In common usage a general rule of thumb has been passed along to determine proper weight:

1. For men, 106 lb (47.7 kg) for the first 5 ft (150 cm), then add 6 lb/in (2.7 kg/2.5 cm), plus or minus 10 lb (4.5 kg).
2. For women, 100 lb (45 kg) for the first 5 ft, then add 5 lb/in (2.25 kg/2.5 cm), plus or minus 10 lb.

For many persons, however, especially women, unrealistically low figures are produced by this method, and it is seldom used in practice.

Weight-for-height tables

Most of the standard tables are based on the Metropolitan Life Insurance Company's "ideal" weight-for-height charts. These charts have been derived from life expectancy data gathered by the company from their policy holders since the 1930s. These data have problems, however, because they come from a self-selected sample not representative of our general population (see Issues and Answers on p. 361). Also, a number of studies have found that health risks are as great, if not greater, in the very thin, low-weight range as for the extremely obese group. Within each age group, extremely thin and extremely fat persons have higher mortality rates.[9] The message seems to be that persons should strive to be neither excessively overweight nor excessively underweight and that the multitude of health problems attributed to *moderate* amounts of overweight are unfounded.

Ideal Weight

Why is the term *ideal weight* difficult to define? Several factors may help to indicate why this is not a useful concept and why some body fat is essential to health.

Individual Variation

The basic problem with the idea of "ideal" weight, as we have seen, is that it really doesn't exist. A person's ideal body weight depends on many different factors, including age, body shape, metabolic rate, genetic makeup, sex, physical activity, among many others. Persons need varying amounts of weight and can carry different amounts of weight in good health.

Necessity of Body Fat

Some body fat is necessary to survival. This has been demonstrated in times of human starvation. Such victims die of fat loss, not protein depletion. For mere survival men require 3% body fat; women require 12%. Especially for reproductive capacity, women require about 20% body fat. Menstruation, **menarche,** begins when the female body reaches a certain size or, more precisely, when the young girl's body fat reaches this critical proportion of body weight, about 20%, the amount needed for ovulation and thus for any potential pregnancy.

Menarche
Onset of menstruation.

Obesity and Health

Many common beliefs about the relation of obesity and health conflict with data available from scientific studies.

Common Beliefs

Common folk knowledge holds that being fat is "bad for you." Also, traditional medical opinion has contended for many years that obesity is an illness and contributes to a wide number of health problems, including hyperlipidemia, carbohydrate intolerance, surgical risk, anesthesia risk, pulmonary and renal problems, pregnancy complications, diabetes, and hypertension.

Conflicting Data

Often in such broad statements a distinction is not made between moderate overweight states and massive or "morbid" obesity, which poses a different problem entirely. Both extremes of weight variance, fatness and thinness, pose medical problems. But the major issue affecting most Americans is a degree of general overweight in the population that requires closer study. In general, studies show clear health risks in *extreme* obesity, but unless a person is at least 30% *overfat*, the relationship of weight to mortality is questionable.

Specific Health Implications

These data, however, might obscure important health implications of obesity. A recent National Institutes of Health (NIH) consensus development conference of experts identified adverse effects of obesity on health in three main areas[5]:

1. **Hypertension, hypercholesterolemia, and diabetes.** The evidence indicates that in these three chronic conditions of essential hypertension, elevated serum cholesterol, and diabetes mellitus, the association with obesity is strong. This association varies directly with the extent of the obesity and is reversible with weight reduction. BMI values at or above 27.8 for men and 27.3 for women (the 85th percentile level), especially for young adults ages 20 to 44, carried the greatest risk. A genetic factor is present in each of these chronic conditions. So early intervention in developing health habits in diet and exercise, especially for children in high-risk families, is important.

2. **Coronary heart disease (CHD).** Although the evidence was not as

strong, the NIH panel agreed that sufficient long-term data do show a direct association of degree of obesity with CHD, independent of other risk factors.[9] In any event, the primary conditions above are all strong risk factors for CHD, thus linking obesity to CHD.

3. **Cancer.** The NIH found strong associations of some types of cancer with obesity. Obese men, regardless of smoking, had a higher mortality from cancer of the colon, rectum, and prostate. Obese women had higher mortality from cancer of the gallbladder, biliary passages, breast, uterus, and ovaries.

Social Images: Fear of Fatness

Recently, a model of thinness, especially for women, has developed in American society with social blame placed upon fatness.

The Thinness Model

Fueled by capital investment in Madison Avenue advertising, a successful attempt has been made to use an exaggerated image of thinness for marketing many products. The "ideal" woman has been remade in the eyes of America. The gaunt, almost cadaverous models adorning the covers of many glamour magazines seem to mock most women's attempts to feel good about themselves and their bodies. This extreme degree of thinness, however, goes against body wisdom and often contributes to marginal health or reproductive capacity.

The Fatness Blame

Strong prejudice exists in the United States against obese persons, regardless of their age, sex, race, or socioeconomic status.[10] But some people, try as they might, simply cannot and do not lose weight, or they live "yo-yo" lives of perpetual ups and downs of weight—an even greater threat to their physical and emotional health. Overweight persons, especially women, don't conform to these social images and are somehow blamed for their condition. Many people still hold to our popular mythology that fat people are (1) *gluttonous*—they eat more than they should; (2) *lazy*—if they wanted to, they would lose weight; (3) *neurotic*—they have an oral fixation caused by arrested development during childhood; or (4) *unhappy*—they eat because they are depressed. However, studies of comparative behavior have shown no evidence for any of these stereotyped beliefs about overweight persons.[11]

Effects of the Thin-Fat Images

Many Americans *are* unhappy. They can never live up to the thinness ideal. This national obsession has devoured the creative energies of many intelligent persons. Unfortunately, in some extreme cases, this obesssion with thinness has resulted in two serious eating disorders: (1) **anorexia nervosa,** a form of self-induced starvation that has reached alarming proportions among adolescent girls, and (2) **bulimia,** a gorging-purging syndrome that creates both emotional and physical problems. Also, many of the fad weight-loss diets produce nutrient deficiences. When they are practiced apart from a wise exercise program, the energy intake is usually too low—less than 1200 kcal/day for women—to provide enough vitamins and minerals. In general, sufficient iron intake is a problem for American women.

Anorexia nervosa
Extreme psychophysiologic aversion to food, resulting in life-threatening weight loss.

Bulimia
Morbidly increased appetite, often alternating with periods of anorexia or purging.

The Problem of Weight Management

Individual Differences and Extreme Practices

Basis of the Problem

How would a person go about losing excess weight, or more correctly, excess fat? Simple, you say—just reverse the process by which you gained it. When energy intake does not equal energy expended, the difference is reflected in weight gain or loss. And about 3500 kilocalories is the equivalent of 0.45 kg (1 lb) of body fat. Well, that's part of the answer, but it isn't altogether quite that simple. Many individual differences often lead to extreme practices, and genetic, physical, and psychosocial factors are involved.

Energy Balance

A number of real factors influence an individual's point of energy balance. Keeping a weight balance score in purely mathematical terms does not answer the whole question. First, it's difficult to know *precisely* how many kilocalories are in the food you are eating. Second, it's even more difficult to know how many kilocalories you are actually burning up. This depends particularly on your basal metabolic rate (BMR), body size, amount of lean body mass, age, sex, and physical activity, among other things. Third, on a genetic basis, it is true that some persons *do* have more metabolic efficiency. Recent work indicates that some people do "burn" food more easily than others (see Chapter 5, Issues and Answers, p. 145).

Extreme Practices

Individual differences in energy needs, combined with social pressures, lead many obese individuals to use various extreme approaches to weight loss, many of which often create problems.

Fad diets. A constant array of various diet books floods the American market. They usually sell briefly and then fade away, largely because their "quick fix" does not work. Nutritional science finds itself caught in the "diet wars" because there are no magic, simple answers to a complex problem.[12] Most of the fad diets fail on two counts: (1) they are based on scientific inaccuracies and misinformation and hence are often nutritionally inadequate, and (2) they do not address the basic behavioral problem involved in life-long food and exercise habit change, actually a new lifestyle, required to maintain a healthy weight for a given individual once it is achieved.[13,14] For some persons the degree of caloric restriction required places impossible demands and they find themselves caught in the "yo-yo dieting" trap, with weight going up and down—again and again and again and weight loss more and more difficult each time—the physiologic effects of which we still do not fully know.[15,16]

Fasting. This drastic approach takes many forms, from literal fasting to use of very-low-calorie diets of special formulas. Effects may be those of semi-starvation: acidosis, postural hypotension, increase in urinary loss of important electrolytes, increase in serum uric acid, constipation, and a decrease in **basal metabolic rate (BMR).** In past use of such extreme practices there has been sufficient loss of heart muscle to cause death.[17] And, at best, more recent programs have failed in the critical period after initial weight loss to help persons maintain the new weight when refeeding began.[18]

Basal metabolic rate (BMR) Rate of internal chemical activity in resting tissue.

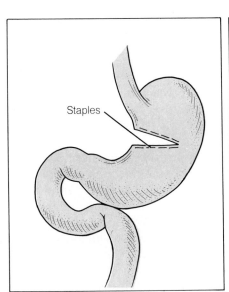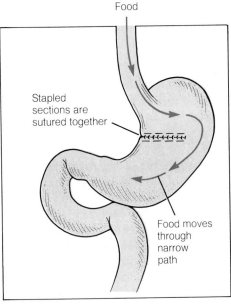

Food

Staples

Stapled
sections are
sutured together

Food moves
through
narrow
path

Figure 15-1
Gastroplasty is a type of restrictive gastric surgical procedure used for treatment of severe obesity.

Special clothing and body wraps. Special "sauna suits" are claimed to help weight loss in specific spots of the body or to help clear up so-called cellulite tissue. To the scientific community "spot reduction" is a fabrication, as is *cellulite*, a word coined some years ago in Europe by a beauty operator and has no factual basis. This mummy-like wrapping is endured by some persons in an attempt to reduce body size. What small weight loss may result is usually caused by temporary water loss. The only way to lose weight is to burn up more kilocalories than are consumed.

Drugs. Amphetamines, commonly called "speed," were once popular in the treatment of obesity. However, they are no longer used because of their danger to health. Common over-the-counter drugs in use today as "appetite depressants" to aid weight loss contain the drug *phenylpropanolamine (PPA)*, a stimulant similar to amphetamine. PPA has been linked to increased blood pressure and damage to the blood vessels in the brain, leading to central nervous system disorders such as confusion, hallucination, stroke, and psychotic behavior.[19]

Surgery. Surgical intervention is usually reserved for medical treatment of severely obese persons after more traditional methods have failed. This extreme approach has included such procedures as wiring the jaws shut, suctioning fat from lipid tissues, and even intestinal bypass, which resulted in serious side effects and is no longer used. Current procedures focus on gastric bypass, including forms of gastroplasty and gastric stapling (Figure 15-1). But these surgeries are not without problems and require skilled nutritional management.[20-22] A recently introduced, less involved procedure is the use of the "gastric bubble." In this method a soft polyurethane sac is inserted into the stomach through a tube, then inflated, and the tube removed. The free-floating "bubble," about the shape and size of a small juice can, remains to give a feeling of fullness and reduce food intake. It is not a permanent fixture and must be removed after 4 months, but another unit can be placed if still needed.

Causes of Obesity

Theories about the cause of obesity vary. From studies in this area, four types of factors have been identified: genetic, psychologic, social, and physiologic.

Genetic Factors

Evidence is increasing that genetic inheritance probably influences a person's chances of becoming fat more than any other basic factor. A genetic base regulates differences in body fat and sex differences in weight. Within families, if one parent is obese, a child has a 40% chance of becoming obese. This chance becomes 80% if both parents are obese and only 7% if neither parent is obese.[23] Studies of twins have shown that **monozygote** (identical) twins reared apart are more similar in percentage of body fat than are **dizygote** (fraternal) twins. Naturally the family, as the primary transmitter of culture, also exerts social pressure and children learn food habits and attitudes that add an environmental influence.[24] But studies of adopted children, whose adoption records were available, show that the children reflect weight patterns of their biologic parents, not of their adoptive parents.[25] These results further reinforce the genetic link to obesity indicated by many other studies in both animals and humans.[26]

Current work seems to indicate an underlying biochemical mechanism of this genetic link, an enzyme that acts as a "signaling molecule" to the body's fat metabolism.[27] In the model of other genetic disease, measurement of such an enzyme might eventually distinguish obesities that arise from genetic or metabolic defects from those that result from overeating. An increasing number of investigators are concluding that we are probably dealing with different "obesities" having different causes, different characteristics, and different indications for treatment.[28]

Psychologic Factors

Fat persons are seen as having less control over their appetites and as being more responsive to external cues than to internal ones. That is, some believe obese persons eat (1) when it's mealtime by the clock or when they're surrounded by tasty foods, instead of when they're really hungry, (2) when they're unhappy, or (3) because as children they associated food with maternal love. Studies have shown that these factors cannot be applied to fat persons as a group.[23] They have no more tendency to these actions and feelings than anyone else. But there is no question about the role that psychology must play in any weight-maintenance program. Our cultural "ideal" thin-body type and resulting social discrimination against obese persons have created psychologic problems in many individuals. Social support, in the form of counselor, support group, friends, or family is critical for a successful weight-maintenance program.

Social Factors

Class values of different social groups also influence obesity. As a person moves upward in a social class, he or she has a tendency to be more highly

Monozygote
Single fertilized ovum; may result in identical twins.

Zygote
Fertilized ovum; the single cell before the division process starts.

motivated to maintain a moderate or acceptable body weight. In lower socioeconomic status groups obesity is fairly common and considered normal. In higher-level groups greater social value is usually placed on the thinner state. The length of exposure to these values and their pressure on individuals in any social class determines reaction to them.

Physiologic Factors

The normal physiology of the growth years contributes to accumulation of fat tissue deposits. There are critical periods during growth for the development of obesity, such as early childhood and early stages of puberty. Early adulthood is another potential period because of reduced physical activity with no adjustment of caloric intake. For women other times may be during pregnancy and after menopause, resulting from hormonal changes. For men a critical period is middle adulthood, generally because of decreasing activity with no change in large food habits formed during the high energy needs of adolescence. Both men and women tend to gain weight after age 50 because of the lowered BMR and decreased physical exercise, with failure to adjust kilocalories accordingly. Two theories of physiologic factors contributing to weight management problems have developed from studies of various age groups.

Fat cell theory. This theory holds that the percentage of body fat an individual carries is determined largely by the number of fat cells in the body, which is partly determined by inheritance and partly by eating patterns (see the box on p. 350). Once the body has added fat cells to accommodate extra fuel storage, these cells remain and can store varying amounts of fat.

A special type of fat cell, so-called *brown fat* because of its high concentration of blood supply and pigment, may be involved and is of particular interest in obesity studies.[29] This small amount of special brown fat, only about 1% of body weight, is scattered over the body in specific places. For example, some is found just above the kidneys, surrounding the heart, along the aorta, and between the shoulder blades. This specialized brown adipose tissue's function is to burn off excess energy as heat, which it does at a much higher rate than ordinary "white fat" cells do. Obesity results when some sort of brown tissue defect interferes with this function. How much such defective energy buffering by brown fat might contribute to human obesity is uncertain.

Set-point theory. Several investigators have proposed a different way of looking at obesity.[30] This view reinforces findings that we are not dealing with a singular condition called "obesity" but with different conditions better termed as "obesities" with different causes, characteristics, and treatments.[28] It has been labeled the "set point" theory because of its basis in individual metabolic regulation of body fat, through an internal mechanism controlling the amount of body fat that an individual will normally have. This physiologic response to individual genetic influence distinguishes obesity from former claims that it is purely a psychologic problem and the obese person is at fault. It provides a basis for understanding why it is so difficult for some obese persons to lose weight and maintain weight at a lower level. The idea of body fat set point is that the individual will eat to regain whatever amount of fat that person's body metabolism is "set" to, or genetically "programmed"

To Probe Further

The Control of Body Fat

Most persons still believe that obesity is largely a psychologic disorder. Continuing research, however, increasingly reveals that its underlying cause is mainly physiologic. A complex set of metabolic and genetic factors controls fat cell development.

Fat cell size and number

Early work by Hirsh and Knittle in the 1970s on fat cell development laid important groundwork in fat cell theory. Their studies indicated that the fat cells of adult-onset obese persons were much *larger* than those of normal-weight controls. In contrast, they found that childhood-onset obese persons had a far greater *number* of fat cells, as much as a fivefold increase. On this basis it was believed that early nutritional and genetic influences led to this increased number of fat cells during growth years, with the number stabilizing in adolescence. The resulting fat cell hypothesis was that weight gain or loss after that growth point could occur only by changes in cell size but not in cell number. Subsequent study, however, has shown that cell number can be changed during adulthood as well. It is now known that the number of fat cells in adults can increase with prolonged excessive dietary intake, that is, positive energy balance. This increase is probably stimulated when the size of the present fat cells reaches an upper limit. Similarly, the number of fat cells can decrease when the person loses a great deal of weight and maintains that weight for an extended period.

Fat cell theory

Current fat cell theory holds that persons are obese because of their many fat cells and that weight loss is difficult because of the natural biologic pressure to keep all of these cells filled with fat for a constant energy supply. In this case the only way such a person could achieve society's unrealistic ideal weight, especially for women, would be to deplete the fat content of all these fat cells and thus reduce their size. The result, however, of this depleted fat cell state is a distressed condition similar to that undergone by normal-weight persons who are starving. Such obese persons are therefore trapped in a no-win situation: they feel the biologic "starvation" pressure to fill (nourish) their many fat cells but are still overweight because of the tremendous number of fat cells demanding such nourishment. Thus cell size sets a biologic limit beyond which weight loss is exceedingly difficult, and fat cell number sets the body weight at the point this limit is reached. Much more research is needed, however, before these theories can be fully validated.

Lipoprotein link

Undoubtedly a complex metabolic chain is involved in all these processes. The work of Schwartz and Brunzell indicates that one possible link is lipoprotein lipase (LPL). The fat cell synthesizes this important enzyme for its crucial work in the uptake of fatty acids for synthesis of fat in the fat cell. Their research shows that adipose tissue LPL activity increases during weight loss, thus making the cell even more efficient in making fats.

Genetic influence

Heredity is a primary factor controlling the number of fat cells in the body, but other factors may influence its expression. In a remarkable experiment with a special genetically obese strain of mice, Stern's group at the University of California, Davis, was able to actually prevent the expression of this genetic trait by exercising the mice just before the time their juvenile-onset obesity would naturally have occurred.

Clinical significance

What does this work on fat cells mean for the clinical practitioner? This may soon be apparent with needed continuing research. One thing is evident thus far: risk for medical problems is related to the size of the fat cells present more than to the number of fat cells or the person's weight per se. An obese person with too many fat cells may reduce any health risk to normal by reducing cells to normal size, even though by society's standard the person may still be overweight. As yet, methods for identifying these persons by determining fat cell size and number are costly and not readily available, but this will change as this issue of weight and health vs weight and society receives greater attention and social values change. In the meantime we *can* emphasize increased physical activity to our clients. Research has clearly shown that exercise influences fat cell metabolism.

REFERENCES

Brownell KD: Obesity and weight control: the good and the bad of dieting, Nutr Today 22(3):4, 1987.

Brownell KD and Foreyt JP: Handbook of eating disorders: physiology, psychology, and treatment of obesity, anorexia, and bulimia, New York, 1986, Basic Books.

Berdanier CR: You are what you inherit, Nutr Today 21(5):18, 1986.

Hirsh J and Knittle JL: Increase in adipose tissue lipoprotein lipase activity with weight loss, J Clin Invest 67:1425, 1981.

Hirsch J and Leibel RL: New light on obesity, N Engl J Med 318:509, February 25, 1988.

Stern JS, Dunn JR, and Johnson PR: Spontaneous activity and adipose cellularity in the genetically obese yellow (Ay/a) mouse, Fed Proc 36:1150, 1977.

for, and will similarly lose weight gained in excess of this internally regulated point. Apparently the major way of lowering this set point is by increasing physical exercise, which in turn raises the BMR and programs the body to store less fat than it did before. These increased levels of physical activity, especially aerobic exercise, will help the body to regulate itself at a lower level of body fat (see the box on p. 353). In combination with a well-balanced moderate diet, increased exercise offers the main support for gradual and sustained loss of excess fat.

The Health Model: A Positive Personal Approach

General Components

Healthful, successful, and lasting weight management can occur through combined wisdom from different areas of research, both nutritional and behavioral. A well-balanced, individually tailored food plan, together with a gradually increased exercise program, can be effective and personally rewarding. In common practice the general approach to simple obesity is based on underlying energy balance and the client's personal situational needs. It focuses on two main aspects: (1) motivation and support and (2) a personalized program.

Motivation and Support

The degree of personal motivation is a prime factor. Through initial interviews the nutrition counselor determines individual needs, attitudes toward food, and the meaning that food has for the client. Recognition is given to emotional factors involved, and support is provided by the nutritionist, together with the nurse and the physician, to meet the client's particular personal needs.

A Personal Program

Such a personal weight management program will include some form of the following parts:

1. **Food behaviors.** Note the usual quantity of food served and eaten. Then use smaller portions, attractively served. Take time to eat *slowly* and savor the food taste and texture. Reduce hidden factors added in food preparation such as fat, sugar, and salt. Increase fiber content. Choose a variety of foods from a basic food guide, such as the exchange system (see the box on p. 355), which can serve as a focus for sound nutrition education. Emphasize whole primary foods and only a minimum of processed foods. Plan a fairly even food distribution each day.

2. **Exercise behaviors.** Plan a regular daily exercise schedule. Start with simple walking, building to a brisk aerobic pace, for about a half hour a day. Add other activities that can have aerobic value, such as swimming, or develop a set of body exercises, including stretching, body and muscle development, aerobic periods, and a cool-down period (see the box on the facing page). Set occasional goals and note progress. Above all, use a variety of activities and enjoy them.

3. **Relaxation exercises.** Practice progressive muscle relaxation and stress-reduction exercises. Learn a simple pattern as a guide, using imagery as a mental focusing devise. Use background tapes or environmental records if they are helpful. Select a suitable time for daily practice and stay with it. Start with a brief 10-minute period, then increase as desired.

4. **Personal interest area.** Develop some creative interest area for intellectual stimulation, personal enjoyment, and fulfillment. Explore various community groups or resources to support such activities.

5. **Follow-up program.** The nutrition counselor and the client need to develop some schedule of follow-up contacts or appointments. On subsequent visits progress can be reviewed, problems discussed, and solutions mutually

Clinical Application

Benefits of Aerobic Exercise in Weight Management

The goal of weight management is to reduce adipose tissue and in most cases to build lean body mass (LBM). Both tissues are lost when a person tries to reach a weight goal by reducing food intake alone.

The optimal body composition can be achieved by combining food restriction with aerobic exercise. This type of exercise consists of activities that are sustained long enough to draw on the body's fat reserves for fuel while increasing oxygen intake (thus the name "aerobic"). Lean body tissue burns fats in the presence of oxygen. Thus aerobic activity is best suited for achieving the ideal high LBM−low fatty tissue balance in the body.

The benefits of aerobic exercise to the overweight person in a weight-management program include the following:

- Lower set point
- Suppressed appetite
- Reduced body fat
- Higher basal metabolic rate
- Increased energy expenditure
- Retention or building of LBM levels

Sometimes clients complain of difficulty or disappointment in a slow rate of weight loss, difficulty in controlling the appetite, or consistent "flabbiness" despite continuing diet management. These persons may welcome the suggestion of aerobic activity to help meet these needs. You may want to recommend a brisk daily walk, jumping rope, swimming, bicycling, jogging, running, or some other activity that they can sustain long enough for it to have an aerobic effect (see Chapter 18). Note carefully the physical stress this activity may place on individuals who have not exercised for some time or who have medical problems related to exertion. Advise these clients to have a physical checkup before beginning such a program on their own or before joining a local gymnasium or other community fitness center.

REFERENCES
Pacy PJ and others: The energy cost of aerobic exercise in fed and fasted normal subjects, Am J Clin Nutr 42:764, Nov 1985.
Pacy PJ, Webster J, and Garrow JS: Exercise and obesity, Sports Medicine 3(2):89, 1986.

explored. Continuing support can be provided. Practical suggestions for dealing with such things as realistic goals, food binges, weight plateaus, meals away from home, and other special situations can be discussed (see the box on p. 357). These guides may help the client anticipate needs, avoid pitfalls, sustain motivation, and deal positively with periods of frustration.

Behavior Modification

Practitioners in a health care setting recognize the need for supportive therapies in weight management that focus on the behavioral aspects of the problem. Food behavior is rooted in many human experiences and varying life situations. These experiences often produce addictive forms of eating response or conditioning. Behavior-oriented therapies help the person change such inappropriate food and eating patterns through increased insight, motivation, and reconditioning techniques.[31-33]

Principles of a Sound Food Plan

On the basis of careful interviewing, body composition measures, and evaluation of available laboratory data, the nutritionist makes a comprehensive assessment of nutritional and health status, food habits and behaviors, and living situation (see Chapter 17). Then on the basis of this individual assessment, personal needs and goals can be established with the client, and a personal food plan is developed to meet nutritional and personal needs. A sound food plan will involve the following components.

Energy Balance

The energy intake level (kilocalories) is adjusted to meet individual weight-reduction requirements. A decrease of about 1000 kcal/day from usual eating habits is necessary to lose about 2 lb/week, a decrease of 500 kcal/day to lose about 1 lb/week. This gradual rate is best for long-term success and health. On the average, for women, a sound diet for energy needs is based on about 1200 kcal/day. For larger women and for men, a diet of about 1500 to 1800 kcal/day would meet weight reduction energy needs.

Nutrient Balance

Basic energy nutrients are outlined to achieve the following nutrient balance:
1. **Carbohydrate.** About 50% to 55% of total kilocalories, with emphasis on complex forms such as starches with fiber and a limit on simple sugars.
2. **Protein.** Approximately 20% of total kilocalories, with emphasis on lean food to curtail fat and small portions.
3. **Fat.** About 25% to 30% of total kilocalories, with emphasis on plant fats, scant use, and alternate seasonings.

In general, this nutrient balance approximates the recommendations of the U.S. Dietary Guidelines for Healthy Americans. Review these guidelines in Chapter 1. They are helpful as a good basic nutrition education tool.

Distribution Balance

Spread food fairly evenly throughout the day to meet energy needs. Consider any daily problem times and plan simple snacks to meet such needs.

Food Guide

Use some type of general food lists from which the client can make a variety of food choices to fulfill the basic food plan. The food exchange system provides such a guide (see the box on the facing page). Table 15-1 shows food plans on several caloric levels; the related food lists are given in Appendix H. This system provides a good general reference guide for comparative food values and portions, variety in food choices, and basic meal planning. Food items can easily be combined into desired dishes. In food preparation use alternate seasonings, such as herbs and spices, onion and garlic, lemon juice, vinegar, wine, fat-free broth, mustard, and other condiments.

To Probe Further

Food Guide: The Exchange System of Dietary Management

The exchange system of dietary management, developed by two professional organizations, the American Dietetic Association and the American Diabetes Association, is based on the concept of nutritional equivalency. Thus its basic food lists are simple groupings of common foods according to their generally equivalent nutritional values. This system may be used for any situation requiring caloric and energy macronutrient control.

The foods are divided into six basic groups (with subgroups), called the "exchange lists." Each food item within a group or subgroup contains about the same food value as other food items in that group, allowing for exchange within groups, thus providing for variety in food choices as well as food value control. Hence, the term *food exchanges* is sometimes used to refer to food choices or servings. The total number of "exchanges" per day depends on individual nutritional needs, based on normal nutrition standards. Although there is some variation in the composition of foods within the exchange groups, for simplicity the following values for carbohydrate, protein, fat, and kilocalories are used.

Exchange Lists

Food groups	Carbohydrate (g)	Protein (g)	Fat (g)	Kilocalories
Starch or bread	15	3	trace	80
Meat				
Lean	—	7	3	55
Medium-fat	—	7	5	75
High-fat	—	7	8	100
Vegetable	5	2	—	25
Fruit	15	—	—	60
Milk				
Skimmed	12	8	trace	90
Low-fat	12	8	5	120
Whole	12	8	8	150
Fat	—	—	5	45

REFERENCE
Franz MJ and others: Exchange lists: revised 1986, J Am Diet Assoc 87(1):28, 1987.

Personal Needs
Individual Adaptations

Throughout the planning remember to focus on the individual client and personal needs. If the plan is unrealistic, it will not be followed. Some per-

Table 15-1
Weight Reduction Food Plans Using the Exchange System of Dietary Control* (Total Kilocalorie Distribution: 50% Carbohydrate, 20% Protein, 30% Fat)

Food exchange groups	1000 kcal	1200 kcal	1500 kcal	1800 kcal
Total number exchanges/day				
Milk (nonfat)	2	2	2	2
Vegetable	3	3	4	4
Fruit	3	3	4	4
Bread	4	5	7	9
Meat	3	4	5	7
Fat	4	4	5	5
Meal pattern of food exchanges				
Breakfast				
Fruit	1	1	1	1
Meat			1	1
Bread	1	1	2	2
Fat	1	1	1	1
Milk	½	½	½	½
Lunch/supper				
Meat	1	1	1	2
Vegetable	1	1	2	2
Bread	1	2	2	3
Fat	1	1	2	2
Fruit	1	1	1	1
Milk	½	½	½	½
Dinner				
Meat	2	2	2	3
Vegetable	2	2	2	2
Bread	1	1	2	3
Fat	2	2	2	2
Fruit			1	1
Milk	½	½	½	½
Snack (afternoon or evening)				
Milk	½	½	½	½
Meat		1	1	1
Bread	1	1	1	1
Fruit	1	1	1	1

*See food exchange lists, Appendix H.

sons find it helpful to keep a daily journal, which can include notes of food intake, environmental food cues, feelings, physical symptoms, and any stress factors related to food behavior. It may also include notes about other activities such as physical exercise or stress-reduction practice. A periodic review of such notes may help in making general observations, determining problem areas, monitoring progress, and gaining insights for setting personal goals to achieve desired health and fitness behavior changes.

Treatment Choices

What is a reasonable guide that practitioners can use to plan an appropriate weight management approach? A simple classification outlined by a leading

Clinical Application

Goals

Be realistic. Don't set your goals too high. Adapt your rate of loss to 450 to 900 g (1 to 2 lb) per week. If visible tools are helpful motivation techniques, use them.

Kilocalories

Don't be an obsessive kilocalorie counter. Simply become familiar with the food exchanges in your diet list and learn the general values of some of your favorite home dishes so that you might occasionally make substitutions.

Plateaus

Anticipate plateaus. They happen to everyone. They are related to water accumulation as fat is lost. During these periods increase your exercise to help you get started again.

Binges

Don't be discouraged when you break down and have a dietary binge. This too happens to most persons. Simply keep them infrequent, and when possible, plan ahead for special occasions. Adjust the following day's diet or remaining part of the same day accordingly.

Special diet foods

There is no need to purchase special low-kilocalorie foods. Learn to read labels carefully. Most special diet foods are expensive, and many are not much lower in kilocalories than regular foods.

Home meals

Try to avoid a separate menu for yourself. Adapt your needs to the family meal, adjusting seasoning or method of preparing family dishes to lower kilocalorie values of added fats and starches.

Eating away from home

Watch portions. When a guest, limit extras such as sauces and dressings and trim meat well. In restaurants select singly prepared items rather than combination dishes. Avoid items with heavy sauces or fat seasoning. Select fruit or sherbet as desserts rather than pastries.

Appetite control

Avoid dependence on appetite-depressant medications. Usually they are only crutches. Beginning efforts to control appetite may be aided by nibbling on food from the free list or by saving over meal items for use between meals, such as the fruit.

Meal pattern

Eat three or more meals a day. If you are used to three meals, then leave it at that. If you are helped by snacks between meals, then plan part of your day's allowance to account for them. The main thing is that you do not take all of your kilocalories at one sitting. Avoid the all-too-common pattern of no breakfast, little or no lunch, and a huge dinner.

researcher in this field, based on the degree of overweight, can provide a wise guide[34]:

1. **Mild**—20% to 40% overweight (about 91% of all obese women). Only a moderate caloric restriction is indicated, along with nutrition education, behavior therapy, and increased physical exercise. Such a program is best provided by nonphysician health professionals or community groups.
2. **Moderate**—41% to 100% (about 9% of all obese women). Special programs, sometimes including medically supervised very-low-calorie formulas and refeeding diets, may be indicated for some persons.[35,36]
3. **Severe**—greater than 100% (0.5% of all obese women). Only special surgical procedures using some sort of gastric restriction appear to have any measure of success.[20]

Essential parts of all programs are nutrition counseling and education, behavior modification, and increased physical activity. Working with persons in the moderate and severe groups defined above requires medical supervision and is best accomplished with a team of health professionals.

Preventive Approach

In the final analysis, it would seem that the most constructive work in weight management would be aimed at *prevention*. Early nutrition education, positive food and fitness behavior and habit formation in the family, with support and guidance for young parents and children before the obese condition develops, will help prevent many problems in later adulthood.

To Sum Up

Body weight has traditionally been used as an indicator of obesity, which may raise the risk of health problems. New methods of determining body weight reveal that the underlying *composition* of that weight, the lean vs fat tissue, is its most important aspect. Weight-management programs have traditionally been designed for obese persons. However, a growing modern obsession with thinness has created a new weight-management problem—eating disorders that result in semistarvation. These disorders are strongly associated with societal pressures, and psychologic counseling is an important part of therapy. Problems involved in planning a weight-management program, either for the obese or malnourished person, include the metabolic and energy needs of the individual, personal food choices and habits, and variations in needs for fat tissues during different stages of the life cycle.

The health model of weight management is based on personal motivation and support for the individual. Aspects of such a program include changing food behaviors, increasing physical activity, learning and practicing relaxation techniques, and developing personal interests. Behavior modification strategies help the individual examine the effect of life situations on eating habits and change those situations that encourage overeating. A sound weight-management plan is based on an adjusted kilocalorie level that allows for (1) a gradual, moderate rate of loss, (2) sound nutrition, and (3) support for food behavior changes. The ideal plan begins with prevention, stressing positive food habits and physical fitness from early childhood to help prevent major problems later in life.

1. What is meant by "ideal weight"? Explain the variables involved in determining this factor. What role does it play in weight management?
2. Describe two major eating disorders associated with America's growing obsession with thinness. What social factors contribute to this obsession? Compare how these factors contribute to the growing tendency toward overweight.
3. Describe the fat cell theory and the set point theory of body fat formation. What implications are presented for the future of weight-management methods?
4. Describe five components of the "health model" for weight management. How does this model differ from the traditional medical model?
5. What are the principles of a sound food plan for weight-management programs?

References

1. Stern JS: Obesity treatment, J Am Diet Assoc 84(4):405, 1984.
2. Andres R: Effect of obesity on total mortality, Int J Obesity 4:381, 1980.
3. Gurin J: What's your natural weight? Am Health 3(3):43, 1984.
4. Williams SR: Body composition. In Williams SR and Worthington-Roberts BS, editors: Nutrition throughout the life cycle, St Louis, 1988, The CV Mosby Co.
5. Burton BT and Foster WR: Health implications of obesity: an NIH consensus development conference, J Am Diet Assoc 85(9):1117, 1985.
6. Lukaski HC: Methods for the assessment of human body composition: traditional and new, Am J Clin Nutr 46:537, Oct 1987.
7. Jequier E: Energy, obesity, and body weight standards, Am J Clin Nutr 45(suppl):1035, May 1987.
8. Stark RET: Body mass index, The Bariatrician 4:20, Winter 1987.
9. Hubert HB and others: Obesity as an independent risk factor for cardiovascular disease: a 26-year follow-up of participants in the Framingham Heart Study, Circulation 67:968, 1983.
10. Wadden TA and Stunkard AJ: Social and psychological consequences of obesity, Ann Intern Med 103(6):1062, 1985.
11. Kannel WB and Gordon T: Physiological and medical concomitants of obesity: the Framingham study. In Bray GA, editor: Obesity in America, DHEW Pub No. (NIH) 79-359, Washington, DC, 1979, U.S. Government Printing Office.
12. Trafford A: America's diet wars, US News and World Report 100(2):62, 1986.
13. Fisher MC and LaChance PA: Nutrition evaluation of published weight-reducing diets, J Am Diet Assoc 85(4):450, 1985.
14. Byerly L and others: Popular diets: how they rate, ed 2, Santa Monica, Calif, 1987, California Dietetic Association, Los Angeles District.
15. Pasulka PS: Is there risk in recurrent dieting? Top Clin Nutr 2(2):1, 1987.
16. Brownell K: The yo-yo trap, Am Health 7(2):78, 1988.
17. Survey of very-low-calorie weight reduction diets, Arch Intern Med 143(7):1423, 1983.
18. Sikand G and others: Two-year follow-up of patients treated with a very-low-calorie diet and exercise training, J Am Diet Assoc 88(4):487, 1988.
19. Bennett W and Gurin J: The dieter's dilemma, New York, 1983, Basic Books.
20. Randell S and Zeffrino WW: Surgical management of the morbidly obese, Top Clin Nutr 2(2):55, 1987.

21. Graney AS, Smith LB, and Hammer KA: Gastric partitioning for morbid obesity: postoperative weight loss, technical complications, and protein status, J Am Diet Assoc 86(5):630, 1986.

22. Priddy MLB: Gastric reduction surgery: a dietitian's experience and perspective, J Am Diet Assoc 85(4):455, 1985.

23. Foreman L: The fat fallacy, Health 15(9):23, 1983.

24. Frankl RT: Obesity a family matter: creating new behavior, J Am Diet Assoc 85(5):597, 1985.

25. Stunkard AJ and others: An adoption study of human obesity, N Engl J Med 314:193, Jan 23, 1986.

26. Berdanier CR: You are what you inherit, Nutr Today 21(5):18, 1986.

27. Moffat AS: Weight control: genetics or gluttony, Am Health 7(7):106, 1988.

28. Brownell KD: Obesity and weight control: the good and the bad of dieting, Nutr Today 22(3):4, 1987.

29. Schultz LO: Brown adipose tissue: regulation of thermogenesis and implications for obesity, J Am Diet Assoc 87(6):761, 1987.

30. Keesey RE and Corbett SW: Metabolic defense of the body weight setpoint. In Stunkard AJ and Steller E, editors: Eating and its disorders, New York, 1984, Raven Press.

31. Nash JD: Maximize your body potential, Palo Alto, Calif, 1986, Bull Publishing Co.

32. Nash JD: Taking charge of your weight and well-being, Palo Alto, Calif, 1978, Bull Publishing Co.

33. Ferguson JM: Habits not diets, Palo Alto, Calif, 1988, Bull Publishing Co.

34. Stunkard AJ: The current status of treatment for obesity in adults. In Stunkard AJ and Steller E, editors: Eating and its disorders, New York, 1984, Raven Press.

35. Fenhouse D: The OPTIFAST Program: a viable treatment for obesity, Top Clin Nutr 2(2):69, 1987.

36. Brownell KD: The psychology and physiology of obesity: implications for screening and treatment, J Am Diet Assoc 84(4):406, 1984.

Further Readings

Berdanier CR: You are what you inherit, Nutr Today 21(5):18, 1986.

Brownell KD: Obesity and weight control: the good and the bad of dieting, Nutr Today 22(3):4, 1987.

These two articles from an excellent journal describe the growing evidence for a genetic "handicap" as a cause of obesity—the bad news—but they encourage persons so predisposed with knowledge of the many nongenetic factors that contribute to body fat that can be managed—the good news.

Caballero B: Absorption and metabolism of sweetening agents, Clin Nutr 3(2):65, 1984.

Fox M: Sweet nothing? Health 19(12):10, 1987.

von Borstel RW: Metabolic and physiologic effects of sweeteners, Clin Nutr 4(6):215, 1985.

These articles describe the nature and effect of both nutritive and nonnutritive sweeteners and explain why sugar substitutes such as aspartame (NutriSweet) fail to fulfill satiety needs.

Nash JD: Maximize your body potential, Palo Alto, Calif, 1986, Bull Publishing Co.

Nash JD: Taking charge of your weight and well-being, Palo Alto, Calif, 1978, Bull Publishing Co.

Ferguson JM: Habits not diets, Palo Alto, Calif, 1988, Bull Publishing Co.

Ikeda J: Winning weight loss for teens, Palo Alto, Calif, 1987, Bull Publishing Co.

This publisher and his winning authors have provided in these little gems excellent guides for the "health" model of weight management, which not only emphasizes sound nutrition but also focuses on physical fitness, behavior modification, and building self-esteem—a winning combination.

The Use and Abuse of Height-Weight Tables

On March 1, 1983, with considerable media coverage, the Metropolitan Life Insurance Company (MLI) issued its "new" weight-height tables. These charts list recommended weight ranges for women and men of varying body frames at different heights. The last time they were revised was in 1959. Now, after analyzing mortality data on 4.2 million people for 22 years, the company statisticians have determined that Americans can weigh from 2 to 13 lbs more than they do now and expect to live longer than their leaner counterparts.

The public may welcome this news, as expressed in the public press with statements such as, "Now it's OK to weigh more." On the other hand, various investigators and practitioners in medicine and nutrition are raising more serious questions about the uses and abuses of these tables over the years. There is evidence from many sides that we are rethinking the relationship of overweight, health, and longevity. Questions are being raised not only about the difference in the two most recent tables, the 1959 and 1983 versions, but also, and more significantly, the conceptual basis of their construction in the first place. Which table is best? Is either one valid as a health standard for clinical practice? How can we deal with weight management issues related both to health dictates and to social demands? A better understanding of how these tables came to be and what current research teaches us concerning their appropriate use in practice will help us use them in a broader and more appropriate manner in our own practice.

Development of Standard Height-Weight Tables

The earliest weight tables appeared in Europe in 1836, simply based on the weights of "a moderate number of Belgians." Through the intervening years, the development of weight-height tables as we have come to know them has been dominated mainly by the insurance industry and used by insurance companies as a guide for evaluating life insurance applicants. Early industry leaders candidly admitted that weight-height concerns had no commercial significance until life insurance came into being. Standards were set by the industry on the assumption that overweight people were bad insurance risks and higher premiums were set for these persons, if they were accepted at all.

Over the last few decades, a leader in the insurance industry, the Metropolitan Life Insurance Company, has taken the lead in revising earlier tables. In 1942 and 1943 MLI challenged the previous tables' use of only average weights as standard. Instead, they sought to relate weight to disease and mortality. They also introduced the idea of body frame size as a factor in appropriate weight but gave no guidelines for determining body type. Their data base for analysis came from a sampling of their policyholders. The weight statistically associated with longevity they called "ideal weight" and so titled their 1942-1943 table. In 1959 they issued a revision of the table, based again on data from policyholders, this time including persons insured by 26 life insurance companies in the United States and Canada—The Build and Blood Pressure Study, 1959. They concluded that the lowest mortality rates were associated with below-average weight and thus used the term "desirable weight" in the title of their 1959 table revision.

Currently, with their new 1983 revision based on data from 25 insurance companies and over 4 million policyholders, MLI statisticians have dropped both "desirable" and "ideal." Instead the new table is simply titled with the date of issue and includes a footnote that weights of persons at age 25 to 59 are based on lowest mortality. Weights are again given in terms of

Continued.

The Use and Abuse of Height-Weight Tables—cont'd

body frame size, with the same three designations. Instructions are included this time for finding your frame size by measuring your elbow bones with fingers and a ruler—not exactly an easy procedure. The designated weights are only slightly higher than those in the 1959 tables, the greatest increases being for shorter men and women.

Changing concepts

Over the past few years, the data and philosophy behind the 1959 tables and, currently, the 1983 revisions have been increasingly questioned by researchers and practitioners. These concerned leaders include such persons from medicine as Reuben Andres, clinical director of the Gerontology Research Center at the National Institute on Aging, and Ancel Keys, a pioneer researcher in the field of nutrition and medicine. Their questions have focused mainly on limitations built into the tables by the nature of their population data base and the factors of age and frame used in the tables' analysis and construction.

Limitations of Population Base

Many persons, even including MLI actuaries and statisticians themselves, have pointed out that insurance policy-holders are not representative of the population at large. Three reasons have been cited: (1) They are persons valuing insurance and able to afford it—largely white, middle-class, adult males. (2) Underwriting practices vary widely from strict to lenient, with weight measurements and health data inaccurate or falsely self-reported—unsuitable for medical or public health purposes. (3) The population of American policyholders does not reflect the general population incidence of chronic disease or acute illnesses because such persons usually do not apply for insurance or may be rejected if they do. Moreover, overweight persons charged higher rates may have been motivated to purchase insurance by fear of a

hidden health problem that could lead to an early death.

Age factor

Andres was among the first to voice concerns about the dangers of thinness and to question the risk of being moderately overweight. He has since analyzed the data himself and found that the new MLI tables were "too liberal for young adults and too restrictive for older people." He has constructed a new table, using the insurance data, that gives safe ranges of weight for different heights *and ages.*

The biologic fact is that most persons get fatter as they get older. Thus, according to Andres, the "safe" range of weight raises with age. Adults who gain about 8 to 10 lbs a decade may actually be helping themselves to keep healthy. Both Andres and Keys conclude that unless an individual has hypertension or diabetes, overweight does not increase mortality or the development of coronary heart disease.

Body frame

The concept of body frame as used in these tables is without scientific foundation. Keys has stated that these frame types were created simply by dividing the weight distribution of the data into thirds and labeling those thirds as "small," "medium," and "large." In fact, Andres calls such distinction of frame size a "fiction." The American Medical Association has also pointed out the difficulties of scientifically determining frame size.

What is the Answer?

So the question remains: Which weight-height standard do we use— 1959 or 1983? The answer is *neither.* These tables may be useful as guides but should not be used as standards for determining "ideal" body weight. How can they? Ideal weight is based primarily on the amount of lean body tissue, from a table. They *might* be able to estimate it, by measuring subcutaneous fat with calipers at designated spots on the body or by submerging the individual in a water tank and gauging the percent fat by the amount of water that is displaced. If they do, they may find that some of their "overweight" clients are, in fact, very lean, with well-developed musculature contributing to excess weight. Conversely, some of their "ideal weight" clients may, in fact, be obese in the true sense of the word—having too much body fat. Worst of all, they might find out that some of their formerly undernourished patients who start to gain weight "quite nicely" are, in fact, edematous and in dire need of nutritional intervention.

It is unfortunate that the medical community and the public have taken these guidelines so seriously for so long. Perhaps the time has come to alleviate the anxiety surrounding weight by taking these charts down from their traditional havens over our scales and placing them in their rightful place on the desk or in the drawer as one of our reference guides. Perhaps then both patient and counselor will be released from "the numbers game." We can then delve further into the physiologic, cultural, economic, and social factors that *really* count in the process of weight management. With this tool in proper perspective, we can focus our clinical concerns on those with "dangerous" weights—the very thin and the extremely obese—and give primary attention from a health care standpoint to those middle-weight persons who have weight-related disease such as diabetes and hypertension.

As for the social issues involved, our weights and our looks remain intensely personal. But many moderately overweight middle adults, unhappy for years with their bodies, will escape from the tyranny of the tables and feel better about themselves. Ultimately, all our ideas about what looks good may gradually change, and we'll discover that we're in better shape than we thought.

REFERENCES

Andres R: Effect of obesity on total mortality, Int J Obesity 4:381, 1980.

Burton BT and Foster WR: Health implications of obesity: an NIH consensus development conference, J Am Diet Assoc 85(9):1117, 1985.

Gurin J: What's your natural weight? Am Health 3(3):43, 1984.

Himes JH, and Bouchard C: Do the new Metropolitan Life Insurance weight-height tables correctly assess body frame and body fat relationships? Am J Pub Health 75:1076, Sept 1985.

Keys A: Overweight, obesity, coronary heart disease and mortality, Nutr Rev 38:297, 1980.

Schultz LO: Obese, overweight, desirable, ideal: where to draw the line in 1986? J Am Diet Assoc 86(12):1702, 1986.

Weigley ES: Average? Ideal? Desirable? A brief overview of height-weight tables in the United States, J Am Diet Assoc 84(4):417, 1984.

16 Nutrition and Stress Management

Chapter Objectives

After studying this chapter, the student should be able to:

1. Identify ways in which stress in our lives acts as a risk factor in health and disease, and describe some of the common life stressors' relation to nutrition.

2. Trace the stages of the body's automatic physiologic response to stress and describe positive adaptive supports to avoid exhaustion and disease.

3. Relate physiologic and psychosocial stress to the life cycle stages.

4. Describe nutritional support that may be provided for the stress of disease, the workplace, or the environment.

5. Describe the high-risk impact of poverty in human lives and realistic ways of meeting nutritional needs.

6. Describe ways of reducing stress and providing nutritional support.

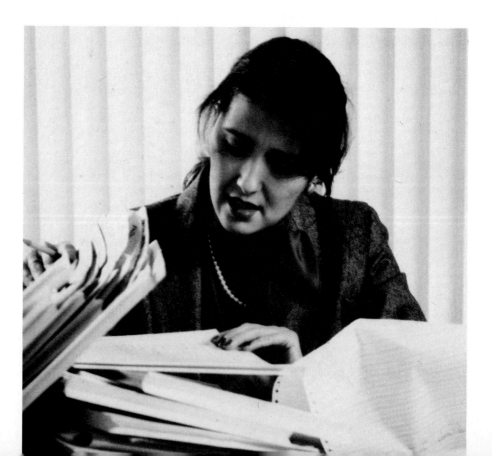

Modern society is fast-paced and competitive. Pressures and problems in this complex age of technology with its rapidly changing environment affect our air, our water, and our food. But our daily lives are affected even more. Modern life's stresses, both physical and psychosocial, cause physiologic waves to wash over our bodies, contributing further to disease and malnutrition.

These automatic physiologic waves that sweep through the body are built-in adaptive responses to stress triggered through our neuroendocrine system. Through some 40,000 or more years of human development this physiologic reaction has protected the body from danger—the familiar "fight or flight" response. But this response is not well adapted to today's high-pressured and unphysical modern society and lifestyle. Often we can neither fight nor flee. Yet the same set of physiologic responses continues to be triggered as if our lives were actually threatened. And indeed they often are, for these repeated physiologic reactions are linked to reduced immune function and the emergence of our so-called diseases of civilization—heart disease, cancer, diabetes, and hypertension.

In this final chapter in our life cycle and health maintenance sequence, we examine some of these issues of modern stress in relation to nutrition and health. We seek first to understand this ever-present underlying physiologic nature of stress and its effects, so that we can better apply these principles to nutritional support needs. Especially is such support needed in high-risk populations. Then we seek ways to manage the inevitable stress in our lives, to move toward more successful coping skills and positive health.

Stress and Nutritional Support

The early classic work of Canadian physician Hans Selye has clearly shown the close relationship of stress to health maintenance and disease.[1] He called stress "the wear and tear in the human machinery which accompanies any vital activity."[2] His basic work indicates that different reactions in different persons depend on *conditioning factors*, which can inhibit or enhance one or more stress effects. These factors may be internal or built-in ones, such as genetic predisposition, age, or sex. Or they may be external or manageable ones, such as poor diet or alcohol and other drug abuse. Based on Selye's important work, stress management has become a necessary consideration in nutrition assessment and support to identify and provide care for individual human needs, both in health promotion and in disease risk-reduction and treatment.

Human Needs: The Process of Life Changes and Events

Constant change and balance are both basic to the ongoing process of life. The changing human body gives evidence of the dynamic interior metabolism interacting with the changing exterior environment. Normal physiologic stress is a vital part of this interaction. For example, during pregnancy nor-

The Role of Stress as a Risk Factor

mal physiologic stress adapts the maternal body to support fetal growth and prepare for birth. Also, normal stress of inserted muscles on bones helps maintain calcium balance, and the general stress of pain warns of injury or illness. But it is severe, prolonged, relentless, uncontrolled stress—be it physical or psychosocial hunger or pain—that contributes to exhaustion of resources and illness. Such debilitating stress may relate to four basic areas of human need, to which health team workers must always be sensitive in order to identify individual stresses requiring assessment and care. The areas are (1) life cycle growth and development, (2) health-disease status, (3) stress-coping balance, and (4) general human needs for self-fulfillment. All of these areas involve nutritional concerns.

Life Cycle Growth and Development

As we have seen in previous chapters, each stage of human life brings unique physical characteristics and psychosocial maturation. Both of these are integral aspects of every person's total life and health. The American psychoanalyst Erik Erikson has provided much insight to help us understand this progressive development of human growth.[3,4] Physical and psychosocial strains along the way confront each individual (see Chapters 12 and 13). Given favorable life circumstances, persons develop positive internal resources to meet life's inevitable crises. Although in periods of increased stress some regression may occur, generally the child and then the adult integrates self-controls and strengths in relation to physical maturation and develops neuromuscular and mental skills. But to the degree that individual life circumstances have not been favorable, stresses multiply and contribute to health problems.

Health-Disease Status

Throughout the life cycle, persons experience varying degrees of health and disease. Many fortunate ones remain in good health because of their "luck of the draw" in genetic heritage. Others less fortunate sustain varying degrees of disease or injury. Individual responses depend on personal resources, physical and mental, as well as psychosocial and economic. Thus any person's health and nutrition status will always involve data from two basic sources:

1. **Subjective data.** Information such as perceived pain, tolerances, feelings about health status or care, and personal perceptions of problems, goals, and priorities is vital for planning valid personal care. This important primary information is gained from talking with and listening to the person and the family.
2. **Objective data.** Also important is quantified information indicating body functions and capacities. This information comes from various technologic sources, such as laboratory or x-ray or other tests, performance measures, nutrition analyses, physical findings, and clinical and behavioral observations and tests.

Too often health professionals may dwell mainly in the area of their modern medical technology and its multitude of procedures and tests (see the box on p. 368), perhaps because they feel more skilled and comfortable and less vulnerable here. But all the while, especially in high-risk populations, significant roots of disease lie in the first subjective area of personal stresses and needs—economic, psychosocial, and mental pressures, as well as physical ones.

Stress-Coping Balance

Stress is a fact of life. So a coping balance must also be present to maintain positive health. In *physiologic stress,* either normal or abnormal, a number of automatic physiologic responses maintain the body in a state of dynamic balance or **homeostasis.** For example, to meet physiologic stress of disease, injury, shock, or physical exertion, various homeostatic mechanisms automatically respond to restore the body's normal metabolism. Similarly, in *psychosocial stress,* a person uses learned mental defense mechanisms, which may or may not be constructive in the circumstances. For example, such defenses as rationalization, compensation, suppression, depression, withdrawal, or substitution are developed during growing years to cope with stress, relieve tension, and preserve the inner self-concept. Often such learned reactions are the only means of making a painful situation psychologically tolerable, but some are less constructive than others.

Homeostasis
State of internal stability of a body or an organism.

Basic Human Needs

Human needs and motives, including nutrition-related ones, are highly personal. People are not the same the world over. Those of differing cultures and life circumstances are not motivated by the same needs and goals. Even primary biologic drives, such as hunger and sex, are modified in their expression by many cultural, social, and personal influences. A hierarchy of human needs, such as that developed by American psychologist Abraham Maslow (see Chapter 9), helps us understand human strivings.[5] Through his classic work with persons showing characteristics of positive mental health behavior, he described five levels of common human needs, each having priority at different times depending on personal circumstances, from basic hunger and safety needs to need for love, self-esteem, and self-fulfillment.

These levels of need overlap, of course, and vary with particular situations and time. Nonetheless, they help us understand basic human needs and plan nutrition and health care accordingly, especially in times of stress, both for our clients and for ourselves.

The Nature of Stress
Perception of Stress

Individual responses to stress vary according to its reality and how it is perceived. The word *perception* comes from the Latin verb *perceptio,* which means literally "to take in" or to comprehend. We constantly receive through our senses a chaotic assortment of impressions. We make sense out of this chaos through our brain's interpretation of it all, which enables us to live in an environment that feels relatively stable. But perception also limits understanding, because everything the outer world offers is understood through a social and personal lens. We perceive every life experience through a blend of three factors: (1) the actual external *reality,* (2) the *message* of the stimulus that is conveyed by the nervous system to the brain's integrative centers where thinking and evaluation go on, and (3) the *interpretation* that we put on every bit of information. A host of subjective elements, such as hunger,

Clinical Application

Signs of Stress in Medical Care

Modern medical technology has placed in physicians' hands a panoply of medical tests, the increasing use of which may well evidence a growing stress for physicians and patients alike. Stressed, overworked physicians, wary of malpractice suits in our increasingly litigious society, often feel compelled to practice defensive medicine with an excessive battery of diagnostic tests. And anxious patients in an ever more complex world often place an unquestioning and demanding faith in such apparently flawless scientific evidence, despite estimates that about 20% of all these tests are unnecessary.

According to current surveys, medical tests may well be excessive—but flawless they are not. Nearly 1400 tests are available to U.S. physicians, from simple blood counts to electrocardiograms to complex expensive CT scans. During the one year of 1987, for example, in the United States some 19 billion tests were performed, nearly 80 for every single person—man, woman, and child. Surely this must make us the most analyzed people on the planet. And the cost of these tests continues to rise. In 1987 the bottom line was more than $100 billion, taking 20% of our nation's total health care bill. Worse yet, the test results can be, and sometimes too often are, wrong or misinterpreted, actually causing harm through failure to detect a serious condition or by indicating nonexistent illness.

The problem of error rates in clinical laboratory tests varies, of course, from one laboratory or procedure to another. But overall, the two procedures most often incorrect are the Papanicolaou (Pap) test for cervical cancer and blood tests for serum cholesterol levels. In the first case, concerned physicians estimate that Pap smears miss 20% to 40% of precancerous or cancerous conditions, often bringing tragedy to lives of the women involved. And the sheer increase in numbers of tests done, with blood tests now packaged and often ordered in blocks of 20 or more rather than singly, cannot help but increase the number of errors and the cost.

Because of the increasing personal, professional, and public concern about the costly trap of excessive medical tests, efforts are being made to curb the stress for both physicians and patients. On the basis of recommendations from the Centers for Disease Control, Congress is investigating the problem with the intent of establishing better and more universal regulation of clinical laboratories with improved proficiency standards. In addition, insurance companies are beginning to create new guidelines for common tests that may involve refusal of payment for unneeded ones. If the reasonable dual goal of curbing laboratory error and preventing useless tests from being ordered in the first place can be achieved, it will be an important step toward reducing some of the stress inherent in the present system for physician and patient alike.

REFERENCE

Grady D, Cronin M, and Garelik G: Going overboard on medical tests, Time, p 80, April 25, 1988.

thirst, hatred, fear, self-interest, values, and temperament influence response to everything the outer world presents.

Common Life Stressors

As indicated, common life stressors are twofold in nature: (1) physical or physiologic stress and (2) psychologic or socioeconomic stress. The first form of stress may come from injury, disability, disease, or physical abuse. The second form may come from emotional pressures, verbal abuse, or lack of financial resources. Undoubtedly, emotional tension from multiple causes is the most common agent of human stress. It can contribute to serious conditions such as cardiovascular and gastrointestinal diseases, diabetes, and cancer, especially if the body is conditioned by malnutrition, faulty diet, or poor housing and homelessness, as is often the case with high-risk families in the grip of poverty. Ultimately, the effect of any life stressor will depend on three influencing characteristics of the stress: (1) its strength, whether it is relatively mild with minor consequences or severe with major results; (2) its duration, whether it is fairly transient or is long term and relentless; and (3) the strength of resisting forces, the personal coping resources, whether they are strong, relatively positive and constructive, or whether they are more negative, pessimistic, and destructive.

When any form of stress occurs, the body automatically responds to defend itself from harm. Selye called this common physiologic response to stress the *general adaptive syndrome*.[2] An understanding of this automatic "cascade of physiologic events" provides an essential base for (1) identifying needs and resources; (2) planning nutritional support, both immediate and long-term; and (3) rebuilding metabolic reserves. This immediate reaction of the body to stress involves actions of the combined neuroendocrine systems through three progressive stages of physiologic response, as illustrated in Figure 16-1.

Physiologic Response to Stress: The General Adaptive Syndrome

Stage I: The Initial Alarm Reaction to Stress
Brain Signals

In this first stage the body's forces are mobilized for action. In response to a perceived threat the brain instantly triggers the release of chemical messengers, **neurotransmitters,** in the brain cortex. These messengers then relay impulses along neuron tracks in the brain's outer edge to the *hypothalamus*, the "primitive" brain at the head of the brainstem that governs autonomic body functions such as breathing, heart rate, blood pressure, digestion, hormonal balance, and many other vital activities. This part of the brain has been called the "automatic pilot" or the "brain's brain." Upon instant receipt of the stress message, the hypothalamus immediately triggers still other chemical messengers and hormones along two separate yet integrated tracks to adapt the body's normal physiology to changes needed to combat the danger.[6] In Figure 16-1 you can trace these brain signals and message relays along their two tracks and note the body's important protective physiologic effects.

Neurotransmitters
Chemical substances that relay messages through the central nervous system.

Stage II: Resistance and Adaptation to Stress

Following the initial alarm reaction, if the particular stress has not been so strong that continued exposure overwhelms the person's coping resources, a

Figure 16-1
Progressive sequence of physiologic events in response to
stress.

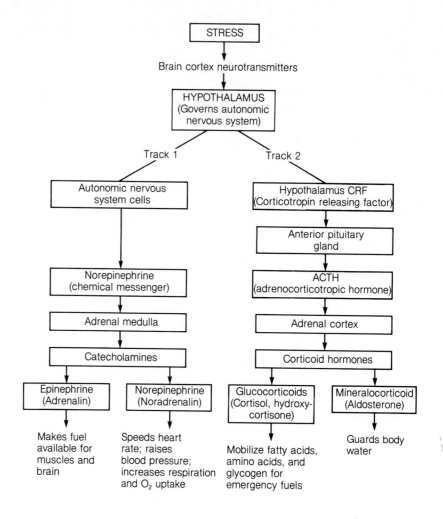

second stage of resistance and adaptation follows. Here energy reserves are adjusted and rebuilt, allowing a certain tolerance to build up.

Hormonal Feedback Mechanism

The body's normal hormonal feedback mechanism now comes into play to shut off continued output of the initiating hormonal agent and thus return blood levels of hormones from various target glands back to their normal levels. For example, during the initial alarm reaction, thyroid hormone and adrenal cortex corticoids, which manage massive immediate metabolic needs, flood the circulation and raise blood levels of these substances. Then, in this second stage of response, these high levels in turn feed back to the controlling master gland, the pituitary, to now shut off or lower its triggering hormones, TSH to the thyroid gland and ACTH to the adrenal glands, for a period of automatic adjustment back to normal balance.

Rebuilding Reserves

As a result of the massive alarm reaction, normal body reserves are rapidly depleted. The blood becomes concentrated with metabolic materials and there is marked loss of body weight. A period of restoration must eventually follow. This period allows the glands and other body tissue reserves to rebuild, the blood dilution to resume normal levels, and the body weight to return toward normal. This vital rebuilding process obviously requires positive nutritional support.[7-9]

Adaptive Homeostasis

The level of this adaptation to the initial or chronic stress depends, of course, on the extent of the stress and the person's coping powers. The stress reaction is generalized throughout the body, always resulting in this general adaptive syndrome identified by Selye.[2] This is true no matter what type of stress is applied. Under the influence of stress, some higher-risk persons may develop such conditions as gastric ulcers, cardiovascular disease, hypertension, headache, or neurosis, depending on the nature of their physical and psychosocial makeup and situation. When stress is superimposed on persons made vulnerable by nutritional deficiency, disorder, or disease, the effect is to make a bad situation worse. Often this is the case, for example, of high-risk populations suffering chronic stress of poverty and malnutrition.

Stage III: Exhaustion of Stress-Coping Resources

After still more prolonged exposure to stress, the adaptation powers of the body weaken and a final stage of exhaustion follows. If the stress is severe enough and applied long enough, particularly if disease compounds it, the person's adaptation energy becomes exhausted and must be restored if life is to continue.

Immunity

Persons under stress of life events experience depressed immune function and increased vulnerability to disease. This is true of both physiologic disease and psychosocial pressure, which can bring crises both large and small. Studies of groups of people under stress have shown measured reduction of immune response and increased episodes of infectious disease.[10] In these measures, one of the immune functions, that of the "natural killer cells" activity, was found to be especially depressed. These important cells are members of the T cell population of lymphoid cells, the **lymphocytes,** a type of white blood cell making up a major component of the body's remarkable defense system.[11,12] Together with a companion B cell population of lymphoid cells, these lymphocytes come from precursor cells in the bone marrow (Figure 16-2).

Lymphocytes
Special white cells from lymphoid tissue that participate in humoral and cell-mediated immunity.

The T cells make up the majority of the circulating pool of small lymphocytes in blood and lymph and in certain areas of the lymph nodes and spleen. A T cell recognizes invading substances by means of specific special receptors on its surface. Upon contact with the *antigen*—any foreign intruder or "nonself," an alien substance such as a virus—the T cells immediately multiply and initiate specific cellular immune responses. They activate the *phagocytes,* special cells that can destroy invaders, and they release chemical mediators to start the inflammatory process. Some T cells can even become "killer cells" themselves and attack antigens directly.

Disease

Researchers studying crisis-related immunity have concluded that heightened and sustained stress can suppress immune function. But whether or

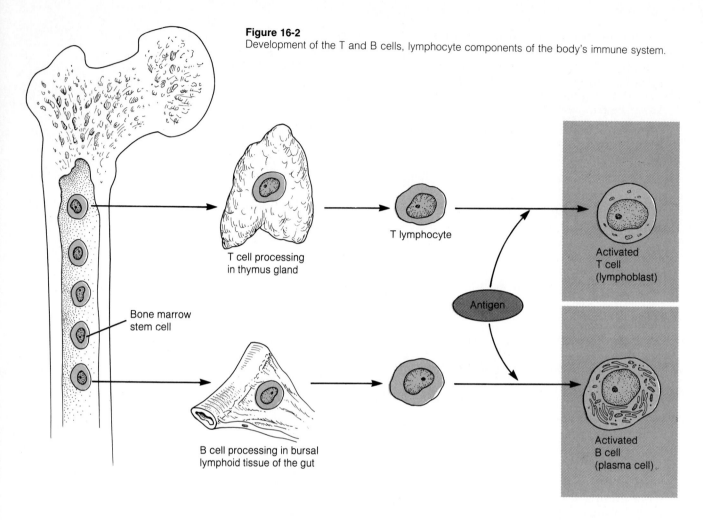

Figure 16-2
Development of the T and B cells, lymphocyte components of the body's immune system.

not this condition leads to disease depends on individual conditioning factors such as poor health and nutrition (see the box on p. 374), exposure to infectious disease, and general physiologic and psychologic resources.[8-10]

Death

The exhaustion stage of response to stress cannot be maintained for long periods of time because body systems begin to wear out in their ability to cope. If resources are not restored and the stress is relentless and prolonged, finally the body's energy sources are depleted and death follows. Intervention must occur earlier to reduce stress, prevent disease, and promote health. A vital part of such intervention is nutritional support.

Life Cycle Stress: High-Risk Population Groups

Life Cycle Stress Periods

At each stage of the human life cycle, specific physiologic and psychosocial developments create nutrition-related stress for both the physical body and the person. In previous chapters we have discussed some of the general stress factors that might intervene along the way, such as poor eating habits, bizarre diets, extreme vegetarianism, substance abuse as with alcohol and drugs, megadoses of food supplements, nutrient imbalances, eating disorders, lack of exercise or extreme exercise, or poor mental attitude. Nutritional needs must be met within the total life context at any particular point. Added stress may be imposed by physical trauma, injury, disease, or disability. Other stress may relate to the workplace, the rapidly changing environment, or increasing social isolation in a profoundly changing society (see Issues and Answers on p. 391). And for many the overriding pain of poverty leads to physical, psychosocial, and mental health problems.

Here, then, we review briefly some of the stress factors through the life cycle and consider approaches to nutritional care. And in the remaining parts of the chapter, we will explore ways of managing high-risk stress as a means of more positive nutritional support and health promotion in general.

Pregnancy
Physiologic and Psychosocial Stress

As indicated in Chapter 11, enormous physiologic changes occur in the pregnant woman's body to sustain and support a healthy pregnancy and its outcome, a healthy baby. But pregnancy also presents added psychologic and socioeconomic stress to both parents as they face changing social and personal roles and financial responsibilities. Many parents have matured physically and emotionally through their own growth and development to meet these changing life needs. But others lack these resources and face greater stress. This is especially true, for example, in teenage pregnancies. Also, cultural and social influences have shaped values and beliefs of both parents about pregnancy. Genetic heritage and previous life experiences and food habits have determined the mother's current health and nutritional reserves to meet the physiologic stress of her pregnancy. All of these conditioning factors are important.

High-Risk Pregnancy: Added Stress Factors

A number of added stress factors can contribute to a high-risk pregnancy and a potential poor outcome. Some of these stresses are present when the pregnancy begins. These include the following: (1) age extremes for reproduction—teenagers aged 15 or younger and women aged 35 or older; (2) frequent pregnancies—3 or more during a 2-year period; and (3) poor obstetric history and fetal performance. These risks are further compounded by the stress of (1) poverty and lack of prenatal care and (2) harmful personal habits. These harmful habits include abuse of alcohol resulting in the well-known fetal alcohol syndrome; abuse of drugs resulting in addicted infants; the smoking of cigarettes, an increasing habit among young women, resulting in low-birth-weight infants; and bizarre or faddist food habits that deny essential nutrients to the fetus. Such behaviors contribute to both fetal damage and to inadequate maternal weight gain and low-birth-weight infants. These preexisting maternal risk factors require special personal counseling and nutritional guidance (see Chapter 11).

High-Risk Pregnancy: Clinical Complications

Still further physiologic and personal stress may be added by clinical complications of the mother's pregnancy. These complications include anemia, pregnancy-induced hypertension, and preexisting maternal disease such as insulin-dependent diabetes mellitus (IDDM) or maternal phenylketonuria (MPKU). Special team care (see Chapter 11) is needed in these complicated pregnancies to provide individual specific nutritional support.

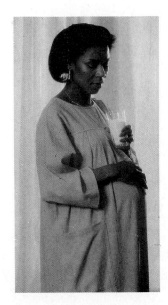

Numerous stress factors can contribute to a high-risk pregnancy, increasing the need for nutritional guidance.

To Probe Further

Interactive Cycle: Stress, Nutritional Status, and Immunity

Stress wears many faces and shows itself in different forms. It imposes an interactive cycle of physiologic events involving nutritional status and the body's line of defense, its all-important immune system. The full effects of stress on nutrient needs and immunity are yet to be completely understood, because both the stress and our responses to it are difficult to measure. But we do know that continued stress is like a run on the metabolic bank, soon exhausting its resources and defenses.

A number of important questions need answers. Precisely how does the neuroendocrine-metabolic cascade triggered by stress affect our need for specific nutrients? How does stress affect our long-term health and well-being? To answer these questions, we need to know just what the role of stress is in our utilization of nutrients, and just what effect our nutrient status has on our response to stress. That they are both related is obvious, but they are conditioned by the nature of the stress and by the individual. And if the stress becomes chronic and is unrelieved, the prolonged hormonal-metabolic toll may be irreversible. The endocrine responses to stress determine the metabolic adjustments that occur in the stressed state. The main purpose of these adjustments is to provide a continuous fuel supply to the central nervous system and the required substrates for function and repair of body tissues.

Although we do not have all the answers yet to questions about the interactive nature of stress, nutritional status, and immunity, we do have enough information at present to emphasize the importance of optimal nutrition in guarding against disease and promoting a rapid recovery when it does occur. The following nutritional factors play lead roles in this overall process:

- **Energy.** Stress may increase the body's basal caloric need as much as 200%. The stress hormones act to increase body heat production, and when this heat is released it is not available to the body as chemical energy for cell metabolism. Then weight loss beyond what could be explained by decreased appetite and food intake occurs. This caloric inefficiency induced by stress accounts for the dramatic increase in energy intake need, which may rise as much as tenfold in severely traumatized persons. And if fat fuel stores are inadequate, the individual may not survive. In this case, thin is not beautiful; thin is dead.
- **Protein.** Stress may increase the body's basal protein need from 60% to as much as 500%. The integrity of body tissues involved in the body's immune system, such as the skin and the mucosal tissue, depends on adequate protein. Mucosal immunity especially depends on the protection of its mucosal secretions, which constantly bathe the body cavities and orifices. These secretions contain a variety of biochemical and immunologic factors. The antibodies formed require protein.
- **Fat.** Dietary fatty acids, notably linoleic and arachidonic acids, influence prostaglandin synthesis by macrophages. In turn these pros-taglandins can stimulate and suppress other cellular and humoral immune functions as needed.

- **Vitamins.** We have long known that vitamin A functions in the maintenance of healthy epithelial tissue such as the outer skin and the inner mucosal tissue. Vitamin A–deficient persons have fewer goblet cells and less protective mucus production with fewer component immunoglobulin factors. Work with vitamin C has shown that it enhances phagocytosis activity by macrophages, and in vitamin C deficiency protective macrophage mobilization and aggregation are impaired. Deficiencies of vitamins A, B_{12}, and folate all impair T cell production response. Antibody production in the spleen after an antigen challenge has been found to be impaired in animals deficient in vitamins A and E and pyridoxine. Megadoses of vitamin E have been associated with suppression of B cell functions. In addition, because of their key functions as coenzymes in energy and protein metabolism, requirements for thiamin, riboflavin, and niacin are increased in response to stress.
- **Minerals.** Deficiencies of zinc impair T cell proliferation and responsiveness. Iron deficiencies affect humoral immunity.

These examples make it clear that nutritional status influences immunity and response to stress. On this foundation we can now build our practice. The challenges of the decade ahead for nutrition scientists are to further define and quantify nutrition's interactive role in both stress and immunity, and to further clarify the exquisite mechanisms involved.

REFERENCES
Barone J: Immunity: a delicate balance, Am Health 6(10):58, 1987.
Berdanier CD: The many faces of stress, Nutr Today 22(2):12, 1987.
Sherman AR: Alterations in immunity related to nutritional status, Nutr Today 21(2):7, 1986.

Infant Growth and Development
Physiologic and Psychosocial Stress

Normal growth demands place both physiologic and psychosocial stress on the infant. Birth itself is a stress. After the period of rapid fetal growth, the full-term neonate moves quickly at birth from a warm, protective, and supportive uterine environment to the stress of the external world, literally cut off from its former umbilical nourishment. Survival depends on immediate adaptation. Not only is physiologic nourishment by either breast-feeding or appropriate formula required, but also psychosocial nurturing by loving care is needed for both physical comfort and emotional support. Indeed, feeding becomes the twofold link to survival by supplying essential nutritional support and the main means of establishing human relationships.

High-Risk Infants

Not all infants are fortunate in their development and growth experience during the stress of these early critical fetal-neonatal-infant periods of life. They carry the additional stress of developmental problems or disease. Tiny babies born prematurely or small for gestational age have low birth weights

(LBW) and suffer some form of intrauterine growth retardation (IUGR). The subgroup IUGR refers to term babies born at 37 or more weeks of gestation, having both weight and length problems. The premature subgroup refers to preterm LBW babies born before week 37 of gestation. In general, the morbidity and mortality rates are significant in these LBW babies.

Other high-risk infants may have birth defects. And still others generally fail to thrive. This growth failure can be attributed to both organic defect possibilities and nonorganic factors contributing to the stress of defective mother-infant interaction.[13] Decreased energy intake causes the lack of appropriate weight gain. But defective mother-infant interaction can cause not only decreased energy intake but also developmental delay and abnormal behaviors. All of these high-risk infants are subjected to greatly increased physiologic and psychosocial stress and bring added emotional stress to their parents and families. All of them require much special care and nutritional support. Careful nutrition and social assessment are needed to identify underlying causes of the associated feeding problems so that appropriate care can be planned.

Childhood Growth and Development
Physiologic and Psychosocial Development

During the period of latent childhood growth between infancy and adolescence, the child's growth rate slows and becomes more erratic, steady but in spurts. Nonetheless, continued growth places metabolic stress demands on the young body that gradually increase the energy and nutrient needs. In the early school years especially, growth rates vary widely as resources are being laid down for the rapid adolescent growth ahead. During these years children need not only physiologic nutrition support but also psychosocial nurturing as they progressively gain personal strengths of autonomy, initiative, and industry through supportive family relationships and other broadening social experiences. Food and mealtimes become an increasingly important means of socialization.

High-Risk Children

Added physiologic and psychosocial stress increase health risks for children. For example, such stresses may be associated with growth failure, developmental disability, or inheritance of chronic disease.

Growth failure. The growth potential of an individual is genetically determined. If conditions are favorable, each child will grow according to his or her own predetermined growth curve, or "canal," giving the name "canalization" to this process of normal individual growth pattern.[14] Unfavorable stressful conditions deflect a child away from this individual predetermined growth curve. The extent of the growth failure depends on the severity of the unfavorable conditions and how long the child is exposed to them without adequate relief, leaving the child stunted and wasted. Depending on the extent of damage and the quality of rehabilitation, the "catch-up" growth may restore a child to his or her growth channel in response to a high-energy diet with appropriate amounts of protein and trace elements. For example, for a weight gain of 20g/kg/day a child requires 174 kcal/kg/day and 4.8 g protein/kg/day to achieve a self-correcting growth response.[14]

Developmental disability. Developmentally disabled children are at high risk for nutritional deficiency and multiple health problems. They have sustained chronic physical or mental impairments during the growth years from numerous causes, including conditions such as cerebral palsy, spina bifida, and Down syndrome. A myriad of psychosocial, economic, and physical stresses face these children and their families. A team of specialists is needed to provide care, with the team nutritionist determining nutritional needs and using available resource persons and agencies as indicated.[15] The development of these children to their highest physical, mental, and emotional potential is based on optimal nutrition.

Inheritance of chronic disease. Children born with various metabolic disorders of genetic origin are now able to develop normally by using from birth a special formula and diet that control the intake of specific nutrients for which the corresponding specific enzyme is missing or inadequate. For example, children screened at birth and found to have phenylketonuria (PKU) cannot metabolize the essential amino acid phenylalanine because of a lack of the cell enzyme phenylalanine hydroxylase. Without treatment the brain would become damaged and severe mental retardation would follow. Now, however, screened at birth and immediately treated with a specific low-phenylalanine diet, including special formulas and foods, they grow normally— but not without stress. The diet is more and more difficult to follow for some children as they grow older, and the stress of feeling "different" often brings strains and relapses in dietary control.

Also, a number of the lipid disorders, as well as essential hypertension, which underlie potential development of coronary heart disease, are familial (see Chapter 20). Children in such genetically high-risk families carry a strong risk for developing these chronic diseases. Thus both pediatricians and nutritionists advise the adoption of prudent family eating patterns that control cholesterol, fat, and sodium intake. Childhood obesity, a growing risk problem, is also receiving more attention.[16]

Adolescent Growth and Development
Physiologic and Psychosocial Development

The flooding hormones of puberty rapidly increase the stress of adolescent growth and sexual maturation. This is an ambivalent period full of stresses and strains as these older children struggle to find their own identities and self-images and reach adult maturity. Individual adolescents vary greatly in response to these stressful tensions, depending on the supportive resources provided for them in their earlier developmental years. The identity crisis of growing up both physically and emotionally is necessary preparation for an adult role in a complex society. There is little wonder that this period is fraught with stress and its problems, many of which are carried into adulthood unresolved. This whole maturation process has never been easy. But in today's rapidly changing world it seems even more profound and produces many psychologic, emotional, and social tensions.

High-Risk Adolescents

A number of young girls, pressured by family and society to maintain the thin "ideal" figure, add the stress of constant dieting to their already increased physiologic demands of accelerated adolescent growth. Some develop a distorted perception of their body image with resulting serious semi-starvation eating disorders of *anorexia nervosa* or *bulimia*. Also, an increasing number of adolescent girls are experiencing the multiple health risks and stresses of teenage pregnancies. Lacking education or skills, they face uncertain futures of rearing their young children as a single parent, unprepared to provide financial or emotional support. The added stress of poverty often results.

Two other sources of physiologic and psychosocial stress bring health risks during the teen years and compromise nutritional status. These are excessive athletic training and abuse of alcohol and other drugs:

1. **Athletics.** The challenge and excitement of team sports sometimes push young preadolescents and adolescents to place added health risks on their bodies. Pressure to be admired by peers, to achieve approval of coach or parents, or to follow in the footsteps of a favored older brother or sister may lead some boys and girls to exceed their physical capacity or sustain serious injury. The constant search for the "competitive edge" may lead to dietary misinformation and exploitation, with consequent nutritional problems.

2. **Alcohol and other drug abuse.** As adolescents approach the drinking age in their community, alcohol becomes a means of appearing more adult and may assume an increasing share of the total energy intake. Pressured by peer groups, some begin to drink at younger and younger ages and reach the stage of addiction by adolescence. Even mild alcohol abuse in the face of the increased nutritional requirements of adolescence can compromise nutritional status; for example, folic acid is destroyed by excessive alcohol. The extent of excessive social drinking, as well as teenage alcoholism in susceptible persons, presents a serious risk to life and health, especially when combined with highway driving, as often occurs after parties. Other drug abuse and addiction have also brought devastating results to many young lives. Many have become addicted as early as elementary school, bringing physical and mental illness, malnutrition, disease, and death. A large part of any alcohol or other drug abuse rehabilitation program must be optimal nutrition support.

Adulthood and Aging
Physiologic Stress of Aging

The biologic changes of aging are general but persons in the advancing years of life experience the physiologic stress of aging in different ways, depending in large measure on their health status. They display a wide variety of individual reactions to normal body stress. They simply get old at different rates and in different ways. On top of individual genetic heritage, each person bears the unique imprint of health and disease experience. This combination has a direct effect on individual aging. But in any case, the body's physical resources gradually decline and risk of disease and dependency increases.

Psychosocial Problems

In young and middle adulthood, personal stress relates mainly to striving to find one's way in the world with family and career.[17,18] Greater stress and risks develop if disease, disability, or poverty is present. The population of older adults aged 85 and older is growing, so individual stress of health concerns and needs of this expanding age group is also increasing. As biologic changes occur there often comes concern about body functions, decreased capacities, increasing social stress and isolation (see Issues and Answers on p. 391), personal losses, and diminished social opportunities to maintain self-esteem. Financial pressures and a decreasing sense of acceptance and accomplishment cause many elderly persons mental stress and loss of personal values. Many feel inadequate. Often they are lonely, restless, unhappy, and uncertain. The greater part of the aging process in any area is culturally determined. Unfortunately, in many instances Western culture imposes a set of negative roles on persons as they reach older age. All of these factors, both physical and psychosocial, increase health risks and vulnerability to disease and malnutrition in the aging population.

At any age, the presence of injury, disease, and disability adds more stress, with increased health and nutrition risks, to the general strains of human growth and development. These high-risk persons are found in hospitals and clinics, medical and rehabilitation centers, community agencies, and homes. In each case special nutritional care and support are needed to help reduce risks and manage stress. Comprehensive nutrition assessment (see Chapter 17) is needed to identify these high-risk patients and plan their care. Extended disabling conditions bring with them still more stress and require continued nutritional support.

Childhood Disease

Growing children are vulnerable to various forms of *protein-calorie malnutrition*, especially children from poor homes and stressed families. The problem of child abuse in some stressed families is a serious one and adds more risk to their physical and emotional health, even to their lives. An underlying malnutrition is easily compounded by the stress of hospitalization and disease. Children with gastrointestinal problems that hinder food intake and utilization are at special risk of growth retardation. For example, inflammatory bowel disease, which often becomes chronic over time, prevents absorption of needed nutrients and stunts growth (see Chapter 19). Metabolic diseases such as insulin-dependent diabetes mellitus (IDDM) and other genetic disorders carry risks of complications involving various organ systems and require special individual management (see Chapter 21). Hypermetabolic diseases such as cancer may threaten life and require vigorous nutritional support (see Chapter 24).

Traumatic Injury and Disability

Persons of any age sustaining critical trauma such as extensive burns (see Chapter 23), spinal cord injury, or other serious injuries and disabilities undergo extreme physiologic and psychosocial stress and are at special risk. They require both immediate care and long-term rehabilitation by a nutrition support team of specialists.[19,20] Three important factors guide this individual nutrition support: (1) need to replenish the large catabolic losses, (2) demand for essential anabolic tissue healing, and (3) need for extensive personal support. The plan of care for these stressed high-risk patients and its outcome depend on (1) age—elderly persons and children are more vulnerable; (2) health condition—any preexisting condition, malnutrition, or dis-

The Stress of Physical Trauma and Disease

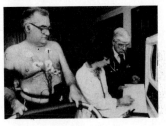

Injury, disease, or disability at any age contributes to stress and increased nutrition risks.

ease such as diabetes or cardiovascular or renal problems complicates care; and (3) wound severity—location, extent, and time elapsed before treatment influence risk and prognosis.

Chronic Diseases of Aging

Added stress and health risks among adults include chronic diseases of aging or any of the multiple risk factors for such diseases. For example, coronary heart disease, the major cause of death in the United States and most other Western societies, is a multifaceted disease with numerous risk factors, as summarized in Table 16-1. Some of these risks involve personal characteristics that we cannot control, such as our genetic heritage. Other are background conditions that can be screened and treated. But in the middle, and most important, are those personal behaviors that we learn and, with motivation, can change. One of these learned behaviors is our degree of ability to cope with life's stresses. Others are harmful habits we can seek to change. Most of these interventions to reduce risk involve in some way food patterns and nutrition.[21] All of these high-risk persons require special nutritional care and support.

Stress Related to Work, Increased Exercise, and Environment

Many persons have increased stress and health risk owing to the nature of their jobs, intensive exercise, and environmental factors. Increasing awareness of these problems, preventive measures to reduce risks, and health care for exposed persons have begun to develop through work-site programs, sports medicine practice, and community health programs.

Stress of the Workplace
Work-Site Hazards

Increased physical risks and stresses occur in labor-intensive jobs and those with safety and health hazards, such as use of heavy machinery or hazardous tools and working at heights. Poor lighting and ventilation, as well as smoking, present health risks in offices and industrial plants. Two special high-risk groups are (1) migrant farm workers whose lives involve multiple physical, psychologic, and socioeconomic stress factors; and (2) workers in electronic and chemical industries, and those handling radioactive materials. Such groups of workers may be exposed to hazardous chemicals or other carcinogenic substances.

Table 16-1

Multiple Risk Factors in Cardiovascular Disease

Personal characteristics (no control)	Learned behaviors (intervene and change)	Background conditions (screen and treat)
Sex	Stress and coping	Hypertension
Age	Cigarette smoking	Diabetes mellitus
Family history	Sedentary life	Hyperlipidemia (especially
	Obesity	hypercholesterolemia)
	Food habits	
	Excess fat	
	Excess sugar	
	Excess salt	

Management-Employee Relations

Also, in positions of business management, the well-known "executive syndrome" of stress-related ills—peptic ulcer, heart disease, hypertension, diabetes, and alcohol and other drug abuse—can result from the competitive pressures of managing a business. Sometimes in today's business world these pressures are reflected in deteriorating management-employee relations and mounting stress from our jobs. A study by the National Center for Health Statistics indicated that more than half of the 40,000 workers surveyed reported increasing job stress.[22] Much of this stress is spilling over to affect workers' personal lives and health. In this business age of dislocation and uncertainty, as we are shifting from the heavy industry of the past to a more technologic service economy of the present and future, many workers are saying "my job is killing me" and naming a tyrannical boss as the main culprit. These job-related ills also affect workers suffering economic hardships, unemployment, or underemployment.

The Stress of Heavy Exercise

Aside from heavy labor on the job, many persons in athletics and intensive physical fitness programs also suffer physical stress and risk injury (see Chapter 14). Heavy athletic exercise places great stress on the body. Heavy body-contact team sports, especially in the big business of professional teams where high stakes in money and competition are involved, carry tremendous pressure and risk of disabling injury. For every "star" there are hundreds of battered bodies who never make top billing or income. And every team member's playing life is short. Also, compulsive persons in individual athletic activities, such as running, or those in strenuous physical fitness programs can be severely injured.

Environmental Stress Factors

Persons exposed to a variety of environmental stress factors carry additional health risks. Air and water pollution is one of the prices we are paying for our advanced technologic society. Health problems accumulate over time, for example, when buried radioactive or chemical wastes leach out into ground water and contaminate public water sources, or when automobile and factory emissions contaminate air and increase respiratory problems. The ever increasing use of pesticides or other potentially dangerous agricultural chemicals (see Chapter 9) has led to accumulated exposure for farm workers and consumers alike. Only recently, after a 14-year stalemate, have chemical companies and public interest groups finally agreed on pesticide law reforms, a significant part of which will speed up the safety review of old pesticides in long use.[23]

The High-Risk Problem of Poverty
Poverty and Hunger

We are made increasingly aware through the daily news or personal contact and experience in our own communities that poverty and its toll in human lives are hard realities for many persons and stand in stark contrast to an otherwise affluent society. As we discussed in previous chapters, extreme poverty and its ever-present companion hunger, even to famine and death, exist in a number of the world's nations, fanned by war and class barriers.

Poverty, Psychosocial Stress, and Mental Health

But the social roots of poverty and its harvest of hunger do not stop at our borders. Even here in the United States, one of the wealthiest countries on earth, many studies document a "growing epidemic" of hunger and malnutrition among the poor.[24,25] The Physician Task Force on Hunger in America has found that in the United States alone, at least 20 million persons, 12 million of whom are children, suffer from hunger. In the past hunger has been viewed mainly as a problem of overpopulation. World population has just passed the 5 billion mark and grows daily. Now, however, hunger is recognized as more than just a problem of numbers of people. It is also seen as a major problem, with economic and social and political roots, of the increasing gap between the rich and the poor, within and between countries.

Poverty and Politics

In recent times hunger in America became extensive and was recognized by official sources. Government responses during the 1960s and 1970s almost eliminated the problem, with special programs to reach and feed poor, high-risk persons such as isolated elderly people, poor pregnant women, mothers, infants, and children. However, government policy changes of a new administration in the early 1980s effectively reduced help to the poor, and more families slipped below the officially declared poverty line. Together with economically depressed areas of unemployment and "new poor," the number of malnourished persons has continued to grow.[26] The most recent report of the Physician Task Force on Hunger in America, based on government figures and the physicians' own survey of 25 depressed areas in 8 states, concluded that despite a gradual national economic growth, 32.4 million people do not share these benefits of an improved life. Instead, they live—barely—on an annual income at or below a federal poverty level of about $9000 for a family of 3.[27]

A number of socioeconomic and political factors have contributed to the plight of the millions of Americans who are living at or below the poverty line. These include economic displacement, underemployment, unemployment, homelessness, marital breakup, poor health, alcoholism and other drug abuse, functional illiteracy, mental illness, and wage discrimination based on sex and race.[28,29] As is true in any system, those holding political power at any given time and place determine the economic, agricultural, and food distribution policies that reflect their ideology and may or may not meet the needs of the people involved. Many of these persons, some of them homeless, must rely regularly on soup kitchens and food banks to supplement their meager diets. This relentless stress of poverty imposes large health risks on individuals and families, especially the growing numbers of young children caught in its grip.

The Psychosocial Stress of Poverty

Tremendous human problems exist among the poor, problems that at times seem almost insurmountable. Often a "culture of poverty" develops and is reinforced and perpetuated by society's values and attitudes. Such attitudes serve to wall off poor persons more completely than do physical barriers. As a result of the extreme pressures and stress caused by their living conditions, poverty-stricken persons become victims of negative attitudes and behaviors that influence their use of community health services.

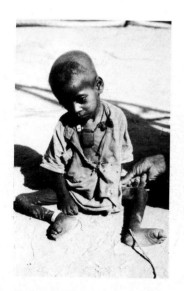

The stress of poverty imposes large health and nutrition risks.

These psychosocial stresses of poverty further increase health risks of persons involved. It is small wonder that they often become frustrated with despair, caught in a vicious cycle of feelings of isolation, insecurity, and powerlessness. As health workers, we must begin with self-awareness of personal social values and attitudes, if we are to be true "helping vehicles" and agents of constructive change. Only then can we establish a genuine rapport within which we can work together. And we must *listen*—positively, actively, and creatively. Refer back to Chapter 9 and reread the discussion about the ecology of human nutrition and the twin problems of poverty and malnutrition. We need to constantly resensitize ourselves to these human problems and never view them in the abstract, but in terms of the human lives they represent.

Mental Health Needs and Problems

Human Needs and Strivings

As indicated, throughout the life cycle, the mature human personality develops through a series of positive responses to normal psychosocial developmental tasks.[3,4] Given the necessary physical and emotional support, children develop into mature adults, with the turbulent teen years yielding the more assured self-identity of adulthood. On this basis, then, the young adult can develop significant personal relationships, rather than become socially isolated. The middle adult can nurture the next generation in turn, rather than withdraw into self-absorption. And the older adult can become a whole integrated person, rather than retreat into bitterness and negative attitudes, poorly equipped to deal with life's necessary adjustment to old age and health problems. These maturing processes blend with all basic human needs and strivings. All persons struggle to meet these human needs, from basic survival necessities of food to appease hunger to higher need levels of safety, love, self-esteem, and self-fulfillment.[5]

Mental Health Problems

For many persons, however, depending on the coping resources they developed through the maturing process, conditioned by any genetic predisposition, life stresses produce increased risk of mental health problems. Many of these problems clinicians see daily in primary health care. A recent National Institute of Mental Health study confirms relatively high rates of mental disorders among medical outpatient services in primary care settings, ranging between 19% and 27%.[30] An increasing number of these disorders were found to be in the substance abuse-dependency category, centering on alcohol and drugs, the most prevalent disorder among male patients. Other categories included phobias and affective disorders such as depression, the two most prevalent among female patients. All of these mental health problems involve a large high-risk population and have implications for public health, food behaviors, and nutritional status.

Long-Term Institutional Care

At special risk are persons in long-term institutional care facilities for both physical and mental disorders. Often increased numbers of patients and inadequate staff personnel result in limited individual attention with increased stress of nutrition and health problems.

Prison Populations

Increased numbers of crimes, many of them drug-related, have led to highly crowded conditions in prisons, making a situation that is bad at best even worse. Such high-stress settings multiply both physical and mental health risks, and individual needs often suffer.

High-Risk Stress Management

As we have seen here, a key factor in the development of disease and risk of poor nutrition is stress, both physiologic and psychosocial. This basic risk factor permeates human life, with both positive and negative effects. The goal of health promotion therefore centers on managing stress in positive ways by (1) identifying high-risk persons, (2) recognizing key elements in daily stress management, and (3) planning appropriate methods of reducing stress and its health risks. This positive approach applies not only to the lives of our clients and patients but also to our own. The familiar "burnout" syndrome is not uncommon.

Key Elements in Daily Stress Management
Personal Approaches

Key coping factors for building positive personal resources to manage daily stress include a sense of being in control of one's own life, developing positive personality characteristics, and being able to do some self-assessment.

Control of personal life. Many studies indicate that stress will be better tolerated and provoke fewer negative physiologic effects if the person has a measure of control over it.[31] Some stressors in life can be changed, many cannot. But the ultimate control lies within: we choose how we will respond.

Role of personality. Positive personality characteristics, such as hopefulness, a positive outlook or general life orientation, and ability to "go with the flow," have been found to correlate with a better ability to deal with life's stressors and with a lowered risk of illness. On the other hand, a rigid, "uptight" approach to life places persons at much higher risk. This high-risk type of person is generally characterized by two basic behaviors: (1) work-compulsion—tries to do too much in one space of time, expects a great deal from self, and has unreasonable expectations about others; and (2) free-floating hostility—loses temper easily, is impatient, and struggles against time and other people.[32] These behaviors may not be easy to change. After all, American business and society reward such single-minded competitive productivity. But for healthier and happier living, some personal change is worth the effort.

Self-assessment. Ask yourself some important questions: Do you know how you typically react? Do you know what level of stress you are operating under? Do you know what direction you seem to be taking? Then seek the following alternative ways of changing your stress pattern: (1) determine your own priorities and values in life; (2) avoid those stressors that can be avoided; and (3) displace stressors that cannot be eliminated with other positive activities to strengthen your coping ability and develop more constructive relaxed behavior. These positive activities include a focus on key elements that help displace and reduce stress: diet, exercise, relaxation, and personal interest areas, as described below.

Social Approaches

Human beings are by nature social beings and need other people in their lives to sustain positive health. Although persons at times cherish quiet times alone, there are no true hermits. Everyone needs some kind of social support system, a network of friends and family to count on when help is needed. Also, meaningful common interest groups may provide additional stimulus and support. These include groups such as church, school, or special courses, community groups, sports teams, personal interest or hobby groups, music groups or choruses, computer clubs, political groups, volunteer work, or social clubs. A sense of belonging can be developed many ways. This feeling, one of having something to contribute and having someone to turn to, is critical as a buffer from unavoidable life stresses.

Methods of Reducing Stress and Health Risks

Positive Health Promotion

The preventive approach of developing positive health means making changes wherever necessary to build positive attitudes and habits. This life style approach includes actions in three main areas—exercise, relaxation, and diet—to reduce stress-related risk factors and promote health.

Physical Activities

A number of activities to build physical fitness are described in Chapter 14, including aerobic exercise for strengthening heart and lung action. But there are many more beneficial effects of physical exercise. As a means of improving both mental and physical health, exercise can do the following:

- Drain off accumulated excess chemical messengers, catecholamines and hormones, triggered by the primitive "fight or flight" response to stress.
- Increase the rate and efficiency of body metabolism.
- Decrease body fat deposits and help maintain a healthy weight.
- Increase blood levels of high-density lipoproteins (HDL), which help control serum cholesterol and decrease risk of coronary heart disease.
- Help dissipate anger and hostility.
- Improve overall health and well-being, decreasing risk of illness and its physiologic and psychologic stress.
- Induce a meditation-like state, bringing a sense of detachment and mental relaxation.
- Brighten the mood and help maintain a positive outlook.

Relaxation Exercises

Relaxation is the needed counterbalance with physical activity as a means of reducing stress and its high-risk effects. The ways persons unwind are as varied as the persons themselves. But a personally satisfying means of relaxing is important to everyone. Even persons with turbulent and demanding lives have learned to find little daily time-out opportunities that create islands of peace to help break the cycle of chronic stress.[33] For many persons, though, this attitude and this ability do not come easily or naturally. Our rigid and fast-paced lifestyle cultivates negative ways in which people physically rein-force stress in their lives, ways in which they "take it out" on others around them and on their own bodies. Muscle tension is a common result, as are headaches, backaches, and leg cramps—all classic symptoms of stress over-load.

A number of useful techniques are available that help people *learn* to relax. With practice, a necessity for any learning, persons not only can re-lax muscle tensions but also help control such autonomic functions as breathing, pulse rate, blood pressure, and peripheral blood circulation. These techniques include biofeedback, progressive muscle relaxation exer-cises, and meditation with visual imagery. A number of medical centers are studying the induced relaxation response, used with meditation and guided imagery to help treat problems.[34] Investigators have found strong evidence that the calming effects of these techniques relieve stress and help support the body's immune system. To build a personal program, individual methods of relaxation will vary, with some techniques being assisted by background tapes. But with regular practice, significant personal results will follow.

Diet

First, a word of warning. Despite the great amount of food misinformation available today from many sources, there is no "wonder cure" for stress. Be-ware the wonder-food or supplement claim, the so-called magic properties of any specific nutrient or food. Instead seek a basic balanced dietary pattern that is both nutritionally sound and personally satisfying.

Nutritional balance. In general, a balanced diet is one that provides suffi-cient energy to maintain a healthy weight and supplies all the necessary ma-cronutrients and micronutrients. As yet, no clear scientific evidence relates specific nutrients to stress, and stress itself is hard to measure because of its many faces. But there is increasing interest and concern among scientists and clinicians working in the area that stress may well affect nutrient needs in ways we do not yet fully understand.[8] It is true, of course, that in cases of debilitation and malnutrition, more nutrient density is needed to replenish stores. But in most instances of usual daily-living stress patterns, a reasonable and regular diet of sound nutrition in satisfying food choices is the need. As we discussed in Chapter 9 and as indicated in Table 16-2, a complex web of many different factors influences food choices. Being aware of these influ-ences may help a person make more positive choices. Whatever the choices may be, the well-nourished person has a much better means of coping with stress, be it severe or mild, and of maintaining strong immune defenses against disease.[9]

Nonetheless, as easy as it sounds to speak of balanced diets, surveys in-dicate that Americans as a whole eat a diet often deficient in basic nutri-ents such as iron, calcium, magnesium, zinc, vitamin A, vitamin C, and folic acid.[35] The simple admonition to "eat right" can allow many variations in food choices and still follow wise health promotion guidelines (see Chapter 1). It is, in fact, a simple prescription that society would do well to incorpo-rate into a new, healthier lifestyle, along with some daily form of exercise and relaxation.

Physical factors	Social factors	Physiologic factors
Food supply available	Advertising	Allergy
Food technology	Culture	Disability
Geography, agriculture, distribution	Education (nutrition and general)	Health-disease status
Personal economics, income	Political and economic policies	Heredity
Sanitation, housing	Religion and social custom	Personal food acceptance
Season, climate	Social class, role	Needs, energy, or nutrients
Storage and cooking facilities	Social problems, poverty, or alcoholism	Therapeutic diets

Table 16-2
Factors Determining Food Choices

Food and mood. We all know from personal experience that mood influences the food that we eat. Sometimes either overeating or loss of appetite is associated with periods of depression or disappointment. "Comfort foods" have a place in dealing with stress. Plan for their wise use in times of need.

Food pattern and pace. Food habits are hard to change. They are always tied to lifestyle. Many persons eat rapidly and irregularly, and suffer both physical and emotional consequences. Persons are better able to deal with stress if they simply slow their eating to savor the food, eat smaller "minimeals" more frequently, and avoid the rich, heavy meals that often make up the typical food pattern. Moderation and variety are the key. Begin with breakfast, needed by the body after the overnight fast, and continue through the day with small amounts of food to refuel the body at regular intervals. Avoid the excesses of fat, salt, sugar, and in some cases caffeine (mostly in the form of coffee) that Americans tend to eat. Over 80% of American adults drink coffee; 75% of these drink 2 or more cups a day, and 16% drink over 6 cups a day.[36] Individual sensitivity to caffeine is highly variable, but it is a stimulant drug that many consider to be abused. In larger intakes, it depletes the body's vitamin C and thiamin stores, and even a mild deficiency of thiamin may create nervousness, irritability, loss of memory, or inability to concentrate.

Socioeconomic Needs

In cases of economic stress, various food assistance programs may help supply needed food (see Chapter 10). Other community programs such as food banks and public meals help fill emergency needs.

Hypermetabolic Needs

Additional energy and nutritive demands are created by the physiologic stress of hypermetabolic conditions such as traumatic injury, surgery, infection, or cancer. The magnitude of the metabolic response varies. But in any case it underscores the importance of good prestress nutritional status on a regular basis.

To Sum Up

The modern world is demanding and complex. It exposes human beings to many stresses and risk factors that affect nutritional status and health, both physical and emotional. Among these risk factors, stress plays a major role. It triggers a cascade of primitive automatic physiologic events, designed as a "fight or flight" mechanism to protect the body through the general alarm and adaptive responses. But in a modern stress-filled world this reaction only compounds the problem and contributes to illness. Throughout life, physiologic and psychosocial stress attends growth and development, with special high-risk persons being pregnant women, infants, young children, adolescents, and elderly persons.

At any age additional stress factors may increase health risks for vulnerable persons. These stress factors include physical trauma and disease, disability, environmental problems, the multiple problems of poverty and general economic stress with greater repercussions in minority populations, and mental problems. High-stress management involves both personal and social approaches, based on identified individual and family needs, goals, and expectations. Methods of reducing stress and health risks focus on positive promotion of health and nutrition and helping to build greater effective coping capacity through sound diet, relaxation, and physical activity, with a strengthened personal support system.

Questions for Review

1. Describe the general adaptive syndrome identified by Selye, which the body activates in response to stress, in terms of the physiologic events in each of its three stages. Why does this response create problems in today's modern society?
2. Identify sources of physiologic and psychosocial stress in each of the growth and development stages of the life cycle. Select several of these problems, describe their nature, and outline general care.
3. Describe additional high-risk stress conditions that may occur throughout the life cycle, giving approaches to planning nutrition and health care. Give special attention to the problem of poverty.
4. Identify and describe key elements in daily stress management and methods of reducing stress and health risks.

References

1. Selye H: The stress of life, New York, 1956, McGraw-Hill Book Co.
2. Selye H: Hunger and stress, Nutr Today 5(1):2, 1970.
3. Erikson E: Childhood and society, New York, 1963, WW Norton & Co, Inc.
4. Hall E: A conversation with Erik Erikson, Psychol Today 17(6):22, 1983.
5. Maslow AH: Motivation and personality, New York, 1954, Harper & Row, Inc.
6. Axelrod J and Reisine TD: Stress hormones: their interaction and regulation, Science 224:452, 1984.
7. Wallis C: Stress—can we cope? Time, p 48, June 6, 1983.
8. Berdanier CD: The many faces of stress, Nutr Today 22(2):12, 1987.
9. Sherman AR: Alterations in immunity related to nutritional status, Nutr Today 21(4):7, 1986.
10. Miller JA: Immunity and crises, large and small, Sci News 129(2):12, 1987.
11. Young JD and Cohen ZA: How killer cells kill, Sci Am 258(1):38, 1988.
12. Cohen IR: The self, the world, and autoimmunity, Sci Am 258(4):52, 1988.

13. Powell GF: Nutrition in nonorganic failure to thrive, Clin Nutr 4(2):54, 1985.

14. Ashworth A and Millward DJ: Catch-up growth in children, Nutr Rev 44:157, May 1986.

15. Wodarski LA: Nutrition intervention in developmental disabilities: an interdisciplinary approach, J Am Diet Assoc 85(2):218, 1985.

16. Kolata G: Obese children: a growing problem, Science 232:20, Apr 4, 1986.

17. Cohen S and Syme SL: Social support and health, New York, 1985, Academic Press.

18. House JS, Landis KR, and Umberson D: Social relationships and health, Science 241:540, July 29, 1988.

19. Brauer PM and Swinamer D: Nutritional support of the critically ill. Part I: Review, J Can Diet Assoc 46:292, Nov 1985.

20. Brauer PM and Swinamer D: Nutritional support of the critically ill. Part II: Guidelines for the clinical dietitian, J Can Diet Assoc 46:304, Nov 1985.

21. Leerhsen C and Namuth T: Alcohol and the family, Newsweek, p 62, Jan 18, 1988.

22. Miller A and others: Stress on the job, Newsweek, p 40, April 25, 1988.

23. Sun M: Antagonists agree on pesticide law reform, Science 232:16, April 4, 1986.

24. Physician Task Force for Hunger in America: The growing epidemic, Cambridge, Mass, 1985, Harvard University School of Public Health.

25. Physician Task Force for Hunger in America: Increasing hunger and declining help, Cambridge, Mass, 1986, Harvard University School of Public Health.

26. Brown JL: Hunger in the U.S., Sci Am 256(2):37, 1987.

27. American notes: The steady hold of hunger, Time, p 63, Nov 9, 1987.

28. Foerster S and Hinton A: Hunger in America: an ADA perspective, J Am Diet Assoc 87(11):1571, 1987.

29. Cross AT: Politics, poverty, and nutrition, J Am Diet Assoc 87(8):1007, 1987.

30. Kessler LG and others: Psychiatric diagnoses of medical service users: evidence from the Epidemiologic Catchment Area Program, Am J Pub Health 77(1):18, 1987.

31. Stein RA: Personal strategies for living with less stress, New York, 1983, John Gallagher Communications, Ltd.

32. Ferguson T: Type A behavior and the Type B solution, Med Self-Care 12:36, Spring 1983.

33. Ferguson T: Dr. Pelletier's guide to do-it-yourself stress management, Med Self-Care 36:46, Sept/Oct 1986.

34. Squires S: The power of positive imagery: visions to boost immunity, Am Health 6(6):56, 1987.

35. Pao EM and Mickle SJ: Problem nutrients in the United States, Food Technology 35:58, Sept 1981.

36. Gelmch WH: A regimen for stress reduction, Supervisory Management 27:16, Dec 1982.

Further Readings

Berdanier CD: The many faces of stress, Nutr Today 22(2):12, 1987.
This author clarifies the many ways that stress may affect nutrient needs, using helpful illustrations and a table showing the effect of stress on the basal requirements for selected nutrients.
Brown JL: Hunger in the U.S., Sci Am 256(2):37, 1987.

Leverett M and others: Governor Cuomo's nutrition education campaign in a low-income urban setting, J Nutr Educ 18(6):247, 1986.
These articles describe the devastating effects of poverty and hunger in American lives and application of this knowledge to a state project in New York to help individuals and families on food stamps achieve better nutrition.

Cross AT: Politics, poverty, and nutrition, J Am Diet Assoc 87(8):1007, 1987.

This sensitive nutritionist-attorney-educator reviews the political background of poverty and nutrition in the United States and makes a strong case for viewing access to adequate food and freedom from hunger and malnutrition as basic human rights.

Ferguson T: Dr. Pelletier's guide to do-it-yourself stress management, Med Self-Care 35:46, Sept/Oct 1986.

This physician-editor of a popular self-care journal provides excellent stress management guidelines from discussions with stress expert Ken Pelletier, clinical psychologist who recently developed such a program for Blue Cross.

Report, Tension—the good, the bad, and the manageable, Univ Calif Berkeley Wellness Letter 3(8):7, 1987.

This brief report lists practical ways of defining stress and dealing with it. For the entire booklet on dealing with tensions, write to the National Mental Health Association, 1021 Prince Street, Alexandria, VA 22314.

Social Isolation Stress and Health

Part of being human is the social activity of eating. Even on the occasions when we eat alone, we are experiencing the social web of our culture in the nature of the food and the meanings it has for us. It is small wonder, then, that food intake and social relationships are inevitably interwoven with nutritional status and health. When deprived of these significant relations, we feel the stress of social isolation and our health suffers.

But, you may well ask, what is new about these associations? We've seen before that isolated persons seem to have more health problems. This is true. Scientists interested in this issue have long noted such associations between social relationships and health. But the reasons behind their observations have been far less clear, raising still more unanswered questions about cause-and-effect relationships. For example, does the lack of satisfying social relationships itself cause people to become ill or die? Or are people with ill health just less likely to establish and maintain significant social relationships? Or is there some other causal factor, such as a *misanthropic* (Greek *miso*, hatred; *anthropos*, man) personality, which predisposes persons to "hate mankind" in general and leads to lowered capacity to form quality social relationships in particular, that makes persons become ill or die? A growing body of evidence, however, is beginning to bring some answers. It is beginning to reveal the significant impact of social isolation stress on health and its role as an important risk factor of growing concern in our rapidly changing society.

Background studies

The concept of "social support" first appeared in the mental health literature of the mid-1970s and was linked to the rapidly developing field of research on stress and its psychosocial and physiologic associations with the causes of health and illness. There was growing recognition that chronic disease in an aging population and changing society was caused not by a single factor such as a microbe—as had often been the case in the past—but rather by multiple behavioral, environmental, biologic, and genetic factors, which combined over time to produce illness or death. Both population studies and clinical research began to bring some answers.

Population studies. Compelling evidence from an early 1965 baseline study of 4775 urban adults in Alameda County, California, aged 30 to 69 years, which surveyed four types of social ties—marriage, extended family and friends, church, and other formal or informal group affiliations—indicated that lack of social relationships constitutes a major risk factor for mortality. Similar population studies followed in other places such as Tecumseh, Michigan; Evans County, Georgia; Gothenberg, Sweden; and rural eastern Finland. Although methods and results varied and raised further questions for study, there was a remarkable consistency in the finding that social relationships do predict mortality for men and women in a wide range of populations, even after adjustment for medical risk factors involved.

Clinical studies. There was also growing evidence from clinical research with both animals and humans that variations in social contacts produce both psychologic and physiologic effects that could, if prolonged, lead to serious illness or death. On the basis of results from a wide range of studies through the 1970s and early 1980s, a psychophysiologic theory was proposed, reinforcing Selye's earlier work on stress, to explain how social relationships and contacts can promote health and protect against disease. This broad base of studies suggests that social relationships and contacts mediate their effect through the *amygdala* (Greek *amygdale*, almond), a small oval complex

Continued.

Social Isolation Stress and Health—cont'd

of nuclei within the tip of the brain's temporal lobe connected through the limbic cortex to the hypothalamus. This mediation acts to (1) activate the anterior hypothalamic zone, stimulating release of human growth hormone; and (2) inhibit the posterior hypothalamic zone, depressing secretion of ACTH, cortisol, catecholamines, and associated sympathetic autonomic nervous system activity. These mechanisms are consistent with the impact of social relations on illness or death from a wide range of causes, as well as adverse effects on the growth and development of infants and young children who are deprived of these early satisfying social contacts and fail to thrive. Overall, the theory and evidence for the impact of social relationships on health are steadily building from both physiologic and psychosocial studies and clinical experience.

Risk factor for health

The growing evidence of social relationships as a cause of risk factor in illness and death from a wide range of diseases is probably stronger than the evidence that led to the designation of Type A behavior pattern as a risk factor for coronary heart disease. The evidence on the relationship between social relationships and health is as strong as that for cigarette smoking established in the Surgeon General's 1964 report. Although the current evidence firmly establishes a lack of social relationships as a risk factor in illness or death, three basic questions require further investigation: What precise mechanisms and processes link social relationships to health? What "levels of exposure" to social relationships determine these effects? How can we lower the prevalence of relative social isolation in our modern society or lessen its harmful effects on health?

Linking mechanisms

Over the past decade, social support research has established the supportive quality of social relationships, especially their capacity to buffer or moderate the harmful effects of stress and other health hazards. But recent experimental studies with animals and humans seem to indicate that social relationships have generally beneficial effects on health, not solely or primarily attributable to their buffering effects, and that there may be aspects of social relationships other than their supportive quality that account for these positive effects. Current investigators point to our need to understand better the social, psychologic, and biologic processes that link quality and quantity of social relationships to health. Social support is only one of these processes, whether it is in the form of emotional nurturing, practical help, or information. But social relationships may also affect health because they regulate or integrate human thought, feelings, motivation, and behavior in ways that promote health. Current views suggest that social relationships affect health by (1) fostering a sense of meaning or wholeness to life; and (2) facilitating health-promoting behaviors such as sound diet, proper sleep, regular exercise, appropriate use of alcohol (if used at all), avoidance of cigarette smoking or the use of other harmful drugs, and adherence to medical regimens or the seeking of appopriate medical care.

Determinants of social relationships

Clearly, both biology and personality affect persons' health and the quality and quantity of their social relationships. Current research shows that social relationships have a predictive, and arguably causal, association with health in their own right. But the quality and extent of persons' social relationships is also a function of broader social forces. Whether we are employed, are married, attend church, belong to organizations, frequently see friends or relatives, and the nature of these contacts, are all determined in part by our positions in the larger social structure. This social structure is further stratified by age, race, sex, and socioeconomic status and is organized in terms of residential communities, work organizations, and larger political and economic structures. Surveys indicate that those persons generally less socially integrated in our society are the poor, the elderly, and blacks. Also, changing social patterns of having fewer children, living longer, and moving frequently affect opportunities for work, marriage, living and working in different settings, making friends, and seeing relatives. And all of these social patterns are themselves subject to larger economic and political change, which can directly affect persons' social relationships.

To verify this research base concerning the significant association of social relationships to health, we have only to look around us at our rapidly changing society and the effects of these changes in people's lives over the past few decades. In contrast with the 1950s, for example, adults today are less likely to be married, more likely to be living alone and to live longer, and less likely to belong to voluntary organizations or visit informally with others. These far-reaching social changes mean that in the twenty-first century, soon to be upon us, we will see a steady increase in the number of older people who lack spouses or children, the very persons to whom they would likely turn for social support.

It is indeed ironic that we are just now learning the full impact of social relationships to our health and well-being, at a time of great social change when we have an increasing likelihood of losing some of our more traditional social supports. The implications of the increasing social isolation stress are obvious for community health care programs and resources to help meet these changing needs.

REFERENCES

Cohen S and Syme SL: Social support and health, New York, 1985, Academic Press.

House JS, Landis KR, and Umberson D: Social relationships and health, Science 241:540, July 29, 1988.

Lazarus RS and Folkman S: Stress, appraisal, and coping, New York, 1984, Springer.

Wietzman LT: The divorce revolution, New York, 1985, Free Press.

Williams RB: Perspectives in behavioral medicine, New York, 1985, Academic Press.

Part III

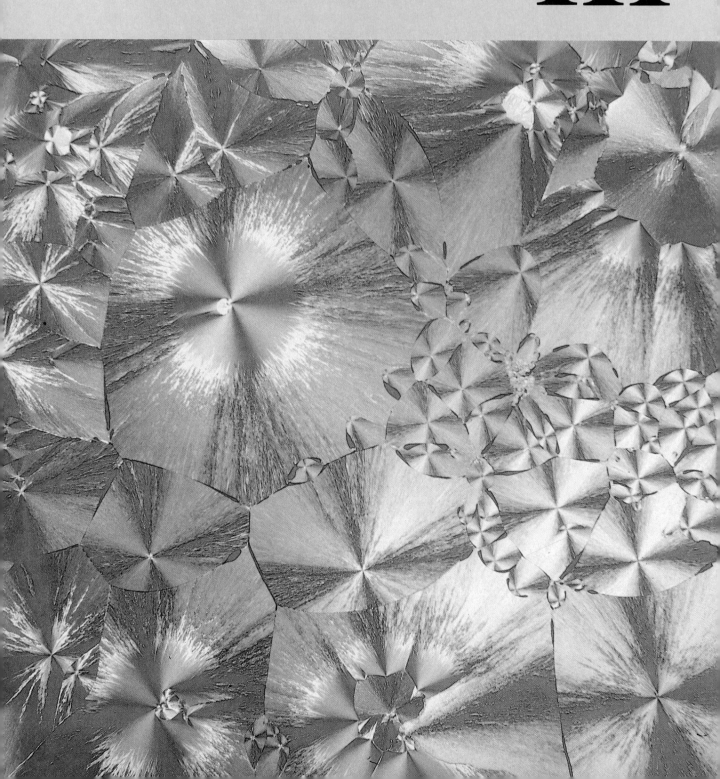

Introduction to Diet Therapy

17 Nutritional Assessment and Therapy in Patient Care

Chapter Objectives

After studying this chapter, the student should be able to:

1. Recognize the aspects of our modern health care system that can create problems in patient care and plan ways of minimizing their effects.
2. Identify and describe the components of the therapeutic process in patient care.
3. Relate methods of basic nutritional assessment to planning sound nutritional care.
4. Plan and carry out quality standards of nutritional care for all patients.

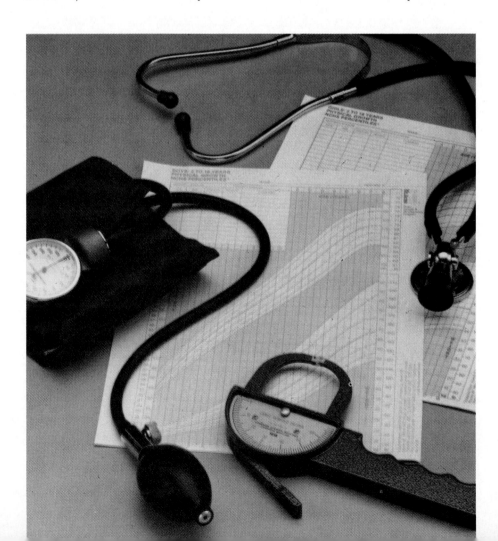

Persons face acute illness or chronic disease and its treatment in a variety of settings: the acute care hospital, the long-term rehabilitation center, the extended care facility, the clinic, the private office, and the home. In all instances nutritional care is fundamental. It is vital support for any medical treatment. Frequently it is the primary therapy in itself.

Comprehensive nutritional assessment provides the necessary data for appropriate nutritional therapy based on identified needs. Clinical nutritionists, all registered dietitians (RDs) with advanced degrees in nutritional science, use their expertise and skills to make sound clinical judgments and work effectively with the clinical care team. Together these professionals provide an essential component for successful medical treatment. They assist the patient in recovery from illness or injury, help the person maintain follow-up care to promote health, and also help to control health care costs.

With this chapter, we begin our final study sequence on clinical nutrition. Here we focus first on the comprehensive assessment and care of the patient's nutritional needs. Wherever the place of care and whatever the need, the health care practitioners, the patient, and the family work together to support the healing process and promote health.

Stress of the Therapeutic Encounter

In the modern hospital setting the therapeutic encounter between health care providers and their patients occurs under stressful conditions at best. Several factors can contribute to added nutritional toll.

Bed Rest

Even though the reason for the hospitalization may indicate the need for bed rest, at the same time the bed rest itself can have detrimental effects on the body's physiology.[1] For example, after just 3 days of lying supine in bed, the body begins to lose its resistance to the pull of gravity and continuing inactivity diminishes muscle tone, bone calcium, plasma volume, and gastric secretions, bringing some impairment of glucose tolerance and shifts in body fluids and electrolytes.

Hospital Malnutrition

Hospital or iatrogenic malnutrition has been widely documented. First, hospitalized patients with hypermetabolic and physiologic stress of illness or injury are at particular risk for malnutrition from their increased needs for nutritional support. Then, in addition, patients may have inadequate nourishment from such ward management problems as (1) highly restricted diets remaining on order and unsupplemented too long, (2) lack of adequate admission nutrition screening or follow-up monitoring to identify high-risk patients and provide essential nutritional support,[2-4] or (3) meals that are missed because of interference of medical ward rounds and clinical test procedures. For example, an audit in a Wisconsin hospital revealed that in 1 week 5% of the patient trays were not served at all, 24% were held back be-

Hospitalized Patients: The Therapeutic Process

cause patients were having medical procedures performed at mealtime, and 15% were served but uneaten because of poor appetite.[5]

Hospital Setting and System

An injured or ill patient, each of whom is a unique person, requires special treatment and care. At the same time a sometimes formidable array of staff persons seek to determine needs and implement what each perceives to be appropriate care. It is no surprise that the course does not always run smoothly or that patients often feel intimidated and powerless.[6] Sometimes our complex system and highly specialized technology get in the way and we lose sight of our reason for being—fulfilling individual human needs and personal care. Constant open and validating communication is essential, both among the health team members and between the health care provider and the patient and family. In this team effort to provide quality nutritional care, the clinical nutritionist or dietitian, who is a clinical nutrition specialist, carries the primary responsibility in collaboration with the physician. The nurse and other primary care practitioners provide essential support.

Focus of Care: The Patient

The primary principle of nutritional practice, then, too often overlooked in the many routine procedures of the hospital setting, should be evident: to be valid, nutritional care must be *person-centered*. It must be based on identified needs, updated constantly with the patient, with continuing results monitored in relation to therapy goals. This is necessary, of course, to provide essential physical care. But it is also necessary to support the patient's personal needs for maintaining self-esteem and control as much as possible.[6] In addition, a second fundamental fact needs emphasis: despite all methods, tools, and technologies described here or elsewhere, *the most therapeutic tool you will ever use is yourself.* It is to this seemingly simple yet profoundly personal healing encounter that you bring yourself and your skills.

The most important tool you can bring to your patient-client encounter is yourself.

Phases of the Care Process
Assessment: Data Base

Nutritional status
Condition or situation related to degree of body nourishment.

A broad base of relative information about the patient's **nutritional status,** food habits, and life situation is necessary for making accurate initial assessments. Useful background information may come from a variety of sources, such as the patient, the patient's chart, family or other relatives and friends, oral and written communication with other hospital personnel or staff, and related research.

Analysis: Problem List

A careful analysis of all data collected determines specific patient needs. Some needs will be immediately evident. Others will develop as the situation unfolds. On the basis of this analysis, a list of problems may be formed to guide continuing care activities.

Planning Care: Needs and Goals

Valid care is based on identified problems. The plan must always be based on personal needs and goals of the individual patient, as well as the identified medical care requirements or options discussed with the patient and family.

Implementing Care: Actions

The patient care plan is put into action according to realistic and appropriate activities within each situation. For example, nutritional care and education will involve decisions and actions concerning an appropriate food plan and mode of feeding, as well as the training and education needs of the patient, staff, and family who will carry it out.

Evaluating and Recording Care: Results

As every care activity is carried out, results are carefully checked to see if the identified needs have been met. Appropriate revisions of the care plan can be made as needed for continuing care. These results are carefully recorded in the patient's medical record. Clear documentation of all activities is essential.

The Purpose and Process of Collecting Nutritional Data

The fundamental purpose of **nutritional assessment** in general clinical practice is to determine (1) the overall nutritional status of the patient; (2) current health care needs, both physical and psychosocial, as well as personal; and (3) related factors influencing these needs in the person's current life situation. The clinical nutritionist, assisted by other health team members as needed, uses several basic types of activities for nutritional assessment of patients' needs. These include (1) A—anthropometric measures, (2) B—biochemical tests, (3) C— clinical observations and physical examination, and (4) D—diet evaluation, based on careful personal history including diet-drug interactions, social and family history, and medical history.

Each of these approaches in some form is important because no single parameter can measure individual nutritional status directly or determine all problems or needs. Further, the overall resulting picture must be interpreted within the context of personal social and health factors that may alter nutritional requirements.[7] Only with this type of comprehensive evaluation can nutrition assessment become the real index to the quality of life that it should be.[8] Since such a comprehensive history is a fundamental tool for planning health care, history-taking is a primary skill for all health professionals. A broad number of tests may be used for research purposes in a large facility with access to highly sophisticated equipment. However, the precedures outlined here provide a good base in general practice.

A—Anthropometric Measures

Skill gained through careful practice is necessary to minimize the margin of error in making body measurements. Selection and maintenance of proper procedures and equipment, as well as attention to careful technique, are essential in securing accurate data.

Weight

Hospitalized patients should be weighed at consistent times, for example, before breakfast after the bladder has been emptied. Clinic patients should be weighed without shoes in light, indoor clothing or an examining gown. For accuracy, use regular clinic beam scales with nondetachable weights. An additional weight attachment is available for use with very obese persons. Metric scales with readings to the nearest 20 g provide specific data. However,

---

Nutritional Assessment and Analysis

Nutritional assessment
To judge or evaluate by measurement of values involved. Evaluation of nutritional status by broad study of nutrition-related measures and values involved—physical, physiologic, psychosocial, personal, cultural, medical, and dietary—and environmental influences affecting them, for the purpose of maintaining health or treating disease.

Methods of nutritional assessment:
  Anthropometric measures
  Biochemical tests
  Clinical observation
  Dietary evaluation

the standard clinic scale is satisfactory. Check all scales frequently and have them calibrated every 3 or 4 months for continued accuracy.

After careful reading and recording of the patient's weight, ask about the usual body weight and compare it with standard height-weight tables.[9,10] Refer back to Issues and Answers in Chapter 15 to avoid misuse of these tables. Interpret present weight in terms of percentage of usual and standard body weight for height. Check for any recent weight loss: 1% to 2% in the past week, 5% over the past month, 7.5% during the previous 3 months, or 10% in the past 6 months is significant. More than this rate can be severe. Values charted in the patient's record should indicate percentage of weight change.

Height

If possible, use a fixed measuring stick or tape on a true vertical flat surface. If such is not available, the movable measuring rod on the platform clinic scales may be used with reasonable accuracy. Have the patient stand as straight as possible, without shoes or cap, heels together, and looking straight ahead. The heels, buttocks, shoulders, and head should be touching the wall or vertical surface of the measuring rod. Read the measure carefully and compare it with previous recordings. Note the growth of children or the diminishing height of adults. Metric measures of height in centimeters provide accurate data.

Body Mass Index (BMI)

The weight and height measures can be used to calculate the patient's body mass index: weight (kg) divided by height (meters)^2. This ratio is commonly used in evaluating obesity states in relation to risk factors. Details of this calculation and its interpretation as a risk factor are described in Chapter 15 on weight management.

Body Frame

Two added measures have recently been developed to answer questions about the arbitrary categories of body frame size for height and weight used in the current tables of the Metropolitan Life Insurance Company.[11] One measure used is that of elbow breadth.[12] The other is a measure of wrist circumference and the ratio of this measure to height: height (cm) divided by wrist circumference (cm).[13,14]

Body Measures

In general clinical practice the clinical nutritionist uses two basic body measurements—the mid–upper-arm circumference and the triceps skinfold thickness—and from these calculates a third measure, the mid–upper-arm muscle circumference. First, using a nonstretchable centimeter tape, the midpoint of the upper arm is located on the nondominant arm, unless it is affected by edema. The circumference is measured at this midpoint and read accurately to the nearest tenth of a centimeter and recorded. The resulting measure is compared with previous measurements to note possible changes. Second, using a standard millimeter skinfold caliper, a measure is taken of the triceps skinfold thickness at this same midpoint of the upper arm. This measure provides an estimate of the subcutaneous fat reserves. Then, together with the midpoint circumference value at this same point, the mid–upper-arm muscle circumference can be calculated. This final derived value gives an indirect measure of the body's skeletal muscle mass, a good indicator of body composition. Finally, to interpret the patient's measurements for monitoring nutritional status, these values are compared as percentages of standards provided in reference tables.

Alternative Measures for Nonambulatory Patients

Three alternative measures can provide values for estimating height and weight of persons confined to bed:

1. **Total arm length.** With the patient holding the arm straight down by the side of the body, and using a nonstretchable metric tape, the arm length is measured from attachment at the shoulder to the end of the arm at the wrist. Reference standards indicate relation of this measure to height equivalents.[15] This is also a useful alternative to standing body height when body conditions distort usual standing height of ambulatory patients. For example, this measure is helpful with older persons, in whom a general thinning of weight-bearing cartilages, the "bent-knee gait," and a possible **kyphosis** of the spine may make standing height measurement inaccurate.

2. **Knee height.** With the patient lying in the supine position and left knee and ankle each bent at a 90-degree angle, the knee height is measured with a special caliper. This measurement is then used to calculate the value for deriving body height equivalent.[16]

3. **Calf circumference.** With the patient in the same supine position and left knee bent at a 90-degree angle, and using nonstretchable metric tape, the calf circumference is measured at the largest point. This measurement is then used with three other values—knee height, midarm circumference, and subscapular skinfold—to derive body weight equivalent.[16,17]

B—Biochemical Tests

A number of laboratory tests are available for studying nutritional status. The most commonly used ones for assessing and monitoring nutritional status and planning nutritional care in clinical practice are listed here. General ranges for normal values are given in standard texts.

Measures of Plasma Protein

Basic measures include serum albumin, hemoglobin, and hematocrit. Additional ones may include serum transferrin or total iron-binding capacity (TIBC) and ferritin.

Measures of Protein Metabolism

Basic 24-hour urine tests are used to measure urinary **creatinine** and urea nitrogen levels. These materials are products of protein metabolism. The patient's 24-hour excretion of creatinine is interpreted in terms of ideal creatinine excretion for height, the creatinine-height index (CHI). Comparison is made with standard values for this index. The patient's 24-hour urea nitrogen excretion is used with the calculated dietary nitrogen intake over the same 24-hour period to calculate nitrogen balance.

Measures of Immune System Integrity—Anergy

Basic measures are made of lymphocyte count. Additional measures may be made by skin testing, observing delayed sensitivity to common recall antigens such as mumps or purified protein derivative of tuberculin (PPD). Skin tests

Kyphosis
An increased, abnormal convexity of the upper part of the spine; hunchback.

Creatinine
Byproduct of creatine metabolism; levels in the urine indicate the amount of lean body mass.

Anergy
Diminished capacity of the immune system.

are read at 24 and 48 hours, with greater than 5 mm considered positive and the presence of one positive test indicating intact immunity.

C—Clinical Observations

Keen observation is made of possible malnutrition signs and those evident through vital signs and physical examination.

Clinical Signs of Malnutrition

Careful attention to physical signs of possible malnutrition provides an added dimension to the overall assessment of general nutritional status (see the box on p. 405). A guide for a general examination of such signs is given in Table 17-1. A careful description of any such observations is documented in the patient's medical record.

Vital Signs and Physical Examination

Other physical data may include pulse rate, respiration, temperature, and blood pressure. A study of the common procedures of a normal physical examination will provide useful background orientation.[18]

D—Diet Evaluation

A careful nutrition history, including nutritional information related to living situation and other personal, psychosocial, and economic problems, is a fundamental part of nutrition assessment. But obtaining accurate information about basic food patterns and actual dietary intake is not a simple matter. However, a sensitive practitioner may obtain useful information by using one or more of the basic tools described here.

Specific 24-Hour Food Record

$$\text{N balance} = \frac{\text{total protein}}{6.25}$$

For hospitalized patients, a record of food intake over a specific 24-hour period may be needed for tests such as a nitrogen balance study or for monitoring energy and nutrient intake. A careful explanation of purpose and procedure for the patient and staff is needed. However, such a brief recall or record in general practice has limited value in determining overall basic food habits.

Diet History

In clinical practice we need general knowledge of the patient's basic eating habits to determine any possible nutritional deficiencies. In conjunction with the patient's usual living situation and related food attitudes and behaviors, social and family history, and medical history with current status and treatment, the nutrition interview (Figure 17-1) provides an essential base for further personal nutrition counseling and planning of care.[19,20] For example, an activity-associated day's food intake pattern, using guides discussed in Chapters 1 and 10, can provide a useful tool for obtaining a fairly valid picture of food habits and eating behaviors (see the box on p. 409). In addition to food and nutrition information, drug therapy data from the medical record or the patient and family is important to determine any possible drug-nutrient interaction involved or any teaching needed by the patient (see Chapter 18). Research carefully *all* prescriptions and over-the-counter drugs the patient is using.

Table 17-1

Clinical Signs of Nutritional Status

Body area	Signs of good nutrition	Signs of poor nutrition
General appearance	Alert, responsive	Listless, apathetic, cachexic
Weight	Normal for height, age, body build	Overweight or underweight (special concern for underweight)
Posture	Erect, arms and legs straight	Sagging shoulders, sunken chest, humped back
Muscles	Well developed; firm, good tone; some fat under skin	Flaccid, poor tone; undeveloped; tender, "wasted" appearance; cannot walk properly
Nervous control	Good attention span; not irritable or restless; normal reflexes; psychologic stability	Inattentive, irritable, confused; burning and tingling of hands and feet (paresthesia); loss of position and vibratory sense; weakness and tenderness of muscles (may result in inability to walk); decrease or loss of ankle and knee reflexes
Gastrointestinal function	Good appetite and digestion, normal regular elimination, no palpable (perceptible to touch) organs or masses	Anorexia, indigestion, constipation or diarrhea, liver or spleen enlargement
Cardiovascular function	Normal heart rate and rhythm, no murmurs, normal blood pressure for age	Rapid heart rate (above 100 beats/minute tachycardia), enlarged heart, abnormal rhythm, elevated blood pressure
General vitality	Endurance, energetic, sleeps well, vigorous	Easily fatigued, no energy, falls asleep easily, looks tired, apathetic
Hair	Shiny, lustrous, firm, not easily plucked, healthy scalp	Stringy, dull, brittle, dry, thin and sparse; depigmented; can be easily plucked
Skin (general)	Smooth, slightly moist, good color	Rough, dry, scaly, pale, pigmented, irritated; bruises; petechiae
Face and neck	Skin color uniform, smooth, pink, healthy appearance, not swollen	Greasy, discolored, scaly, swollen; skin dark over cheeks and under eyes; lumpiness or flakiness of skin around nose and mouth
Lips	Smooth, good color, moist, not chapped or swollen	Dry, scaly, swollen, redness and swelling (chelosis), or angular lesions at corners of the mouth or fissures or scars (stomatitis)
Mouth, oral membranes	Reddish pink mucous membranes in oral cavity	Swollen, boggy oral mucous membranes
Gums	Good pink color, healthy, red, no swelling or bleeding	Spongy, bleed easily, marginal redness, inflamed, gums receding
Tongue	Good pink color or deep reddish in appearance, not swollen or smooth, surface papillae present, no lesion	Swelling, scarlet and raw, magenta color, beefy (glossitis), hyperemic and hypertrophic papillae, atrophic papillae
Teeth	No cavities, no pain, bright, straight, no crowding, well-shaped jaw, clean, no discoloration	Unfilled caries, absent teeth, worn surfaces, mottled (fluorosis), malpositioned
Eyes	Bright, clear, shiny; no sores at corner of eyelids; membranes moist and healthy pink color, no prominent blood vessels or mount of tissue or sclera; no fatigue circles beneath	Eye membranes pale (pale conjunctivas), redness of membrane (conjunctival injection), dryness, signs of infection; Bitot's spots, redness and fissuring of eyelid corners (angular palpebritis), dryness of eye membrane (conjunctival xerosis), dull appearance of cornea (corneal xerosis), soft cornea (keratomalacia)

Williams SR: Nutritional assessment and guidance in prenatal care. In Worthington-Roberts BS and Williams SR,: Nutrition in pregnancy and lactation, ed 4, St Louis, 1989, Times-Mirror/Mosby College Publishing.

Continued.

Table 17-1

Clinical Signs of Nutritional Status—cont'd

Body area	Signs of good nutrition	Signs of poor nutrition
Neck (glands)	No enlargement	Thyroid enlarged
Nails	Firm, pink	Spoon shaped (koilonychia), brittle, ridged
Legs, feet	No tenderness, weakness, or swelling, good color	Edema, tender calf, tingling weakness
Skeleton	No malformations	Bowlegs, knock-knees, chest deformity at diaphragm, beaded ribs, prominent scapulas

Figure 17-1
Interviewing of patient to plan personal care.

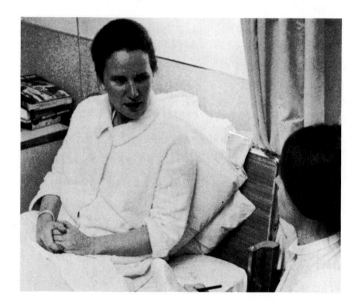

Periodic Food Records

At various times, a 3- to 7-day food record is a helpful tool for assessing food patterns, especially when used to follow up a comprehensive initial diet history or counseling instructions for a required special therapeutic diet. A 3-day record is generally sufficient for determining overall food, energy, and nutrient intake.[20]

Analyzing Nutritional Data

Valid patient care planning requires analysis of all nutritional data collected. On this basis problems requiring solutions can be identified. A detailed analysis of the nutrition information helps determine nutritional diagnosis, any primary or secondary nutritional disease, and any underlying nutrition-related conditions.

Nutritional Diagnosis

All the various nutritional data for each patient, collected by the clinical nutritionist and other team members through the broad assessment activities

To Probe Further

Nutritional Assessment: When Being Objective Does Not Always Mean Being Objective

Nutritionists, as do other health professionals, like numbers. They monitor serum levels of liver-secreted plasma proteins, such as albumin and transferrin, and anthropometric measurements, creatinine-height index, and cell-mediated immunity to identify malnutrition. One study now suggests that these numbers don't add up to the accuracy of the clinical examination in determining a patient's nutritional status.

Researchers from the University of Toronto and Toronto General Hospital suggest that objective measurements may sometimes be inaccurate because they are influenced by several factors: (1) the effects of the disease process itself (rather than the distinct issue of malnutrition) on changes in nutrient levels; (2) delayed response to nutritional depletion (or repletion) because of the relatively long half-lives of such indices as serum albumin and transferrin; and (3) the wide range of confidence limits in nutritional measurements.

These workers found that two clinical evaluators, who were physicians, were able to agree on the nutritional status of 81% of 59 surgical patients examined independently. The history, emphasizing weight loss, edema, anorexia, unusual food intakes, and so on, and physical examination, stressing jaundice, muscle wasting, edema, conditions of oral structures, and similar findings, provided enough information for them to come to conclusions that agreed with objective evaluations.

Does this mean that laboratory tests should be placed in "semiretirement," limited to use in epidemiologic surveys instead of in evaluating individuals? These researchers think so, but they do acknowledge that accurate assessment tests do exist, such as total body nitrogen and total body potassium, although these are not generally available. They also suggest the possibility of combining several known indices to make a more sensitive one, even though this lends itself to the possibility of leaving out one measurement that could have an important effect on the calculations.

However, they do emphasize an important point: nutritional status is as dependent on what you *see* of the patient's status, as well as what you read on a laboratory sheet.

REFERENCES
Baker JP and others: Nutritional assessment: a comparison of clinical judgment and objective measurements, N Engl J Med 306:969, 1982.
Burggaf V and Donlon B: Assessing the elderly: Part one of two parts system by system, Am J Nurs 85:974, Sept 1985.
Detsky AS and others: What is subjective global assessment of nutritional status? J Parental Enteral Nutr 11:8, Jan/Feb 1987.

described, must be carefully analyzed to reach a valid nutritional diagnosis and plan of care. The nutritional diagnosis will require information about all aspects related to the patient's needs: nutrient deficiencies, underlying disease requiring a modified nutrient or food plan, any personal cultural and ethnic needs, or economic needs, as well as mode of feeding and dietary mangement.

Primary and Secondary Nutritional Disease

The clinical nutritionist coordinates these nutrition activities and carries a major responsibility on the health care team for interpreting nutrition-related data and for making decisions and recommendations concerning any primary or secondary nutritional states. *Primary* deficiency disease results from a lack of essential nutrient in the diet, for whatever reason. *Secondary* deficiency disease results from one or more barriers to the use of the nutrients after they are consumed in food. This inability to use a given nutrient may stem from digestive or malabsorption problems or from lack of specific cell enzymes. Such problems may be caused by conditions such as lactose intolerance, celiac disease, inflammatory bowel disease, cell metabolism defects in genetic disease, or **chemotherapy** or radiation treatments.

Nutrition-Related Conditions

Related chronic disease problems with nutrition involvement will also be considered. These include such conditions as heart disease, hypertension, cancer, diabetes, liver, and renal disease. Surgery also imposes nutrition demands and modifications. Any quantifiable data collected can be analyzed by computer. Two major nutritional tasks in which the computer excels are (1) baseline screening to identify persons at risk of malnutrition because of their disease, injury, or lifestyle; and (2) analysis of intake to monitor effectiveness of ongoing treatment.[21,22] Laboratory data may be handled in a similar manner, with general patterns of change monitored over time. Careful appraisal of medical and personal data from histories, records, reports, and interviews will help focus on various needs and problems and provide a realistic picture of nutritional and eating difficulties.

Problem List

On the basis of this careful analysis, a problem list is usually developed. Around such a list, realistic and relevant personal care may be planned. Every aspect of the patient's needs is considered. In conference with the health care team, the patient, family, and any other significant persons, personal goals are determined for care. These goals help establish priorities for immediate and long-term care.

Basic Concepts of Diet Therapy
Normal Nutrition Base

A therapeutic diet is always based on the normal nutritional requirements for a particular patient. It is modified only as the specific disease in the specific individual necessitates. In planning and counseling for nutritional care this is an important initial fact to grasp and impart to patients and clients. For example, it is a great source of encouragement to the parents of a newly diagnosed diabetic child to know that the food plan will be based on individual growth and development needs and will make use of regular foods.

Disease Application

The principles of a special therapeutic diet will be based on modifications of the nutritional components of the normal diet as a particular disease condition may require. These changes may include the following types of modifications: (1) *nutrients*: modification of one or more of the basic nutrients—protein, carbohydrate, fat, minerals, and vitamins; (2) *energy*: modification in

---

Chemotherapy
Treatment of disease with chemicals that destroy unhealthy tissue (see Chapter 24).

Nutritional Intervention: Care Plan and Management

energy value as expressed in kilocalories; and (3) *texture*: modification in texture or seasoning, such as liquid or low residue.

Individual Adaptation

A therapeutic diet may be theoretically correct and have well-balanced food plans, but if these plans are unacceptable to the patient, they will not be followed. A workable plan for a specific person must be based on individual food habits within the specific personal life situation. This can be achieved only through careful planning *with the patient,* or with the parents of a child requiring a special diet, based on an initial interview to obtain a diet history, knowledge of personal food habits, living conditions, and related factors. In this way, diet principles can be understood and motivation secured to follow through. Whatever the problems, nutritional care is valid only to the extent that it involves this kind of knowledge, skills, and insights. Individual adaptations of the diet to meet individual needs are imperative for successful therapy.

Routine House Diets

A schedule of routine "house" diets, based on some type of cycle menu plan, is usually followed in hospitals for those patients not requiring a special diet modification. According to general patient need and tolerance, the diet order may be liquid (clear liquid or full liquid, with milk used on the full liquid diet), soft (no raw foods, generally somewhat bland in seasoning), and regular (a full, normal-for-age diet). Occasionally an interval step between soft and regular may be used (a light diet). Sample menus from hospital staff dietitians may be compared to note differences.

Managing the Mode of Feeding

Depending on the patient's condition, the clinical nutritionist may manage the diet by using any one of four feeding modes.

Enteral: Oral Diet

As long as possible, of course, regular oral feeding is preferred. Supplements are added if needed. According to the patient's condition, assistance in eating may also be needed (Figure 17-2).

Enteral: Tube Feeding

If a patient is unable to eat but the gastrointestinal tract can be used, tube feeding may provide needed nutritional support. A number of commercial formulas are available or a blended formula may be calculated and prepared.

Parenteral: Peripheral Vein Feeding

If the patient cannot take in food or formula by way of the gastrointestinal tract, intravenous feeding will be needed. Solutions of dextrose, amino acids, vitamins, and minerals, with intermittent lipid formula, can be fed through peripheral veins when the need is not extensive or long-term.

Parenteral: Total Parenteral Nutrition (TPN)

If the patient's nutritional need is great and support therapy may be required for a longer time, feeding through a large central vein is needed. Placement of this tube is a special surgical procedure. More concentrated

Total parenteral nutrition (TPN)
Feeding of a nutritionally complete solution through a large central vein (see Chapter 23).

Figure 17-2
Child with fractured arm is assisted in eating by student nurse.

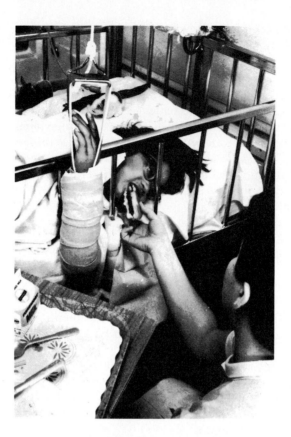

special solutions can be used and monitored by a nutrition support team. The formulas are determined by the nutritionist and the physician, prepared by trained pharmacists, and administered by specially trained nurses. This skilled nutritional support team is essential for successful therapy.

Details of these various modes of feeding are given in Chapters 23 and 24, as they apply to different conditions.

Evaluation: Quality Patient Care

General Considerations

When the nutritional care plan is carried out, patient care activities need to be considered in terms of the nutritional diagnosis and treatment objectives, and the extent to which each of the care activities helps to meet the particular goals of the patient and the family. This evaluation is both continuous and terminal. It seeks to validate care while it is being given, as well as to determine the effectiveness of a particular course of care. Various areas need to be investigated.

Estimate the Achievement of Nutritional Therapy Goals

What is the effect of the diet or mode of feeding on the illness or the patient's situation? Is any change needed in the nutrient ratios of the diet or formula as originally calculated, in the meal-distribution pattern, or in the feeding mode?

Judge the Accuracy of Intervention Actions

Is there need to change any of the nutritional care plan components? For example, is a change needed in the type of food or feeding equipment, envi-

Clinical Application

Name _____ Date _____
  Height _____ Weight (lb) _____ (kg) _____ Age _____
                 Ideal weight _____

Referral
Diagnosis
Diet order
Members of household
Occupation
Recreation, physical activity

Nutrition History: Activity-Associated General Day's Food Pattern

Present food intake

	Place	Hour	Frequency, form, and amount checklist
Breakfast			Milk
			Cheese
			Meat
			Fish
			Poultry
Noon meal			Eggs
			Cream
			Butter, margarine
			Other fats
Evening meal			Vegetables, green
			Vegetables, other
			Fruits (citrus)
			Legumes
Extra meals			Potato
			Bread—kind
			Sugar
			Desserts
			Beverages
Summary			Alcohol
			Vitamins
			Candy

ronment for meals, procedures for counseling, or types of learning activities for nutrition education and self-care procedures?

Determine the Patient's Ability to Follow Prescribed Nutritional Therapy

Do any hindrances or disabilities prevent the patient from following the treatment plan? What is the impact of the nutritional therapy on the patient, the family, or the staff? Were the necessary nutrition assessment procedures for collecting nutrition data carried out correctly? Do the patient and family understand the information given for self-care? Have the community resources required by the patient and family been available or convenient for use? Has any needed food assistance program been sufficient to meet needs for the patient's ongoing care?

Quality Patient Care
PSROs

Since the establishment of Professional Standards Review Organizations (PSROs) in 1972, there has been an increased emphasis on setting practice standards and forming hospital patient care review committees to monitor the delivery of quality patient care. In addition, at present an increased focus on cost control in health care settings requires that mechanisms be developed for effectively evaluating patient care programs on the basis of (1) cost effectiveness and (2) provision of nutritional services by the most qualified personnel.

Quality Care Models

Within clinical nutrition practice, standards for both professional and support level staff have been developed in a number of medical care settings.[23] These models of quality care have established specific standards for (1) identifying patients who require increased nutritional support or nutrition education, (2) determining patient care priorities and spelling out the degree of care required, and (3) defining role responsibilities for carrying out each part of the care plan. These models have been applied to specific patient care needs, such as a standard of practice for quality assurance in nutritional care for patients with cancer.[24]

DRGs

With increasing concerns about health care costs, a system of preset payment for hospitalized Medicare patients according to specific diagnosis-related groups (DRGs) was developed in 1981.[25] This prospective payment control plan was first applied to government funded Medicare patients, but in today's world of economic realities some form of this management scheme is fast becoming a part of practice for the majority of hospitalized patients.[26] Such increasing inevitable emphasis on cost containment brings a new demand for accountability by all health care professionals and managers.

Collaborative Roles of the Nutritionist and Nurse

The clinical nutritionist or dietitian works closely with the nurse in managing the nutritional care of patients. At varying times, depending on need, the nurse may provide valuable nutrition assistance as coordinator, interpreter, or teacher. Skills in consultation and referral are therefore essential.

Coordinator

Nurses can coordinate special services or treatment required because of their close relationship to patients and their constant attendance. The nurse may help schedule activities to prevent conflicts or secure needed consultation for the patient with the dietitian, social worker, or other health team member. Sometimes hospital malnutrition exists simply because meals are constantly being interrupted by various procedures, staff interviews, or medical rounds.

Interpreter

Because of a close relationship with the patient, the nurse can help reduce tension by careful, brief, easily understood explanations concerning various treatments and plans of care. This will include basic interpretation of the therapeutic diet from the clinical nutritionist or the physician and of the resulting food selections on the tray. The nurse may sometimes assist the patient in making appropriate selections from the menus provided.

Teacher or counselor

One of the nurse's most significant roles is that of health care educator and counselor. Innumerable informal opportunities occur during daily nursing care for planned conversation about sound nutrition principles, reinforcing the counseling of the clinical nutritionist. In addition, according to patient situations, the nurse may work with the clinical nutritionist during periods of instruction about principles of the patient's diet therapy in relation to the disease process. The nurse will work in close cooperation with the clinical nutritionist and the physician to coordinate nutritional and medical management of the patient's illness into overall nursing care. At all times the nurse will work closely with the hospital's clinical nutrition staff to support and reinforce primary nutrition education. These nutrition experts will always be excellent resources for needed nutrition consultation and referral.

Clearly, learning about the hospitalized patient's nutritional needs is a continuing activity beginning with admission. It should follow through and include plans for continuing application in the home environment. Follow-up care may be provided by the hospital's clinic dietitian, by consultation with clinical nutritionists in community private practice, by public health nutritionists and nurses, or by referrals to community agencies and resources.

To Sum Up

The basis for an accurate assessment of the patient's nutritional needs begins with the individual patient and family. Physical and psychologic, social, economic, and cultural factors in and out of the clinical setting all play a role in evaluating the patient's health status and any possible problems with adherence to a nutritional care plan.

Nutritional assessment is based on a broad foundation of pertinent data, including food and drug uses and values. The effectiveness of an assessment based on analysis of these data depends in turn on effective communication with the patient, family members, and "significant others" in the development of an appropriate care plan, as well as with other members of the health care team. The patient's medical record is a basic means of communication among health care team members.

Nutritional therapy, based on a combination of the personal and physiologic needs of the patient, requires a close working relationship among nutrition, medical, and nursing staff in the health care facility. The nurse's schedule offers many opportunities to reinforce nutritional principles of the diet. Nutritional therapy doesn't end with the patient's discharge. Outpatient nutrition services, appropriate social services, and food resources in the community help meet continuing needs of patients and their families.

Questions for Review

1. Identify and discuss the possible effects of various psychologic factors on the outcome of nutritional therapy.
2. Outline a procedure for assessing the nutritional needs and building a care plan for a 65-year-old widower hospitalized with coronary heart disease (refer to Chapter 20, if necessary). Include community agencies the patient could be referred to for follow-up care, services, and information.
3. List and describe five commonly used anthropometric measures, five serum and two urinary tests for nutritional information, and six clinical signs used to assess nutritional status.
4. Describe the nature and purpose of quality assurance plans for standards of nutritional care.

References

1. Rubin M: The physiology of bed rest, Am J Nurs 88(1):50, 1988.
2. Christensen KS and Gstundter KM: Hospital-wide screening improves basis for nutrition intervention, J Am Diet Assoc 85(6):704, 1985.
3. Kamath SK and others: Hospital malnutrition: a 33-hospital screening study, J Am Diet Assoc 86(2):203, 1986.
4. Noel MB and Wojnaroski SM: Nutrition screening for long-term care residents, J Am Diet Assoc 87(11):1557, 1987.
5. Kared FA, Becker DS, and Finkelestein G: Unreceived meals a source of malnutrition, Hospitals 56(2):47, 1982.
6. Smith FB: Patient power, Am J Nurs 85(11):1260, 1985.
7. Underwood BA: Evaluating the nutritional status of individuals: a critique of approaches, Nutr Rev 44(suppl):213, May 1986.
8. Paige DM and Davis LR: Nutritional assessment: an index to the quality of life, Clin Nutr 7(2):77, 1988.
9. Weigley ES: Average? Ideal? Desirable? A brief overview of height-weight tables in the United States, J Am Diet Assoc 84(4):417, 1984.
10. Schultz LO: Obese, overweight, desirable, ideal: where to draw the line in 1986? J Am Diet Assoc 86(12):1702, 1986.
11. Himes JH and Bouchard C: Do the new Metropolitan Life Insurance weight-height tables correctly assess body frame and body fat relationships? Am J Pub Health 75(9):1076, 1985.
12. Frisancho AR: Nutritional anthropometry, J Am Diet Assoc 88(5):553, 1988.
13. Grant JP: Handbook of total parenteral nutrition, Philadelphia, 1980, WB Saunders Co.
14. Nowak RK and Schultz LO: A comparison of two methods for the determination of body frame size, J Am Diet Assoc 87(3):339, 1987.
15. Mitchell CO and Lipschitz DA: Arm length measurement as an alternative to height in nutritional assessment of the elderly, J Parenteral Enteral Nutr 6(3):226, 1982.
16. Chumlea WC, Roche AF, and Mukherjee D: Nutritional assessment of the elderly through anthropometry, Columbus, Ohio, 1987, Ross Laboratories.
17. Chumlea WC and others: Prediction of body weight for the nonambulatory elderly from anthropometry, J Am Diet Assoc 88(5):564, 1988.
18. Rosenfeld I: The complete medical exam, New York, 1978, Simon & Schuster.
19. Swan E and Rohrback C: Nutritional assessment—an investigative interview, Nutr Support Serv 1(5):14, 1982.
20. Bingham SA: The dietary assessment of individuals: methods, accuracy, new techniques, and recommendations, Nutr Abstr and Rev 57(10):705, 1987.
21. Hannaman KN and Penner SF: A nutrition assessment tool that includes diagnosis, J Am Diet Assoc 85(5):607, 1985.

22. Bunton PW: Using the computer as a referral source to find the patient at nutritional risk, J Am Diet Assoc 86(9):1232, 1986.
23. Ometer JL and Oberfill MS: Quality assurance. I. A levels of care model, J Am Diet Assoc 81(2):129, 1982.
24. Ometer JL and Oberfill MS: Quality assurance. II. Application of oncology standards against a levels of care model, J Am Diet Assoc 81(2):132, 1982.
25. Yale University School Of Organization and Management: The new ICD-9-CM diagnosis related groups classification scheme, New Haven, Conn, 1981, Yale University Press.
26. Huyck NI and Fairchild MM: Provision of clinical nutrition services by diagnosis-related groups (DRGs) and major diagnostic categories (MDCs), J Am Diet Assoc 87(1):69, 1987.

Further Readings

Clay G, Bouchard C, and Hemphill K: A comprehensive nutrition case management system, J Am Diet Assoc 88(2):196, 1988.

This article describes an excellent nutrition assessment and management system model featuring (1) decreased charting time, (2) precise documentation, (3) nutritional diagnosis tool for intervention therapy, (4) quality care standard, (5) computer adaptation, and (6) quality assurance audits.

Dikovics A: Nutritional assessment: case study methods, Philadelphia, 1986, George F. Stickley Co.

This small paperback packs a great deal of nutrition assessment information into a variety of case studies, with numerous reference materials, making it a good supplemental reference for beginning level courses.

Dwyer JT and others: Changes in relative weight among institutionalized elderly adults, J Gerontology 42:246, May 1987.

Matthews LE: Using anthropometric parameters to evaluate nutritional status, J Nutr Elderly 5:67, Winter 1985/1986.

Tramposch TS and Blue LS: A nutrition screening and assessment system for use with the elderly in extended care, J Am Diet Assoc 87(9):1207, 1987.

These three articles discuss special assessment needs of elderly persons in extended care facilities with adapted methods and standard reference norms, especially for nonambulatory residents.

Frisancho AR: Commentary: Nutritional anthropometry, J Am Diet Assoc 88(5):553, 1988.

Chumlea WC, Roche AF, and Steinbaugh ML: Prediction of body weight for the nonambulatory elderly from anthropometry, J Am Diet Assoc 88(5):564, 1988.

Falciglia G, O'Connor J, and Gedling E: Upper arm anthropometric norms in elderly white subjects, J Am Diet Assoc 88(5):569, 1988.

These three articles in a single journal issue provide good background for using anthropometry to assess nutritional status, especially in elderly persons.

"How Fat Am I Really?" A Summary of Methods of Measuring Body Fat

When a client asks you this question, you could simply weigh the person on a scale and compare the resulting figure with a standard weight/height table. This will only tell you the total weight, however, and not the amount of *fat*, which is a true indicator of obesity.

Several methods of estimating body fat are available, though none are perfect. Some have the advantage of being simple to perform, are inexpensive, and are convenient for use in most clinical settings:

Skinfold thickness

This method involves the use of calipers (or **ultrasound**) to measure the amount of fat lying underneath the skin at specific body sites: biceps, triceps, and subcapsular and suprailiac areas. This method has its drawbacks in use with the individual client because it fails to account for differences in age, the compressibility of fat in each area, skin thickness, and the fact that fat-free mass (FFM) may not be constant in all individuals. However, it is a cheap assessment method and tends to work well in epidemiologic studies and in clinical work—if done accurately.

Muscle metabolites

Levels of two metabolites in the urine are measured to estimate tissue: creatinine and 3-methyl histidine. The latter may be a more accurate indicator of fat-free weight, though its use is limited in a disease state because of a higher turnover rate in its levels in muscular tissue. creatinine is easier to measure. However, urine levels fluctuate with menstruation, age, infection, fever, trauma, and disease.

Body density

Another method of estimating body fat is growing in popularity, despite its inconvenience and expense. Body density measurement involves underwater weighing in a closed container to estimate body fat by the amount of water such fat displaces. Two methods are used: (1) total immersion, in which results can be affected by residual air in the gut (calculations account for residual air in the lungs) and (2) use of the plethysmograph, a vessel that requires the subject to stand in water only up to the neck, with the air in the lungs, gut, and surrounding spaces measured by a special pump. The latter method tends to be the more accurate of the two.

Other more exotic methods involve the use of traceable radioactive or non-radioactive **isotopes** of natural elements, which diffuse throughout the body:

Total body water

This method involves giving a dose of a special **isotope** of water and measures the amount of isotope given off after it has reached an equilibrium with regular body water, a process that takes only 3 to 4 hours. This test assumes that the water content of nonadipose tissue—or fat-free mass (FFM)—remains constant. If this is true, the amount of FFM could be subtracted from the entire body weight to estimate the amount of body fat. This assumption fails, however, in light of the fact that (1) water levels rise when muscle-wasting occurs, and (2) adipose tissue itself contains water, which is not accounted for in this test. Both facts indicate that this test will underestimate the amount of water in the body.

Ultrasound
Sound waves at a frequency above that which can be heard by the human ear (20 kilocycles/second); in controlled doses, can be used as a therapeutic or diagnostic tool (e.g., to determine skinfold thickness).

Isotope
An element that has the same number of protons (atomic number) as another element but which has a different number of neutrons (atomic number).

Total body potassium

This method uses a naturally occurring isotope of potassium, ^{40}K, to measure lean body tissue. Results match those of other tests very closely for healthy, non-obese subjects 20 to 29 years of age. However, this test overestimates the amount of fat in patients suffering from **cachexia** and underestimates the amount of lean in obese subjects. The lean tissue of obese persons apparently has less potassium, and their excess adipose tissue may inhibit the measurement of ^{40}K in lean tissue.

Total body nitrogen

This measure reflects total body protein in muscle and nonmuscle lean tissue. Estimating fatty tissue is simply a matter of subtracting this amount from the total body weight. Because it measures more than muscle, it is less likely to underestimate lean body mass in individuals with muscle-wasting conditions (e.g., cancer). The main drawback, however, is cost of the test and accessibility of equipment.

Fat-soluble gases

Another method based on diffusion, but not using radioactive elements, uses fat-soluble gases, such as those used in anesthesia. These gases should be good indicators of body fat when they are absorbed into it. Unfortunately, they take a long time to be absorbed and are not absorbed evenly throughout all body fat.

Whole body conductivity

This new technique takes advantage of the fact that lean tissue conducts electricity better than fat. Tests based on this theory have worked well on farm animals. It is believed that they will work equally well on humans.

Perhaps in the near future, technology will have developed a simple, inexpensive, and accurate method of measuring body fat. The nutrition counselor could then at long last answer more accurately the most frequently asked question and work with the client to develop a truly effective strategy for weight reduction.

Cachexia
General poor health and malnutrition, usually indicated by an emaciated appearance.

REFERENCES
Heymsfield SB and others: Measurement of muscle mass in humans: validity of the 24-hour urinary creatinine method, Am J Clin Nutr 37(3):478, 1983.
Lukaski HC: Methods for the assessment of human body composition: traditional and new, Am J Clin Nutr 46:537, 1987.
Seidell JC and others: Assessment of intra-abdominal and subcutaneous abdominal fat: relation between anthropometry and computed tomography, Am J Clin Nutr 45(1):7, 1987.

18 Drug-Nutrient Interactions

Chapter Objectives

After studying this chapter, the student should be able to:

1. Describe ways in which food and its nutrients affect the use of drugs in the body.
2. Identify effects of drugs on appetite, nutrient absorption, vitamins, and minerals.
3. Identify effects of food nutrients and cooking methods on drug distribution and metabolism in the body.
4. Identify points along the gastrointestinal tract where foods just consumed might affect the efficiency of drug action.
5. Relate food intake to whether it either helps or hinders the body's use of particular drugs.

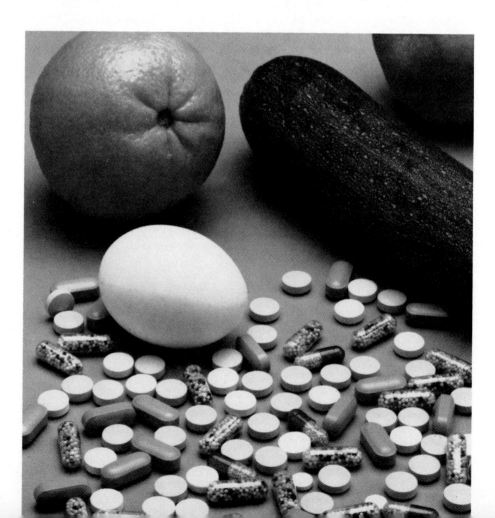

PREVIEW

Today consumers are generally better informed about misuse of drugs, both prescription and over-the-counter nonprescription ones. However, in our overmedicated society, many persons are often dangerously uninformed or misinformed about the specific drugs they may be taking, especially in relation to the food they eat.

The influence of food and dietary patterns on drug absorption and bioavailability is complex. All members of the health care team must have basic knowledge of both drug action and related nutrition effects to guide patients in making the wisest and most effective use of their drug and nutritional therapies.

In this chapter, continuing our clinical nutrition sequence, we look briefly at some major effects of combining food and nutrients with drugs. We will see how these interactions affect nutritional therapy and education, and understand why this knowledge is an important aspect of all patient care, especially nutritional care.

Our Medicated Society: Extent of the Problem

The field of nutrient-drug interaction is both complex and confusing. We face a drug-oriented medical environment and a bewildering array of drug items. Every year American physicians prescribe and pharmacists dispense a total amount of drugs sufficient to provide seven individual medications for each woman, man, and child in the United States. To this amount we can then add the large volume of nonprescription drugs that Americans purchase over the counter. Some concerned persons have come to view our overmedicated society with alarm. Knowledgeable and concerned pharmacologists indicate that outside of extremely serious illness, most general medical problems can be treated with less than 25 drugs. The World Health Organization (WHO) has estimated that only some 150 to 200 drugs are actually needed to take care of almost all ordinary illnesses around the world. Yet on our American market there are about 54,000 drugs, many of them only slight variations of other drugs, the so-called "me to" drugs.

Possible Cause and Effect

The modern medical world is increasing in complexity and specialization because of advancing technology. Specialty areas or disciplines can easily become isolated from the many other important interacting factors when the care of patients falls outside their primary area of expertise. Physicians who prescribe medications, pharmacists who fill these prescriptions, or nurses who administer them may not be fully aware of a particular drug's impact on an individual patient's nutritional state. They may be unaware of the patient's diet and how it may influence the effects of medication. Similarly a clinical nutritionist may provide a diet prescription and food plan yet not be fully aware of the patient's medication program and its implications for sound nutritional care.

Drug-Nutrient Problems in Modern Medicine

Drug Use and Nutritional Status
Elderly Persons at Risk

All of us, at any age, risk harmful drug or drug-nutrient interactions. However, elderly persons are particularly vulnerable.[1,2] Several things contribute to this increased risk among the elderly: (1) they are likely to be taking more drugs for longer periods of time to control chronic diseases and (2) illness, mental confusion, or lack of drug information may increase errors in self-care.[3-6] As a result, concerned physicians, nutritionists, pharmacists, and nurses are working more and more together as a team to provide drug and nutritional education and therapy on a sounder basis. A number of drug-nutrient interactions demand this type of team work in patient care. To meet this need, team process guides are being developed for various conditions.[7,8]

General Hospital Malnutrition

Studies of hospital malnutrition indicate that there are a number of possible mechanisms of nutrient-drug interaction. Results of these studies give us information on contributing causes to this general malnutrition. Such causes are especially prevalent in hospitalized patients and require informed therapy.[9,10] These nutrient-drug mechanisms that influence nutrition status include those affecting the following:

- Decreased intestinal absorption
- Increased renal excretion
- Competition or displacement of nutrients for carrier protein sites
- Interference with synthesis of necessary enzyme, coenzyme, or carrier
- Hormonal effects on genetic systems
- The drug delivery system
- Components in drug formulation

In this chapter we will briefly review various effects of drugs on food and nutrients and, conversely, effects of food and nutrients on drugs, with some examples in each case.

Effects of Drugs on Food and Nutrients

Drug Effects on Food Intake
Increased Appetite

A number of drugs have the effect of increasing appetite.[1,11] These drugs include the following:

1. **Antihistamines.** These drugs can lead to marked increase in appetite and subsequent weight gain. One of these agents, both an antihistamine and a serotonin antagonist, is cyproheptadine hydrochloride (Periactin).

2. **Psychotropic drugs.** Some of the tranquilizers may lead to **hyperphagia** (the opposite of **hypophagia**). Tranquilizers that lead to weight gain when given to psychotic patients may have the opposite effect on geriatric patients. Some of these drugs include chlordiazepoxide hydrochloride (Librium), diazepam (Valium), chlorpromazine hydrochloride (Thorazine), and meprobamate (Equanil). As with the tranquilizers (see Issues and Answers on p. 432), other types of antidepressant drugs such as amitriptyline hydrochloride (Elavil) may promote appetite and lead to marked weight gain.

3. **Steroids.** Anabolic steroids, including testosterone, promote nitrogen retention, increased lean body mass, and subsequent weight gain. Some athletes and body builders form habits of drug abuse with steroids to obtain these characteristic effects but harm their bodies in the process.

Hyperphagia
Eating or ingesting more food than necessary for optimal body function.

Hypophagia
Eating less than necessary for optimal health.

Decreased Appetite

A number of drugs have the opposite effect of decreasing appetite.[1,11] Some examples of these drugs include the following:

1. **Amphetamines.** These drugs act as stimulants to the central nervous system and have the effect of depressing the desire for food, thus leading to marked loss of weight. For this reason they have been used in the past as appetite-depressant drugs in the treatment of obesity. However, long-term use of these drugs in such treatment has caused problems, including addiction, since in most cases appetite itself is not the primary cause of the excess weight. For this reason, amphetamines are rarely used now for this purpose.

2. **Insulin.** A rapid drop in blood sugar, *hypoglycemia*, can be induced by insulin. This effect is not marked by hunger but often causes nausea, weakness, and aversion to foods. The hypoglycemic reaction is distinct from the effect of general insulin use in the management of diabetes, which may bring a feeling of hunger as nutrient metabolism is improved.

3. **Alcohol.** Abuse of alcohol can lead to loss of appetite, reduced food intake, and malnutrition.[12] This *anorexia*—loss of appetite—can stem from various effects of alcoholism, such as gastritis, lactose intolerance, hepatitis, cirrhosis, ketosis, pancreatitis, alcoholic brain syndrome, drunkenness, and withdrawal symptoms. The resulting reduced food intake can then lead to malnutrition, which further complicates the anorexia by causing deficiencies of thiamin, zinc, or protein.

Taste Changes

A loss of taste, **dysgeusia,** may be caused by a number of drugs. For example, the **chelating agent** D-penicillamine may be used in the treatment of conditions such as heavy metal poisoning, rheumatoid arthritis, or cystinuria. The side effect of taste loss occurs as the agent also binds zinc and causes a drug-induced zinc deficiency. Other drugs affecting taste acuity include **diuretics,** and anticancer agents such as methotrexate and doxorubicin hydrochloride (Adriamycin), as well as agents used to treat Parkinson's disease. Even a 1-g dose of aspirin can increase perception of a bitter taste. Sodium lauryl sulfate, a substance often used in toothpaste to make it clean teeth better, can make orange juice taste bitter. A number of other drugs can also affect taste and smell (see the box on p. 422). Thus when any of these drugs are used, discussion of these sensory effects with the patient and use of food seasonings to enhance taste and smell will be useful.

Nausea

Many drugs have the effect of decreasing appetite because they contribute to nausea and vomiting. For example, cardiac glycosides, digitalis, and related drugs can produce nausea if used in relatively large amounts. A number of drugs used in cancer chemotherapy (see Chapter 24) have similar effects and can contribute to malnutrition and weight loss.

Bulking Effects

Various agents, such as methylcellulose and other dietary fiber products, can interfere with absorption of nutrients and contribute to their loss.[13] These bulking agents can also contribute to decreased intake of food by creating a

Dysgeusia
Altered sense of taste.

Chelating agent
Substance that combines with a metal, firmly binding it; chemotherapeutic use for metal poisoning.

Diuretic
A substance that increases or promotes urine excretion.

sense of fullness and lack of desire for food intake. For this reason they have sometimes been used as adjunct therapy in weight management.

Drug Effects on Nutrient Absorption and Metabolism

Increased Nutrient Absorption

A number of drugs can increase nutrient absorption and thus benefit nutritional status. For example, cimetidine (Tagamet) and ranitidine (Zantac), gastric antisecretory agents, have helped patients with many different gastrointestinal problems. The drugs reduce gastric acid and volume output, lower duodenal acid load and volume, reduce jejunal flow, maintain pH of secretions, decrease fecal fat, nitrogen, and volume and thus improve absorption of protein and carbohydrate. Therefore these drugs are widely used in the treatment of peptic ulcer disease (see Chapter 19) and other gastrointestinal disorders.

Decreased Nutrient Absorption

A number of drugs contribute to primary malabsorption of nutrients. Colchicine, for example, a drug used in the treatment of gout, can lead to vitamin B_{12} deficiency, causing megaloblastic anemia. Alcohol abuse can provoke malabsorption of thiamin and folic acid, causing peripheral neuritis and anemia. Laxatives can produce severe malabsorption, leading to conditions such as osteomalacia. Secondary malabsorption may also be drug-induced. Some drugs inhibit vitamin D absorption, leading to malabsorption and consequent deficiency of calcium. For example, the antibiotic neomycin causes tissue changes in the intestinal villi, which precipitate bile salts, prevent fat breakdown by inhibiting pancreatic lipase, and decrease bile acid absorption. These effects lead to **steatorrhea** and failure to absorb fat-soluble vitamins A, D, E, and K. Malabsorption of vitamin D in turn leads to a calcium deficiency. Other drugs cause malabsorption of folic acid or impair its utilization, causing malabsorption of still other nutrients. Methotrexate, for example, is a folic acid antagonist and impairs the intestinal absorption of calcium. Summaries of the drugs causing primary and secondary nutrient malabsorption are given in Tables 18-1 and 18-2.

Steatorrhea
Excessive fat amounts in the feces, often due to malabsorption syndromes.

Mineral Depletion

Certain drugs can lead to mineral depletion through induced gastrointestinal losses or renal excretion.

1. **Diuretics.** Diuretic drugs are intentionally used to reduce levels of excess tissue water and sodium. But they can also result in loss of other minerals, such as potassium, magnesium, and zinc.[14] Potassium deficiency is marked by weakness, anorexia, nausea, vomiting, listlessness, apprehension, and sometimes diffuse pain, drowsiness, stupor, and irrational behavior. Conversely, use of potassium-retaining diuretics, such as spironolactone, as well as overuse of potassium supplementation, can cause the opposite effect of hyperkalemia.[15]

2. **Chelating agents.** Penicillamine attaches to metals and binds them, thus possibly leading to deficiency of such key trace elements as zinc and copper.

3. **Alcohol.** The abuse of alcohol can lead to diminished levels of potassium, magnesium, and zinc.

4. **Antacids.** These commonly used over-the-counter medications are of concern because they can produce phosphate deficiency, with symptoms of

Table 18-1

Drugs Causing Primary Nutrient Malabsorption

Drug	Use	Nutrients lost	Action
Cholestyramine	Holds bile acid; hypo-cholesterolemic agent	Fat; fat-soluble vitamins A, D, and K; vitamin B_{12}; iron	Binding agent for bile salts and nutrients
Colchicine	Antigout agent	Fat; vitamin B_{12}; provitamin A (carotene); lactose; sodium, potassium	Enzyme damage; inhibits cell division; structural defect
Methyldopa	Antihypertensive agent	Vitamin B_{12}, folic acid; iron	Unclear; possible autoimmune action
Mineral oil	Laxative	Fat-soluble vitamins A, D, and K; provitamin A (carotene)	Nutrients dissolve in oil and are lost in feces
Neomycin	Antibiotic	Fat; vitamin B_{12}; nitrogen; lactose, sucrose; sodium, potassium, iron, calcium	Binds bile salts; lowers pancreatic lipase; structural defect
Para-aminosalicylic acid	Antituberculosis agent	Fat; folic acid, vitamin B_{12}	Blocks mucosal uptake of vitamin B_{12}
Phenolphthalein	Laxative	Calcium, potassium; vitamin D	Rapid intestinal transit; loss of structural tissue integrity
Potassium chloride	Potassium replacement	Vitamin B_{12}	Lowered ileal pH
Salicylazosulfapyridine (Azulfidine)	Antiinflammatory agent (ulcerative colitis)	Folic acid	Blocks mucosal uptake of folic acid

Adapted from Roe DA: Interactions between drugs and nutrients, Med Clin North Am 63(5):985, 1979.

Table 18-2

Drugs Causing Secondary Malabsorption of Calcium

Drug	Use	Action
Phenytoin, phenobarbital, primidone	Anticonvulsant agents	Accelerated vitamin D metabolism
Diphosphonates	Paget's disease (increased bone resorption and deformity)	Vitamin D hormone $[1,25,(OH)_2D_2]$ formation decreased
Glucocorticoids, such as prednisone	Collagen disease; allergies	Calcium transport decreased
Glutethimide	Sedative	Impaired calcium transport
Methotrexate	Leukemia	Folic acid antagonist—acute deficiency of the vitamin

Adapted from Roe DA: Interactions between drugs and nutrients, Med Clin North Am 63(5):985, 1979.

Clinical Application

The Proof of the Pudding . . .

The senses of taste and smell greatly affect our responses to various foods. The loss of these senses can drive persons to constantly seek elusive satisfaction by overeating, or it may stop them from eating entirely. In either case the pleasure of eating has gone and nutritional status suffers. Patients taking drugs that affect taste and smell will need counseling concerning food choices, combinations, and seasonings that can help overcome this difficulty. Some of these drugs include the following:

Anesthetics, local: benzocaine, cocaine, procaine

Antibiotics: amphotericin B, ampicillin, griseofulvin, lincomycin, streptomycin, tetracyclines

Anticoagulant: phenindione

Antihistamine: chlorpheniramine maleate

Antihypertensive agents: captopril, diazoxide, ethacrynic acid

Anti-infectious agent: clofibrate

Cholesterol-lowering agent: clofibrate

Hypoglycemic agent: glipizide

Psychoactive agents: carbamazepine, lithium carbonate, phenytoin, amphetamines

Toothpaste ingredient: sodium lauryl sulfate

Indeed, the proof of the pudding—the "pudding" being our food—*is* in the taste thereof, which can easily be affected by a variety of drugs, resulting in diminished appetite and needed food intake. Patients on these drugs can benefit from counseling about these taste effects and ways of counteracting them in food selection, seasoning, and serving.

REFERENCES

Barley B: Taste killers, Am Health 3(1):22, 1984.

Garabedian-Ruffalo SM, and Ruffalo RL: Drug and nutrient interactions, Am Fam Physician 33:165, 1986.

Roe DA: Dimensions of risk assessment for drug and nutrient interactions, Nutr Today 22(6):20, 1987.

Paresthesia
Abnormal sensations such as prickling, burning, "crawling" of skin, etc.

anorexia, malaise, **paresthesia,** profound muscle weakness, and convulsions, as well as calcification of soft tissues from the prolonged hypercalcemia.[16]

5. **Aspirin.** Salicylates such as aspirin (acetylsalicylic acid—ASA) can induce iron deficiency by causing low-level blood loss from erosions in the stomach or intestinal tissue when taken incorrectly (see the box on p. 429).

Vitamin Depletion

Certain drugs act as metabolic antagonists and cause deficiencies of the vitamins involved.

1. **Vitamin antagonists.** Various drugs have been used successfully to treat disease because they are antagonists of certain vitamins and thus can control key metabolic reactions in which that vitamin is involved. For example, coumarin anticoagulants inhibit regeneration of vitamin K, which is necessary for blood clotting (see Chapter 7). Also, some cancer chemotherapy

Target vitamin	Drugs
Vitamin K	Coumarin anticoagulants
Folic acid	Methotrexate
	Pyrimethamine
	Triamterene
	Trimethoprim
Vitamin B_6	Cycloserine
	Hydralazine
	Isoniazid
	Levodopa

Table 18-3

Examples of Drugs that Act as Vitamin Antagonists

Adapted from Roe DA: Interactions between drugs and nutrients. Med Clin North Am 63(5):985, 1979.

Nutrient affected by OCA	Effect	Clinical result
Vitamins		
Retinol (vitamin A)	Impairs liver storage; increases plasma binding	Unclear
Pyridoxine (vitamin B_6)	Alters metabolism of tryptophan and vitamin B_6	Abnormal protein metabolism; mood changes
Cobalamin (vitamin B_{12})	Reduces vitamin B_{12} serum levels	Unclear
Folic acid	Reduces red cell concentration; increases folate-binding protein	Megaloblastic anemia
Minerals		
Copper	Increases plasma levels of ceruloplasmin	Unclear
Iron	Increases serum levels of transferrin	Unclear
Zinc	Reduces serum levels of zinc	Unclear

Table 18-4

Interactions Between Oral Contraceptive Agents (OCA) and Vitamins and Minerals Affecting Nutritional Status

Data adapted from Butterworth CE Jr and Weinser RL: Malnutrition in hospital patients: assessment and treatment. In Goodhart RS and Shills ME, editors: Modern nutrition in health and disease, ed 6, Philadelphia, 1980, Lea & Febiger.

drugs such as methotrexate have multiple antagonist effects on folic acid metabolism, thus inhibiting the synthesis of cell reproduction substances—DNA, RNA, and protein. In a similar manner, the antimalaria drug pyrimethamine inhibits the action of folic acid in protein synthesis. A list of vitamin-antagonist drugs is given in Table 18-3.

2. **Hypovitaminosis from use of oral contraceptives.** Some women using oral contraceptive agents (OCA) have developed subclinical deficiencies of folic acid, riboflavin, pyridoxine, cobalamin, and ascorbic acid. OCAs induce a greater demand for these vitamins. Table 18-4 includes a list of some of these effects on nutritional status.

Special Adverse Reactions

Several reactions are related to specific drug interactions with particular nutrients (Table 18-5).

1. **Monoamine oxidase inhibitors (MAOIs).** These antidepressant drugs increase the vascular effect of simple **vasoactive** amines, such as tyramine and dopamine, in certain foods in the diet. The resulting *tyramine syndrome* is marked by headache, pallor, nausea, and restlessness. With increased absorption, symptoms may escalate to apprehension, sweating, palpitations, chest pain, fever, and increased blood pressure, at times to the extent of hypertensive crisis and stroke. A low tyramine food list is provided in Table 18-6 for use by any patient taking one of these antidepressant drugs.

2. **Flushing reaction.** A number of drugs react with alcohol to produce a **flushing reaction** along with **dyspnea** and headache. Central nervous system depressants, including hypnotic sedatives, antihistamines, phenothiazines, and narcotic analgesics, may cause a loss of consciousness if taken in combination with alcohol.

3. **Hypoglycemia.** Drugs such as chlorpropamide (Diabinese) and similar oral medications used to control noninsulin-dependent diabetes mellitus (NIDDM) (see Chapter 21) are hypoglycemic agents. They precipitate a rapid release of insulin, which may provoke a hypoglycemic reaction. This response of a rapidly reduced blood glucose level is especially strong when the drugs are used with alcohol. The symptoms of hypoglycemia include weakness, mental confusion, and irrational behavior. If not treated, loss of consciousness can follow.

Vasoactive
Having an effect on the diameter of blood vessels.

Flushing reaction
Short-term reaction resulting in redness of neck and face.

Dyspnea
Labored, difficult breathing.

Table 18-5

Adverse Drug Reactions Caused by Alcohol and Specific Foods

Type of reaction	Drugs	Alcohol/foods	Effects
Flushing	Chlorpropamide (diabetes) Griseofulvin Tetrachloroethylene	Alcohol	Dyspnea, headache, flushing

Disulfiram reaction	Aldehyde dehydrogenase inhibitors:
	  Disulfiram (Antabuse)
	  Calcium carbimide
	  Metronidazole
	  Nitrofurantoin
	  Sulfonylureas
		Alcohol
		Foods containing alcohol
			Abdominal and chest pain, flushing, headache, nausea and vomiting

Hypoglycemia	Insulin-releasing agents: Oral hypoglycemic drugs	Alcohol Sugar, sweets	Mental confusion, weakness, irrational behavior, unconsciousness

Tyramine reaction	Monoamine oxidase inhibitors (MAOI):
	  Antidepressants such as phenelzine
	  Procarbazine
	  Isoniazid (isonicotinic acid hydrazide)
		Foods containing large amounts of tyramine:
		  Cheese
		  Red wines
		  Chicken liver
		  Broad beans
		  Yeast
			Cerebrovascular accident (CVA), flushing, hypertension

Adapted from Roe DA: Interactions between drugs and nutrients, Med Clin North Am 63(5):985, 1979.

Table 18-6
Tyramine-Restricted Diet

General directions

- Designed for patients on monoamine oxidase (MAO) inhibitors, drugs that have been reported to cause hypertensive crises when used with tyramine-rich foods. These include foods in which aging, protein breakdown, and putrefaction are used to increase flavor. Studies indicate that as little as 5 to 6 mg of tyramine can produce a response, and 25 mg is a danger dose.
- Food sources of other pressor amines such as histamine, dihydroxyphenylalanine, and hydroxytyramine are also avoided.
- Avoid all foods listed. Limited amounts of foods with a lower tyramine amount such as yeast bread may be included in a specific diet.
- Avoid over-the-counter drugs such as decongestants, cold remedies, and antihistamines.

Foods to avoid		Additional foods to avoid
(Representative tyramine values in μg/g or ml)		Other aged cheeses
		Blue
Cheeses		Boursault
N.Y. state cheddar	1416	Brick
Gruyère	516	Cheddars (other)
Stilton	466	Gouda
Emmentaler	225	Mozzarella
Brie	180	Parmesan
Camembert	86	Provolone
Processed American	50	Romano
Wines		Roquefort
Chianti	25.4	Yeast and products made with yeast
Sherry	3.6	Homemade bread
Riesling	0.6	Yeast extracts such as soup cubes, canned meats, and marmite
Sauterne	0.4	Italian broad beans with pod (fava beans)
Beer, ale—varies with brand		Meat
Highest	4.4	Aged game
Average	2.3	Liver
Least	1.8	Canned meats with yeast extracts
		Fish (salted dried)
		Herring, cod, capelin
		Pickled herring
		Other
		Cream, especially sour
		Yogurt
		Soy sauce, vanilla, chocolate
		Salad dressings

4. **Disulfiram reaction.** The drug **disulfiram,** commonly called Antabuse, is used in the treatment of alcoholism. It combats alcohol consumption by producing extremely unpleasant side effects when taken with alcohol. Within 15 minutes flushing ensues, followed by headache, nausea, vomiting, and chest or abdominal pain. Other drugs, including aldehyde dehydrogenase inhibitors, may have this similar disulfiram effect.

Disulfiram
A white to off-white, crystalline powder antioxidant; inhibits oxidation of the acetaldehyde metabolized from alcohol.

Effects of Food and Nutrients on Drugs

Food Factors Affecting Drug Absorption

The absorption of drugs is a complex matter. Food can affect eventual drug absorption in a number of ways.

Solution

Before an orally administered tablet or capsule can dissolve, it must first disintegrate. The drug's absorption, either from solution in acid gastric secretions or in the more alkaline medium of the intestine, may be more or less complete depending on its degree of solubility. The drug then passes through the intestinal mucosa and liver circulation before entering systemic circulation. Here it may be subject to metabolism, deactivation, and elimination through the so-called first-pass mechanism. Food may affect eventual drug absorption at any of these points.

Stomach-Emptying Rate

The composition of the diet affects the rate at which the food enters the small intestine from the stomach. Fats, high temperatures, and solid meals prolong the time the food stays in the stomach. Food usually increases secretion of bile, acid, and gut enzymes. It also enhances intestinal motility and **splanchnic** blood flow. Drugs may adsorb to certain food particles.

Splanchnic
Pertaining to the large interior organs of the body, especially those located in the abdomen.

Clinical Significance

Any clinical significance of these food effects depends on the extent of the effect and the nature of the drug. A small change in absorption may be critical for a drug with a steep dose-response curve, but unnoticeable for a drug with a wide range of effective concentration. In general the amount of absorption is clinically more important than the rate, since it has more impact on the steady-state plasma concentration of the drug after multiple doses. Table 18-7 gives some examples of drugs whose amount and rate of absorption is influenced by food.

Food Effects on Drug Absorption
Increased Drug Absorption

Various circumstances contribute to increased absorption of a drug.

1. **Dissolving characteristics.** When a drug does not dissolve rapidly after it has been taken, the time it remains in the stomach with food is prolonged. This increased time in the stomach may increase its effective dissolution and consequent absorption.

2. **Gastric-emptying time.** Delayed emptying of food from the stomach can have the effect of doling out small portions of a drug, creating more optimal saturation rates on the absorptive sites in the small intestine.

3. **Nutrients.** Some nutrients promote absorption of certain drugs. For example, high-fat diets increase absorption of the antifungal drug griseofulvin. This drug is fat-soluble, and high-fat diets stimulate secretion of bile acids, which aid in the absorption of the drug. Vitamin C, as well as gastric acid, enhances iron absorption.

4. **Blood flow.** Food intake increases splanchnic blood flow. This increased circulation increases absorption.

5. **Nutritional status.** In addition to the presence of specific nutrients, nutritional status may also affect bioavailability of certain drugs. For example,

Absorption reduced by food	Absorption delayed by food
Amoxicillin	Acetaminophen
Ampicillin	Amoxicillin
Aspirin	Aspirin
Demethyl chlortetracycline	Cephalexin
Doxycycline	Cephradine
Isoniazid	Digoxin
Levodopa	Furosemide
Methacycline	Potassium ion
Oxytetracycline	Sulfadiazine
Penicillin G, V(K)	Sulfamethoxine
Phenethicillin	Sulfamethoxypyridazine
Phenobarbital	Sulfanilamide
Propantheline	Sulfasymasine
Rifampicin	Sulfisoxazole
Tetracycline	

Table 18-7

Food Effect on Drug Absorption

Adapted from Roe DA: Interactions between drugs and nutrients, Med Clin North Am 63(5):985, 1979.

chloramphenicol is absorbed more slowly in children with protein-energy malnutrition, but elimination of the drug is also slower in well-nourished children, resulting in a net increased bioavailability of the drug.

Decreased Drug Absorption

The absorption of some drugs is delayed or reduced by the presence of food.

1. **Aspirin.** The absorption of aspirin is reduced or delayed by food. So it should be taken on an empty stomach with ample water, preferably cold (see the box on p. 429).

2. **Tetracycline.** Nutrition status may also have an impact on drug absorption. For example, tetracycline absorption is impaired in malnourished individuals. Absorption of this commonly used antibiotic is also hindered when it is taken with milk, as well as with antacids or iron supplements. The drug combines with these materials to form new insoluble compounds that the body cannot absorb.[19]

3. **Phenytoin.** The presence of protein inhibits the absorption of phenytoin. Carbohydrate increases its absorption, but fat has no impact.

Food Effects on Drug Distribution and Metabolism
Carbohydrate and Fat

Dietary carbohydrate and fat, especially their relative quantities, influence liver enzymes that metabolize drugs. For example, the presence of fat increases the activity of diazepam (Valium). Fat increases the concentration of the unbound active drug by displacing it from binding sites in plasma and tissue protein.

Indole
Compound produced in the intestines by the decomposition of tryptophan; obtained from indigo and coal tar.

Cruciferous vegetables
Vegetables belonging to the botanical family *Cruciferae* or *Brassicaceae*, whose members have cross-like, four-petaled flowers; e.g., broccoli, cabbage, brussels sprouts, cauliflower.

Indoles

The **indoles** in **cruciferous vegetables** (cabbage, brussels sprouts, broccoli, cauliflower) can speed up the rate of drug metabolism. They apparently induce mixed-function oxidase enzyme systems in the liver.

Cooking Methods

The method of cooking foods may alter the rate of drug metabolism. Charcoal broiling, for example, increases hepatic drug metabolism through enzyme induction.

Changes in Intestinal Microflora

Changes in intestinal microflora related to the amount of dietary protein or fiber, for example, may influence intestinal drug metabolism.

Vitamin Effects on Drug Action
Effects of Vitamin Megadoses on Drug Effectiveness

Pharmacologic doses of vitamins can decrease blood levels of drugs when vitamins interact with drugs. For example, large doses of folic acid or pyridoxine can reduce blood level and effectiveness of such anticonvulsive drugs as phenytoin (Dilantin) or phenobarbital that are used for seizure control. Unwise self-medication with large drug-level doses of vitamins can cause severe toxic complications.[20] On the other hand, vitamins themselves may become important medications when used as part of the medical treatment for a secondary deficiency induced by a childhood genetic or metabolic disease. Such is the case with biotin in treating certain organic acidemias, or riboflavin in treating certain defects in fatty acid metabolism.[21]

Control of Drug Intoxication

Riboflavin can be useful in treating boric acid poisoning. Boric acid combines with the ribityl side-chain of riboflavin and is excreted in the urine. Also, vitamin E combats pulmonary oxygen toxicity. Premature human infants at risk for development of bronchopulmonary dysplasia by oxygen treatment have been protected by vitamin E administration during the acute phase of respiratory distress requiring oxygen treatment.

To Sum Up

The field of nutrient-drug interaction is in its infancy. More research is needed to sort out complicated relationships and possible effects. Drugs can have multiple effects on the body's absorption, metabolism, retention, and nutrient status. They can provoke adverse reactions in combination with certain foods and can influence appetite, either repressing it or artificially stimulating it. Drugs can either increase an individual's absorption of nutrients or, more commonly, decrease absorption, sometimes leading to clinical deficiencies. Drugs can also induce mineral and vitamin deficiencies by their mode of action.

Just as drugs affect our use of food, food affects our use of drugs. Food can affect the absorption of drugs in a variety of ways. Foods also have an effect on subsequent distribution and metabolism of drugs. Vitamins may interfere with drug effectiveness, especially if they are taken in large doses. On the other hand, large doses of specific vitamins can be effective in countering certain toxicity conditions or a specific secondary deficiency induced by a genetic disease.

Aspirin has a venerable history. Being a buffered form of salicylic acid, it is a modified version of an ancient folk-remedy, willow bark, used for many hundreds of years for fever, aches, and pain. The acetyl group in acetylsalicylic acid makes aspirin easier on the stomach than willow bark.

Aspirin is an analgesic agent used for relief of minor aches and pains. Its mechanism of action is through inhibition of certain **prostaglandins** (see Chapter 3), which have a profound influence on a spectrum of physiologic functions, including blood clotting, blood pressure, the inflammatory process, contraction of voluntary muscles, and transmission of nerve impulses.

Studies implicate aspirin in alleviating many disorders, dangers, and discomforts, including the following:

- The risk of repeated *transient ischemic attacks (TIAs)*, or little strokes, is reduced by 50% in men (but *not* women) who have already had one.
- Many studies indicate that aspirin is effective in reducing risk for *myocardial infarction*, or heart attack.
- Aspirin is one of the most effective antiinflammatory drugs and is effective in the long-term treatment of *arthritis*.
- Aspirin may play a role in inhibiting the spread of some *cancers* through its action of inhibiting production of prostaglandin E_2.
- Aspirin's effect as an anticoagulant is important in the treatment of *phlebitis* and other clot-related disorders.
- Aspirin may be effective in promoting *sleep*. Many scientists now believe aspirin is as effective as most prescription sedatives, and it has far fewer and less serious side effects.
- Diabetic patients who take aspirin may have lower risk of developing *retinopathy*.

It is important to remember that aspirin is a *drug*. Many of the benefits of aspirin stem from its systemic, wide-reaching effects on metabolism, which may have unforeseen short- and long-term detrimental results. We do know that aspirin is to be strictly *avoided* by persons with hemophilia. Also, allergic reactions to aspirin can be severe. Aspirin seems to be implicated in asthma. Children are especially vulnerable to side effects and should not be given aspirin without a physician's instructions.

Aspirin is an irritant to the stomach and gut. Its continuous use is associated with low-level chronic loss of iron caused by mucosal erosion of the stomach and gut. This can lead to iron-deficiency anemia.

Aspirin has been linked to birth defects, especially when it is taken later in the course of pregnancy. It increases risk of infant and neonatal mortality, low birth weight, and intracranial hemorrhage.

The best way to take aspirin is on an empty stomach with a full glass of water. This is important: the absorption of aspirin is facilitated by a large volume of liquid and inhibited by the presence of food. In addition, taking aspirin—especially on an empty stomach—without a large fluid intake invites erosion of the stomach lining.

The Pain Reliever Doctors Recommend Most

Prostaglandins
Small hormone-like biochemicals that are derivatives of fatty acids.

REFERENCES
Griffith HW: Complete guide to prescription and non-prescription drugs, ed 5, Los Angeles, 1988, The Body Press, Price Stern Sloan, Inc.
Koch PA and others: Influence of food and fluid ingestion on aspirin bioavailability, J Pharm Sci 67(11):1533, 1978.
Ribakove BM: Aspirin, Health 14(2):40, 1982.

Questions for Review

1. Name four ways food may affect drug use and give examples of each.
2. If your patient were using a prescribed MAOI such as Parnate, what foods would you instruct him/her to avoid?
3. What is the most effective way to take aspirin, with what type of liquid, and with or without food? Why?
4. What foods would you suggest to a hypertensive patient on the diuretic drug hydrochlorothiazide as good sources of potassium replacement?
5. Outline suggestions you would discuss with a patient experiencing a drug-induced taste loss. How would you explain the taste loss?
6. How do cimetidine (Tagamet) or ranitidine (Zantac) help improve the nutritional status of persons with gastrointestinal disease?

References

1. Roe DA: Diet, nutrition and drug reaction. In Shils ME and Young VR, editors: Modern nutrition in health and disease, ed 7, Philadelphia, 1988, Lea & Febiger.
2. Roe DA: Geriatric nutrition, ed 2, Englewood Cliffs, NJ, 1987, Prentice-Hall, Inc.
3. Welling P: Nutrient effects on drug metabolism and action in the elderly, Drug-Nutrient Interactions 4(1/2):173, 1985.
4. Munro HN: Nutrient needs and nutritional status in relation to aging, Drug-Nutrient Interactions 4(1/2):55, 1985.
5. Garattini S: Drug metabolism and actions in the aged, Drug-Nutrient Interactions 4(1/2):87, 1985.
6. Lamy PP: Nutrition, drugs, and the elderly, Clin Nutr 2(6):9, 1983.
7. Roe DA: Process guides on drug and nutrient interactions for health care providers and patients. I. An overview, Drug-Nutrient Interactions 5(3):131, 1987.
8. Roe DA: Process guides on drug and nutrient interactions in arthritics, Drug-Nutrient Interactions 5(3):135, 1987.
9. Kamath SK and others: Hospital malnutrition: a 33-hospital screening study, J Am Diet Assoc 86(2):203, 1986.
10. Torum B and Viteri FE: Protein-energy malnutrition. In Shils ME and Young, VR, editors: Modern nutrition in health and disease, ed 7, Philadelphia, 1988, Lea & Febiger.
11. Griffith HW: Complete guide to prescription and nonprescription drugs, Los Angeles, 1988, The Body Press, Price Stern Sloan, Inc.
12. Seitz HK: Alcohol effects on drug-nutrient interactions, Drug-Nutrition Interactions 4(1/2):143, 1985.
13. Roe DA, Kalkwarf H, and Stevens J: Effect of fiber supplements on the apparent absorption of pharmacological doses of riboflavin, J Am Diet Assoc 88(2):212, 1988.
14. Dorup I and others: Reduced concentrations of potassium, magnesium, and sodium-potassium pumps in human skeletal muscle during treatment with diuretics, Br Med J 296:455, 1988.
15. Russell RP: Potassium supplementation, potassium-retaining diuretics, and hazards of hyperkalemia, Clin Nutr 6(2):70, 1987.
16. Tolstoi LG and Fosmire G: Milk-alkali syndrome revisited: a review of 63 years, Nutr Today 22(2):22, 1987.
17. McCabe BJ: Dietary tyramine and other pressor amines in MAOI regimens: a review, J Am Diet Assoc 86(8):1059, 1986.
18. Lippman S: Monoamine oxidase inhibitors, Am Fam Physician 34:113, July 1986.
19. Avors J: Why Tums don't go with tetracycline, Am Health 1(2):74, 1982.
20. Evans CD and Lacey JH: Toxicity of vitamins: complications of a health movement, Br Med J 292:509, 1986.
21. Marshall MW: The nutritional importance of biotin—an update, Nutr Today 22(6):26, 1987.

Diet pills and stroke, Am J Nurs 87:1070, Aug 1987.

Tolstoi LG and Fosmire G: Milk-alkali syndrome revisited: a review of 63 years, Nutr Today 22(2):22, 1987.

Here are two reviews of the possible dangers in abuse of two popular over-the-counter nonprescription drugs—pheylpropanolamine (PPA), the fifth most frequently used drug product in the United States, found in many diet pills; and antacids, used by 27% of the adult United States population, who spend $500 million a year for these products.

Marshall MW: The nutritional importance of biotin—an update, Nutr Today 22(6):26, 1987.

This article provides a good illustration of a nutrient used in drug dosages as medical treatment for inborn errors of metabolism in children.

McCabe BJ: Dietary tyramine and other pressor amines in MAOI regimens: a review, J Am Diet Assoc 86(8):1059, 1986.

This nutritionist-author provides a critical review of the literature and rational guidelines for diet planning and counseling of patients on monoamine oxidase inhibitor (MAOI) drugs, with many tables and references.

Roe DA: Dimensions of risk assessment for drug and nutrient interactions, Nutr Today 22(6):20, 1987.

Here Dr. Roe, prolific physician-author-editor and leading authority on drug-nutrient interactions, discusses the professional health team's joint responsibilities for assessment of a patient's risk of drug-nutrient interactions.

Smith CH and Bidlack WR: Dietary concerns associated with the use of medications, J Am Diet Assoc 84(8):901, 1984.

This comprehensive review article provides excellent reference material, including large tables and extensive cited references, for planned patient education and counseling to avoid harmful drug-nutrient interactions.

Further Readings

The Calming of America?

American medicine has many names for the psychoactive drugs that act on the mind to dull its reactions. But all these drugs interact dangerously with alcohol and in some cases with commonly eaten foods. Perhaps the name that best fits the effect of these drugs is *tranquilizer*, from a Latin root meaning "calm, quiet, stillness." This meaning signifies the escape many persons seek from a turbulent, confusing world.

We live in an age of stress, often called the "era of anxiety." We also live in a culture committed to "instant" cures and the avoidance of discomfort. Often instead of probing the causes of our problems and striving to alter the conditions that produce them, we feel somehow that we must never feel uncomfortable. And if we do, we take something for it. We seek the "magic potion" to ease the pain and often the symptoms.

To what extent do we actually use such antianxiety drugs in our search for relief? According to the National Academy of Sciences, some 8.5 million Americans take prescription sleeping pills at least once a year. Two million take them every night for periods of at least 2 months at a time. A study conducted by the National Institute on Drug Abuse indicated that 17 million Americans have used stimulants, 28 million have taken sedatives, and 51 million—nearly 1 out of every 4 Americans—have taken tranquilizers.

America's single most widely prescribed tranquilizer drug is *diazepam (Valium)*. For example, in one recent year, 3.2 billion pills were sold legally, up 50% from the year before, enough to provide every man, woman, and child in the United States with 145 pills a year. Today Valium remains the country's most widely prescribed drug, although a similar antianxiety agent *lorazepam (Ativan)*, is close on its heels. It is difficult to explain just why Valium is the most frequently prescribed psychoactive drug in the United States.

Certainly from a scientific or a pharmacologic viewpoint, no superior effectiveness has been proved. Its popularity may be explained by an aggressive marketing program, leading more physicians to prescribe it, and increased quantities of the drug that are being manufactured. In turn, the increased availability of the drug has led to increased black market exposure and easy street usage. Also, probably the pale blue Valium tablets were more appealing than the dark green capsules or yellow tablets of some of its competitors.

Valium belongs to a group of psychoactive drugs, first introduced in 1960, called *benzodiazepines*. These antianxiety drugs bind to specific receptor sites in the brain. Their clinical effects are mediated through the central nervous system. For some time scientists have sought the identity of the body's natural compound that occupies these receptor sites in the brain. Now pharmacologists report purification of this natural substance. Paradoxically, they have discovered that this new 104-amino acid brain peptide not only blocks the receptor-binding action of the antianxiety drugs but also appears to induce anxiety, indicating that it is not a natural tranquilizer, but has just the opposite effect. Thus this newly identified compound has been named *diazepam-binding inhibitor (DBI)*. These scientists suggest that the naturally occurring DBI acts to trigger anxiety-associated behavior. Apparently, then, drugs such as Valium achieve their antianxiety effect by getting in the way of this naturally occurring anxiety-producing brain peptide.

Along with its desired effect, a drug usually causes some unwanted side effects. In the case of antianxiety drugs such as Valium, several interactions and side effects relate to nutrition counseling needs.

- **Alcohol.** Tranquilizers and alcohol do not mix. These drugs enhance the effects of alcohol and other central nervous system (CNS) depressant drugs that slow down the nervous system. In addition to alcohol, other CNS depressant drugs include over-the-counter antihistamines or medicine for hay fever, other allergies, or colds, as well as prescribed anticonvulsants (e.g., Dilantin), pain medications, or narcotics. Long-term use of alcohol also induces liver enzyme changes leading to more rapid metabolism, reducing the effect of drugs that are detoxified by the liver. Thus in the alcoholic, benzodiazepines may be metabolized more rapidly and the person may use larger and larger doses to achieve the desired effect.

- **Weight gain.** Persons on these antianxiety drugs often have a marked increase in appetite with subsequent weight gain. This may bring added concern and require general weight management counseling.

- **Gastrointestinal problems.** Some general side effects interfere with food intake and use. These problems range from heartburn, nausea, and vomiting to constipation or diarrhea. Individual counseling relating to food choices, combinations, and forms may be needed.

- **Pregnancy and lactation.** Some cases of birth defects from benzodiazepine use during the first 3 months of pregnancy have been reported. In addition, continued use during pregnancy may cause fetal dependency with withdrawal side effects after birth. During lactation these drugs may pass into the breast milk and cause unwanted effects in the infant.

Such widespread use—and abuse—of tranquilizers means that we will frequently encounter them in clinical practice. Nutrition counseling must involve assessment of all possible food, drug, and alcohol interactions, with related guidance concerning dietary management.

REFERENCES

Griffith HW: Complete guide to prescription and non-prescription drugs: Side effects, warnings and vital data for safe use, ed 5, Los Angeles, 1988, The Body Press, Price Stern Sloan, Inc.

Hughes R and Brewin R: The daze of our lives, Fam Health (11(10):28, 1979.

Miller JA: Brain peptides in a chemistry of anxiety, Sci News 123(5):388, 1983.

19 Gastrointestinal Problems

Chapter Objectives

After study of this chapter, the student should be able to:

1. Identify food-related problems that occur in the mouth and esophagus and describe the general nutritional therapy needed in each case.
2. Describe the current nutritional therapy for peptic ulcer disease and contrast it with previous traditional therapy.
3. Describe the rationale for current nutritional treatment of diverticulitis in contrast to former therapy.
4. Relate nutritional therapy for inflammatory bowel disease to the underlying problems involved and outline a specific patient's nutritional care plan.
5. Describe the food intolerance problem in phenylketonuria and its related nutritional therapy.
6. Compare the underlying problem in both galactosemia and lactose intolerance and the nutritional therapy in each case.
7. Identify basic food allergy or sensitivity problems and develop realistic plans for nutritional therapy.
8. Compare liver functions and nutritional problems in hepatitis, cirrhosis, and hepatic encephalopathy, relating the therapy in each case.
9. Relate gallbladder and pancreatic functions to nutritional therapy for disease in each organ.

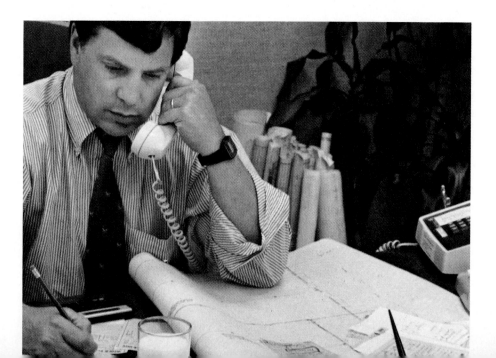

Surrounding every stomach there is a person. The gastrointestinal tract is a sensitive mirror of the individual human condition. Its physiologic function reflects both physical and psychologic conditioning.

In adapting nutritional therapy to treat patients with gastrointestinal disorders, we have to focus our care on the person. We deal not so much with a specific food item per se as with the state of the body that receives it.

Ingestion, digestion, and absorption of the food begin in the mouth and esophagus and end in the remaining gastrointestinal tract, supported by secretions from important accessory organs such as the liver, gallbladder, and pancreas. All along the way a series of intimately related secretory and neuromuscular mechanisms accomplish these vital tasks.

In this chapter of our continuing clinical nutrition study, we consider the nature of clinical problems that may occur in this fundamental body system and its adjacent accessory organs. These problems of necessity govern our related nutritional therapy in each case. But also, in each case, we seek to apply this clinical background knowledge to the individual patient involved and focus on personal needs. As always, our primary concern is the *person* with the problem and how we might best provide needed nutritional support for healing.

Mouth Problems
Cleft Palate and Cleft Lip

Cleft palate in infants and younger children results from abnormalities in the structure of the mouth. When parts of the upper jaw and palate separating the mouth and nasal cavity do not fuse properly during fetal development, the anatomic abnormality creates difficult feeding problems. The premaxillary and maxillary processes normally fuse early in gestation, between the fifth and eighth weeks of intrauterine life. Fusion of the palate is completed about 1 month later. If this fusion fails to occur, cleft lip (hairlip) or cleft palate results. Nutritional problems relate mainly to general feeding difficulties and follow-up surgical repair.

1. **Feeding difficulties.** The infant with cleft palate or lip is unable to suck adequately, so feedings are tiring and lengthy. A softened nipple with an enlarged opening helps the infant obtain milk by a chewing motion. In some instances a medicine dropper or gavage feedings may be used initially. Holding the infant in an upright position and feeding slowly avoids aspiration of milk into the airway. Brief rest periods and frequent burping help expel the large amount of air swallowed.

2. **Surgical repair.** Corrective surgery is usually done at about 6 months of age. Follow-up work is done as needed, depending on the extent of the deformity and the growth of the child. During the surgery period the child is usually cared for by a team of specialists. Preparation for surgery demands good nutritional status (see Chapter 23). Following surgery, special nutritional support and nursing care are essential. The infant or child is usually fed a fluid or semifluid diet by use of a syringe or large dropper in the cor-

Problems of the Mouth and Esophagus

ner of the mouth. Great care must be exercised to protect the suture line and avoid any strain.

Dental Caries

Over the past few decades there has been a significant continuing decline in the caries rate. Some of this decline results from increased use of fluoridated public water supplies and fluoridated toothpastes as well as better dental hygiene. However, during this same period the use of sugar in foods consumed by children has not declined. There has been a downward trend in the consumption of refined cane and beet sugar, but this has been compensated for by an increase in the use of high-fructose corn sweeteners in processed foods. The net result is that the use of sugars is relatively unchanged, and gradually increasing. The large amount of dietary sugar consumed by children is still a nutritional concern.

Although the problem of dental caries has decreased in recent years, it is by no means solved. However, two nutritional factors are apparent: (1) adhesive simple carbohydrates, such as sweets, candy bars, and caramels, consumed at frequent intervals do increase dental caries, but simple carbohydrates in liquid form are less cariogenic than those in solid form; and (2) fluoridated public water supplies do decrease dental caries rates, although this practice still remains a source of controversy in some communities.

Dentures

In some older persons, loss of teeth or ill-fitting dentures may cause problems with chewing and hence digestion of foods. The health of the gums on which the dentures rest is imperative for successful fit and use. Vitamins A and C are particularly related to the integrity of gum tissue and may need special attention in the diet when healing or strengthening is necessary. When dental problems exist or when dentures are not available, a *mechanical soft diet* may be used. In this diet all foods are soft-cooked. Meats are ground and sometimes mixed with sauces or gravies to require less chewing and make eating easier.

Fractured Jaw

A fractured jaw or other surgical procedure on the mouth or neck can pose obvious eating problems. After the initial jaw injury has been corrected with surgical wiring, the resulting immobility prevents normal eating. A liquid diet high in protein and energy, taken through a straw, is needed to provide healing nutrients. A typical high-protein, high-caloric blended formula is given in Table 19-1. As healing continues, semisolid soft foods requiring little chewing can be introduced at first, with gradual advance to regular foods.

Esophageal Problems
Nature of Problems

After food is taken into the mouth, chewed, and swallowed, it passes down the esophagus to the stomach aided by peristalsis and gravity. At the entry to the stomach, the *gastroesophageal sphincter muscle* forms a controlling valve. It relaxes to receive the food, then closes to hold each **bolus** for digestive action of enzymes in the gastric acid mix. A number of conditions may interfere with this normal food passage and create problems. These conditions vary

Bolus
A rounded mass of food that is ready to be swallowed.

Ingredients	Amount	Approximate food value	
Milk	1 cup	Protein	40 g
Eggs	2	Fat	30 g
Skim milk powder	6 to 8 tbsp	Carbohydrate	70 g
or Casec	2 tbsp	Calories	710
Sugar	2 tbsp		
Ice cream	2.5 cm (1 in) slice or 1 scoop		
Cocoa or other flavoring	2 tbsp		
Vanilla	Few drops, as desired		

Table 19-1
High-Protein, High-Calorie Formula

widely from brief periods of functional discomfort—**dysphagia** ("indigestion")—to serious disease and complete obstruction. In any case, choice of food and feeding mode are adapted to the degree of dysfunction. Several types of esophageal problems encountered in general clinical practice are briefly described here.

Dysphagia
Difficulty in swallowing.

Reflux Esophagitis

Regurgitation of the acid gastric contents into the lower part of the esophagus creates tissue irritation. The hydrochloric acid and pepsin cause tissue erosion, with symptoms of substernal burning, cramping, pressure sensation, or severe pain. These symptoms are aggravated by lying down or by any increase in abdominal pressure, such as that caused by tight clothing. This condition is related to: (1) an incompetent gastroesophageal sphincter muscle; (2) frequency and duration of the acid reflux; and (3) the inability of the esophagus to produce normal secondary peristaltic waves to prevent prolonged contact of the esophageal mucosa with the acid and pepsin. A *hiatal hernia* may or may not be present. In addition, the acid reflux may be caused by the upward pressure of advancing pregnancy or obesity or by pernicious vomiting or nasogastric tube. The most common symptom is **pyrosis.** It is frequently severe, occurring 30 to 60 minutes after eating. Sometimes pain radiates into the neck and jaw or down the arms. Other symptoms include iron-deficiency anemia, with chronic tissue bleeding, or aspiration, which may cause cough, dyspnea, or pneumonitis. The most common complications are **stenosis** and *esophageal ulcer.* Also, significant **gastritis** in the herniated portion of the stomach may cause *occult bleeding* and anemia. Treatment centers on the often associated or precipitating factor of obesity. Thus weight reduction is essential. The patient should avoid lying down immediately after meals and should sleep with the head of the bed elevated. Frequent use of antacids helps control the symptoms. From 85% to 90% of persons with esophagitis respond to weight reduction and conservative measures.

Pyrosis
Heartburn.

Stenosis
Narrowing or closing of a canal or duct.

Gastritis
Inflammation of the stomach.

Hiatal Hernia

Normally the lower end of the esophagus enters the chest cavity at the **hiatus,** an opening in the diaphragmatic membrane, and immediately joins the

Hiatus
An opening or gap.

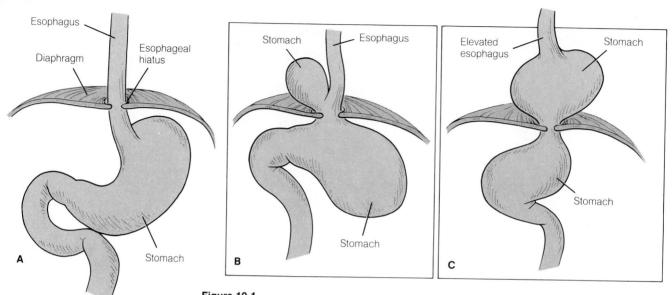

Figure 19-1
Hiatal hernia in comparison with normal stmach placement. **A,** Normal stomach. **B,** Paraesophageal hernia (esophagus in normal position). **C,** Esophageal hiatal hernia (elevated esophagus).

upper portion of the stomach. A hiatal hernia occurs when a portion of the upper part of the stomach at this entry point protrudes through the hiatus alongside the lower portion of the esophagus (Figure 19-1). Food is easily held in this herniated area of the stomach and mixed with acid and pepsin, then it is regurgitated back up into the lower portion of the esophagus. Gastritis can occur in this herniated portion of the stomach, as indicated, and cause bleeding and anemia. The reflux of acid gastric contents causes symptoms similar to those described above. Since obesity is frequently associated with hiatal hernia, weight reduction is a primary need. Avoiding tight clothing helps relieve discomfort. Patients will need to avoid leaning over or lying down immediately after meals and should sleep with the head of the bed elevated. Antacids help relieve the burning sensation. Large hiatal hernias or smaller sliding hernias may require surgical repair.

Diverticula

Small outpouchings in the gastrointestinal tract are called *diverticula*. These pouches may occur in the esophagus and the lower intestine. Esophageal diverticula cause general dysphagia with regurgitation of undigested or partially digested food. If the diverticula are located in the upper part of the esophagus, the main symptoms are dysphagia, regurgitation, coughing, bad breath, and a foul taste in the mouth. Difficulty in swallowing increases, and eating becomes more difficult. Weight loss and impaired nutrition follow. If the diverticula are in the middle or lower portion of the esophagus, the symptoms are more delayed after beginning to eat. Ultimately, however, the condition produces dysphagia and pain. Nutritional therapy centers on selecting foods according to tolerance and developing habits of eating slowly and chewing food well. Surgical removal of large, symptom-producing diverticula may be indicated.

Peptic Ulcer Disease

Incidence

Throughout the world peptic ulcer disease affects about 10% of the population. It is the subject of millions of dollars of research and causes the loss of many productive work hours. It can occur at any age, but the highest incidence is in middle adulthood, between ages 45 and 55. Gastric and duodenal ulcers, along with the complication of perforation, occur more often in men than in women, but related frequencies vary with the patient's age and the type of ulcer involved. Peptic ulcers may occur with other diseases or with injuries such as burns—the so-called stress ulcer.

Causes

The exact cause of peptic ulcer is unclear. There is some evidence that a genetic factor may be involved, since close relatives of patients with ulcers have approximately three times as many ulcers as members of the general population. It is evident, however, that both physical and psychogenic factors are involved and that there is an imbalance between two basic factors: (1) gastric acid and pepsin and (2) tissue resistance.

Physical Factors

Peptic ulcer is the general term given to an eroded mucosal lesion in the central portion of the gastrointestinal tract. Areas affected include the lower portion of the esophagus, the stomach, and the first portion of the duodenum, the "duodenal bulb." Esophageal and gastric ulcers are less common. Most ulcers occur in the duodenal bulb, where gastric contents emptying into the duodenum through the pyloric valve are most concentrated. Gastric ulcers occur usually along the lesser curvature of the stomach. Peptic ulcer itself is a **benign** disease. Gastric ulcers, however, are more prone to develop into **malignant** disease. The underlying lesion results from an imbalance between the gastric acid and pepsin secretions and the degree of tissue resistance to these secretions.[1]

Benign
Not malignant or recurring.

Malignant
Not improving, worsening; resulting in death.

1. **Gastric acid and pepsin.** In ulcer formation, large amounts of hydrochloric acid and the strong gastric enzyme pepsin are secreted. Although much research is being done on this hypersecretion of acid, little is understood about its underlying causes.

2. **Tissue resistance.** The balancing factor in the development of the disease is the degree of mucosal tissue resistance to withstand the erosive and digestive action of these secretions. Several factors seem to influence the tissue's ability to withstand such destructive action: (a) the integrity of the mucosal cells, (b) the ability of the epithelial cells to regenerate themselves, (c) the mucosal barrier, and (d) the blood supply. Various topical irritants interfere with normal function of this tissue, including aspirin, alcohol, certain drugs, caffeine, or bile acids that may come in contact with the mucosa. Thus factors that contribute to weakened mucosa resistance in patients with gastric ulcers revolve around poor nutrition, diminished mucosal blood flow, and a defect in the inhibition of gastric acid and pepsin secretion. In the development of gastric ulcers, although the presence of acid is essential, the degree of tissue sensitivity seems to be the paramount factor. In the development of duodenal ulcers, excess production of acid and pepsin is the primary factor. In either case, gastric hydrochloric acid is the necessary factor in the development and recurrence of peptic ulcer.

Psychogenic Factors

The influence of psychologic factors in the development of peptic ulcer is highly variable. Such stress factors may well play some role, but there is no distinct personality type that is free from the disease. Men are affected two to three times more frequently than are women, and the average age of incidence has increased. These are the adult years when career and personal strivings are at a peak. Also, stress ulcers occur in conjunction with emergency injuries such as burns or long-term rehabilitation processes.

Symptoms and General Management
Clinical Symptoms

Basic symptoms of peptic ulcer are increased gastric tone and painful hunger contractions when the stomach is empty. In duodenal ulcer, the amount and concentration of hydrochloric acid are increased. In gastric ulcer it may be normal. Nutritional deficiencies are evident in low plasma protein levels, anemia, and loss of weight. Hemorrhage may be the first sign in some patients. Diagnosis is based on clinical findings, x-ray tests, or visualization by gastroscopy.

General Medical Management

The prime objective in medical management is to provide psychologic rest and support tissue healing. Three factors form the basis of care:

1. **Drug therapy.** Antacids buffer excess acid present. Other drugs inhibit gastric acid secretion, which is normally stimulated by the presence of food and the local hormone *gastrin* in the lower part of the stomach. Two commonly used drugs to inhibit gastric acid secretion are *cimetidine* (Tagamet) and *ranitidine* (Zantac). These drugs are antihistamines that act as antagonists to block histamine-stimulated gastric acid secretion.

2. **Rest.** Both physical and mental rest are required for healing. This rest is aided as needed by sedative therapy and stress-reduction relaxation techniques (see Chapter 16).

3. **Diet.** Nutritional therapy for peptic ulcer has changed considerably in recent times. Its basic objective is to support healing and prevent further tissue damage.

Dietary Management
Traditional "Bland" Diets

The so-called "bland" diets used in the past for treatment of peptic ulcer have proved to be unwarranted and ineffective. A more liberal individual approach prevails today in modern clinical practice.

Basis for change. The development of more liberal approaches in the care of persons with peptic ulcer is based on recognition of individual need and use of a sound nutritional base for healing. Over the past few decades an accumulation of clinical experience and research has reinforced this approach and refuted many food dogmas of the past.

1. **Protein foods.** Milk and other protein foods have been considered effective buffering agents because of their amphoteric nature (acting as both acids and bases). However, although they do have some buffering effect, they also induce gastric secretions, as do all foods ingested. Recent studies indicate that a diet with a high milk content has an adverse effect on the healing rate

of the ulcer, because the high calcium content may also stimulate excess acid production; therefore, the use of milk should be limited.[2] Some investigators have questioned the effect of milk on gastric acid secretion, whereas other clinicians express opposing views. In general, proteins influence gastric secretions even more than do carbohydrates and fats. Volume of any food sufficient to exert pressure against the lower stomach wall stimulates gastric acid secretion through the gastrin mechanism. Any form of fat tends to suppress gastric secretion and motility through the enterogastrone mechanism (see Chapter 2), accounting for some of the effect of whole milk. Milk continues to be a source of needed nutrients for healing purposes.

2. **Seasonings.** Other studies indicate that herbs and spices and other condiments have had little or no irritating effect on the majority of persons with ulcers. The sight, smell, and taste of most food normally initiate gastric secretion.[3] But no significant change in gastric pH has been noted with the use of any particular items, except *alcohol, caffeine, black pepper,* and *meat extractives.* No food is sufficiently acid of itself to effect a significant pH change or cause direct irritation of an ulcer.

3. **Food texture.** The routine omission of any fiber in the diet to treat ulcers seems to have no basis in fact. A regular diet, including good food sources of dietary fiber, has proved to be beneficial.[4]

4. **Gas formers.** Routinely omitting a number of foods because of their reputation for being "gas formers" has also been questioned. Clinical observations show that tolerance for a variety of standard foods is highly individual. Patients with gastrointestinal disease have shown no greater intolerance for such foods than have persons without disease.

Current Liberal Management

Sound nutritional management is essential in the total medical care of the person with peptic ulcer disease. The individual must be the focus of treatment. The patient is not "an ulcer"; he or she is a *person* with an ulcer. The course of the disease is conditioned by the patient's unique makeup and life situation, and its presence in turn affects his or her life. Therefore two basic principles guide the current liberal approach:

1. **The individual must be treated as such.** A careful initial history will give information about daily living situations, attitudes, food reactions, and tolerances. On the basis of such a history a reasonable and adequate nutritional program *that can be followed* may be worked out with the patient.

2. **The activity of the ulcer will influence dietary management.** During acute periods of active ulceration more modified treatment may be needed to control acidity and initiate healing. However, when pain disappears, feedings can be liberalized according to individual tolerance and desire, using a variety of foods. Sound nutritional support and improved emotional outlook hasten recovery. During quiet periods, and for long-term preventive measures when the person has no symptoms, judicious choices from a wide range of foods and regular, unhurried eating habits will provide the best course of action.

Summary of General Nutritional Therapy for Peptic Ulcer

1. **Sound total nutrition.** There must be optimal overall nutritional intake to support recovery and maintain healthy tissue, based on individual needs and food tolerances.

2. **Protein.** Since protein provides the necessary amino acids for synthesis of tissue protein, there must be adequate dietary protein for tissue-healing needs, but not excessive amounts that stimulate more gastric secretion. This means that adequate carbohydrate is needed to supply energy requirements and spare protein for the necessary tissue healing.

3. **Fat.** Moderate amounts of fat help to suppress gastric secretion and motility. If cardiovascular disease is a concern, reduction of saturated fats and cholesterol is indicated, with substitution of mono- and polyunsaturated fat (see Chapter 20).

4. **Meal pattern.** Meals and snacks at regular intervals in small proportions will help maintain individual control of gastric secretions. These may be frequent, small feedings during more active stress periods. Regular meals, moderate in size and sufficient in number for individual need, should be established as a regular habit.

5. **Individual need.** Positive individual needs and a flexible program guide food planning. Individual counseling that meets personal needs forms the keystone of wise peptic ulcer therapy.

A general dietary guide incorporating these liberal nutritional therapy principles to control peptic ulcer disease is provided here (see box, p. 444).

Intestinal Diseases

General Functional Disorders
Irritable Bowel Syndrome

This general stress-related functional disorder of the intestine may occur at any age but is more frequent in women. It may be caused by irritation of the mucous membrane, with symptoms varying between spastic constipation and "nervous" diarrhea. These harried individuals develop patterns of irregular eating and bowel habits. They often resort to excessive use of laxatives, cathartics, enemas, and a variety of medications. In general, individual education and reassurance, along with sound diet counseling, are paramount factors in management of the condition.[5] Dietary measures are designed to provide optimal nutrition and regular bowel motility. There should be additional amounts of bulk foods, such as fruits, vegetables, and whole grains. However, during alternate periods of diarrhea or excess flatulence, the fiber content may need to be decreased. Supportive therapy is needed to help reduce stress factors involved.

Constipation

A common disorder, usually of short duration, constipation is characterized by retention of feces in the colon beyond the normal emptying time. It is a problem Americans spend a quarter of a billion dollars to relieve each year but hardly ever discuss. However, the "regularity" of elimination is highly individual, and it is not necessary for health to have a bowel movement every day. Usually this common short-term problem results from various sources of nervous tension and worry and changes in social setting, such as vacations with altered routines. Also, it may be caused by prolonged use of laxatives or cathartics, low-fiber diets, or lack of exercise, all of which can contribute to a decreased intestinal muscle tone. Improved exercise, dietary, and bowel habits are usually sufficient to remedy the situation. The diet should include increased dietary fiber and naturally laxative fruits, such as dried prunes and figs, as well as increased fluid. If chronic constipation persists, however, agents that increase stool bulk may be necessary. These bulking agents include bran, cellulose, and hemicellulose materials. Taking any laxative on a regular basis should be avoided.

Diarrhea

Functional diarrhea occurs in different types and from different causes, but all forms create nutritional imbalances (see Issues and Answers, p. 471). Diarrhea may result from general dietary excesses, with fermentation of sugars involved, or excess fiber stimulation of intestinal muscle function. In other cases it may result from a specific food-borne infectious organism or from acute food poisoning.[6] In still other instances it may be due to intolerance of specific food or nutrient factors.[7] For example, *lactose intolerance* is a rather widespread condition in which the milk sugar lactose cannot be digested because of a lactase deficiency (see p. 455). Diarrhea in infants is a serious problem, especially if it is prolonged and associated with infection. The infant's relatively high body water content and large area of intestinal mucosa in proportion to body surface area cause rapid fluid and electrolyte loss.

Organic Intestinal Diseases

Organic diseases of the intestine may be classified in three general groups, based on their underlying cause:

1. **Anatomic changes:** for example, the development of diverticula, a condition called *diverticulosis*, and their infectious process *diverticulitis*.
2. **Malabsorption syndromes:** for example, *celiac syndrome* in children, commonly called *sprue* in adults.
3. **Infectious mucosal changes:** for example, *inflammatory bowel disease*, which includes both ulcerative colitis and Crohn's disease (regional enteritis).

In each one of these types of intestinal disease, we will discuss the representative disease indicated in terms of (1) nature of the disease process, (2) its clinical symptoms, and (3) the resulting nutritional therapy required.

Diverticulosis

Nature of the disease. Diverticula (from the Latin verb *diverticulare*, meaning "to turn aside") are small tubular sacs branching off from a main canal or cavity in the body. The formation of these small sacs protruding from the intestinal lumen, usually the colon, produces the condition *diverticulosis*. More often diverticulosis occurs in older adults and develops at points of weakened musculature in the bowel wall. The condition causes no problem unless the small diverticula become infected and inflamed. This diseased state is called *diverticulitis*, which in some cases can lead to complicating perforation.

Clinical symptoms. The condition is usually without symptoms unless the diverticula become infected. Fecal residue causes increased irritation as the infection and inflammation spread. Increased *hypermotility* and intraluminal pressures from **luminal segmentation** cause pain. The pain and tenderness are usually localized in the lower left side of the abdomen and are accompanied by nausea, vomiting, distension, diarrhea, intestinal spasm, and fever. If the disease process continues, intestinal obstruction or perforation may necessitate surgical intervention.

Luminal segmentation
Formation of divisions, or segments, along the alimentary canal. In diverticulitis, this may occur at the site of diverticuli and increase the motility of the gastrointestinal tract, promoting diarrhea.

Liberal Food Guide for Peptic Ulcer

General directions
- Respect individual responses or tolerances to specific foods experienced at any given time, remembering that the same food may evoke different responses at different times depending on the stress factor.
- Eat smaller meals more often, eat slowly, and savor your food in a calm environment as much as possible.
- Try to avoid caffeine beverages such as coffee, cola, and tea; also avoid alcohol.
- Cut down on or quit smoking cigarettes—not only to help the ulcer but also to help food taste better.
- Avoid excessive pepper on food or concentrated meat broths and extractives.
- Avoid frequent use of aspirin or other drugs that may damage the stomach lining.

Foods	Recommended foods	Controlled foods
Bread, cereals (at least 4 servings daily)	Any whole-grain or enriched bread, cereals, crackers, pasta	None
Vegetables (at least 2 servings daily)	Any vegetable, raw or cooked; vegetable juices	None
Potatoes, other starches	White potatoes, sweet potatoes, or yams; enriched rice, brown rice; corn, barley, millet, bulgur; pasta	Fried forms
Fruits (at least 2 servings daily)	Any fruit, raw or cooked; fruit juices	None
Milk, milk products (2 servings daily as desired)	Any form of milk or milk drink; yogurt; cheeses	None
Meat or substitutes (2 servings daily)	Poultry, fish and shellfish, lean meats; eggs, cheeses; legumes—dried beans and peas, lentils, soybeans; smooth peanut butter	Fried forms or too highly seasoned or fatty
Soups, stews	Mildly seasoned, less concentrated meat stock base; any cream soups	More highly seasoned or concentrated base
Desserts	Any desserts tolerated	Items containing nuts or coconut; fried pastries
Beverages	Decaffeinated coffee, cocoa, fruit drinks, mineral waters, noncola soft drinks; less strong tea with milk	Regular coffee, strong tea; colas, alcohol
Fats (use in moderation)	Margarine; butter, cream; vegetable oils; mild salad dressings, mayonnaise, oil and vinegar with herbs	Highly seasoned dressings
Sauces, gravies	Mildly flavored, less strong meat bases	Strongly seasoned, especially with pepper, hot peppers, and sauces
Miscellaneous	Salt in moderation (iodized); flavorings; herbs, spices; mustard, catsup, vinegar in moderation, as tolerated	Strongly flavored condiments; popcorn; nuts, coconut as tolerated

Nutritional therapy. Current studies and clinical practice have demonstrated better management of chronic diverticular disease with an increased amount of dietary fiber than with the former practice of restricted residue. In acute episodes of active disease, however, the amount of dietary fiber may need to be reduced. The type of fiber used apparently also plays a part. Some studies have indicated that fibers of a coarse type have a more significant effect on stool weight, increased intestinal transit, and reduced intraluminal pressure in the colon than do the fine types of bran. Thus, in its use as dietary fiber, the texture of bran may be important in relationship to its clinical effectiveness. The relationship of dietary fiber and diverticular disease has recently been further reinforced by studies of populations, such as in Japan since the current "westernizing" of its culture. An extended discussion of dietary fiber and its relation to health and disease, with application to clinical needs, is found in Chapter 3.

Malabsorption Syndrome—Celiac Disease

Nature of the disease. Malabsorption syndrome may have multiple causes, either damage to the mucosal villi and absorbing surface itself or conditions that interfere with normal absorption processes.[8] In the condition of **celiac disease,** the specific offending agent is the *gliadin* fraction in the plant protein *gluten.* The syndrome is therefore more specifically named **gluten-sensitive enteropathy.** The gliadin fraction of gluten is particularly toxic to sensitive individuals. As little as 3 g/day can produce diarrhea and steatorrhea in celiac patients who are in remission. When these peptides of gliadin, derived from digestion of wheat protein, enter the mucosal epithelial cells, they cannot be further broken down. Thus they accumulate in the cells and interfere with normal cell metabolism. The damaged mucosa becomes permeable to other wheat and milk proteins. In turn these substances act as antigens, foreign invaders that stimulate antigen-antibody reactions (see Chapters 16 and 24). In some cases, this process may diffusely involve the entire intestinal mucosa, with more severe effect on the upper small bowel. As a result, the absorption area is greatly impaired for all nutrients, especially fat. Adult celiac syndrome, often called **sprue,** is similar in nature to the related childhood celiac disease. Most adult patients with sprue give a history of having had such episodes of celiac disease as a child.

Clinical symptoms. The characteristic diarrhea consists of multiple foamy, malodorous, bulky, and greasy stools. Poor absorption of fat is evident in the large amounts appearing in the stools as fatty acids and soaps (fatty acids saponified with calcium salts). Poor absorption of iron produces a microcytic-hypochromic anemia. In some persons a lack of folic acid produces a macrocytic anemia. Poor absorption of vitamin K may lead to hemorrhagic tendencies. Poor calcium absorption may produce a disturbed serum calcium/phosphorus ratio with resulting tetany (see Chapter 8). The condition varies widely in severity of symptoms and nature of treatment.

Nutritional therapy. General care of the patient with malabsorption focuses on nutritional support to counteract lost nutrients and fluids and provide nutritional support for the medical treatment. Depending on the severity of the condition and its resulting malnutrition, parenteral as well as enteral modes

Celiac disease
Malabsorption syndrome brought on by eating gluten-rich foods (wheat, rye, barley, and oats). Characterized by steatorrhea, distention, flatulence, weight loss, and malnutrition because of poor absorption associated with damage to the mucosal villi. May be a hereditary condition.

Gluten-sensitive enteropathy
A disorder characterized by the inability to absorb *gluten,* a protein found in wheat, barley, oats, and rye. Commonly found in *celiac disease* and *sprue.*

Sprue
Alternate term for adult celiac disease, a malabsorption syndrome.

of supplemented feeding may be needed.[8,9] In cases of a specific biochemical defect such as with the gluten-induced enteropathy, for example, special nutritional therapy centers on the gluten-free diet. Removal of the offending agent, the gliadin fraction of gluten, brings marked remission of symptoms. Gluten is a protein found mainly in wheat, with additional amounts in rye and oat. General guidelines for restricting food sources of gluten are provided here (see box on facing page).

Inflammatory Bowel Disease

Nature of the disease. The term *inflammatory bowel disease* is used to apply to both *ulcerative colitis* and *Crohn's disease*. Their related condition, *short-bowel syndrome*, results from repeated surgical removal of sections of the intestine as the disease process progresses. The incidence rate of these diseases, especially Crohn's disease, has increased worldwide.[10] The two diseases have similar clinical and pathologic features. Crohn's disease is especially prevalent in industrialized areas of the world, suggesting that pathogenic agents in the environment play a significant role. Its incidence is highest among teenagers, with a secondary peak at ages 55 to 60.

Both ulcerative colitis and Crohn's disease have severe, often devastating nutritional consequences, but they can be distinguished by two main differences: (1) *anatomic distribution* of the inflammatory process and (2) the *nature of tissue changes* involved.[10] First, Crohn's disease can occur in any part of the intestinal tract, but ulcerative colitis is confined to the colon and rectum. Second, in Crohn's disease, the inflammatory tissue changes become chronic and can involve any part of the intestinal wall and may penetrate the entire wall. Often this extensive tissue involvement leads to partial or complete obstruction and to *fistula* formation. The tissue changes in ulcerative colitis, on the other hand, are usually acute, lasting for brief periods, and are limited to the mucosal and submucosal tissue layers of the intestinal wall.

Clinical symptoms. A chronic bloody diarrhea is the most common clinical symptom, occurring at night as well as during the day (see Issues and Answers, p. 471). Ulceration of the mucous membrane of the intestine leads to various associated nutritional problems such as anorexia, nutritional edema, anemia, avitaminosis, protein losses, negative nitrogen balance, dehydration, and electrolyte disturbances. Clinicians have observed evidence of specific deficiencies of zinc and vitamin E, with improvement occurring when supplements of the particular nutrients involved are taken. There is general weight loss, often general malnutrition, fever, skin lesions, and arthritic joint involvement.[11]

Nutritional therapy. Nutritional support is essential to medical management with various drugs. Drug therapy includes antibacterial and antiinflammatory medication such as adrenal corticosteroids or immunosuppressive agents such as mercaptopurine or azathioprine in continuing Crohn's disease (see box, p. 448). Recent studies also suggest that the potent immunosuppressive drug cyclosporin, well known for its ability to prevent transplanted organ rejection, can help heal severe ulcerative colitis and prevent surgical intervention.[12] Two goals are paramount in this essential nutritional therapy: (1) supporting the tissue-healing process and (2) avoiding nutritional deficiency states that can be caused by both the disease and its medical drug therapy. In

---

U.S. incidence rates of Crohn's disease are 4 to 6/100,000 adults/year, with prevalence rates of 40 to 100/100,000. Incidence is highest among teenagers, with a secondary peak at ages 55 to 60.

Corticosteroid
A steroid (hormonal substance) secreted by the adrenal cortex that influences the metabolism of nutrients, electrolytes, and water. Clinically, corticosteroids are given to reduce (among other things) inflammation, as in inflammatory bowel disease such as Crohn's disease or ulcerative colitis.

Gluten-Free Diet for Adult Celiac Disease (Sprue)

Characteristics
- All forms of wheat, rye, oat, buckwheat, and barley are omitted, except gluten-free wheat starch.
- All other foods are permitted freely, unless specified otherwise by the physician.
- The diet should be high in protein, calories, vitamins, and minerals.

Foods	Allowed	Not allowed
Milk (2 glasses or more)	As desired	
Cheese	Any, as desired	
Eggs (1 or 2 daily)	As desired	
Meat, fish, fowl (1 or 2 servings)	Any plain meat	Breaded, creamed, or with thickened gravy; no bread dressings
Soups	All clear and vegetable soups; cream soups thickened with cream, cornstarch, or potato flour only	No wheat flour–thickened soup; no canned soup except clear broth
Vegetables (2 servings of green or yellow daily, at least)	As desired, except creamed	No cream sauce or breading
Fruits (at least 2 or 3 daily, including 1 citrus)	As desired	
Bread	Only that made from rice, corn, or soybean flour, or gluten-free wheat starch	All bread, rolls, crackers, cake, and cookies made from wheat and rye, Ry-Krisp, muffins, biscuits, waffles, pancake flour, and other prepared mixes, rusks, Zwiebach, pretzels; any product containing oatmeal, barley, or buckwheat; no breaded food or food crumbs
Cereals	Cornflakes, cornmeal, hominy, rice, Rice Krispies, Puffed Rice, precooked rice cereals	No wheat or rye cereals, wheat germ, barley, buckwheat, kasha
Pastas		No macaroni, spaghetti, noodles, dumplings
Desserts	Jell-O, fruit Jell-O, ice or sherbet, homemade ice cream, custard, junket, rice pudding, cornstarch pudding (home-made)	Cakes, cookies, pastry; commercial ice cream and ice cream cones; prepared mixes, puddings; homemade puddings thickened with wheat flour

CAUTION: Read labels on all packaged and prepared foods.

serious conditions, nutritional management includes use of elemental formulas composed of absorbable isotonic preparations of amino acids, glucose, fat, minerals, and vitamins. In patients who tolerate these supplements, there is diminished gastrointestinal protein loss and improved nutrition, accompanied by clinical remission. In cases where the small bowel has been shortened

Clinical Application

Effects of Drug Therapy on the Nutritional Status of the Patient with Crohn's Disease

Corticosteroids
Steroids (hormonal substance) secreted by the adrenal cortex to influence the metabolism of nutrients, electrolytes, and water. Clinically they are given to reduce, among other things, inflammation, as in inflammatory bowel disease such as Crohn's disease or ulcerative colitis.

Osteomalacia
Softening of bone caused by impaired mineral uptake; usually resulting from calcium and vitamin D deficiency.

The nutritionist involved in the care of patients with Crohn's disease should consider the effect of drug therapy on their nutritional status, as well as the effects of malabsorption caused by the disease itself. Commonly used medications with significant effects on patient nutrition include prednisone, salicylazosulfapyridine, and cholestyramine.

Prednisone is a **corticosteroid** and thus triggers gluconeogenesis. As a result, it stimulates an increased appetite, protein catabolism, and fluid retention. Prednisone has an antagonistic effect on vitamin D, resulting in reduced calcium transport and ultimately **osteomalacia.** The drug also inhibits collagen synthesis, a function of vitamin C, and the complete breakdown of tryptophan, a function of B_6, thereby increasing the patient's needs for these nutrients as well.

Salicylazosulfapyridine (SAS) is an effective treatment for Crohn's disease, although its metabolic activity is unclear. SAS affects nutrition status by inducing nausea, vomiting, and anorexia. Folate deficiency is associated with this drug, either because of the mild hemolysis or because of decreased absorption induced in many patients. Iron needs are sometimes increased during SAS therapy, also as a result of hemolysis.

Cholestyramine is an anion exchange resin used to treat diarrhea. It is associated with malabsorption of fat and fat-soluble vitamins. Iron and vitamin B_{12} requirements are sometimes increased as well because of reduced absorption.

To correct specific nutrient deficiencies during drug therapy, first identify each specific deficiency, then plan to correct it by food, oral supplementation, or formula. Although there are several elemental and chemically defined formulas available for tube feeding, the oral route is preferred. Most patients can consume a nutritious diet as long as levels of fat and lactose, both poorly absorbed in Crohn's disease, are carefully monitored. In addition, you may want to confer with the physician and pharmacist about the possibility of reducing the medication dosage to enhance the patient's recovery from damage caused by malabsorption or nutrient antagonist effects of the drug.

REFERENCES

Fuchs GJ, Grand RJ, and Motil KJ: Malnutrition and nutritional support in inflammatory bowel disease, Nutr Supp Serv 5(6):28, June 1985.

Hodges PE, and Thomson ABR: Nutritional status of patients with Crohn's disease, J Can Diet Assoc 43(3):194, 1982.

Parenteral
Not through the alimentary canal. Given by injection through a subcutaneous, intramuscular, intravenous, or other route.

or the disease process is extensive, as in Crohn's disease, **parenteral** feeding (TPN) is most effective (see Chapters 17 and 23). Such TPN feeding through a large central vein is particularly important in childhood to prevent severe growth retardation.[11] Nutritional repletion improves symptoms dramatically. There is diminished gastrointestinal secretion and motility, decreased disease activity, relief of partial intestinal obstruction, occasional closure of enteric fistulas, and renewed immunocompetence. Nutritional supplements are usually necessary to avoid deficiencies in agents such as zinc, copper, chromium, selenium, and other nutrients.

General continuing dietary management. Emphasis of treatment should be on restoring optimal nutrient intake, removing deficits, preventing local trauma to inflamed areas, and controlling less easily absorbed material such as fats. To help secure additional kilocalories, medium-chain triglycerides (MCT), as in the commercial preparation MCT oil, may be used instead of regular fats. The focus of the diet centers on protein and energy, minerals and vitamins, and texture.

1. **High protein.** In inflammatory bowel disease, there are large losses of protein from the intestinal mucosal tissue by exudations and bleeding, as well as losses associated with impaired intestinal absorption. Healing can occur only if adequate protein is provided. Through elemental formulas or protein supplements with food as tolerated, the diet must supply adequate protein—about 100 g/day—for needed tissue synthesis and healing. Tasteful ways of including protein foods of high biologic value (eggs, meat, cheese) can be devised to tempt poor appetites. Milk often causes difficulty with many patients, so it is usually omitted at first, then gradually added in cooked forms.

2. **High energy.** About 2500 to 3000 kcal/day are needed to restore nutritional deficits from daily losses in the stools and consequent weight loss. Also the negative nitrogen balance can be overcome only if sufficient kilocalories are present to spare protein for tissue building.

3. **Increased minerals and vitamins.** When anemia is present, iron therapy is used. Sometimes oral iron preparations are poorly tolerated, and blood transfusions may be used during critical periods. Extra vitamins needed for healing and the increased protein and energy metabolism should be added. These are thiamin, riboflavin, niacin, and ascorbic acid. Trace minerals such as zinc, which participate in tissue synthesis, are needed along with vitamin E, which contributes to tissue integrity. Supplements of these vitamins and minerals are routine. Potassium therapy may be indicated if undue losses from diarrhea and tissue destruction occur causing hypokalemia.

4. **Low residue.** To avoid irritation of the mucosal lining until healing is well established, the diet should be fairly low in residue. In acute stages the diet may need to be almost residue free through the use of elemental formulas and residue-free foods. A low-residue diet (see box, p. 450) may be used initially, with additional protein and kilocalories given in interval feedings. As soon as tolerated, a regular diet with high-protein feedings is indicated. Only heavy roughage need be avoided. The primary concern is supplying the necessary nutrition in as appetizing a manner as possible.

Perhaps no other condition better illustrates the need for a close working relationship among the team of physician, clinical nutritionist, nurse, and patient than does inflammatory bowel disease. The patient's appetite is poor, but adequate nutritional intake is imperative. In creative ways, individually explored and implemented, the fundamental therapeutic needs must be met. This can be done through vigorous nutritional care using a range of feeding modes, combined with constant supportive warmth and encouragement.

Low-Residue Diet

Foods	Allowed	Not allowed
Beverages	Only 2 glasses of milk, if allowed, boiled or evaporated; fruit juices, coffee, tea, carbonated beverages	Alcohol
Eggs	Prepared in any manner, except fried	Fried eggs
Cheese	Cottage, cream, milk American, Tillamook (use in small amounts)	Highly flavored cheeses
Meat or poultry	Roasted, baked, or broiled tender beef, bacon, ham, lamb, liver, veal, fish, chicken, or turkey	Tough meats, pork; no fried or highly spiced meats
Soup	Bouillon, broth, strained cream soups from the foods allowed	Any others
Fats	Butter, margarine, oils, 30 ml (1 oz) cream daily	None
Vegetables	Canned or cooked strained vegetables, such as asparagus, beets, carrots, peas, pumpkin, squash, spinach, young string beans, tomato juice	Raw or whole cooked vegetables
Fruits	Strained fruit juices, cooked or canned apples, apricots, Royal Anne cherries, peaches, pears; dried fruit puree; ripe banana and avocado; all without skins or seeds	All other raw fruits, other cooked fruits
Bread and crackers	Refined bread, toast, rolls, crackers	Pancakes, waffles, whole-grain bread or rolls
Cereals	Cooked cereal such as Cream of Wheat, Maltomeal, strained oatmeal, cornmeal, cornflakes, puffed rice, Rice Krispies, puffed wheat	Whole-grain cereals; other prepared cereals
Potatoes or substitute	Potatoes, white rice, macaroni, noodles, spaghetti	Fried potato, potato chips, brown rice
Desserts	Gelatin desserts, tapioca, angel food or sponge cake, plain custards, water ice or ice cream without fruit or nuts, rennet or simple puddings	Rich pastries, pies, anything with nuts or dried fruits
Sweets	Sugar, jelly, honey, syrups, gumdrops, hard candy, plain creams, milk chocolate	Other candy; jam, marmalade
Miscellaneous	Cream sauce, plain gravy, salt	Nuts, olives, popcorn, rich gravies, pepper, spices, vinegar

Food Allergies and Sensitivities

Immunocompetence
The ability to produce antibodies in response to an antigen.

General Nature of Allergies

A number of conditions may cause certain food allergies or sensitivities. These may be conditions of **immunocompetence** or of specific genetic origin. The resulting difficulty in handling certain foods may lie at the point of digestion and absorption in the intestine or at the metabolic level in the cell.

The word "allergy" comes from the Greek words, *allos* (other) and *ergon* (work). Thus the name implies an unusual or inappropriate response to a stimulus, usually an environmental factor. An allergic condition results from a disorder of the immune system. It is immunity gone wrong.[13]

Food Allergy
Definition

The term **food allergy** should be used only for hypersensitivity that is caused by immunologic reaction to specific food constituents or their digestive products. The term **food sensitivity** is a general nonspecific term more correctly used for nonallergic food sensitivities, though it is sometimes used synonymously with food allergies. Food allergy is distinct from other food intolerances or sensitivities, which are caused by nonimmunologic mechanisms, such as lack of digestive enzymes or cell enzymes. In general, the process of diagnosis and treatment of adverse reactions to foods includes clinical assessment, dietary manipulation, and laboratory tests.

Food allergy
Specific term for immunologic sensitivity reactions.

Food sensitivity
General term for adverse nutrient reactions.

Common Food Allergens

A wide variety of environmental, emotional, and physical factors influence reaction, and a suitable regimen is sometimes difficult to find. Since sensitivity to protein substances is a common basis for food allergy, the early foods of infants and children are frequent offenders. Children tend to become less allergic to these foods as they become older.

1. **Milk.** Cow's milk has long been a common cause of allergic response in infants. In sensitive children it may cause gastrointestinal difficulties, such as vomiting, diarrhea, and colic, or respiratory and skin problems. The problem is generally identified by clinical symptoms, family history, and a trial on a milk-free diet, using an appropriate substitute formula such as a soybean preparation. Freedom from symptoms on a milk-free diet is then followed by a retrial on milk to determine if it causes the symptoms to reappear. Only then is the diagnosis of milk allergy established. Often symptoms appear and disappear spontaneously, regardless of dietary changes. But they tend to be more often caused by food if gastrointestinal problems are present.

2. **Eggs, wheat, and other foods.** Solid food is added to the infant's diet at about 6 months of age. Since the albumin in egg white is a potential allergen, it is usually added later, following earlier use of other foods and egg yolk. Wheat is also a fairly common food allergen among allergic children, so a rice cereal is often the first grain introduced. The specific biochemical sensitivity to gluten, a protein found in wheat, in the child with gluten-induced celiac disease may be considered an example, although the biochemical defect in the mucosal cells in this disease represents a different sensitivity mechanism.

Nutritional Management
Elimination Diets

In an allergic child's diet, solid foods are usually added slowly to the original formula, with common offenders excluded in early feedings. The following foods that have been frequent offenders may be avoided initially and added cautiously as the child grows older:

eggs	bacon
fish	citrus fruits
wheat	nuts
strawberries	peanut butter
tomatoes	chocolate
pork	pineapple
milk or milk products	

In some cases, a series of specific diagnostic food elimination diets are used to identify offending foods. A core of less-often offending foods is used initially, with gradual addition of other single foods one at a time to test the response. If a given food causes return of the allergy, the food is then identified as an allergen and eliminated from use. It may be retested later to determine if it is still an allergen. Guidance in the substitution of special food products and in the use of special recipes can be provided. In some cases, certain additives used in food processing may be the offending agents.

Family Education and Counseling

Knowledge and understanding of the allergic state and the many factors that may influence it are essential. If specific foods have been definitely identified as allergens, careful guidance is needed to eliminate these from the diet. Common uses of the offending food in daily meal patterns and its occurrence in a number of commercial products and other hidden sources should be discussed. Label reading and recipe adaptation are important. As an allergic child grows older, reaction to a given food may wane, and it can gradually be added to the diet.

Food Intolerances from Genetic-Metabolic Disease

Nature of Genetic Disease

Certain food intolerances may also stem from underlying genetic disease that affects the metabolism of one or more specific nutrients. Genetic disease results from the individual's specific gene inheritance. The gene pattern of the original chromosomes we receive from our parents at our conception determines our inherited physical traits or genetic disease pattern. Genes in each cell control not only common hereditary characteristics but also the metabolic functions of the cell. They regulate the synthesis of some 1000 or more *specific* cell enzymes that control metabolism within the cell. Each of these enzymes is a *specific* protein synthesized by a *specific* DNA pattern in a *specific* gene. When a specific gene is abnormal (mutant), the enzyme whose synthesis that gene controls cannot be made. In turn, then, the specific metabolic reaction controlled by that specific missing enzyme cannot take place. The specific genetic disease caused by this metabolic block then manifests clinical symptoms connected with resulting abnormal metabolic products. As primary examples here, we will look briefly at two such genetic diseases: (1) *phenylketonuria,* which affects amino acid metabolism, and (2) *galactosemia,* which affects carbohydrate metabolism. Both are detected by newborn screening procedures, mandatory now by law.

Phenylketonuria (PKU)

Metabolic defect. PKU results from the missing cell enzyme, *phenylalanine hydroxylase,* which oxidizes *phenylalanine,* an essential amino acid, to tyrosine, another amino acid. Phenylalanine then accumulates in the blood, and its alternate metabolites, the phenyl acids, are excreted in the urine. One of these urinary acids, *phenylpyruvic acid,* is a phenylketone, hence the name of the disease *phenylketonuria (PKU).* The condition may exist as classic PKU or as one of several *hyperphenylalanemia variants (HPV).* More recent work over the past decade has shown that phenylalanine hydroxylase is not a single enzyme but a combination of four factors, one or more of which may be active. Untreated PKU can produce devastating effects, but present nutritional therapy can avoid these results.[14]

Clinical symptoms. In past years, before current newborn screening laws and dietary treatment practices from birth, the most profound effect observed in persons with *untreated* PKU was severe mental retardation. The IQ of affected persons was usually below 50 and frequently less than 20. Central nervous system damage caused irritability, hyperactivity, convulsive seizures, and bizarre behavior.

Nutritional therapy. PKU can now be well controlled by special diet therapy. After screening at birth, a special low-phenylalanine diet effectively controls the serum phenylalanine levels so that they are maintained at appropriate amounts to prevent clinical symptoms and promote normal growth and development.[14] Since phenylalanine is an essential amino acid necessary for growth, it cannot be totally removed from the diet. Blood levels of phenylalanine are constantly monitored, and the metabolic team nutritionist calculates the special diet for each infant and child to allow only the limited amount of phenylalanine tolerated. Based on extensive studies, guidelines for dietary management of PKU are currently being used effectively to build lifetime habits, since research now indicates that there is no safe age at which a child may discontinue the diet.[14-16] This dietary management is built on two basic components: (1) a substitute for milk, a special formula now called a "medical food" since it is continued past infancy and childhood into adolescence and adulthood, and (2) guidelines for adding solid foods, both regular and special low-protein products, and then building continuing food habits.

Family counseling. Initial education and continuing support of parents are essential, since dietary management of PKU is the only known effective method of treatment and maintaining the diet becomes more difficult as the child grows older.[17] Parents must understand and accept the necessity of the diet, and this requires patience, understanding, and continued reinforcement. The PKU team, together with wise parents, provides initial and continuing care so that the PKU child will grow and develop normally (Figure 19-2). Such a child, diagnosed at birth by widespread screening programs, can have a healthy and happy life, instead of the profound disease consequences experienced in the past.

Maternal PKU. The current practice of long-term dietary management is especially critical for young women who are reaching the age of potential high-risk pregnancies with maternal PKU (see Chapter 11). A large study is now underway in both the United States and Canada to investigate the effects of maternal PKU on pregnancy outcome. This Maternal PKU Collaborative Study is evaluating the effectiveness of the phenylalanine-restricted

Figure 19-2
PKU. This child is a delightful, perfectly developed 2-year-old. Screened and diagnosed at birth, she has eaten a carefully controlled low-phenylalanine diet and is growing normally.

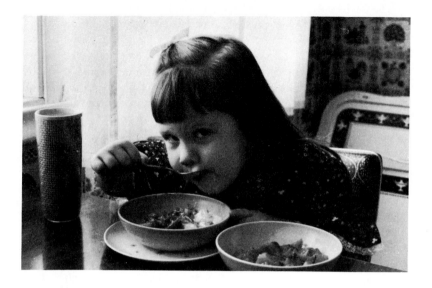

diet in reducing the poor reproductive outcome generally associated with maternal PKU in the past.[18,19]

Galactosemia

Metabolic defect. This genetic disease, also caused by a missing cell enzyme, affects carbohydrate metabolism. The missing enzyme controls the conversion of *galactose,* which is derived from lactose, to glucose. Milk, the infant's first food, contains a large amount of the precursor lactose (milk sugar). After galactose is initially combined with phosphate to begin the metabolic conversion to glucose, it cannot proceed further in the galactosemic infant. Galactose rapidly accumulates in the blood and in various body tissues.

Hepatomegaly
Enlargement of the liver.

Ascites
Accumulation of fluid in the abdominal cavity.

Clinical symptoms. In the past the excess tissue accumulations of galactose caused rapid damage to the untreated infant. The child failed to thrive, and clinical symptoms appeared soon after birth. Continued liver damage brought jaundice, **hepatomegaly** with cirrhosis, enlargement of the spleen, and **ascites.** Without treatment, death usually resulted from liver failure. If the infant survived, continuing tissue damage and hypoglycemia in the optic lens and the brain caused cataracts and mental retardation. Now, however, with newborn screening programs, these infants are diagnosed at birth and started on special dietary management. With this vital nutritional therapy, they continue to grow and develop normally.

Nutritional therapy. The main indirect source of dietary galactose is the lactose in milk. Therefore *all* forms of milk and lactose must be removed from the diet. In this instance a *galactose-free diet* is used. Any needed amount of galactose for certain body structures can be synthesized by the body. A soy-base formula, such as Isomil or Prosobee, is used. Breast-feeding, of course, cannot be used. Later, as solid foods are added to the infant's diet at about 6 months of age, careful attention must be given to avoiding lactose from other food sources. Parents quickly learn to check labels carefully on all commercial products to detect any lactose or lactose-containing substances.

Lactose Intolerance

A deficiency of any one of the disaccharidases in the small intestine mucosal cells—lactase, sucrase, or maltase—may produce a wide range of gastrointestinal problems and abdominal pain because the specific sugar involved cannot be digested (see Chapter 2). Of these, lactose intolerance is the most common. It is frequently seen in adults and may also occur in children. The accumulated concentration of undigested lactose in the intestine creates osmotic pressure that draws fluid into the gut, thus stimulating **hypermotility** and resulting in abdominal cramping and diarrhea. Milk treated with lactase enzyme, lactose-hydrolyzed milk, can be tolerated by these persons without the difficulty encountered with regular milk. A diet similar to that used for galactosemia is required, although the underlying cause of the difficulty is quite different. Milk, unless treated with lactase enzyme, and all products containing lactose are carefully avoided. Soy milk products are used for children.

Hypermotility
Excessive peristaltic activity along the alimentary canal.

Three major accessory organs lie adjacent to the gastrointestinal tract and produce important digestive agents that enter the intestine and aid in the handling of food substances. Specific enzymes are produced for each of the major nutrients, and bile is added to assist in the enzyme digestion of fats. These three major organs are the liver, gallbladder, and pancreas. Diseases of these organs can easily affect gastrointestinal function and cause problems in the normal handling of specific types of food.

Problems of the Accessory Organs

Hepatitis

Nature of the disease. Acute hepatitis is usually a self-limiting inflammatory condition. It can be caused by various agents such as viruses, alcohol, drugs, or toxins. A main form results from viral infection (virus A hepatitis and virus B hepatitis). The term *viral hepatitis* usually refers to both forms. In infectious hepatitis the viral agent is transmitted by the oral-fecal route, a common one for many epidemic diseases. The usual entry is through contaminated food or water. In other cases the virus may be transmitted in infected blood used for transfusions or contaminated instruments, such as syringes or needles. Another main form results from alcohol abuse. *Alcoholic hepatitis* is a serious precirrhotic form of alcohol injury of the liver affecting its tissue structures and functions (Figure 19-3). It is frequently accompanied by protein-calorie malnutrition, which increases the risk for clinical severity and poor prognosis.[20]

Clinical symptoms. The viral agents of hepatitis, as well as the toxicity caused by alcohol abuse, produce diffuse injury to essential functional liver cells. In milder cases the liver injury is largely reversible, but with increasing severity more extensive **necrosis** occurs. In some cases massive necrosis may lead to liver failure and death. A cardinal symptom of hepatitis is *anorexia*, contributing to the risk of malnutrition. Varying clinical symptoms appear, depending on the degree of liver injury. *Jaundice*, a major symptom, may be obvious or not, depending on the severity of the disease, and can have both nutritional and psychologic effects (see box, p. 456). There is evidence that malnutrition and impaired immunocompetence contribute to spontaneous infections and continuing liver disease. General symptoms, in addition to the

Necrosis
Cell death.

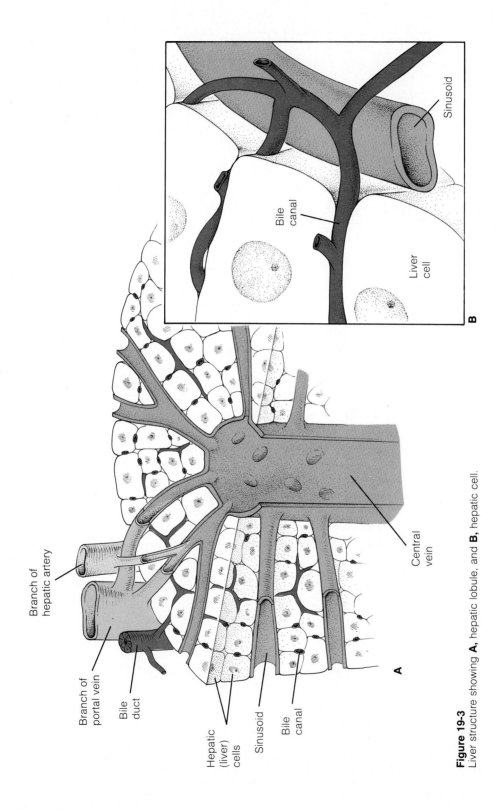

Figure 19-3
Liver structure showing **A,** hepatic lobule, and **B,** hepatic cell.

To Probe Further

Jaundice: When to Expect It, What to Do About It

Since jaundice is not usually a life-threatening condition, it is easy for health workers to take it lightly. After all, the yellow-to-orange skin color that arises in this disorder is harmless, so it would seem. But it reflects an accumulation of excessive bile pigments in the blood that results from a rise in *bilirubin,* a product of heme that is released when red blood cells are destroyed. The underlying condition causing the hemolysis is the major issue of medical treatment.

In a broader psychologic sense, however, the condition can be devastating. The embarrassment of an altered body image, with accompanying depression and withdrawal, can affect appetite and willingness to comply with therapy recommended for the underlying illness. To promote a healthy recovery, health workers must treat jaundice as seriously as these effects dictate. Several actions are helpful:

Explain the reason for jaundice

Jaundice can be discussed in three phases—prehepatic, hepatic, and posthepatic:

- **Prehepatic jaundice.** Most often this phase is caused by a massive breakdown in red blood cells. It is seen most often in Rh factor sensitization, hemolytic anemias, sickle cell anemia, massive lung infarctions, transfusion reactions, and septicemia. The result is an excessive amount of bilirubin in a form that cannot be excreted—i.e., fat-soluble. The body's bilirubin transport system, based on albumin, then deposits the excess in the patient's skin.

- **Hepatic jaundice.** In this case, the liver cannot convert fat-soluble bilirubin into the water-soluble form required for its removal from the blood. This condition is seen in hepatitis, cirrhosis, metastatic cancer, and prolonged drug use, especially of drugs broken down by the liver.

- **Posthepatic jaundice.** This phase occurs when the flow of bile into the duodenum is blocked. Since bile carries water-soluble excretable bilirubin, this blockage can cause it to back up, resulting in a backlog of bilirubin in the blood. Blockage often occurs with inflammation, scar tissue, stones, or tumors in the liver, bile, or pancreatic systems.

Identify nutrition-related problems

Jaundice is often associated with anorexia, indigestion, nausea, and vomiting.

Help resolve nutrition-related problems

To overcome indigestion or anorexia, recommend small meals providing some of the patient's favorite foods. To overcome nausea or vomiting, simple foods may be necessary. Foods rich in fat and caffeine should also be avoided.

Encourage the patient to discuss personal feelings and concerns

Such information is essential to develop a treatment plan designed to meet each patient's unique needs. Counseling helps the patient feel psychologically stronger and ready to help the health care process.

Continued.

To Probe Further

Jaundice: When to Expect It, What to Do About It—cont'd

Discuss pertinent patient needs with family and/or friends

Often "significant others" avoid the patient with discolored skin out of embarrassment or a lack of understanding. A discussion of the patient's need for support may help other persons accept the patient socially and support efforts to resolve underlying health problems.

Make referrals to outside agencies, as needed

If jaundice is caused by alcohol or drug abuse, the patient and family may require special counseling. Referral to community programs after hospital discharge may help provide continuing support.

REFERENCE
Gannon RB, and Pickett K: Jaundice, Am J Nurs 83:404, 1983.

---

main sign of anorexia, include malaise, weakness, nausea and vomiting, diarrhea, headache, fever, enlarged and tender liver, and enlarged spleen. When jaundice develops, it usually occurs for an initial period of 5 to 10 days, deepens for 1 to 2 weeks, then levels off and decreases. After this crisis point there is a sufficient recovery of injured cells and convalescence of 3 weeks to 3 months follows. Optimal care during this time is essential to avoid relapse.

General treatment. Bedrest is essential. Physical exercise increases both severity and duration of the disease. A daily intake of 3000 to 3500 ml of fluid guards against dehydration and gives a general sense of well-being and improved appetite. However, optimal nutrition is the major therapy.[21] It provides the essential foundation for recovery of the injured liver cells and overall return of strength.

Nutritional therapy. The principles of diet therapy relate to the liver's function in metabolizing each of the nutrients:

1. **Adequate protein.** Protein is essential for liver cell regeneration. It also provides lipotropic agents such as methionine and choline (see Chapter 2) for the conversion of fats to lipoproteins and removal from the liver, thus preventing fatty infiltration. The diet should supply from 75 to 100 g/day of high-quality protein.

2. **High carbohydrate.** Sufficient available glucose must be provided to restore protective glycogen reserves and meet the energy demands of the disease process. Also, adequate glucose for energy ensures the use of protein for vital tissue regeneration. The diet should supply from 300 to 400 g/day of carbohydrate.

3. **Moderate fat.** A moderate amount of fat makes the food more palatable and therefore encourages the anorexic patient to eat. Some easily used fat, such as whole milk, cream, butter, margarine, mayonnaise, and vegetable oil, is beneficial. The diet should supply about 100 to 150 g/day of such fat.

4. **High energy.** From 2500 to 3000 kcal/day are needed to furnish energy

High-Protein, High-Carbohydrate, Moderate-Fat Daily Diet

1 L (1 qt) of milk

1 to 2 eggs

224 g (8 oz) lean meat, fish, poultry

4 servings vegetables
   2 servings potato or substitute
   1 serving green leafy or yellow vegetable
   1 to 2 servings of other vegetables, including 1 raw

3 to 4 servings fruit (include juices often)
   1 to 2 citrus fruits (or other good source of ascorbic acid)
   2 servings other fruit

6 to 8 servings bread and cereal (whole grain or enriched)
   1 serving cereal
   5 to 6 slices bread, crackers

2 to 4 tbsp butter or fortified margarine

Additional jam, jelly, honey, and other carbohydrate foods as patient desires and is able to eat them

Sweetened fruit juices increase both carbohydrate and fluid

---

demands of the tissue regeneration process, to compensate for losses from fever and debilitation, and to renew strength and recuperative powers.

5. **Meals and feedings.** The problem of supplying a diet adequate to meet the increased nutritive demands for a patient whose illness makes food almost repellent calls for creativity and supportive encouragement. The food may need to be in liquid form at first, using concentrated commercial or blended formulas for frequent feedings (Table 19-1). As the patient improves, appetizing and attractive food is needed. Since nutritional therapy is the key to recovery, a major nutrition and nursing responsibility requires devising ways to encourage the increased amounts of food intake needed (see box, above). The clinical nutritionist and the nurse will work together closely to achieve this goal.

Cirrhosis

Nature of the disease. Liver disease may advance to the chronic stage of cirrhosis (Figure 19-4). Some forms of cirrhosis result from biliary obstruction or liver necrosis from undetermined causes. In some cases it results from previous viral hepatitis. The most common problem, however, is fatty cirrhosis associated with malnutrition and alcoholism. This relentless malnutrition, together with impaired immunocompetence, accounts for the frequent infectious relapses. An increasingly poor food intake, as the alcoholic person continues to drink excessively, leads to multiple nutritional deficiencies. However, alcoholism can cause cirrhosis and death not only because it promotes malnutrition but also because alcohol and its metabolic products disturb liver metabolism and damage functional liver cells directly. Damage to liver cells

The French physician Laennec first named the disease, from the Greek word *kirrhos,* meaning "orange," because the cirrhotic liver has a firm, fibrous mass and orange-colored nodules projecting from its surface. The nutritional or alcoholic form of cirrhosis bears his name, *Laennec's cirrhosis.*

Figure 19-4
Comparison of normal
liver and liver with
cirrhotic tissue changes.
A, Anterior view of organ,
B, cross section, **C,** tissue
structure.

Normal liver

Liver with alcoholic cirrhosis

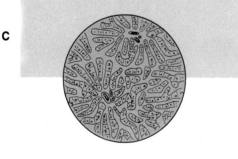
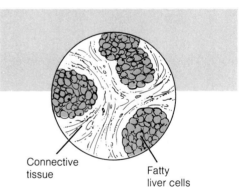

Nodules

A

B

Liver tissue

Liver
tissue
(nodule)

C

Connective
tissue

Fatty
liver cells

occurs as fatty infiltration causes cellular destruction and fibrotic tissue
changes.

Clinical symptoms. Early signs of cirrhosis include gastrointestinal disturbances such as nausea, vomiting, loss of appetite, distention, and epigastric
pain. In time jaundice may appear. There is increasing weakness, edema, ascites, and anemia from gastrointestinal bleeding, iron deficiency, or hemorrhage. A specific **macrocytic anemia** from folic acid deficiency is also frequently observed. Steatorrhea is a common symptom. Essentially, the major
symptoms are caused by a basic protein deficiency and its multiple metabolic
problems: (1) plasma protein levels fall leading to failure of the capillary
fluid shift mechanism (see Chapter 8), causing ascites; (2) lipotropic agents
are not supplied for fat conversion to lipoproteins and damaging fat accumulates in the liver tissue; (3) blood clotting mechanisms are impaired since
factors such as prothrombin and **fibrinogen** are not adequately produced;
and (4) general tissue catabolism and negative nitrogen balance continue the
overall degenerative process.

As the disease progresses, the increasing fibrotic scar tissue impairs blood

Macrocytic anemia
An anemia characterized by red
cells that are larger and paler
than normal.

Fibrinogen
A fraction of human plasma
given via transfusion to increase
coagulation of the blood.

circulation through the liver, and portal hypertension follows. Contributing further to the problem is the continuing ascites. The impaired portal circulation with increasing venous pressure may lead to esophageal **varices,** with danger of rupture and fatal massive hemorrhage.

Varices
Enlarged veins.

Nutritional therapy. When alcoholism is the underlying problem, treatment is difficult. Each patient requires supportive care. Therapy is usually aimed at correcting fluid and electrolyte problems and providing nutritional support for hepatic repair as much as possible. Nutritional therapy for cirrhosis should include the following principles:

1. **Protein according to tolerance.** In the absence of impending hepatic coma, about 80 to 100 g/day of protein is needed to correct severe undernutrition, regenerate functional liver tissue, and replenish plasma protein. However, if signs of hepatic coma appear, protein must be adjusted to individual tolerance.

2. **Low sodium.** Sodium is usually restricted to 500 to 1000 mg/day (see Chapter 20) to help reduce fluid retention.

3. **Texture.** If esophageal varices develop, it may be necessary to give soft foods that are smooth in texture to prevent danger of rupture and hemorrhage.

4. **Optimal general nutrition.** The remaining overall diet principles outlined for hepatitis are continued for cirrhosis for the same reasons. Kilocalories, carbohydrates, and vitamins are supplied according to individual need and deficiency. Moderate fat is used. Alcohol is strictly forbidden.

Hepatic Encephalopathy

Nature of the disease. As cirrhotic changes continue in the liver, the portal blood circulation diminishes and liver functions begin to fail. The normal liver has a major function of removing ammonia from the blood by converting it to urea for excretion. The failing liver can no longer inactivate or detoxify substances or metabolize others. A key factor involved in the progressive disease process is an elevated blood level of ammonia. The resulting hepatic **encephalopathy,** sometimes called *hepatic coma,* brings changes in consciousness, behavior, and neurologic status.

Encephalopathy
Any degenerative disease of the brain.

Clinical symptoms. Typical response involves disorders of consciousness and alterations in motor function. There is apathy, confusion, inappropriate behavior, and drowsiness, progressing to coma. The speech may be slurred or monotonous. A coarse, flapping tremor is observed in the outstretched hands. The breath may have a fecal odor.

Basic treatment objectives. The fundamental objective of treatment is twofold: (1) removal of the sources of excess ammonia and (2) provision of nutritional support. Medical and nutritional therapy are involved. Parenteral fluid and electrolytes are used to restore normal balances. Two drugs may be used to control ammonia—lactulose and neomysin. Lactulose is a nonabsorbable synthetic disaccharide that reduces the absorption of intestinal ammonia.[22] Neomysin is an antibiotic that reduces the population of urea-splitting organisms within the bowel that produce ammonia. To stop bleeding into the intestine as another source of intestinal ammonia, a Sengstaken-Blakemore tube may be used.

Nutritional therapy. Special parenteral and enteral nutritional support may include use of *branched-chain amino acids.* These three essential amino acids—leucine, isoleucine, and valine (see Chapter 6)—are not catabolized by the liver but are taken up by other tissues. Thus they can be metabolized without depending on healthy liver tissue, as is the case with other amino acids. Solutions of these branched-chain amino acids, for example, hepatamine, have therefore been used successfully to maintain adequate nitrogen balance and reduce the encephalopathy.

General nutritional support for hepatic encephalopathy is based on the following principles of dietary management:

1. **Low protein.** Protein intake is reduced as individually necessary to restrict the dietary sources of nitrogen in amino acids. The amount of restriction will vary with the circumstances. The unconscious patient will receive no protein, but the usual amounts given range from 15 to 50 g/day, depending on whether symptoms of ammonia intoxication are severe or mild. A simple method for controlling dietary protein uses a base meal pattern containing approximately 15 g protein, adding small items of protein foods according to the level of protein desired (see box on facing page).

2. **Kilocalories and vitamins.** Adequate energy intake is crucial to the patient's recovery, especially through the impact of caloric intake on liver glycogen reserves and their protective role in the healing process. The amounts of kilocalories and vitamins are prescribed according to need. About 2000 kcal/day is needed to prevent tissue catabolism, which would be a source of more amino acids and available nitrogen and urea. Sufficient carbohydrate is essential as the primary energy source, with some fat as tolerated. Vitamin K is usually given parenterally, along with other vitamins and minerals that may be deficient.

3. **Fluid intake.** Fluid intake-output balance is carefully controlled.

Gallbladder Disease

Function of the gallbladder. The basic function of the gallbladder is to concentrate and store the bile produced in its initial watery solution by the liver. The liver secretes about 600 to 800 ml/day of bile, which the gallbladder normally concentrates fivefold to tenfold to accommodate this daily bile in its small capacity of 40 to 70 ml. Through the *cholecystokinin (CCK) mechanism* (see Chapter 2), the presence of fat in the duodenum stimulates contraction of the gallbladder with the release of concentrated bile into the common duct and then into the small intestine.

Nature of disease: cholecystitis and cholelithiasis. Inflammation of the gallbladder is called *cholecystitis*. It usually results from a low-grade chronic infection. Normally bile's main ingredient cholesterol, which is insoluble in water, is kept in solution by the other bile ingredients. However, when the absorbing mucosal tissue of the gallbladder is inflamed or infected, changes occur in the tissue. The absorptive powers of the gallbladder may be altered, affecting the solubility of the bile ingredients. Excess water may be absorbed, or excess bile acids may be absorbed. Under these abnormal absorptive conditions, cholesterol may precipitate, forming gallstones composed of almost pure cholesterol. This condition is called *cholelithiasis*. Excessive use of dietary fat over a long period of time predisposes a person to gallstone formation

The liver produces daily about 600 to 800 ml of bile, which the gallbladder normally concentrates fivefold to tenfold and stores in its small 40- to 70-ml capacity.

Low-Protein Diets—15 g, 30 g, 40 g, and 50 g Protein

General description
- The following diets are used when dietary protein is to be restricted.
- The patterns limit foods containing a large percentage of protein, such as milk, eggs, cheese, meat, fish, fowl, and legumes.
- Meat extractives, soups, broth, bouillon, gravies, and gelatin desserts should also be avoided.

Basic meal patterns (contain approximately 15 g of protein)

Breakfast	Lunch	Dinner
½ cup fruit or fruit juice	1 small potato	1 small potato
½ cup cereal	½ cup vegetable	½ cup vegetable
1 slice toast	Salad (vegetable or fruit)	Salad (vegetable or fruit)
Butter	1 slice bread	1 slice bread
Jelly	Butter	Butter
Sugar	1 serving fruit	1 serving fruit
2 tbsp cream	Sugar	Sugar
Coffee	Coffee or tea	Coffee or tea

For 30 g protein	Examples of meat portions	
Add: 1 cup milk 28 g (1oz) meat, 1 egg, or equivalent	28 g (1 oz) meat = 1 thin slice roast, 4 × 5 cm (1½ × 2 in) 1 rounded tbsp cottage cheese 1 slice American cheese	

For 40 g protein		
Add: 1 cup milk 70 g (2½ oz) meat, or 1 egg and 42 g (1½ oz) meat	70 g (2½ oz) meat = Ground beef patty (5 from 448 g [1 lb]) 1 slice roast	

For 50 g protein		
Add: 1 cup milk 112 g (4 oz) meat, or 2 eggs and 56 g (2 oz) meat	112 g (4 oz) meat = 2 lamb chops 1 average steak	

because of the constant stimulus to produce more cholesterol as a necessary bile ingredient to metabolize fat.

Clinical symptoms. When inflammation, stones, or both are present in the gallbladder, contraction from the cholecystokinin mechanism causes pain. Sometimes the pain is severe. There is fullness and distention after eating and particular difficulty with fatty foods.

General treatment. Surgical removal of the gallbladder, *cholecystectomy,* is usually indicated (see Chapter 23). If the patient is obese, some weight loss before surgery is advisable if surgery can be delayed. Supportive therapy is largely nutritional. The drug chenodiol and ultrasound have been used to dissolve small stones and may prove to be effective alternatives to surgery in some cases.

Nutritional therapy. Basic principles of nutritional therapy for gallbladder disease include the following:

1. **Fat.** Because dietary fat is the principal cause of contraction of the diseased organ and subsequent pain, it is poorly tolerated. Energy should come primarily from carbohydrate foods, especially during acute phases. Fat in the diet should be limited to 20 to 30 g/day. Later the patient may tolerate 50 to 60 g/day, so that the diet can be made more palatable. Control of fat will also contribute to weight control, a primary goal because obesity and excess food intake have been repeatedly associated with the development of gallstones.[23] Although some hospitals may not serve a special diet labeled "low fat" for patients with gallbladder disease, nonetheless attention is needed to moderate the fat intake and curtail foods causing pain or discomfort. Certainly a limit of fat to 25% to 30% of the total kilocalories is prudent. A diet plan for a general low-fat regimen is given here (see box, p. 466).

2. **Kilocalories.** If weight loss is indicated, kilocalories will be reduced according to need. Principles of weight management are discussed in Chapter 15. Usually such a diet will have a relatively low fat ratio and meet the needs of the patient for fat restriction.

3. **Cholesterol and "gas formers."** Two additional modifications usually found in traditional diets for gallbladder disease concern restriction of foods containing cholesterol and foods labeled "gas formers." Neither modification has a valid rationale. The body synthesizes daily several times more cholesterol than is present in an average diet. Thus restriction of dietary cholesterol has little effect in reducing gallstone formation. Total dietary fat reduction is more to the point. As for the use of so-called "gas-formers," such as legumes or cabbage or fiber, blanket restriction seems unwarranted, since food tolerances in any circumstances are highly individual.

Diseases of the Pancreas

Pancreatitis

Nature of the disease. Acute inflammation of the pancreas, *pancreatitis,* is caused by the digestion of the organ tissues by the very enzymes it produces, principally trypsin. Normally enzymes remain in the inactive form until the pancreatic secretions reach the duodenum through the common duct. However, gallbladder disease may cause a gallstone to enter the common bile duct and obstruct the flow from the pancreas or cause a reflux of these secretions and bile from the common duct back into the pancreatic duct. This mixing of digestive materials activates the powerful pancreatic enzymes within the gland. In such activated form, they begin their damaging effects on the pancreatic tissue itself, causing acute pain. Sometimes infectious pancreatitis may occur as a complication of mumps or a bacterial disease. Mild or moderate pancreatitis may subside completely, but it has a tendency to recur.

General treatment. Initial care consists of measures recommended for acute disease involving shock. These measures include intravenous feeding at first, replacement therapy of fluid and electrolytes, blood transfusions, antibiotics and pain medications, and gastric suction.

Nutritional therapy. In early stages, nutritional support is maintained by parenteral feeding; oral feedings are withheld because entry of food into the intestines stimulates pancreatic secretions. As healing progresses and oral feedings are resumed, a light diet is used to avoid excessive stimulation of pancreatic secretions. Alcohol and caffeine should be avoided to decrease pancreatic stimulation.

Cystic Fibrosis of the Pancreas

Nature of the disease. Cystic fibrosis is a generalized hereditary disease of children that involves the exocrine glands, particularly the pancreas, and thus affects many tissues and organs. With a frequency of about 1 in every 2000 live births, cystic fibrosis is the most common life-threatening disorder in children, occurring mainly in whites. It is a devastating illness that afflicts some 30,000 children and young adults in the United States alone.[24,25] It is now known to be inherited as an autosomal recessive trait, with 1 in 20 whites as carriers; the specific gene for its transmission has recently been discovered in a highly competitive race among research groups in Canada, England, and the United States.[26,27] In past years its prognosis was poor. Few children with an early onset survived past 10 years of age. However, with better knowledge of the disease, improved diagnostic tests, clinical treatment, and antibiotic therapy, prognosis has improved.

Clinical symptoms. Cystic fibrosis usually produces characteristic clinical symptoms: (1) pancreatic deficiency with greatly diminished digestion of food caused by absence of pancreatic enzymes; (2) malfunction of mucus-producing glands with accumulation of thick viscid secretions, causing respiratory problems and chronic pulmonary disease; (3) abnormal secretions of the sweat glands, containing high electrolyte levels; and (4) possible cirrhosis of the liver arising from biliary obstruction, malnutrition, and infection.

General treatment. Treatment is based on three factors: (1) control of respiratory infections, (2) relief from the effects of the extremely thick bronchial secretions, and (3) maintenance of sound nutrition. The digestive deficiency and malabsorption are evident in the child's stools. They are similar to those in celiac disease, typically bulky, greasy, and foamy, but they also contain more undigested food. Only about half of the child's food is broken down and absorbed, with the rest passing through the body unused. Thus the child with cystic fibrosis has a much more voracious appetite.

Low-Fat and Fat-Free Diets

Low-fat diet
General description
- This diet contains foods that are low in fat.
- Foods are prepared without the addition of fat.
- Fatty meats, gravies, oils, cream, lard, and desserts containing eggs, butter, cream, nuts, and avocados are avoided.
- Foods should be used in amounts specified and only as tolerated.
- The sample pattern contains approximately 85 g protein, 50 g fat, 220 g carbohydrate, and 1670 kilocalories.

Foods	Allowed	Not allowed
Beverages	Skim milk, coffee, tea, carbonated beverages, fruit juices	Whole milk, cream, evaporated and condensed milk
Bread and cereals	All kinds	Rich rolls or breads, waffles, pancakes
Desserts	Jell-O, sherbet, water ices, fruit whips made without cream, angel food cake, rice and tapioca puddings made with skim milk	Pastries, pies, rich cakes and cookies, ice cream
Fruits	All fruits, as tolerated	Avocado
Eggs	3 allowed per week, cooked any way except fried	Fried eggs
Fats	3 tsp butter or margarine daily	Salad and cooking oils, mayonnaise
Meats	Lean meat such as beef, veal, lamb, liver, lean fish and fowl, baked, broiled, or roasted without added fat	Fried meats, bacon, ham, pork, goose, duck, fatty fish, fish canned in oil, cold cuts
Cheese	Dry or fat-free cottage cheese	All other cheese
Potato or substitute	Potatoes, rice, macaroni, noodles, spaghetti, all prepared without added fat	Fried potatoes, potato chips
Soups	Bouillon or broth, without fat; soups made with skimmed milk	Cream soups
Sweets	Jam, jelly, sugar, sugar candies without nuts or chocolate	Chocolate, nuts, peanut butter
Vegetables	All kinds as tolerated	The following should be omitted if they cause distress: broccoli, cauliflower, corn, cucumber, green pepper, radishes, turnips, onions, dried peas, and beans
Miscellaneous	Salt in moderation	Pepper, spices; highly spiced food, olives, pickles, cream sauces, gravies

Suggested menu pattern

	Breakfast	Lunch and Dinner
	Fruit	Meat, broiled or baked
	Cereal	Potato

Toast, jelly	Vegetable
1 tsp butter or margarine	Salad with fat-free dressing
Egg 3 times per week	Bread, jelly
Skim milk, 1 cup	1 tsp butter or margarine
Coffee, sugar	Fruit or dessert, as allowed
	Skim milk, 1 cup coffee, sugar

Fat-free diet
General description
The following additional restrictions are made to the low-fat diet to make it relatively fat free.
1. Meat, eggs, and butter or margarine are omitted.
2. A substitute for meat at the noon and evening meal is 84 g (3 oz) of fat-free cottage cheese.

Table 19-2

Principles of Dietary Management for Children with Cystic Fibrosis

Principle	Reason
High calorie	Energy demands of growth and compensation for fecal losses; large appetite usually ensures acceptance of increased amounts of food
High protein	Usually tolerated in large amounts; excess above normal growth needs required to compensate for losses
Moderate carbohydrate	Starch less well tolerated, simple sugars easily assimilated
Low to moderate fat, as tolerated	Fat poorly absorbed, but tolerance varies widely
Generous salt	Food generously salted to replace sweat loss; salt supplements in hot weather
Vitamins	Double doses of multivitamins in water-soluble form (vitamin E supplements sometimes used as low blood levels of the vitamin have been observed); vitamin K supplements with prolonged antibiotic therapy
Pancreatic enzymes	Large amounts given by mouth with each meal (may be mixed with cereal or applesauce for infants) to compensate for pancreatic deficiency— powdered pancreas extract containing steapsin, trypsin, and amylopsin (Pancreatin, or other pancreatic extracts such as Cotazym or Viokase)

Nutritional therapy. The basic objective is to compensate for the loss of nutrient material resulting from insufficiency of pancreatic enzymes.[24,28] Protein hydrolysates, emulsified fats, and simple sugars are used more easily. There is a wide variation, however, in tolerance for fat, and the amount of fat is usually prescribed according to the character of the stools. A more readily absorbed fat preparation, a vegetable oil made of short- and medium-chain triglycerides (MCT), can be used for food preparation. Large increases in protein seem to be well tolerated and are needed for the replacement of losses and for growth. Enteral tube feeding as adjunct therapy helps combat malnutrition, and predigested formulas such as Pregestimil have sustained early growth.[29,30] Diet guides for cystic fibrosis are similar to those outlined for celiac disease, except that gluten sources need not be restricted and there is greater emphasis on quantity of food. The important principles of dietary management for children with cystic fibrosis are summarized in Table 19-2.

To Sum Up

The nutritional management of gastrointestinal disease is based on careful consideration of four major factors: (1) *secretory functions,* providing the chemical agents and environment necessary for digestion; (2) *neuromuscular function,* required for motility and mechanical digestion; (3) *absorptive function,* transporting nutrients into the circulatory system; and (4) *psychologic factors,* reflected by changes in gastrointestinal function.

Esophageal problems vary widely from simple dysphagia to serious disease or obstruction. Nutritional therapy varies according to degree of dysfunction.

Peptic ulcer, a common gastrointestinal problem, is an erosion of the mucosal lining of the duodenum and less commonly the stomach. It results in such nutritional problems as low plasma protein levels, anemia, and weight loss. Management consists of drug therapy, rest, and individual nutritional therapy.

Intestinal diseases include anatomic changes as in diverticulosis and malabsorption problems, such as found in celiac disease, ulcerative colitis, and Crohn's disease. Nutritional therapy involves modification of the diet's protein and energy content, food texture, increased vitamins and minerals, and fluid and electrolyte replacement, with continuous dietary adjustment according to need. Allergic responses to common food allergens, as well as missing cell enzymes in genetic disease, may also contribute to gastrointestinal and metabolic problems from related food intolerances.

Accessory organs to the gastrointestinal tract—liver, gallbladder, and pancreas—have important functions related to nutrient digestion, absorption, and metabolism, and their diseases interfere with these normal functions. Common liver disorders include hepatitis, usually caused by viral infection, and cirrhosis, an inflammatory condition resulting from tissue damage by such toxins as excessive alcohol. Uncontrolled cirrhosis leads to hepatic encephalopathy and progressive liver failure. Nutrient and energy levels required vary with each condition.

Diseases of the gallbladder include cholecystitis, inflammation that interferes with the absorption of water and bile acids, and cholelithiasis, or gallstone formation. Treatment involves a generally reduced fat diet and surgical removal of the gallbladder. Diseases of the pancreas include pancreatitis, which may relate to gallstones or other causes of pancreatic enzyme reflux with self-digestion of pancreatic tissue by its own enzymes, and cystic fibrosis, an inherited disease of children in which the pancreatic enzymes are missing.

Questions for Review

1. What is the basic principle of diet planning for patients with esophageal problems? Outline a general nutritional care plan for a patient with reflux esophagitis caused by a hiatal hernia.

2. What are the basic liberalized principles of diet planning for patients with peptic ulcer disease? How do these principles differ from traditional therapy?

3. Outline a course of nutritional management for a person with peptic ulcer disease, based on the liberal individual approach. How would you plan nutrition education for continuing self-care and avoidance of recurrence?

4. Describe the nature, clinical signs, and treatment of each of the following diseases: diverticulitis, celiac disease, and inflammatory bowel disease.

5. Compare the basis of food intolerances due to food allergy and a specific genetic disease such as PKU.

6. What is the rationale for treatment of the spectrum of liver disease—hepatitis, cirrhosis, and hepatic encephalopathy?

7. Develop a 1-day food plan for a 45-year-old man, 183 cm (6 ft, 1 in) tall, weighing 66 kg (145 lb), with infectious hepatitis; another plan for a similar patient with cirrhosis of the liver; and another for a similar patient with hepatic encephalopathy. What principles of diet therapy apply for each?

8. What are the principles of nutritional therapy for gallbladder disease? Write a 1-day meal plan for a 30-year-old woman, 165 cm (5 ft, 6 in) tall, weighing 81 kg (180 lb), who has an inflamed gallbladder with stones and is awaiting a cholecystectomy.

9. Describe the nature of cystic fibrosis and compare its symptoms and nutritional therapy with that of celiac disease.

References

1. Desai MB, and Jeejeebhoy KN: Nutrition and diet in management of disease of the gastrointestinal tract. In Shils ME, and Young VR (editors): Modern nutrition in health and disease, ed 7, Philadelphia, 1988, Lea & Febiger.

2. Kumar N, et al: Effect of milk on patients with duodenal ulcers, Br Med J 293:666, 1986.

3. Feldman M, and Richardson CT: Role of sight, smell, and taste of food in the cephalic phase of gastric acid secretion in humans, Gastroenterology 90:428, 1986.

4. Rydning A, et al: Healing of benign gastric ulcer with low-dose antacids and fiber diet, Gastroenterology 91:56, 1986.

5. Goldsmith G, and Patterson M: Irritable bowel syndrome: treatment update, Am Fam Physician 31:191, 1985.

6. DuPont HL: Food-borne infections and poisonings leading to diarrhea, Clin Nutr 3(1):14, Jan/Feb 1984.

7. Lifshitz F, and Carrera E: Food sensitivity and intolerance leading to diarrhea, Clin Nutr 3(1):5, Jan/Feb 1984.

8. Hermann-Zaidins MG: Malabsorption in adults: etiology, evaluation, and management, J Am Diet Assoc 86(9):1171, Sept 1986.

9. Moore FD: Current thoughts on malabsorption: parenteral, enteral, and oral feeding, J Am Diet Assoc 86(9):1169, Sept 1986.

10. Farthing MJG: Gastrointestinal dysfunction in inflammatory bowel disease, Clin Nutr 2(4, Suppl):5, 1983.

11. Fuchs GJ, and Grand RJ: Malnutrition and nutritional support in inflammatory bowel disease, Nutr Supp Serv 5(6):28, June 1985.

12. Fackelmann KA: Cyclosporin therapy heals colon ulcers, Sci News 135(20):310, May 20, 1989.

13. Buisseret PD: Allergy, Sci Am 247(2):86, 1982.

14. Elsas LJ, and Acosta PB: Nutrition support of inherited metabolic dis-

ease. In Shils ME, and Young VR (editors): Modern nutrition in health and disease, ed 7, Philadelphia, 1988, Lea & Febiger.

15. Schuett VE, Brown ES, and Michals K: Reinstitution of diet therapy in PKU patients from twenty-two US clinics, Am J Pub Health 75(1):39, Jan 1985.

16. Michals K: Diet therapy for phenylketonuria: new challenges, Top Clin Nutr 2(3):40, July 1987.

17. Jahn D: Inside, looking out: one mother's view on phenylketonuria, Top Clin Nutr 2(3):87, July 1987.

18. Rohr FJ: Maternal phenylketonuria: a new challenge in the dietary treatment of phenylketonuria, Top Clin Nutr 2(3):44, July 1987.

19. Friedman EG, and Koch R: Report from the Maternal PKU Collaborative Study, Metabolic Currents 1(1):4, 1988.

20. Mendenhall CL, et al: VA cooperative study on alcoholic hepatitis: prognostic significance of protein-calorie malnutrition, Am J Clin Nutr 43:213, Jan 1986.

21. Mezitis NH: Nutritional management in liver disease, Nutr Clin Prac 3(3):108, June 1988.

22. Fraser CL, and Arieff AI: Hepatic encephalopathy, N Engl J Med 313:865, 1985.

23. Hurley RS, and Mekhijian HS: Dietary habits of patients with cholithiasis: do we need to instruct? J Am Diet Assoc 87(2):209, Feb 1987.

24. Michel SH, and Mueller DH: Practical approaches to nutrition of patients with cystic fibrosis, Top Clin Nutr 2(1):10, Jan 1987.

25. Klass P: Shattered dreams, Discover 9(7):34, July 1988.

26. Roberts L: The race for the cystic fibrosis gene, Science 240:141, April 8, 1988.

27. Roberts L: Race for the cystic fibrosis gene nears end, Science 240:282, April 15, 1988.

28. Vaisman N, et al: Energy expenditure of patients with cystic fibrosis, J Pediatr 111:496, 1987.

29. Moore MC, et al: Enteral-tube feeding as adjunct therapy in malnourished patients with cystic fibrosis: a clinical study and literature review, Am J Clin Nutr 44:33, 1986.

30. Farell PM, et al: Predigested formula for infants with cystic fibrosis, J Am Diet Assoc 87(10):1353, Oct 1987.

Further Readings

Butkus SN, and Mahan LK: Food allergies: immunological reactions to food, J Am Diet Assoc 86(5):601, May 1986.

This article provides background for the immunologic basis of allergies and contrasts food allergy and food intolerance.

Fuchs GJ, Grand RJ, and Motil KJ: Malnutrition and nutritional support in inflammatory bowel disease, Nutr Supp Serv 5(6):85, June 1985.

Imes S, Pinchbeck BR, and Thompson ABR: Diet counseling modifies nutrient intake of patients with Crohn's disease, J Am Diet Assoc 87(4):457, April 1987.

These articles provide background for a review of Crohn's disease and the vital role of nutritional support and counseling.

Gitlin N, and Heyman MB: Nutritional support in liver disease, Nutr Supp Serv 4(6):14, June 1984.

Mezitis NHE: Nutritional management in liver disease, Nutr Clin Pract 3(3):108, June 1988.

These articles provide good reviews of the nutritional management of liver disease, with focus by Dr. Mezitis on a case report of alcoholic hepatitis complicated by severe malnutrition.

Hermann-Zaidins MG: Malabsorption in adults: etiology, evaluation, and management, J Am Diet Assoc 86(9):1171, Sept 1986.

This comprehensive article provides a full picture of the causes, assessment, and care of patients with multiple forms of malabsorption and its resulting malnutrition requiring maximal nutritional support.

Klurfield DM: The role of dietary fiber in gastrointestinal disease, J Am Diet Assoc 87(9):1172, Sept 1987.

This article provides a good review of fiber, soluble and insoluble, in health problems, especially in gastrointestinal disease.

Nutritional Aspects of Diarrhea

Gastrointestinal diseases often present barriers to efficient nutrient absorption. So nutritional deficiencies are automatically planned for. But these conditions also lead frequently to diarrhea, which only compounds the problem of nutrient loss. All types of diarrhea result in loss of fluids and electrolytes, with replacement therapy an initial primary concern. However, different types of diarrhea also present other problems that require different modes of treatment related to the disease the diarrhea accompanies. We will examine first three common types of diarrhea: watery, fatty, and small volume.

Types of diarrhea. Watery diarrhea occurs when the amount of water and electrolytes moving into the intestinal mucosa exceeds the amount absorbed into the bloodstream. This movement of water and electrolytes may be secretive or osmotic. *Secretive* movement of water and electrolytes into the mucosa may be active or passive: (1) *Active movement* occurs with excessive gastric hydrochloric acid secretion or enterotoxic infections (e.g., **cholera**) and (2) *passive movement* occurs with a rise in hydrostatic pressure that accompanies such infectious diseases as salmonellosis or tuberculosis, nonbacterial infections, fungal infections, renal failure, irradiation **enteritis,** and inflammatory bowel disease. Other conditions that are associated with watery diarrhea include hyperthyroidism and thyroid carcinoma and hypermotility of the gastrointestinal tract. *Osmotic* movement of water and electrolytes into the mucosa occurs when nutrients are not absorbed because intolerable levels of nonabsorbable particles are present in the intestinal **chyme.** Such particles include: (1) *lactose* in lactase-deficient individuals, (2) *gluten* in persons with gluten-sensitive enteropathy, (3) large amounts of *magnesium* frequently used in antacid therapy for individuals with peptic ulcers, or (4) *iron.* It also occurs in people with a reduced gastrointestinal transit time caused by the removal of part of the intestine.

Fatty diarrhea, or *steatorrhea,* occurs with maldigestion or malabsorption. *Maldigestion* involves a lack of enzymatic activity required to completely digest food, e.g., reduced pancreatic exocrine activity (release of intestinal enzymes from the pancreas) caused by pancreatic insufficiency. *Malabsorption* means that digested materials do not make it across the intestinal mucosa to enter the bloodstream. This failure occurs in conditions in which the intestinal villi are destroyed (e.g., radiation therapy, celiac disease).

Small volume diarrhea occurs mainly when the rectosigmoid area of the colon is irritated, e.g., in inflammatory bowel disease (Crohn's disease or ulcerative colitis). It also occurs when inflammatory conditions affect areas adjacent to the colon, as in pelvic inflammatory disease, diverticulitis, appendicitis, or hemorrhagic ovarian cysts.

Specific nutritional therapy. If uncontrolled, each of these types of diarrhea bring similar metabolic results: **syncope, hypokalemia,** *acid-base imbalances,* and *hypovolemia* with resulting *renal failure.* They may also be accompanied by low levels of fat-soluble vitamins, B_{12} or folic acid, or eventually lead to protein-energy malnutrition. But in addition to these general conditions, each type also manifests specific problems associated with the specific disorders they accompany, requiring differing treatment in each case.

Watery diarrhea often accompanies inflammatory bowel conditions, such as Crohn's disease, for which diet therapy involves: (1) increased protein and kilocalories, (2) low-residue fats and lactose, and (3) avoidance of foods that stimulate gastric acid secretion, and all types of watery diarrhea can be avoided by reducing the motility of the gastrointestinal tract. In other conditions in which *osmotic diarrhea* occurs, e.g., **dumping syndrome,** this

Continued.

Issues and Answers

Cholera
An acute infectious disease characterized by severe diarrhea, acidosis, vomiting, muscle cramps, and prostration. Associated with drinking contaminated water.

Enteritis
Inflammation of the intestine.

Chyme
A semifluid, creamy, hemogeneous material that forms when gastric secretions digest food.

Syncope
A brief loss of consciousness associated with, among other things, reduced levels of extracellular fluid, as occurs during uncontrolled diarrhea.

Hypokalemia
Low potassium levels in the blood.

"Dumping" syndrome
A number of physical problems (nausea, vomiting, sweating, palpitations, syncope, diarrhea, etc.) that occur when stomach contents are emptied at an abnormally fast rate. Occurs when part of the stomach or intestinal tract is removed.

Nutritional Aspects of Diarrhea—cont'd

problem is avoided by giving fluids *between* meals to avoid any extreme difference in osmotic pressures on either side of the intestinal wall. Small frequent meals also help prevent this problem as well as any painful distention.

Fatty diarrhea frequently accompanies conditions associated with maldigestion, such as chronic pancreatitis. The dietary management of this disease involves: (1) frequent meals, high in protein and carbohydrate, low in fat; (2) consumption of medium-chain triglycerides (MCT), which are more easily absorbed under adverse conditions; and (3) avoidance of gastric stimulants (especially caffeine and alcohol). Fatty diarrhea also accompanies conditions of malabsorption, such as gluten-sensitive enteropathy. In addition, this type of diarrhea also requires the removal of items that will damage the mucosal villi, items such as lactose and gluten and products containing them. Sometimes it requires

restricting fat. In both cases, the primary need is to monitor fats that would otherwise appear in the feces. As the therapy progresses, the fat content of the meal can be increased, as tolerated, to normal levels to improve palatability.

Small volume diarrhea may accompany diverticulosis of the colon. A high-residue diet is recommended to increase fecal bulk, thereby preventing diarrhea. To prevent flatulence and distention, however, the fiber (such as wheat bran, fruits, vegetables) should be added to the diet gradually.

All types of diarrhea can result in malnutrition because of loss of electrolytes and fluids. But it is also important to identify the *type* of diarrhea occurring with each patient. Only then can an effective nutritional management strategy be designed to (1) replace fluid-electrolyte losses and (2) eliminate or prevent other possible nutrition-related problems specific for each case.

REFERENCES

Chernoff R, and Dean JA: Medical and nutritional aspects of intractable diarrhea, J Am Diet Assoc 76:161, Feb 1980.

DuPont HL: Food-borne infections and poisonings leading to diarrhea, Clin Nutr 3(1):14, Jan/Feb 1984.

20 Coronary Heart Disease and Hypertension

Chapter Objectives

After study of this chapter, the student should be able to:

1. Identify the factors related to heart disease and account for their effect on the underlying disease process involved.

2. Describe the relationship of hypertension to heart disease.

3. Describe the possible nutrition factors in heart disease.

4. Relate current knowledge of heart disease to a reasonable plan for nutritional care in its prevention and treatment.

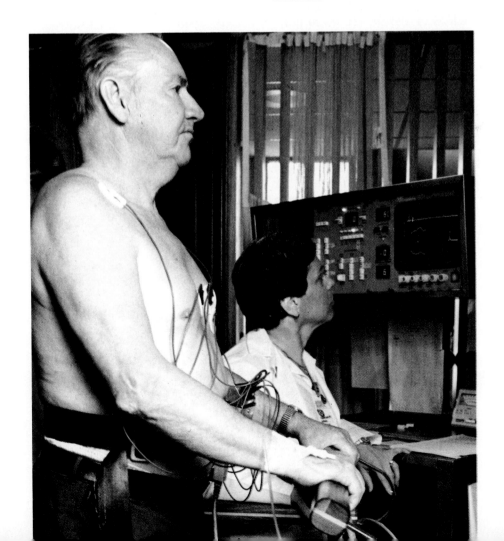

Arteriosclerosis
Group of cardiovascular diseases characterized by a thickening of the arterial walls and a loss of elasticity.

Atheroma
Tumor-type growths on inside lining of blood vessels, composed of lipid material (largely cholesterol) and cellular debris.

Plaque
A patch or flat area forming on a tissue.

Intima
Innermost layer of a blood vessel.

Atherosclerosis
A form of heart disease in which blood vessels are blocked by atheroma (plaque) deposits on the inner lining.

PREVIEW

For the past 50 years diseases of the heart and blood vessels have been the major cause of death in the United States and in most other Western societies. The magnitude of this health care problem is enormous, not only in terms of its human toll but also in the social and economic burdens it represents.

Every day an estimated 3400 Americans, more than two each minute, suffer a heart attack. Every day approximately 1600 persons suffer cerebrovascular accidents—strokes. Every day more than 100,000 children and 1.7 million adults continue to suffer from various forms of rheumatic and congestive heart disease.

Despite a decline in general cardiovascular mortality during the past decade, the leading cause of death in the United States remains coronary heart disease. As more and more is learned about this disease process, the underlying problem of *atherosclerosis*, it is now clear that not one but many factors, including hypertension, are involved and increase a person's risk of developing heart disease.

In this chapter in our continuing sequence of study in clinical nutrition, we will explore this underlying disease process and its risk factors. Then we will relate the nature of this clinical process and its contributing risk factors to preventive approaches of risk reduction, as well as to nutritional therapy and support in disease.

Coronary Heart Disease: The Problem of Atherosclerosis

Embolus
A circulating blood clot, which may come to lodge in a blood vessel, causing an *embolism*.

Ischemia
Deficiency of blood to a body part because of constriction or actual obstruction of a blood vessel.

Infarct
The death of tissue caused by a loss of blood flow to that area, usually caused by a thrombus (clot) clogging the artery feeding the area.

Myocardial infarction (MI)
Death of heart tissue caused by blockage preventing the flow of blood to or through its coronary arteries.

Coronary
Referring to the arteries that carry nutrients and oxygen to the heart muscle.

The Underlying Disease Process

Atherosclerosis, the major **arteriosclerosis** disease and underlying pathologic process in coronary heart disease, remains a major problem in modern medicine. The characteristic lesions involved, **atheromas,** are raised fibrous **plaques** (Figure 20-1). They appear on the interior surface, the **intima,** of the blood vessel as discrete lumps, elevated above the unaffected surrounding area. The plaque usually contains fatty material, such as lipoproteins, the carriers of cholesterol in the blood, which are found both inside and outside of the cells. Crystals of cholesterol can be seen with the unaided eye in the softened cheesy debris of advanced lesions.

It is this fatty debris that suggested the original name **atherosclerosis,** from the Greek words *athera*, meaning "gruel," and *sclerosis,* meaning "hardening." This fatty degeneration and thickening narrows the vessel lumen and may allow a blood clot, an **embolus,** to develop from its irritating presence. Eventually the clot may cut off blood flow in the involved artery. If the artery is a critical one, such as a major coronary vessel, a heart attack occurs. The tissue serviced by the involved artery is deprived of its vital oxygen and nutrient supply, a condition called **ischemia,** and the cells die. The localized area of dying or dead tissue is called an **infarct.** Since the artery is one supplying the cardiac muscle, the *myocardium*, the result is called an acute **myocardial infarction.** The two major **coronary** arteries, with their many branches, are so named because they lie across the brow of the heart muscle and resemble a crown.

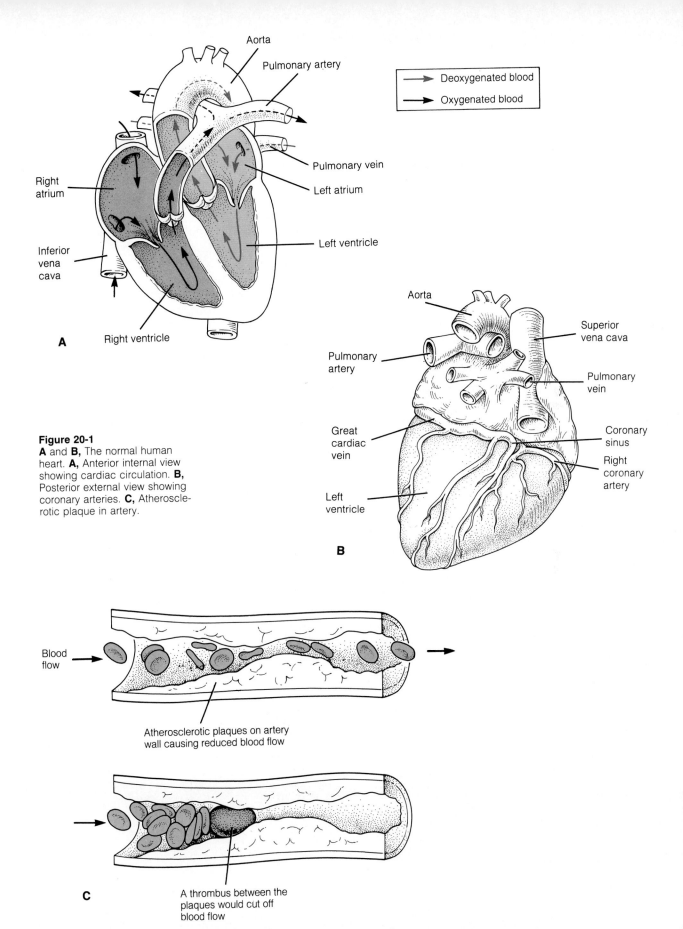

Aorta

Pulmonary artery

→ Deoxygenated blood
→ Oxygenated blood

Right
atrium

Pulmonary vein

Left atrium

Inferior
vena
cava

Left ventricle

A

Right ventricle

Aorta

Superior
vena cava

Pulmonary
artery

Pulmonary
vein

Great
cardiac
vein

Coronary
sinus

Right
coronary
artery

Left
ventricle

B

Figure 20-1
A and **B,** The normal human
heart. **A,** Anterior internal view
showing cardiac circulation. **B,**
Posterior external view showing
coronary arteries. **C,** Atherosclerotic plaque in artery.

Blood
flow

Atherosclerotic plaques on artery
wall causing reduced blood flow

A thrombus between the
plaques would cut off
blood flow

C

On the basis of major investigations over the past decade, three major theories have developed to help explain the cause of these fatty plaques that characterize the underlying disease process:

Injury and Blood Clot

Injury to the blood vessel wall occurs from some mechanical damage or physical condition, leading to rupture of small capillary blood vessels and formation of a blood clot or **thrombosis.** This physical injury may result from elevated blood pressure, chemical damage from cigarette smoking and resulting carbon monoxide in the blood, or some mechanical trauma.[1]

Genetic Factors

Genetic and environmental factors cause mutation of a single smooth muscle cell from near the side of the plaque, and the cells of the plaque are its offspring. The plaque is comparable, then, to a benign tumor of the artery wall. The same kinds of agents or conditions may be involved that transform cells and initiate cancers in a similar process.[2]

Lipid Disorder

Serum lipids, especially serum cholesterol, are the chief cause of the plaque formation and thus of coronary heart disease. Since the fatty plaques involved in the underlying disease process consist mainly of lipid material, especially cholesterol crystals, main investigation has focused on lipid metabolism. A growing mass of evidence from large clinical trials relate these lipids, especially cholesterol, and other lifestyle risk factors (Table 20-1) to incidence of the disease process in numerous population groups.[3] In this chapter we will look mainly at lipid disorders as the basis for current nutritional therapy for persons with heart disease and at the role of hypertension as a major risk factor.

Relation to Lipid Metabolism

In the frustrating search for the cause of atherosclerosis, a number of nutrient factors have been investigated and found to have varying association with the disease process. Several large-scale studies have demonstrated a definite relationship between types of dietary fat and elevated blood lipid levels, especially cholesterol.[3,4] This key relationship has been demonstrated repeatedly. In just the past decade the work of many investigators has brought us

Table 20-1

Multiple Risk Factors in Cardiovascular Disease

Personal characteristics (no control)	Learned behaviors (intervene and change)	Background conditions (screen-treat)
Sex	Stress/coping	Hypertension
Age	Smoking cigarettes	Diabetes mellitus
Family history	Sedentary life	Hyperlipidemia (especially
	Obesity	hypercholesterolemia)
	Food habits	
	Excess fat	
	Excess sugar	
	Excess salt	

much more understanding about the mechanisms for synthesis, transport, and catabolism of cholesterol, and thus the control of blood cholesterol level. It is clear that three lipid substances are involved in the disease process:

Dietary Fat (Triglycerides)

As indicated, these studies have repeatedly shown a definite relationship between the amount and types of fat in the diet and elevated blood lipid levels. Dietary substitution of plant foods with **polyunsaturated** fatty acids for foods high in saturated animal fats has produced a lowering of blood cholesterol.

Polyunsaturated
A carbon chain containing more than one double bond.

Cholesterol

A fat-related compound, cholesterol is synthesized by animal bodies and found in our diet only in animal food sources. Elevated blood cholesterol has been shown to be a primary key to the development of the disease process atherosclerosis.

Lipoproteins

Increased concentrations of certain cholesterol-carrying **lipoproteins,** the low-density lipoproteins (LDL), in the plasma have been shown repeatedly to be related to an increased risk of atherosclerotic heart and peripheral vascular disease.[3] Lipoproteins are the major transport form of lipids in the blood (see Chapter 4). An increase in one or more of these plasma lipoproteins creates the condition called **hyperlipoproteinemia.** A more general term referring to elevated blood lipids is *hyperlipidemia.*

Lipoprotein
Complex of lipids and protein carriers.

Hyperlipoproteinemia
Elevation of lipoproteins in the blood.

Ongoing studies continue to bring us increasing knowledge about the mechanisms involved in these definite relationships between lipids, especially cholesterol, and coronary heart disease. A broad international consensus has emerged for a concerted effort to control cholesterol as a major means of controlling heart disease. The cholesterol-lowering guidelines of the U.S. Consensus Conference and the National Cholesterol Education Program, as well as the recent report of the U.S. Surgeon General, reflect this focus.[5-7] At this point, then, in our advancing research knowledge, we *do* know three things about atherosclerosis: (1) it is a multiple-risk factor disease process; (2) elevated serum cholesterol *is* a major contributor to the disease process; and (3) dietary fat, especially saturated animal fat, *can* affect serum cholesterol level. These findings give impetus to our nutrition intervention efforts.

Classes of Lipoproteins

The lipoproteins in the blood are produced mainly in two places: (1) the *intestinal wall* after initial ingestion, digestion, and absorption of dietary fat from a meal; and (2) the *liver,* from endogenous fat sources. These endogenous lipoproteins carry fat and cholesterol to the tissues for use in energy production and for interchange with other products in cell metabolism. The five types of lipoproteins are classified according to their fat content and thus their density, with those having the highest fat content possessing the lowest density.

Chylomicrons. Highest lipid content, lowest density, composed mostly of dietary triglycerides (TG), with a small amount of carrier protein. They accumulate in portal blood following a meal and are efficiently cleared from the blood by the specific enzyme **lipoprotein lipase.**

Chylomicron
Lowest density lipoprotein; contains the highest amount of fat, mainly triglycerides.

Lipoprotein lipase
An enzyme that helps remove triglycerides from chylomicrons.

Very-low-density lipoprotein (VLDL)
A lipoprotein whose name is derived from its position in electrophoresis, a method used in analyzing lipoprotein fractions in the blood.

Intermediate-density lipoprotein (IDL)
Lipoprotein that is approximately 30% cholesterol; it carries triglycerides to body cells.

Low-density lipoprotein (LDL)
A lipoprotein that carries at least 66% of the total amount of cholesterol in plasma.

Familial hypercholesterolemia
Presence of defective low-density lipoprotein (LDL) receptors, resulting in an increase in LDL-cholesterol.

Very-low-density lipoproteins (VLDL). Still carry a large lipid (TG) content but include about 10% to 15% cholesterol. These lipoproteins are formed in the liver from endogenous fat sources.

Intermediate-density lipoproteins (IDL). Continue the delivery of endogenous triglycerides (TG) to cells and carry about 30% cholesterol.

Low-density lipoproteins (LDL). Carry in addition to other lipids about two thirds or more of the total plasma cholesterol; formed in the serum from catabolism of VLDL. Because LDL carries cholesterol to the cells for deposit in the tissues, it is considered the main agent of concern in elevated serum cholesterol levels, the so-called "bad" cholesterol.

High-density lipoproteins (HDL). Carry less total lipid and more carrier protein. They are formed in the liver from endogenous fat sources. Because HDLs carry cholesterol from the tissues to the liver for catabolism and excretion, higher serum levels of this so-called "good" cholesterol form are considered protective against cardiovascular disease. The "normal" (statistical) range for HDL-cholesterol is 30 to 80 mg/dL, and a value of 75 mg/dL or above contributes definite protection and decreased risk.

The characteristics of these classes of lipoproteins are summarized in Table 20-2. Note the comparative functions of LDL and HDL. Because LDL carries cholesterol to the peripheral cells, for example, it contributes the "cholesterol of concern" in **familial hypercholesterolemia** and is a more valid measure of risk status than is the total cholesterol value.

Classification of Lipid Disorders

Traditional Descriptive Typing System

Based on laboratory designations, an initial *descriptive* typing system for lipid disorders was proposed by Frederickson and others[8]:

Type I	Chylomicrons elevated, rare
Type IIa	LDL elevated, common
Type IIb	LDL and VLDL elevated, common
Type III	IDL elevated, uncommon
Type IV	VLDL elevated, common
Type V	LDL and chylomicrons elevated, uncommon

However, this descriptive classification was limited and not accepted by all clinicians, as one "tongue-in-cheek" report confessed.[9] As more research began to focus on the protein fractions of the lipoprotein molecules, a more comprehensive *functional* classification has developed.

Current Functional Classification

Current clinical practice is based on the more useful functional classification, which concentrates on the important role of carrier protein fractions of the lipoprotein molecules in relation to lipid disease.[10,11] In comparison with the former descriptive typing system, it reveals two additional important factors: (1) increased recognition of the genetic factors involved and (2) increased focus on the role of *apoproteins* in the course of lipoprotein formation, transport, or destruction.

Table 20-2

Characteristics of the Classes of Lipoproteins

Characteristic	Chylomicrons	Very-low density (VLDL)	Intermediate density (IDL)	Low density (LDL)	High density (HDL)
Composition					
Triglycerides (TG)	80%-95%; diet, exogenous	60%-80%; endogenous	40%; endogenous	10%-13%; endogenous	5%-10%; endogenous
Cholesterol	2%-7%	10%-15%	30%	45%-50%	20%
Phospholipid	3%-6%	15%-20%	20%	15%-22%	25%-30%
Protein	1%-2%	5%-10%	10%	20%-25%	45%-50%
Function	Transport dietary TG to plasma and tissues, cells	Transport endogenous TG to cells	Continue transport of endogenous TG to cells	Transport cholesterol to peripheral cells	Transport free cholesterol from membranes to liver for catabolism
Place of synthesis	Intestinal wall	Liver	Liver	Liver	Liver
Size, density					
Description	Largest, lightest	Next largest, lightest	Intermediate size, lighter	Smaller, heavier	Smallest, most dense, heaviest
Density	0.095	0.095-1.006	1.00-1.03	1.019-1.063	1.063-1.210
Size in nanometers (nm)	75-100	30-80	25-40	10-20	7.5-10
Electrophoretic equivalent	Origin (nonmigrating)	Prebeta	Broad beta	Beta	Alpha

Apoproteins. The term **apoprotein** refers to the separate protein part of a combined protein (from the Greek *apo*, meaning "from"). As described in Chapter 4, it is this separate covering of water-soluble protein that allows fats and fat-soluble substances such as cholesterol to travel in the water-based blood circulation. These various apoproteins are genetically determined. Their synthesis is controlled by specific genes, as are all protein substances (see Chapters 6 and 19). It is these genetically controlled apoprotein parts that influence the structure, receptor binding, and metabolism of their related lipoproteins. Currently, apoprotein determination is a useful laboratory tool for identifying persons at high risk for coronary heart disease.[11]

A number of these important apoproteins and their corresponding *apolipoproteins* have been identified. The class designations in common use are apoprotein A, B, C, and E. In turn, each class consists of several different proteins, for example, A-I, A-II, A-III, and A-IV and C-I, C-II, and C-III. All of the classes of apoproteins are made by the liver, and the intestinal mucosa can also make A and B apoproteins. Table 20-3 lists these various classes of apoproteins with their related lipoproteins and functions.

Apoprotein
Protein part of a compound, such as a lipoprotein.

Apo-
Prefix implying separation or being derivative from.

Table 20-3

Apoproteins in the
Structure of Human
Plasma Lipoproteins

Apoprotein	Related lipoprotein	Functions
A-I	HDL, chylomicrons, intestinal VLDL	Activates the plasma enzyme lecithin-cholesterol acyltransferase (LCAT)
A-II	HDL	Transports HDL
A-III	Subfraction of HDL	Catalyzes transfer of cholesterol esters among lipoproteins
B	LDL, VLDL, IDL, chylomicrons, chylomicron remnants	Unclear
C-I	VLDL, HDL, chylomicrons	Activates LCAT
C-II	VLDL, HDL, chylomicrons	Activates lipoprotein lipase
C-III	VLDL, HDL, chylomicrons	Several different forms and functions, depending on structure
E (rich in arginine)	VLDL, HDL, chylomicrons, chylomicron remnants	Excess amount present in beta-VLDL of persons with type III hyperlipoproteinemia

Defects in synthesis of apolipoproteins. This current functional approach classes lipid disorders in four major groups based on the underlying functional problem: (1) defects in apoprotein synthesis, (2) enzyme deficiencies, (3) LDL-receptor deficiency, and (4) other inherited hyperlipidemias. The summary of these lipid disorders in Table 20-4 provides a review of these basic related conditions and nutritional therapies.

Nutritional Therapy—Fat-Controlled Diets
Basic Guidelines

The two major concerns in a fat-controlled diet are: (1) the total amount of fat and (2) the kind of fat used in terms of cholesterol and saturated fats. These two principles were first applied in the generally used approach of the "prudent" food pattern, as originally proposed in 1982 by the American Heart Association (Table 20-5).[12] The initial AHA prudent diet has been revised to meet current lipid-lowering recommendations (Table 20-6). The 1987 report of the Expert Panel on Detection, Evaluation, and Treatment of High Blood Cholesterol in Adults, based on overwhelming evidence reviewed by the NIH Consensus Conference for a causal relationship between blood cholesterol and coronary heart disease, further refined these principles with specific guidelines for practitioners.[13] These current dietary recommendations are shown in Table 20-7. This stepwise approach calls first for a vigorous dietary effort to lower the elevated serum cholesterol before drugs are added. This effort presents special opportunities and challenges for all health care team members, especially for clinical dietitians and public health nutritionists.[14-16]

Table 20-4

Functional Classification of Lipid Disorders

Type of defect	Lipid disorder	Abnormal lipid pattern	Clinical characteristics	Nutritional therapy	Corresponding type in former descriptive classification (Frederickson)
Defective synthesis of apolipoproteins	Apolipoprotein A deficiency	Decreased HDL Increased tissue cholesterol Decreased serum cholesterol Increased serum triglyceride (TG)	Rare Genetic Tangier disease	Low cholesterol Low fat	
	Apolipoprotein B deficiency	High mucosal tissue fat No lipoprotein synthesis possible	Rare Genetic Serious prognosis for child Malabsorption Steatorrhea	Very low fat	
	Apolipoprotein E deficiency	Increased chylomicron remnants Decreased serum LDL Increased cholesterol Increased TG	Relatively uncommon Genetic Xanthomas Premature atherosclerosis	Low cholesterol (<300 mg) Low saturated fat Increased substitution of polyunsaturated fat Weight reduction	Type III
Enzyme deficiency	Lipoprotein lipase deficiency	Increased chylomicrons	Rare Genetic Early childhood Abdominal pain (pancreatitis) Lipemia, retinalis Xanthomas Hepatosplenomegaly	Very low fat (20 g) High carbohydrate Medium-chain triglycerides (MCT)	Type I
	Lecithin-cholesterol acyltransferase (LCAT) deficiency	Overall abnormal lipid pattern: all lipoproteins have low amounts of cholesterol esters and high concentrations of free cholesterol and lecithin Accumulation of large LDL particles rich in unesterified cholesterol	Rare Genetic Abnormal cornea Anemia Kidney damage	Low cholesterol Low fat	

Continued.

Table 20-4

Functional Classification of Lipid Disorders—cont'd

Type of defect	Lipid disorder	Abnormal lipid pattern	Clinical characteristics	Nutritional therapy	Corresponding type in former descriptive classification (Frederickson)
LDL-receptor deficiency	Familial hyper cholesterolemia	Increased LDL Increased total cholesterol Increased VLDL	Common Genetic Increased athero-sclerosis All ages Xanthomas	Low cholesterol (<300 mg) Low saturated fat Substitution of polyunsatu-rated fat	Type II
Other inherited hyperlipidemias	Familial hyper-triglyceridemia	Increased VLDL Increased TG Increased choles-terol Sometimes in-creased blood sugar	Common Genetic Glucose intoler-ance Possible type II (noninsulin-dependent) diabetes melli-tus Obesity Accelerated ath-erosclerosis	Weight reduction Low, simple car-bohydrates Low saturated fat Low cholesterol	Type IV
	Familial multiple hyperlipopro-teinemia	Increased VLDL Increased LDL	Fairly common Genetic Adult Xanthomas; vas-cular disease	Low cholesterol (<300 mg) Low saturated fat Substitution of polyunsatu-rated fat Weight reduction	Type IIb
	Familial type V hyperlipopro-teinemia	Increased chylo-microns Increased VLDL Increased choles-terol Increased TG	Rare Glucose intoler-ance Obesity Abdominal pain (pancreatitis) Hepatospleno-megaly	Weight reduction Controlled carbo-hydrate and fat High protein	Type V

Amount of fat. Almost half of the kilocalories of the average American's diet is contributed by fat. It is recommended that this excess be moderated to at most 30% of the total kilocalories or lowered further to 20% for higher levels of serum cholesterol. Limiting the total amount of fat is, of course, especially indicated when weight reduction is also needed.[17]

Kind of fat. Due largely to the high status of meat and dairy products in the traditional American diet, about two thirds of the total fat in the American diet has been of animal origin and therefore mainly saturated fat. The re-

	Prudent diet	Usual American diet
Total kilocalories	Sufficient to maintain ideal body weight	Often excessive for need
Cholesterol	300 mg	600-800 mg
Total fats (% of kilocalories)	30%-35%	40%-45%
Saturated	10% or less	15%-20%
Monounsaturated	15%	15%-20%
Polyunsaturated	10%	5%-6%
P/S ratio (polyunsaturated/saturated fat in the diet)	1-1.5 = 1	0.3 = 1
Carbohydrate (% of kilocalories)	50%-55%	40%-45%
Starch (complex CHO)	30%-35%	20%-25%
Simple sugars	10%	15%-20%
Proteins (% of total kilocalories)	12%-20%	12%-15%
Sodium	130 mEq	200-250 mEq

Table 20-5

The Prudent Diet as Compared with the Usual American Diet

	Step 1 % total kcalories	Step 2 % total kcalories
Total fat	<30	<30
Saturated	<10	<7
Monounsaturated	10-15	10-15
Polyunsaturated	10	10
Carbohydrate	50-60	50-60
Protein	15-20	15-20
Cholesterol	<300 mg/day	<200 mg/day

Table 20-6

American Heart Association Revised Prudent Diet Guidelines for Lowering Elevated Blood Lipid Levels

maining one third has come from vegetable sources and is mainly unsaturated fat. However, this ratio has gradually been changing over the past few years with the use of less animal and more plant fat. This has been the general goal of the prudent diet (Table 20-5), illustrated by its breakdown of total fat according to degree of saturation with emphasis on unsaturated fats reflected in the **polyunsaturated/saturated (P/S) ratio.**

Cholesterol

The current stepwise guidelines place greater emphasis on the control of cholesterol and total fat and its degrees of saturation, according to serum lev-

Polyunsaturated/saturated (P:S) ratio
Ratio of polyunsaturated to saturated fat (fatty acids) in a diet.

Table 20-7

Step 1 and Step 2 Diets for Treating High Plasma Cholesterol (NCEP)*

Nutrient	Step 1 % total kcalories	Step 2 % total kcalories
Total fat	30	30
Saturated	10	7
Monounsaturated	10 to 15	10 to 15
Polyunsaturated	10	10
Carbohydrates	50 to 60	50 to 60
Protein	10 to 20	10 to 20
Cholesterol	300	200
Total kcalories	Sufficient to achieve and maintain desirable weight	Sufficient to achieve and maintain desirable weight

*National Cholesterol Education Program, adult treatment panel guidelines.

Table 20-8

Evaluation Criteria for Screening and Monitoring Persons for Treatment of Elevated Blood Cholesterol (NCEP)*

Type of test	Blood level classifications (mg/dL)
Total plasma cholesterol	
Desirable level	<200
Borderline-high level	200-239
High level	≥240
LDL cholesterol	
Borderline high-risk	130-159
High-risk	≥160

*National Cholesterol Education Program, adult treatment panel guidelines.

els of LDL cholesterol and presence of heart disease history and other risk factors (Table 20-7). The step 1 diet guide used in the National Cholesterol Education Program is shown here (see box, on facing page). The serum cholesterol values used in the program as guidelines for testing and monitoring are shown in Table 20-8.

Additional Dietary Factors

Several additional dietary factors are involved in nutritional therapy for heart disease. These include dietary fiber, omega-3 fatty acids, and sodium. Each of these factors may need consideration along with the primary focus on fat and cholesterol (see box, p. 487).

The Problem of Acute Cardiovascular Disease: Myocardial Infarction (MI)

Objective

In the initial acute phase of cardiovascular disease, following a heart attack or myocardial infarction (MI), the basic clinical objective is *cardiac rest* to allow the healing process to begin. This needed rest and healing of the heart muscle tissue require close attention to dietary modifications. All care is directed toward this basic need for cardiac rest so that the damaged heart can be restored to normal functioning.

Step 1 Diet Guide: Modifications to Lower Plasma Cholesterol (NCEP)*

Food groups	Choose	Decrease
Fish, chicken, turkey, and lean meats (3-oz cooked portions)	Fish, poultry without skin, lean cuts of beef, lamb, pork, or veal, shellfish	Fatty cuts of beef, lamb, pork, spare ribs, organ meats, regular cold cuts, sausages, hot dogs, bacon, sardines, roe
Skimmed and low-fat milk, cheese, yogurt, and dairy substitutes	Skimmed or 1%-fat milk (liquid, powdered, evaporated), buttermilk	Whole milk: (4% fat) regular, evaporated, condensed; cream, half and half, 2% milk, imitation milk products, most nondairy creamers, whipped toppings
	Nonfat (0% fat) or low-fat yogurt	Whole-milk yogurt
	Low-fat cottage cheese (1% or 2% fat)	Whole-milk cottage cheese (4% fat)
	Low-fat cheeses, farmer or pot cheeses (all of these should be labeled no more than 2 to 6 g fat per oz)	All natural cheeses (eg, blue, Roquefort, Camembert, cheddar, Swiss)
		Low-fat or "light" cream cheese, low-fat or "light" sour cream
		Cream cheeses, sour cream
	Sherbet, sorbet	Ice cream
Eggs	Egg whites (2 whites = 1 whole egg in recipes), cholesterol-free egg substitutes	Egg yolks
Fruits and vegetables	Fresh, frozen, canned, or dried fruits and vegetables	Vegetables prepared butter, cream, or other sauces
Breads and cereals	Homemade baked goods using unsaturated oils sparingly, angel food cake, low-fat crackers, low-fat cookies	Commercially baked goods: pies, cakes, doughnuts, croissants, pastries, muffins, biscuits, high-fat crackers, high-fat cookies
	Rice, pasta	Egg noodles
	Whole-grain breads and cereals (e.g., oatmeal, whole wheat, rye, bran, multigrain)	Breads in which eggs are major ingredient
Fats and oils	Baking cocoa	Chocolate
	Unsaturated vegetable oils: corn, olive, rapeseed, safflower, sesame, soybean, sunflower	Butter, coconut oil, palm oil, palm kernel oil, lard, bacon fat
	Margarine or shortenings made from one of the unsaturated oils listed above	
	Diet margarine	
	Mayonnaise, salad dressings made with unsaturated oils listed above	Dressings made with egg yolk
	Low-fat dressings	
	Seeds and nuts	Coconut

*National Cholesterol Education Program.

Nutritional Therapy

To meet the basic clinical requirement for cardiac rest, the diet will be modified in *energy value* and *texture,* as well as continuing modifications in fat, cholesterol, and sodium.

Energy—Kilocalories

A brief period of undernutrition during the first few days after the attack is advisable. The metabolic demands for digestion, absorption, and metabolism of food require a generous cardiac output volume. Small intakes of food at a time, spread over the day, decrease the metabolic work load to a level that the weakened heart can accommodate. The patient can progress to more food as healing occurs. During the initial recovery stages the diet may be limited to about 1200 to 1500 kilocalories to continue cardiac rest from metabolic work loads. If the patient is obese, as is frequently the case, this kilocalorie level may be continued for a longer period to help the patient begin very gradually to lose some of the excess weight.

Texture

Early feedings will generally include foods soft in texture or easily digested to avoid excess effort in eating. Smaller meals served more frequently may give needed nutrition without undue strain or pressure. Temperature extremes in foods, both solids and liquids, should be avoided.

Fat and Cholesterol

The general "prudent" diet (Tables 20-5 and 20-6) will control amount and kind of fat, as well as cholesterol, for most patient needs. Individual modifications may be used to meet any additional needs. Other food factors such as caffeine may need to be avoided (see box, p. 488).

Sodium

A moderately reduced sodium content in the foods selected is also emphasized. This will help control any tendency to fluid accumulation in the body tissues. Added tissue fluid causes more work for the heart to maintain an increased blood volume circulation.

The Problem of Chronic Heart Disease: Congestive Heart Failure

Pulmonary edema
Fluid accumulation in the lungs.

In chronic coronary heart disease, a condition of *congestive heart failure* may develop over time. The progressively weakened heart muscle, the myocardium, is unable to maintain an adequate cardiac output to sustain normal blood circulation. The resulting fluid imbalances cause *edema*, especially **pulmonary edema,** to develop. This condition brings added problems in breathing and places more stress on the laboring heart.

Cardiac Edema: Sodium and Water Metabolism
Imbalance in Capillary Fluid Shift Mechanism

As the heart fails to pump out the returning blood fast enough, the venous return is retarded. This causes a disproportionate amount of blood to accumulate in the vascular system working with the right side of the heart. The venous pressure rises, a sort of "backup" pressure effect, and overcomes the balance of filtration pressures necessary to maintain the normal *capillary fluid shift mechanism* (see Chapter 8). Fluid that would normally flow between inter-

Clinical Application

Primary focus of nutritional therapy for coronary heart disease (CHD) centers on control of lipid factors, including cholesterol and saturated fats. Two other food factors, however, play a different role. In varying ways they help to protect us from CHD development.

Added Food Factors in CHD Therapy

Dietary fiber

Studies indicate that water-soluble types of dietary fiber have significant cholesterol-lowering effect. Soluble fiber includes gums, pectin, certain hemicelluloses, and storage polysaccharides. Foods rich in soluble fiber include oat bran and dried beans, with additional amounts in barley and fruits. Oat bran, for example, contains a primary water-soluble gum, beta-glucan, which is a lipid-lowering agent. Soluble dietary fiber:

- Delays gastric emptying
- Increases intestinal transit time
- Slows glucose absorption
- Is fermented in the colon into short-chain fatty acids that may inhibit liver cholesterol synthesis and help clear LDL-cholesterol

On the other hand, insoluble dietary fiber—cellulose, lignin, and many hemicelluloses—found in vegetables, wheat, and most other grains, does not have these lipid-lowering effects. Thus an increased use of soluble fiber food sources, especially oat bran and legumes, would have beneficial effects.

Omega-3 fatty acids

Studies indicate that the omega-3 fatty acids, *eicosapentaenoic acid (EPA)* and *docosahexaenoic acid (DHA)* (see Chapter 4), which are found mostly in seafood and marine oils, also have protective functions. They can:

- Change the pattern of plasma fatty acids to alter platelet activity and reduce platelet aggregation that causes blood clotting, thus lowering risk of coronary thrombosis
- Decrease synthesis of very-low-density lipoproteins (VLDL)
- Increase antiinflammatory effects

It would seem, then, that factors in foods such as oats, dried beans, and fatty fish would provide valuable lipid-lowering additions to our diets.

REFERENCES

Anderson JW, and Tietyen-Clarke J: Dietary fiber: hyperlipidemia, hypertension, and coronary heart disease, Am J Gastroenterol 81:907, 1986.

Anderson JW, and Gustafson NJ: Dietary fiber and heart disease: current management concepts and recommendations, Top Clin Nutr 3(2):21, April 1988.

Hepburn FN, Exler J, and Weihrauch JL: Provisional tables on the content of omega-3 fatty acids and other fat components of selected foods, J Am Diet Assoc 86(6):788, June 1986.

Simopoulos AP: Omega-3 fatty acids in growth and development, Part II: The role of omega-3 fatty acids in health and disease: dietary implications Nutr Today 23(3):12, May/June 1988.

To Probe Further

**Recent Risk Factor
Findings**

Recent research findings regarding past and current risk factors for coronary heart disease may affect the advice you give clients about foods and other ingested items. Some formerly forbidden items have been given a reprieve and others need even stricter control.

Use these items

Fish and shellfish. Fish and marine oils are major sources of omega-3 fatty acids, which have been found to have numerous protective functions against coronary heart disease. The long-chain unsaturated fatty acids help prevent platelet aggregation and blood clot formation and lead to production of protective substances such as prostaglandins.

It is also now "safe" to include shrimp, crab, and other edible crustaceans in a low-cholesterol diet. These foods were assigned high cholesterol levels in the 1940s, when the analysis techniques were still very crude. More efficient methods indicate that the cholesterol level of the oyster, for example, has "dropped" from about 200 to 50 mg/98 g (3½ oz). With these new findings, plus a knowledge that shellfish are rich in polyunsaturated fats, you can now reassure shrimp-loving clients that their favorite seafood is no longer taboo.

Milk. Low-fat (2% butterfat) milk, skimmed milk, and fermented milks in the forms of yogurt, buttermilk, and sweet acidophilus milk have not been found to affect serum lipid levels in healthy persons. Only yogurt has resulted in a small rise in triglyceride levels. Studies have shown, however, that skimmed milk has the greatest cholesterol lowering effect. With this in mind, you will want to advise high-risk clients with heart disease to make the switch to skimmed milk. Clients with normal blood lipid levels who are concerned mainly with prevention could be told that moderate use of whole milk probably won't increase their chances of developing disease.

Tighten control of these items

Coffee. Heavy coffee-drinking *does* have an effect on blood cholesterol levels. It also disrupts normal heart rhythms. Serious effects have been seen even in healthy persons after drinking nine or more cups of coffee or tea. These same effects were seen in patients with a history of abnormal heart rhythms after only two cups. The basic recommendation is that persons with coronary heart disease should avoid caffeine. Clients concerned with prevention should be advised to reduce their intake as much as possible.

Alcohol. Several studies have indicated that a moderate alcohol intake raises HDL cholesterol levels, which in turn reduces the risk of developing atherosclerotic plaque. However, in animal studies it was found that taking large amounts of alcohol over an 18-month period interrupts heart rhythms. You may advise clients who want to drink to do so in moderation. Few problems have been found in research subjects who drank less than 6 oz/day of low-alcohol drinks such as beer or wine.

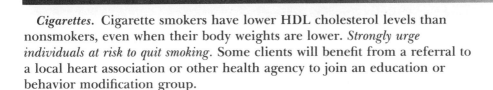

Cigarettes. Cigarette smokers have lower HDL cholesterol levels than nonsmokers, even when their body weights are lower. *Strongly urge individuals at risk to quit smoking.* Some clients will benefit from a referral to a local heart association or other health agency to join an education or behavior modification group.

REFERENCES

Criqui MH, et al: Lipoproteins as mediators for the effects of alcohol consumption and cigarette smoking on cardiovascular mortality: results from the Lipid Clinics Follow-up Study, Am J Epidemiol 126:629, 1987.

Dobmeyer DL, et al: The arrhythmogenic effects of caffeine in human beings, N Engl J Med 308:814, 1983.

McMurtrey JJ, and Sherwin R: History, pharmacology, and toxicology of caffeine and caffeine-containing beverages, Clin Nutr 6(6):249, Nov/Dec 1987.

Simopoulos AP: Omega-3 fatty acids in growth and development and health, Part II: The role of omega-3 fatty acids in health and disease: dietary implications, Nutr Today 23(3):12, May/June 1988.

Thompson LU, et al: The effect of fermented and unfermented milks on serum cholesterol, Am J Clin Nutr 36:1106, 1982.

stitial spaces and blood vessels is held in the tissue spaces rather than being returned to circulation.

Hormonal Mechanisms

Two hormonal mechanisms are involved in fluid balance in the normal circulation. In this instance, both contribute to cardiac edema.

1. **Aldosterone mechanism.** This mechanism, described more completely by its full name **renin-angiotensin-aldosterone** mechanism, is normally a life-saving sodium- and, hence, water-conserving mechanism to ensure essential fluid balances. In this case, however, it only compounds the edema problem. As the heart fails to propel the blood circulation forward, the deficient cardiac output effectively reduces the blood flow through the kidney nephrons. The decreased renal blood pressure triggers the renin-angiotensin system. Renin is an enzyme from the renal cortex that combines in the blood with its substrate, *angiotensinogen,* which is produced in the liver, to produce in turn **angiotensin** I and II. Angiotensin II acts as a stimulant to the adrenal glands to produce aldosterone, the hormone that in turn effects a reabsorption of sodium in an ion exchange with potassium in the distal tubules of the nephrons, and water reabsorption follows. Ordinarily this is a life-saving mechanism to protect the body's vital water supply. In congestive heart failure, however, it only adds to the edema problem. The mechanism reacts as if the body's total fluid volume is reduced, when in truth the fluid is excessive. It simply is not in normal circulation but is being retained in the body's tissues.

2. **ADH mechanism.** This water-conserving hormonal mechanism also adds to the edema. The cardiac stress and the reduced renal flow cause the

Aldosterone
Hormone secreted by the adrenal cortex to regulate sodium, potassium, and water balance.

Renin
Enzyme secreted by the juxta-glomerular cells of the kidney.

Angiotensin
Powerful vasopressor hormone and stimulator of the hormone aldosterone from the adrenal cortex.

Antidiuretic hormone (ADH)
Hormone produced by the pituitary to reduce urine formation.

Vasopressin
Hormone secreted by the hypothalamus to stimulate muscular contraction, raise blood presse, and concentrate urine.

release of the **antidiuretic hormone (ADH),** also known as **vasopressin,** from the pituitary gland. ADH then stimulates still more water reabsorption in the nephrons of the kidney, further increasing the problem of edema.

Increased Cellular Free Potassium

As the reduced blood circulation depresses cell metabolism, cell protein is broken down and releases its bound potassium in the cell. As a result, the amount of free potassium inside the cell is increased, which increases intracellular osmotic pressure. Sodium ions in the fluid surrounding the cell then also increase in number to balance the increased osmotic pressure within the cell and prevent cell dehydration. The increased sodium outside the cell in time causes still more water retention.

Nutritional Therapy—Sodium-Restricted Diet

Because of the role of sodium in water balance, the diet used to treat cardiac edema restricts the sodium intake. Over the past years, four levels of dietary sodium restriction have been outlined by the American Heart Association as guidelines, each level progressively restrictive from mild to severe. The first three of these are in common use, but the final one is too severely restricted to be realistic or useful. Compare these dietary sodium levels with sodium in the general diet.

Sodium in the General Diet

The taste for salt is an acquired one. Some persons salt food heavily and habituate their taste to high salt levels. Others acquire a taste for less salt and use smaller amounts. Use of table salt and an increasing use of processed foods with more salt and other sodium compounds provide the main sources of sodium in the American diet. Common adult intakes of sodium range widely, according to taste habit, from about 3 to 4 g/day with light use to as high as 10 to 12 g/day with heavy use. Salt (NaCl) intakes would be approximately twice these amounts, because sodium (Na) makes up 40% of the NaCl molecule. The large amount of salt in the American diet, estimated to contribute about 6 to 15 g sodium/day (260 to 656 mEq), is largely due to the increased use of many processed food products.

Table salt—sodium chloride (NaCl)—is about 40% (actually 39.34%) sodium (Na).

Sodium Levels in Restricted Diets

As indicated, the main source of dietary sodium is common table salt—sodium chloride. Many other lesser-used sodium compounds, such as baking powder and baking soda, and especially the large amounts of sodium compounds in processed foods, contribute still more. Otherwise, the remaining dietary source is sodium occurring in foods as a natural mineral. In each of these sodium-restricted food lists, these sources of sodium are progressively deleted.

    1. **Mild sodium restriction: 2 to 3 g sodium/day (70 to 130 mEq).** Salt may be used *lightly* in cooking, but no *added* salt is used. Foods in which salt is used as a preservative or a flavoring agent are removed as well. These include such items as pickles, olives, bacon, ham, chips, and many other high salt processed foods (see box, on facing page).

    2. **Moderate sodium restriction: 1 g sodium/day (43.5 mEq).** To maintain this level of restriction, no salt is used in cooking, no salt is added to the

Restrictions for a Mild Low-Sodium Diet (2 to 3 g sodium)

Do not use
- Salt at the table (use salt lightly in cooking)
- Salt-preserved foods such as salted or smoked meat (bacon and bacon fat, bologna, dried or chipped beef, corned beef, frankfurters, ham, kosher meats, luncheon meats, salt pork, sausage, smoked tongue); salted or smoked fish (anchovies, caviar, salted and dried cod, herring, sardines), sauerkraut, olives
- Highly salted foods such as crackers, pretzels, potato chips, corn chips, salted nuts, salted popcorn
- Spices and condiments such as bouillon cubes,* catsup,* chili sauce,* celery salt, garlic sauce, onion salt, monosodium glutamate, meat sauces, meat tenderizers,* pickles, prepared mustard, relishes, Worcestershire sauce, soy sauce
- Cheese,* peanut butter*

*Dietetic low-sodium kinds may be used.

food, and no salty foods are eaten. Beginning with this level, there is some control of natural sodium foods. Vegetables with higher sodium content are somewhat limited, salt-free canned vegetables are substituted for regular canned ones, salt-free baked products are used, and meat and milk are limited to moderate portions (see box, p. 492).

3. **Strict sodium restriction: 0.5 g sodium/day (22 mEq).** To maintain this strict level, in addition to the deletions already made, foods with higher natural sodium content are avoided. These foods include meat, milk, and eggs, which are used only in small portions, and certain vegetables, which are not used at all (see box, p. 493).

4. **Severe sodium restriction: 0.25 g sodium/day (11 mEq).** This level is rarely used because it is too highly limited to be practical or nutritionally adequate, and it is not needed now with available drug therapy. A deletion list for this level would be the same as for the strict 500 mg level, with further limits: only low-sodium milk can be used and meat and eggs are allowed only occasionally.

Incidence

High blood pressure presents a health problem in the lives of some 60 million Americans. At least 95% of these persons have **essential hypertension,** meaning that its cause is unknown. However, since essential hypertension tends to be familial, often beginning in young teen years, a genetic influence may underlie the condition. It has become the fourth largest public health problem in America. It has often been called the "silent disease" because it carries no overt signs, but it can have serious implications if not treated and controlled. Both treatment and control can be accomplished with better individual care available today. Still, despite a wealth of research in past years, there are few clues to its cause and our lack of information sometimes leaves us more confused than enlightened.

Sodium restricted diets: Conversion of mg to mEq Equivalent weight (Eq) of an element equals its atomic weight or gram-molecular weight (mol wt) divided by its valence. (Consult the periodic table of elements in any chemistry book for atomic weights and valences.) Thus for sodium (Na) and potassium (K):

$$1 \text{ Eq Na} = \frac{23 \text{ g (mol wt of Na)}}{1 \text{ (valence of Na)}} = 23 \text{ g}$$

or

$$1 \text{ mEq Na} = 23 \text{ mg}$$

$$1 \text{ Eq K} = \frac{39 \text{ g (mol wt of K)}}{1 \text{ (valence of K)}} = 39 \text{ g}$$

or

$$1 \text{ mEq K} = 39 \text{ mg}$$

The Problem of Essential Hypertension

Essential hypertension
High blood pressure of unknown cause.

Restrictions for a Moderate Low-Sodium Diet (1000 mg sodium)

Do not use
- Salt in cooking or at the table
- Salt-preserved foods such as salted or smoked meat (bacon and bacon fat, bologna, dried or chipped beef, brains, corned beef, frankfurters, ham, kosher meats, luncheon meats, salt pork, sausage, smoked tongue, kidneys), salted or smoked fish (anchovies, caviar, salted and dried cod, herring, sardines, frozen fish fillets, canned salmon,* tuna*), sauerkraut, olives
- Highly salted foods such as crackers, pretzels, potato chips, corn chips, salted nuts, salted popcorn
- Spices and condiments such as bouillon cubes,* catsup,* chili sauce,* celery salt, garlic salt, onion salt, monosodium glutamate, meat sauces, meat tenderizers,* pickles, prepared mustard, relishes, Worcestershire sauce, soy sauce
- Cheese,* peanut butter*
- Buttermilk (unsalted buttermilk may be used) instead of skim milk
- Canned vegetables* or canned vegetable juices*
- Frozen peas, frozen limas, frozen mixed vegetables, or any frozen vegetables to which salt has been added
- More than one serving of any of these vegetables in one day—artichokes, beet greens, beets, carrots, celery, dandelion greens, kale, mustard greens, spinach, Swiss chard, turnips (white)
- Regular bread, rolls,* crackers*
- Dry cereals,* except puffed rice, puffed wheat, and shredded wheat
- Quick-cooking Cream of Wheat
- Shellfish (clams, crab, lobster, shrimp); oysters may be used
- Salted butter, salted margarine, commercial French dressings,* mayonnaise,* or other salad dressings*
- Regular baking powder,* baking soda or anything containing them; self-rising flour
- Prepared mixes (pudding,* gelatin,* cake, biscuit)
- Commercial candies

*Dietetic low-sodium kinds may be used.

Public Awareness

In the past few years, two major events have stimulated increased research interest and public concern about hypertension. First, the National Heart, Lung, and Blood Institute of the National Institutes of Health (NIH) conducted an educational campaign to inform Americans about the serious problem of hypertension. But this effort reached only a limited number of persons; many others remained uninformed and untreated. Nonetheless, it was a significant stimulus to needed follow-up work. Second, clinical trials of the Hypertension Detection and Follow-up Program clearly demonstrated that high blood pressure can effectively be treated, even in its milder forms.[18]

Nondrug Approaches

A significant result of these studies has been a renewed focus on nonpharmacologic approaches to the control of hypertension. The U.S. National

Restrictions for a Strict Low-Sodium Diet (500 mg sodium)

Do not use

- Salt in cooking or at the table
- Salt-preserved foods such as salted or smoked meat (bacon and bacon-fat, bologna, dried or chipped beef, brains, corned beef, frankfurters, ham, kosher meats, luncheon meats, salt pork, sausage, smoked tongue, kidneys), salted or smoked fish (anchovies, caviar, salted and dried cod, herring, sardines, frozen fish fillets, canned salmon,* tuna*), sauerkraut, olives
- Highly salted foods such as crackers, pretzels, potato chips, corn chips, salted nuts, salted popcorn
- Spices and condiments such as bouillon cubes,* catsup,* chili sauce,* celery salt, garlic salt, onion salt, monosodium glutamate (MSG, Accent, and so on), meat sauces, meat tenderizers,* pickles, prepared mustard, relishes, Worcestershire sauce, soy sauce
- Cheese,* peanut butter*
- Buttermilk (unsalted buttermilk may be used) instead of skim milk
- More than 2 cups skim milk a day, including that used on cereal
- Any commercial foods made of milk (ice cream, ice milk, milk shakes)
- Canned vegetables* or canned vegetable juices*
- Frozen peas, frozen limas, frozen mixed vegetables, or any frozen vegetables to which salt has been added
- Artichokes, beet greens, beets, carrots, celery, dandelion greens, kale, mustard greens, spinach, Swiss chard, turnips (white)
- Regular bread,* rolls,* crackers*
- Dry cereals,* except puffed rice, puffed wheat, and shredded wheat
- Quick-cooking Cream of Wheat
- Shellfish (clams, crab, lobster, shrimp); oysters may be used
- Salted butter, salted margarine, commercial French dressings,* mayonnaise,* or other salad dressings*
- Regular baking powder,* baking soda or anything containing them; self-rising flour
- Prepared mixes (pudding,* gelatin,* cake, biscuit)
- Commercial candies

*Dietetic low-sodium kinds may be used.

Heart, Lung, and Blood Institute of NIH has increased its emphasis on nondrug therapies.[19] The NIH report urged that these therapies—diet, exercise, and behavior modification—be "pursued aggressively" not only in treating mild hypertension but also as an important adjunct in more severe cases. Subsequent studies have continued to show the effectiveness of nondrug nutritional therapy.[20-22] The goal of all therapies is to reduce as much as possible the quantity of drugs needed. Thus nutritional therapy has a fundamental role in the care of persons with hypertension (Figure 20-2).

> The trend in treatment of hypertension whenever possible is toward nondrug therapy: diet, exercise, and behavior modification.

Blood Pressure Controls
Arterial Pressure

As commonly measured, blood pressure is an indication of the arterial pressure in the vessels of the upper arm. This measure is obtained by an instru-

Figure 20-2
Monitoring blood pressure. This patient has successfully used nonpharmacologic therapy to control her hypertension.

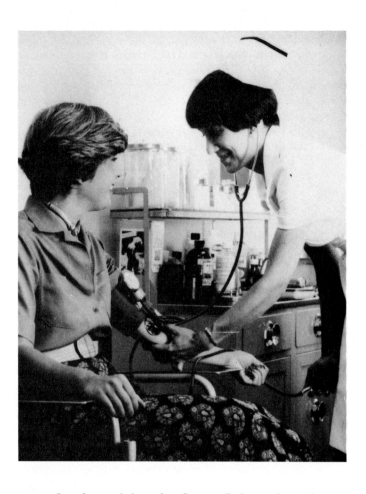

Systolic
Referring to the heart's period of contraction.

Diastolic
Referring to the heart's period of dilation; the "relaxation" phase of the heartbeat.

ment for determining the force of the pulse. This instrument is called a *sphygmomanometer,* from the Greek words *sphygmos,* meaning "pulse," *manos,* meaning "thin," and *metron,* meaning "measure." The pulse pressure is measured in terms of millimeters of mercury (mm Hg) rise in thin contained tubes or in equivalent values read on gauges or digital indicators. The higher or upper value recorded is the **systolic** pressure from the contraction of the heart muscle. The lower value recorded is the **diastolic** pressure, produced during the relaxation phase of the cardiac cycle. Thus the upper limit of a normal adult blood pressure would be recorded 150/89.

Several factors contribute to maintaining the fluid dynamics of normal blood pressure: (1) increased pressure on the forward blood flow; (2) increased resistance from the containing blood vessels; and (3) increased viscosity of the blood itself, making movement through the vessels more difficult. Of these factors, increased viscosity is a rare event. Thus in discussing high blood pressure in general terms, we are dealing with the first two factors, the pumping pressure of the heart muscle propelling the blood forward and the resistance to this forward flow presented by the blood vessel walls normally or by any abnormal added constriction or thickening.

Muscle Tone of Blood Vessel Walls

In hypertension the body's finely tuned mechanisms designed to maintain fluid dynamics are not operating effectively. Normally, these systems include several agents that act to variously dilate and constrict the blood vessels to meet whatever need is present at a given time. In a hypertensive person, however, the dilation or constriction of blood vessels does not occur in the normal manner. If not effectively treated, uncontrolled elevated blood pressure results. The body systems that operate to help maintain normal blood pressure include: (1) neuroendocrine functions of the sympathetic nervous system, mainly mediated by chemical neurotransmitters such as *norepinephrine* (see Chapter 16); (2) hormonal systems such as the renin-angiotensin-aldosterone mechanism and its *vasopressor* effect; and (3) enzyme systems such as the *kallikrein-kinin* mechanism, sometimes operating with *prostaglandins*, which controls substances that act to dialate or constrict smooth muscle as needed.[23]

Step-Care Treatment Approach

Based on national studies and widespread community screening programs, current medical treatment centers on an improved "step-care" method of identifying types of blood pressure levels and matching standard treatment programs to these diagnosed types. Increased emphasis is given to nondrug therapies and to limited use of drugs. The identification of persons with hypertension according to degree of severity has improved the basic approach to care. These steps of care are termed mild, moderate, or severe.

1. **Mild hypertension.** Diastolic pressure (relaxed phase of the cardiac cycle; the lower value) is 90 to 104 mm Hg. Initial consideration is given to other risk factors such as weight or stress. Individual treatment is started with nondrug approaches and centers on nutritional therapies of weight control, sodium restriction, and behavioral techniques for habit changes.

2. **Moderate hypertension.** Diastolic pressure is 105 to 119 mm Hg. Prompt evaluation and treatment is indicated. A combination of drugs may be used: (1) a diuretic agent to decrease the blood volume and (2) a blocking agent to decrease muscle constriction of blood vessel walls. The basic nutritional therapy described above continues as vital support, with the goal of reducing the amount of medication required.

3. **Severe hypertension.** Diastolic pressure is 120 to 130 mm Hg and above. Immediate evaluation and vigorous drug therapy is demanded. Diuretic and blocking agents are continued and a third drug may be added, a peripheral vasodialator to assist in reducing arterial resistance to blood flow. In all cases the implications for diet therapy revolve around: (1) potassium replacement and the use of diuretics and (2) nutritional support for weight management and sodium modification, as well as physical exercise and stress reduction.

Principles of Nutritional Therapy

There is no question that nutritional therapy plays a large role in the treatment of hypertension. Most hypertensive persons respond to some degree of sodium restriction and are called "sodium sensitive."[24,25] Adequate potassium levels relate to blood pressure control mainly through its electrolyte balance with sodium and its replacement need when potassium-losing diuretics are used.[26,27] Studies of the influence of calcium on hypertension show variable results (see Issues and Answers, p. 502). In general, the current focus of nutritional therapy is on weight management, sodium control, general nutrient balance, and an individualized food plan.[28]

Current medical treatment centers on identifying types of blood pressure levels and matching standard treatment programs to the diagnosed types.

Weight Management

Body weight reflects an individual's energy balance. The energy input in food is balanced with the energy output in physical activity, with a desirable lean weight indicating this balance. In practice, weight management is not quite this simple. But because the overweight state has been closely associated with hypertension risk factors, a careful and wisely planned program to maintain a desirable lean weight is a cornerstone of therapy. Guidance for developing such a personal program can be found in Chapter 15.

Sodium Control

Recently there has been an increased public awareness of the effectiveness of lowering our relatively high sodium diet as a general health measure. A moderately reduced daily intake of about 2 to 3 g (90 to 120 mEq) is a reasonable health promotion goal. Persons in a high-risk category for the development of hypertension should reduce their sodium intake as a preventive measure. Persons with diagnosed hypertension should certainly reduce their sodium intake according to the step-care treatment recommendations.

General Energy Nutrient Balance

The ratio of the energy nutrients protein, carbohydrate, and fat in the overall diet for a person with hypertension is an important consideration. Because these three energy nutrients contribute kilocalories, they are important in the overall goal of weight management. The relative ratio suggested by the U.S. Dietary Guidelines (see Chapter 1) provides a reasonable basis for planning the diet: (1) carbohydrate should have the largest allowance, 50% to 55% of the total kilocalories, with a large portion of complex carbohydrate; (2) protein should make up about 15% to 20%, with monitoring of excess protein intake, which usually carries animal fat with it; and (3) fat should be modified to take up only about 25% to 30% of the total kilocalories, with the focus on unsaturated food fat forms. In addition, it would be wise to limit the intake of cholesterol to 300 mg/day.

Personal Food Plan

A realistic and effective individual food plan must provide persons with assistance and guidance in food preparation and selection of food products:

1. **Food preparation.** Numerous guides for preparation of primary foods with alternative seasonings to salt are available. Several are included here in the Appendix; become familiar with them and use them as resources. The use of appropriate spices and herbs can help persons develop a taste for less salt (see box, on facing page).

2. **Food products.** Close attention to food product labeling is important in a person's effort to control sodium. Current labeling regulations, although not perfect, do provide additional information for the consumer who wishes to control the intake of sodium and other food additives. The food industry has responded to current consumer and FDA concerns about the sodium content of food products and is providing more needed information.

Education and Prevention

Both coronary heart disease and hypertension have more or less a chronic nature. Thus an important responsibility of the health care team is educating the patient and family concerning continuing self-care needs for maintaining

Clinical Application

If you counsel with persons on sodium-restricted diets, you probably spend a lot of time answering the question "Is there life without salt?" To which the standard reply is something like, "Of course there is. You'll just have to get used to the natural flavor of foods." This answer usualy falls flat.

We learn to like the taste of salt. It is a taste that "accumulates" over the years. That's why it's unreasonable, for example, to expect a middle-aged man who just discovered he has hypertension to suddenly give up the seasoning habits of a lifetime. It's overly optimistic to expect anyone raised on hot dogs, potato chips, and TV dinners to fall in love with the flavor of fresh broccoli overnight. There is hope, however. Subjects in one study developed a lower tolerance for salty foods after following a low sodium diet for 5 months. So if you can convince clients to reduce their salt intake for a significant period of time, you might get them to fall out of love with the taste of salt.

There is still the problem of getting clients to use less salt to begin with. Answer: introduce them to the world of salt-free seasonings. Some persons are already familiar with a variety of alternative seasonings and only need some recipes that who how to use them creatively. Others think gourmet cooking means just using pepper instead of salt. These individuals need a little extra help in selecting and using salt-free seasonings successfully. Here are some suggestions for guidelines:

- Stop adding salt at the table. It's pure habit. Get rid of the shaker—throw it away, hide it, or get it out of sight—anything to remove the reminder.
- If food tastes too fresh without added salt, sprinkle them with fresh lemon juice—not salt.
- When cooking, cut the amount of salt in the recipe in half and avoid other sodium-rich seasonings.
- If you're already a good cook, or even if you're not, refer to guides for hints on spicing up old favorites without salt.
- If you're not the world's greatest chef, enroll in a basic cooking class at a local adult education center or community college and use these guidelines when preparing meals at home. You may also want to check the Foods section of your local newspaper for listings of special low-sodium cooking classes offered by local health organizations.
- Relax for a moment while dinner is simmering on the stove and enjoy the wonderful new aromas filling your kitchen. Sodium reeduction can introduce you to a flavorful new adventure with food.

The Spice of Life: Breaking Up the Salt Monopoly

REFERENCES
Bertino M, Beauchamp GK, and Engleman K: Long-term reduction in dietary sodium alters the taste of salt, Am J Clin Nutr 36:1134, 1982.
Wylie-Rossett J: Spices to the rescue, Prof Nutr 14:4, 1982.

health. Also, since genetic factors play a large role, early screening of children in high-risk families is significant in prevention of problems.

Start Early

Education for the person with coronary heart disease should not begin with so-called discharge instructions for the hospitalized patient. Such a process is like a mere after-thought. It fails to build sound knowledge for personal decision making or to provide stress-reducing support. Rather, the postcoronary learning experience should begin early in convalescence to give the patient and family a clear knowledge of positive needs and focus on realistic behavior changes. Such an approach will reinforce sound and vigorous self-care within the limits of individual capability and will help avoid the negative view of self as a "cardiac cripple."

Use a Variety of Resources

Many excellent resources for individual and family education are provided by the American Heart Association (AHA) through its national and regional offices. Practical discussions need to center on such aspects as food buying and preparation to make diets palatable and enjoyable. Many helpful suggestions are included in the AHA booklets, spread sheets, and their excellent book, *The American Heart Association Cookbook*. In fact, an increasing number of popular cookbooks are also available. A survey of local markets will give guidance concerning commercial products and label reading.

Build Family Health Habits

In the final analysis, the wisest approach to the control of both coronary heart disease and hypertension is that of prevention of problems and positive health promotion and maintenance. Real contributions begin in childhood, especially in families with strong histories of familial lipid disorders and essential hypertension. In these early developmental years families can build sound health habits with a general focus on good nutrition, including attention to food behaviors related to fat and cholesterol, salt, and sugar and promotion of a physically active life.

Good food habits must be developed early.

To Sum Up

Coronary heart disease remains the leading cause of death in the United States. *Atherosclerosis,* its underlying pathology, involves the formation of plaque, a fatty substance that builds up along the interior surfaces of blood vessels, interfering with blood flow and damaging blood vessels. If this buildup becomes severe, it cuts off blood supplies of oxygen and nutrients to tissue cells, which in turn begin to die. When this occurs in a coronary artery, the result is a *myocardial infarction,* or heart attack.

The risk for atherosclerosis increases with the amount and type of blood lipids (lipoproteins) available. The *apoprotein* portion of lipoproteins is an important genetically determined part of the disease process. Elevated *serum cholesterol* is a primary factor in atherosclerosis development.

Initial dietary recommendations for *acute cardiovascular disease* (heart attack) include caloric restriction, soft-textured foods, and small, frequent meals to reduce the metabolic demands of digestion, absorption, and metabolism of foods and their nutrients. Maintenance of a lean body weight is important. Also fat, saturated fat, cholesterol, and sodium should be restricted.

Persons with *chronic coronary heart disease* (congestive heart failure) and those with *essential hypertension* benefit from weight control, exercise, and sodium restriction to overcome cardiac edema and help control elevated blood pressure.

Current dietary recommendations to help prevent coronary heart disease involve reducing weight, limiting fats to 25% to 30% of all kilocalories with the majority being unsaturated food forms, limiting sodium intake to 2 to 3 g/day, and increasing exercise.

Questions for Review

1. Which types of hyperlipoproteinemia occur most often? Identify the lipids that are elevated in each case, as well as predisposing factors. Describe the types of diet recommended for each.
2. Identify four dietary recommendations that should be made for the person with a heart attack. Describe how each recommendation helps recovery.
3. Discuss the four levels of sodium restriction, describing general food choices and preparation methods.
4. What dietary changes could the average American make to reduce saturated fats and to substitute unsaturated fats?
5. What does the term *essential hypertension* mean? Why would weight management and sodium restriction contribute to its control? What other nutrient factors may be involved in hypertension?

References

1. Ross R, and Glomset JA: Pathogenesis of atherosclerosis, N Engl J Med 295:369, 1976.
2. Beneditt EP: The origin of atherosclerosis, Sci Am 236(2):74, 1977.
3. Grundy SM: Cholesterol and coronary heart disease: a new era, JAMA 256:2849, 1986.
4. Lipid Research Clinics Program: The Lipid Clinics Coronary Primary Prevention Trial results: reduction in incidence of coronary heart disease, JAMA 251:351, 1984.
5. Lowering blood cholesterol to prevent heart disease, Consensus Conference, JAMA 253:2080, 1985.
6. Cleeman JI, and Lenfant C: New guidelines for the treatment of high blood cholesterol in adults from the National Cholesterol Education Program: from controversy to consensus, Cirulation 76:960, 1987.
7. Byrne G: Surgeon general takes aim at saturated fats, Science 241:651, Aug 5, 1988.
8. Frederickson DS, et al: Dietary management of hyperlipoproteinemia, DHEW Pub No (NIH) 76-110, Washington, DC, 1975, US Government Printing Office.
9. Grouse LD: A medical misdemeanor: I harbored evil thoughts about the Frederickson fat classification, JAMA 244:2090. 1980.
10. Kolata, G: Cholesterol-heart disease link illuminated, Science 221:1164, 1983.
11. Ball M, and Mann JI: Apoproteins: predictors of coronary heart disease? Br Med J 293:769, 1986.
12. American Heart Association Nutrition Committee: Rationale of the diet-heart statement of the American Heart Association, Arteriosclerosis 4:177, 1982.
13. National Cholesterol Education Program: Report of the Expert Panel on Detection, Evaluation, and Treatment of High Blood Cholesterol in Adults, Bethesda, MD, 1987, National Heart, Lung, and Blood Institute.

14. Grundy SM: Therapeutic approaches to elevated cholesterol levels: recommendations of the Adult Treatment Panel, National Cholesterol Education Program Newsletter: Cholesterol and Coronary Disease...Reducing the Risk, supplement:7, July 1988.

15. Farrand ME: National Cholesterol Education Program guidelines: new opportunities and challenges for dietitians, Top Clin Nutr 3(2):9, April 1988.

16. Van Horn LV: Meeting the demands of the National Cholesterol Education Program: some ideas from the field, J Am Diet Assoc 88(2):161, Feb 1988.

17. Braunstein NS: Weight management in cardiac rehabilitation patients, Top Clin Nutr 2(2):75, April 1987.

18. Friedwald WT: Current nutrition issues in hypertension, J Am Diet Assoc 80(1):17, Jan 1982.

19. Disten HP, et al: The 1984 report of the Joint National Committee on Detection, Evaluation, and Treatment of High Blood Pressure, Arch Intern Med 144:1045, 1984.

20. Flamenbaum W, and Cohen NS: The decision to "unmedicate," JAMA 253:687, 1985.

21. Langford HG, et al: Dietary therapy slows the return of hypertension after stopping prolonged medication JAMA 253:657, 1985.

22. Stamler R, et al: Nutritional therapy for high blood pressure, final report of a four-year randomized controlled trial—The Hypertension Control Program, JAMA 257:1484, 1987.

23. Frohlich ED: Physiologic observations in essential hypertension, JAMA 80:18, 1982.

24. McGregor GA: Sodium is more important than calcium in essential hypertension, Hypertension 7:628, 1985.

25. National Institutes of Health, USDHHS: Nonpharmacological approaches to the control of high blood pressure, final report of the Subcommittee on Nonpharmacological Therapy for the 1984 Joint National Committee on Detection, Evaluation, and Treatment of High Blood Pressure, National Heart, Lung, and Blood Institute, Bethesda, MD, 1986, US Government Printing Office (Pub No 1986-491-292:41147).

26. Whelton PK, and Klag MJ: Potassium in the homeostasis and reduction of blood pressure, Clin Nutr 6(2):76, March/April 1987.

27. Russell RP: Potassium supplementation, potassium-retaining diuretics, and hazards of hyperkalemia, Clin Nutr 6(2):70, March/April 1987.

28. Wassertheil-Smoller S, et al: Effective dietary intervention in hypertensives: sodium restriction and weight reduction, J Am Diet Assoc 85(4):423, April 1987.

Ernst ND: NIH Consensus Development Conference on lowering blood cholesterol to prevent heart disease: implications for dietitians, J Am Diet Assoc 85(5):586, May 1985.

Van Horn LV: Meeting the demands of the National Cholesterol Education Program: some ideas from the field, J Am Diet Assoc 88(2):161, Feb 1988.

These articles provide background experiences from nutritionists helping develop current national programs for controlling blood cholesterol as a major effort in controlling coronary heart disease.

Poindexter SM, Dear WE, and Dudrick SJ: Nutrition in congestive heart failure, Nutr Clin Prac 1(2):83, 1986.

These clinicians provide background for the role of nutrition in treatment of congestive heart failure, with case history examples.

Simopoulos AP: Omega-3 fatty acids in growth and development and in health and disease, Part I: The role of omega-3 fatty acids in growth and development, Nutr Today 23(2):10, March/April 1988.

Simopoulos AP: Omega-3 fatty acids in growth and development and in health and disease, Part II: the role of omega-3 fatty acids in health and disease, Nutr Today 23(3):12, May/June 1988.

This nutrition scientist in the field of lipid research applies current knowledge of omega-3 fatty acids to the control of heart disease.

Winterfeldt E: Diet and coronary heart disease, Top Clin Nutr 3(2):1, April 1988.

This lead article introduces a series of articles in this issue of a useful journal, *Topics in Clinical Nutrition,* on the subject of heart disease and cardiac care, with discussions on various aspects of nutritional therapy and national programs designed to educate the public about the role of cholesterol in coronary heart disease.

Further Readings

Is Calcium a New Risk Factor in Hypertension Control?

If you had high blood pressure, what would you do—give up salt or drink more milk? This question may sound absurd to anyone familiar with traditional methods of hypertension control, which includes a low-sodium diet. To them giving up salt is the obvious reply. However, in the general public the question is being taken seriously, because a growing number of popular news articles state that persons with high blood pressure may need more calcium.

These reports are based on a number of studies showing that persons with hypertension drink less milk than those with normal blood pressure levels and also have lower serum calcium levels. These studies contradict the findings of earlier studies in which high serum calcium levels were observed in persons with high blood pressure. The latter results are to be expected because of calcium's known contractive effect on smooth muscle tissue such as blood vessels. Large amounts of calcium should cause blood vessels to contract, thus squeezing on the blood flow and bringing a build-up of pressure against arterial walls. The "new" research claims that persons with hypertension don't handle calcium normally. Some of these researchers believe there is a defect in the sodium-calcium exchange system through which the calcium enters the cell when the sodium leaves it. They tend to discredit the sodium theory because sodium reduction doesn't work for everyone with hypertension; even traditionalists realize that only about 30% of those with high blood pressure can control it through sodium reduction alone. Nonetheless there are problems with the new calcium research:

- Most of the studies are based on a small number of subjects. For example, McCarron and Moris's study at the University of Oregon was based on only 23 subjects. Another study finding a different correlation of high blood pressure with high serum cholesterol was based on studies of 9321 subjects.
- Although calcium researchers found low serum calcium levels in subjects with hypertension, total blood calcium levels did not vary with variable blood pressure readings in their study.
- In conditions characterized by high calcium levels, such as hyperparathyroidism, blood pressure levels are also high. As the condition improves and the serum calcium levels fall, blood pressure readings also fall.
- The calcium intake of subjects in the new studies was based on oral 24-hour recall information on diet, which is not generally considered the most accurate method of determining nutrient intake.
- Assuming that the dietary information obtained is accurate, it indicated that subjects with hypertension may have consumed less milk but still obtained *adequate* amounts of calcium.

Another important point to remember is that most calcium-rich foods have higher than average sodium levels per serving. For example, 1½ oz American cheese may provide 250 to 300 mg calcium, but it also provides more than 400 mg sodium.

Many unanswered questions remain about the effects of sodium, calcium, potassium, and many other factors on blood pressure. In any event the American Heart Association and other health organizations still advise the general public to (1) limit sodium intake and (2) take in enough calcium to meet various needs for growth, bone and tooth maintenance, and muscle function.

REFERENCES

Carter CA: Calcium: a new risk factor in hypertension control? High Blood Pressure News 1(1):2, 1983.

McCarron DA, and Morris CD: Blood pressure response to moderate hypertension, Ann Intern Med 103:825, 1985.

MacGregor GA: Sodium is more important than calcium in essential hypertension, Hypertension 7:628, 1985.

21 Diabetes Mellitus

After study of this chapter, the student should be able to:

1. Describe the nature and extent of diabetes mellitus in the population according to type of diabetes, and identify contributing causes and symptoms.

2. Identify the basic goals of current diabetes management and describe the forms of treatment necessary to achieve these goals.

3. Help persons with diabetes plan and maintain good self-care with sound management and practical tools and resources.

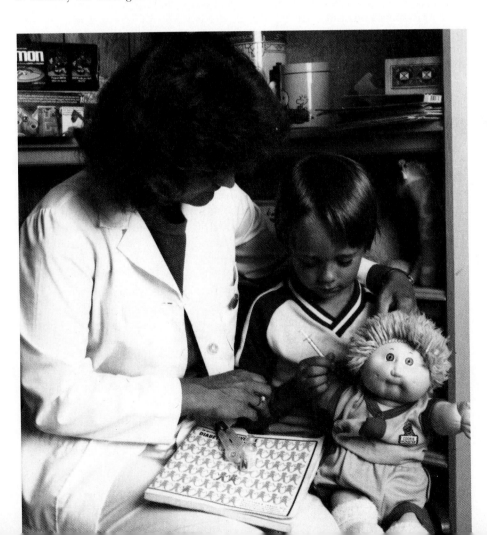

PREVIEW

About 11 million Americans have diabetes, about one in 20 persons. Of this total, 15% are insulin dependent and 85% are noninsulin-dependent. Diabetes complications have become the fifth ranking cause of death from disease in the North American population.

The metabolic disease *diabetes mellitus* has both ancient roots and a rapidly expanding modern research base. Many current studies are helping to explain early observations of its nature and develop better means of care. During the past few years newer information about diabetes indicates that the disease has multiple causes. The current concept held by investigators is that diabetes is not a single disease but a syndrome consisting of many disorders characterized by hyperglycemia and, in a large number of persons, various complications.

Sound nutritional therapy remains the fundamental base of management for all persons with diabetes. Newer forms of insulin and self-monitoring of blood glucose have become indispensable tools of control for many.

In this chapter of our continuing study sequence on clinical nutrition, we will look first at the general nature of diabetes mellitus and its abnormal metabolic pattern. We will see that energy balance, between food intake and energy output with insulin as the controlling agent, forms the essential foundation of good care. Then we will examine the principles of nutritional therapy and daily self-care management that maintain this balance and help avoid symptoms of imbalance and development of complications.

The Nature of Diabetes

Diabetes mellitus
(From Greek *dia,* through, *bainein,* to go *diabetes,* siphon; from Latin *mellitus,* honey, sweet) is a metabolic disorder in which the ability to oxidize the primary fuel glucose is more or less lost, thus also affecting metabolism of the other energy nutrients, fat and protein, because of a lack of available insulin, the pancreatic islet hormone. Glucose accumulates in the blood and is lost in the urine, causing excessive urination, thirst, and hunger, and, over time, multiple system complications.

History

The metabolic disease we know today as **diabetes mellitus** has been with us for a long time. Ancient records describe its devastating effects as observed by early healers. In the first century AD the Greek physician Aretaeus wrote of a malady in which the body "ate its own flesh" and gave off large quantities of urine. He gave it the name *diabetes,* from the Greek word meaning "siphon" or "to pass through." Much later, in the seventeenth century, the word *mellitus,* from the Latin word for "honey," was added because of the sweet nature of the urine. This addition also distinguished it from **diabetes insipidus** ("insipid," meaning tasteless, or *not* sweet), another disorder in which the passage of copious amounts of urine had been observed.

As medical knowledge began to grow, early clinicians such as Rollo in England and Boushardat in France observed that diabetes became less severe in overweight patients who lost weight. Later another French physician, Lancereaux, and his students described two kinds of diabetes: *diabete gras* ("fat diabetes") and *diabete maigre* ("thin diabetes").[1] All these observations preceded any knowledge about insulin or any relation to the pancreas. Throughout these times, which have aptly been called the "Diabetic Dark Ages," persons with diabetes had short lives and were maintained on a variety of semistarvation diets.[2]

Later evidence began to point to the pancreas as a primary organ involved in the disease process. Paul Langerhans (1847-1888), a young German medical student, found special clusters, or islets, of cells scattered about the human pancreas that were different from the rest of the tissue. Although their function was still unknown, these special islet cells were named for their young discoverer: the islets of Langerhans. Research focus then centered on the pancreas. Finally, in 1921-1922 a University of Toronto team discovered and successfully used the controlling agent from the "island cells," naming it **insulin** for its source (see box, p. 507).

Contributory Causes
Insulin Activity

For some time, insulin assay tests developed to measure the level of insulin activity in the blood found insulin-like activity in early diabetes to be two or three times the normal insulin levels. Investigators postulated that the insulin was present but bound with a protein, making it unavailable. It is now evident that diabetes is a condition with multiple forms, resulting from: (1) lack of insulin, as in *insulin-dependent diabetes mellitus (IDDM);* or (2) insulin resistance, as in *noninsulin-dependent diabetes mellitus (NIDDM).*

Weight

Diabetes has long been associated with weight, since early observations of differences in "fat diabetes" and "thin diabetes."[1] Current research has reinforced the relation of the overweight state to NIDDM. Apparently, the obesity interacts with an underlying genetic predisposition to trigger the noninsulin-dependent form of diabetes.

Heredity

Diabetes has usually been defined in terms of heredity. But increasing evidence indicates that there is considerable *genetic variation* between the two main types of diabetes, IDDM and NIDDM. Environmental factors apparently play a role in unmasking the underlying genetic susceptibility, a "thrifty" diabetic genotype that probably developed from primitive times for survival.

The "Thrifty Gene" Hypothesis

This theory indicates that diabetes may be associated with past genetic modifications for survival during varying periods of food availability. In the past this state of diabetes was a saving, or "thrifty," trait that provided better storage and metabolism of food during times when our ancestors lived under more primitive and difficult survival conditions. As food supplies became more plentiful, the negative aspects of the diabetic trait began to appear. Such is indeed the case, for example, with the experience of the Pima Indians in Arizona.[3] In earlier times this group ate a limited diet, mainly of carbohydrate foods harvested by heavy physical labor in a primitive agriculture. Now, however, with the "progress" of civilization, the Pimas have become obese, and *half* of the adults have NIDDM, the highest reported rate of this type of diabetes in the world. This same pattern is seen among populations of now unbanized Pacific Islanders, as well as migrant Asian Indians. Thus evidence suggests that these groups have a genetic susceptibility to NIDDM (diabetic genotype) and that the disease is triggered by environmental fac-

Diabetes insipidus
Condition that shares some of the symptoms of diabetes mellitus: large urine output, great thirst, and, sometimes, a large appetite. But in diabetes insipidus these are symptoms of a specific *injury,* not a collection of metabolic disorders. The impaired pituitary gland produces less *antidiuretic hormone,* a substance that normally helps the kidneys retain water.

tors, including obesity. Just as obesity may result from more than one genetic error, so too may diabetes.[4] As we commonly observe, diet can indeed interact with genetics to develop adult-onset diabetes.

Classification

Increasing evidence indicates differences between insulin-dependent and noninsulin-dependent diabetes, and epidemiologic studies in various population groups have provided newer clinical and pathogenic information. With this growing evidence, an international work group sponsored by the National Institutes of Health (NIH) proposed a basic classification for the diabetes syndrome according to the need of insulin for control. This basis is now used to designate the two main types—IDDM and NIDDM.

Insulin-Dependent Diabetes Mellitus (IDDM)

In its insulin-dependent form, diabetes develops very rapidly and is more severe and unstable. This form occurs mainly in children, and the child is usually underweight. Acidosis is fairly common.

Noninsulin-Dependent Diabetes Mellitus (NIDDM)

In the noninsulin-dependent form, diabetes develops more slowly and is usually milder and more stable. This form occurs mainly in adults, and the person is usually overweight. Acidosis is infrequent. The majority of patients improve with weight loss and are maintained on diet therapy alone. Sometimes there is a need for an oral hypoglycemic medication.

Symptoms

Initial observations. Early signs of diabetes include: (1) increased thirst (polydipsia); (2) increased urination (polyuria); (3) increased hunger (polyphagia); and (4) weight loss with IDDM or obesity with NIDDM.

Laboratory test results. Various clinical laboratory tests taken at this time reveal: (1) glycosuria (sugar in the urine); (2) hyperglycemia (elevated blood sugar); and (3) abnormal glucose tolerance tests.

Other possible symptoms. Additional signs that may appear include: (1) blurred vision; (2) skin irritation or infection; and (3) weakness and loss of strength.

Results of uncontrolled diabetes. Continued symptoms that can occur as an uncontrolled condition becomes more serious include: (1) fluid and electrolyte inbalance; (2) acidosis (ketosis); and (3) coma.

The Metabolic Pattern of Diabetes

Overall Energy Balance and the Energy Nutrients

Because the initial symptoms of glycosuria and hyperglycemia are related to excess glucose, diabetes has been called a disease of carbohydrate metabolism. However, as more becomes known about the intimate interrelationships of carbohydrate, fat, and protein metabolism, we now view it in more general terms. It is a metabolic disorder resulting from a lack of insulin (absolute, partial, or unavailable) affecting more or less each of the basic energy nutrients. It is especially related to the metabolism of the two fuels, carbohydrate and fat, in the body's overall energy system.

Insulin: Saga of a Success Story

On first glance, looking at numbers only, it would appear that the development of insulin was a causal factor in changing the status of diabetes mellitus from a rare disease to one that affects over 10 million Americans. Closer inspection of the facts, however, reveals that the disease was thought to be rare only because its victims died young—there were fewer persons around who had the disease. Today insulin enables over 2 million insulin-dependent individuals to live longer and enjoy productive lives.

The success story behind insulin lies not only in its ability to extend the life span of the person with diabetes, but also in its own resilience. Insulin was discovered during the summer of 1921 at the University of Toronto by Frederick Banting, a surgeon who, according to newspaper accounts of the day, solved the mystery of insulin in his sleep, and Charles Best, a college graduate who was not yet enrolled in medical school. They developed insulin by tying off pancreatic ducts of dogs and waiting for the organ to "die." They then made an extract of the remaining tissue.

The extract worked fairly well in their tests with dogs. An extract that worked in humans was not developed for another 6 months, partly because their extract was originally given by mouth. Even when injected, their formula failed, which indicated that faulty purification methods may have been involved.

Finally, in January of 1922, a successful extract was developed by a new member who joined the research team, J.B. Collip. Its effect on one patient's diabetic condition was not enough to counteract the effect of the treatment of the day—a diet that derived almost *71% of its kilocalories from fat*. The patient died at age 27 with atherosclerosis and coronary heart disease. However, the team was successful with their third patient. The young girl, who was first diagnosed as having diabetes when she was 11 years old, lived to be 73 years of age. After insulin therapy was initiated, she was taken off the popular "starvation" diet of the day, gained weight, and led a normal life.

Ironically, despite Collip's successful extraction procedure, his subsequent actions almost stopped their project. Jealousies developed and, with the permission of the head of the university's physiology department, Collip refused to share his purification methods with Banting. Then, after his extraction product was a success, Collip conveniently "forgot" how to make it! As a result of this foolish battle, at least one patient died because the researchers ran out of the original extract.

Fortunately, Collip miraculously "remembered" how to make his extract the following May. Soon after, insulin was mass produced and made available to the growing number of persons who depended on it for their very survival.

REFERENCES

Altman LK: The tumultuous discovery of insulin: finally, hidden story is told, New York Times, September 14, 1982, pp. C-1, C-6.

Bliss M: The discovery of insulin, Chicago, 1982, University of Chicago Press.

Nestle M, et al: A case of diabetes mellitus, N Engl J Med 81:127, Oct 1982.

Figure 21-1
Sources of blood glucose (food and stored glycogen) and normal routes of control.

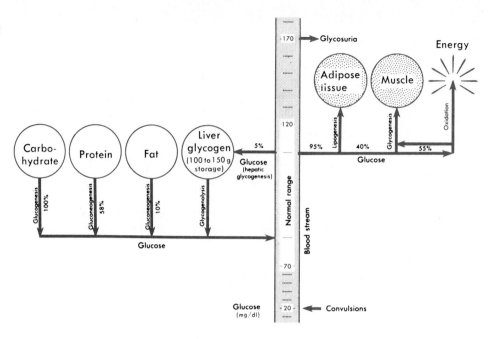

Normal Blood Glucose Controls

Control of blood glucose within its normal range of 70 to 120 mg/dL (3.9 to 6.7 mmol/L) is vital to life. A knowledge of these controls in maintaining a normal blood glucose level is essential to understanding the impairment of these controls in diabetes (see Chapters 2 and 3). An overview of these normal balancing controls is given in Figure 21-1.

Sources of Blood Glucose

To ensure a constant supply of the body's primary fuel, there are two sources of blood glucose: (1) *diet*—the energy nutrients in our food, dietary carbohydrate, protein, and fat; and (2) **glycogen**—the backup source from constant turnover of "stored" liver glycogen by a process called **glycogenolysis.**

Uses of Blood Glucose

To prevent a continued rise of blood glucose above normal limits, there are several basic uses for blood glucose that are constantly available according to need. These include: (1) **glycogenesis**—conversion of glucose to glycogen for "storage" in liver and muscle; (2) **lipogenesis**— conversion of glucose to fat and storage in adipose tissue; (3) **glycolysis**—cell oxidation of glucose for energy.

Pancreatic Hormonal Controls

Three types of islet cells scattered in clusters throughout the pancreas (islets of Langerhans) provide hormones closely interbalanced in regulating blood glucose levels. This specific arrangement of human islet cells is illustrated in Figure 21-2.

    1. **B cells.** The largest portion of the islets is occupied by B cells filling the central zone or about 60% of the gland. These primary cells synthesize *insulin.*

Glycogen
A long, branched chain of glucose units that serves as the storage form of glucose in animals.

Glycogenolysis
Breakdown of stored glycogen to yield glucose.

Glycogenesis
Formation of *glycogen,* the storage form of carbohydrates in animals.

Lipogenesis
Conversion of carbohydrates and protein into body fat.

Glycolysis
Breakdown of glucose to pyruvate and lactate by enzymes.

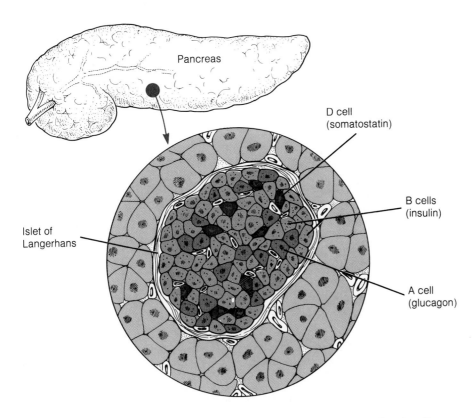

Pancreas

D cell
(somatostatin)

B cells
(insulin)

Islet of
Langerhans

A cell
(glucagon)

Figure 21-2
Islets of Langerhans, located in
the pancreas.

2. **A cells.** Arranged around the outer rim of the islets are the A cells, one to two cells thick, making up about 30% of the total cells. These cells synthesize *glucagon.*

3. **D cells.** Interspersed between the A and B cells, or occasionally between A cells alone, are the D cells, the remaining 10% of the total cells. These cells synthesize *somatostatin.*

Interrelated Hormone Functions

Juncture points of the three types of islet cells act as sensors of the blood glucose concentration and its rate of change. They constantly adjust and balance the rate of secretion of insulin, glucagon, and somatostatin to match whatever conditions prevail at any time. Each one of the three hormones has specific interbalanced functions.

1. **Insulin.** Although all the precise mechanisms are not entirely clear, **insulin** has a profound effect on glucose control. It functions extensively in the metabolism of all three of the energy nutrients:

- Facilitates transport of glucose through cell membranes by way of special insulin receptors. New knowledge of these special receptors shows that they mediate all the metabolic effects of insulin.[5] Weight loss in obese individuals and physical exercise increase the number of these receptors.
- Aids in conversion of glucose to glycogen with its consequent storage in the liver.
- Stimulates conversion of glucose to fat for storage as adipose tissue.
- Inhibits fat breakdown and the breakdown of protein.
- Promotes the uptake of amino acids by skeletal muscles thus increasing protein synthesis.

Insulin
Hormone formed in the beta cells of the pancreas. It is secreted when blood glucose and amino acid levels rise and assists their entry into the cells.

- Influences glucose oxidation through the main glycolytic pathway

2. **Glucagon.** The hormone **glucagon** functions as a balancing antagonist to insulin. It rapidly breaks down liver glycogen, and to a lesser extent fatty acids from adipose tissue, to serve as body fuel. This action raises blood glucose levels to protect the brain and other body tissues. It helps maintain normal blood glucose levels during fasting hours of sleep. A lowering of the blood glucose concentration, increased amino acid concentrations, or sympathetic nervous system stimulation triggers glucagon secretion.

3. Somatostatin. Although the pancreatic islet D cells are the major source of **somatostatin,** this hormone is also synthesized and secreted in different regions of the body, including the hypothalamus. It acts in balance with insulin and glucose to inhibit their interactions as needed to maintain normal blood glucose levels. It also helps regulate blood glucose levels by inhibiting the release of a number of other hormones as needed.

Metabolic Changes in Diabetes

In uncontrolled diabetes, insulin is lacking to facilitate the operation of normal blood glucose controls. Abnormal metabolic changes occur that affect glucose, fat, and protein and account for symptoms.

Glucose. The blood glucose cannot be oxidized properly through the main glycolytic pathway in the cell to furnish energy. Therefore it builds up in the blood.

Fat. The formation of fat is curtailed, and fat breakdown increases. This leads to excess formation and accumulation of ketones, bringing ketoacidosis. The appearance of one of these ketones, **acetone,** in the urine indicates the development of ketoacidosis.

Protein. Tissue protein is also broken down in an effort to secure energy. This causes weight loss and nitrogen excretion in the urine.

General Management of Diabetes

Diagnosis
Glucose-Tolerance Testing

The guiding principles for treating diabetes are early detection and prevention of complications. The former traditional glucose tolerance test is no longer used in regular practice. Instead, in the current procedure, a 75 g dose of glucose is used and two blood tests are taken: fasting and a 2-hour plasma glucose. A 2-hour plasma glucose value of 200 mg/dL (11.0 mmol/L) or above indicates diabetes, and 140 mg/dL (7.8 mmol/L) is the upper level of normal. Those values falling between 140 and 200 mg/dL are labeled *impaired glucose tolerance.* Clinical experience indicates that persons in this latter group tend to progress toward diabetes at a rate about four times that of normal persons. Thus those diagnosed as diabetic and those with impaired glucose tolerance should have follow-up diet therapy and monitoring for glucose management.

Glycosylated Hemoglobin A_1c

This is an additional test used in diabetes screening and monitoring. Glycohemoglobins are relatively stable molecules within the red blood cell. During the life of the cell, about 120 days, glucose molecules attach themselves to the hemoglobin. This irreversible glycosylation of hemoglobin depends on the concentration of blood glucose. The higher the level of circulating glucose over the life of the red blood cells, the higher the concentration of glycohemoglobin. Thus the measurement of hemoglobin A_1c relates to the level of blood glucose over a longer period of time. It provides an effective tool for evaluating long-term management of diabetes and degree of control.

Treatment Goals

Basic Objectives

The health team is guided by three basic objectives in the care of a person with diabetes:

1. **Maintenance of optimal nutrition.** The first objective is to fulfill the basic nutritional requirement for health, growth and development, and a lean body weight.

2. **Avoidance of symptoms.** This objective is designed to keep the person relatively free of symptoms, such as hyperglycemia and glycosuria.

3. **Prevention of complications.** The third objective recognizes the increased risk a person with diabetes faces for developing problems in tissues such as eyes **(retinopathy),** nerve tissues **(neuropathy),** and renal tissues **(nephropathy).** In addition, coronary artery disease occurs in persons with diabetes about four times as often as in the general population. Peripheral vascular disease occurs about 40 times as often.

In all of these areas there is evidence that consistent well-planned food habits and exercise, balanced as needed with early aggressive insulin therapy, through multiple daily injections or continuous subcutaneous infusion by pump, and constantly guided by self-monitoring of blood glucose levels, can significantly reduce risks of these potentially serious complications.[6,7] Current nutritional recommendations of the American Diabetes Association recognize the added risk of vascular disease for persons with diabetes and include revised lipid-lowering diet guidelines.[8]

Self-Care Role of the Person with Diabetes

To control diabetes effectively, the person with diabetes must of necessity have a central position. Daily self-discipline and informed self-care, supported by a skilled and sensitive health care team, are required for sound diabetes management. Ultimately, in the final analysis all persons with diabetes must treat themselves. This is especially true with the tighter normal blood sugar control currently being used with frequent self-monitoring of blood glucose and multiple insulin injections. Thus there is even greater need now for comprehensive diabetes education programs that encourage self-monitoring and self-care responsibility.

The Core Problem

The core problem in diabetes is energy balance, the regulation of the body's primary fuel, blood glucose. Based on this concept of balance, three main principles of nutritional therapy emerge: (1) total energy balance, (2) nutrient balance, and (3) food distribution balance. The fundamental underlying principle may be stated simply: *The diet for any person with diabetes is always based on the normal nutritional needs of that individual.* The personal diet, then, is expressed in terms of: (1) total requirement of kilocalories for en-

Retinopathy
Noninflammatory disease of the retina. In diabetes, it is characterized by small hemorrhages from broken arteries; yellow, waxy discharge; and retinal detachment.

Neuropathy
Two kinds: (1) presence of disease and/or change in function of the peripheral nervous system, (2) noninflammatory injury to the peripheral nervous system; a complication of diabetes.

Nephropathy
Disease of the nephrons in the kidneys; a complication of diabetes.

Principles of Nutritional Therapy: The Balance Concept

ergy needs; (2) a balanced ratio of these kilocalories in grams of carbohydrate, protein, and fat; and (3) a general food distribution pattern for the day.

Total Energy Balance
Weight Management

Since insulin-dependent diabetes mellitus (IDDM) usually begins during childhood (average age is 11), the weight-height measure for children is an index to adequate growth. In their adult years, maintaining a lean weight is a continuing goal (see Chapter 15). Since noninsulin-dependent diabetes mellitus (NIDDM) usually occurs in overweight adults, the major goal is losing excess weight with a sound diet and maintaing a healthy body weight.

Kilocalories

The energy value of a diabetic diet should be expressed in terms of kilocalories sufficient to meet individual needs for normal growth and development, physical activity, and maintenance of a desirable lean weight.

Nutrient Balance

The ratio of carbohydrate, protein, and fat in the diet is based on current recommendations for ideal glucose regulation and lipid-lowering modifications to reduce risks of cardiovascular complications (Table 21-1).

Carbohydrate

A more liberal use of carbohydrates, mainly in complex forms, is needed for smoother blood sugar control. About 50% to 55% of the total kilocalories of the diet is assigned to carbohydrates. Several characteristics of carbohydrate foods need to be examined:

1. **Complex carbohydrates.** The majority of the carbohydrate kilocalories, about 40% to 50% of the total diet kilocalories, should be used as complex carbohydrates—starches. In most cases these complex carbohydrates break down more slowly than simple sugars and release their available glucose over time.

Table 21-1

Distribution of Major Nutrients in Normal and Diabetic Diets (as percentages of total calories)

	Starch and other Polysaccharides* (%)	Sugars† and Dextrins (%)	Fat (%)	Protein (%)	Alcohol (%)
Typical American diet	25-35	20-30	35-45 ⅔ unsaturated	12-19	0-10
Traditional diabetic diets	25-30	10-15‡	40-45	16-21	0
Newer diabetic diets: current therapy	30-45	5-15‡	25-35 less than ½ saturated	12-24	0-6

*A substantial majority of these calories are starch, but complex carbohydrates also include cellulose, hemicellulose, pentosans, and pectin.
†Monosaccharides and disaccharides, mainly sucrose, but also included are fructose, glucose, lactose, and maltose.
‡Almost exclusively natural sugars, mainly in fruit and milk (lactose).

Clinical Application

Meals based on the diabetic exchange lists may some day have to incorporate into food choice instructions a new dimension—special effects of certain foods on blood sugar levels apart from their individual carbohydrate content. But is this reasonable? And is this day soon?

Some thought-provoking research indicates that the rise in blood sugar may be related not only to the type of carbohydrate (i.e., simple or complex) or to the total amount of carbohydrate each food contains, but also to additional factors that are as yet unknown. A *glycemic index* developed through this research indicates that foods within the same food exchange group, especially the bread exchange group, may vary dramatically in their effect on the level of glucose in the blood.

Before the exchange system is drastically revised to accommodate the glycemic index, clinicians must remember that this index applies to single foods tested under laboratory conditions—not to the mixed diet that the average person consumes. They must also consider other nutrients that affect health problems for which persons with diabetes are at risk. For example, according to the index, ice cream raises blood sugar levels by only 30% to 39%, as compared to carrots, which result in a large 80% to 90% rise. However, two factors are significant in the case of diabetes: (1) accompanying increases in fat and cholesterol may increase the risk for atherosclerosis and (2) reduction in fiber may also hinder diabetes control. In Western society, when the average intake of 7 g of fiber per 1000 kcal is raised to 25 to 30 g/1000 kcal, even persons with IDDM may be able to control blood sugar levels with lower insulin dosages.

In planning a diet with each client, the nutritionist must always take into account the entire nutritional value of the plan, the factors that affect conditions to which the person is susceptible, the total caloric value of the plan, and the person's acceptance of the foods discussed. Perhaps a method of diabetic meal-planning that incorporates these factors with the glycemic index will be developed in the future. But current research shows results that conflict with the initial studies, which seem now to have raised more questions than they answered.

Thus for now, the answer to our own question here is, "No, not now." Our knowledge at this point is just too limited to have practical application. And as is often the case, it is a long way from the isolated test setting of the laboratory to the multiple food mix of the dinner table.

But still, it's a fascinating thought.

Should Glycemic Index Be Incorporated into the Exchange System of Diabetic Meal-Planning?

REFERENCES

Coulston AM, and Hollenbeck CB: Source and amount of dietary carbohydrate in patients with noninsulin-dependent diabetes mellitus, Top Clin Nutr 3(1):17, Jan 1988.

Crapo PA, and Olefsky JM: Food fallacies and blood sugar, N Engl J Med 309:44, July 1983.

2. **Glycemic index.** Modification of carbohydrate food to take into account the glycemic index of single foods and food combinations, at least in the light of our current knowledge, provides little clinical assistance in designing meals for persons with diabetes (see box, p. 513).[9] Research in this area is in its early stages and answers to questions of its practical use are incomplete at present. But with more knowledge these considerations may influence groupings and selections of foods in the future.

3. **Dietary fiber.** The degree to which dietary fiber is present in complex carbohydrates such as grains, legumes, vegetables, fruits, and other starches will influence the rate of absorption of the food mix components and alter their effect on the blood glucose level (see box, below). An increased dietary fiber content, especially of soluble dietary fiber forms such as those found in oats, barley, legumes, and fruits, appears to have beneficial effects, particularly in lowering plasma lipids. But there is some controversy about the degree of effect of fiber on blood glucose levels.[9] About 40 g/day of dietary fiber or 25 g/1000 kcal is a reasonable goal.

To Probe Further

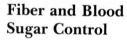
Fiber and Blood Sugar Control

Dietary fiber contributes to diabetes control. Patients using dietary fiber in the form of supplements of high-fiber food, especially soluble fiber such as gums in oats and lentils, have exhibited reductions in fasting blood sugar levels and glycosuria and improved sensitivity to insulin. Precisely how fiber affects the metabolism of glucose is unknown, but several mechanisms have been postulated. Persons with actual NIDDM, but treated with insulin or oral hypoglycemic agents in their obese state, have been able to discontinue or dramatically reduce their dosages on a high-fiber diet. Even persons with IDDM have controlled blood sugar levels with reduced insulin dosages while following a high-fiber diet.

In Western society, the average intake of 7 g of fiber per 1000 kcal can be increased to 25 to 30 g/1000 kcal for better diabetes control by incorporating more dried beans and peas, as well as vegetables, whole grains, and fruits, in the diet. Although this type of diet has many health benefits, it should be introduced with care for the following reasons:

- Insulin-dependent persons on high-fiber diets have experienced hypoglycemic reactions more frequently than those receiving regular meals.
- Palatability sometimes is a problem. However, this objection may be overcome with the use of appropriate food products and methods of preparation.
- Flatulence may be an embarrassing side effect. This problem can be minimized by adding fiber to the diet gradually and following the correct cooking procedures with legumes.

REFERENCES

Anderson JW, et al: Dietary fiber and diabetes: a comprehensive review and practical application, J Am Diet Assoc 87(9):1189, Sept 1987.

Burgess BE: Rationale for changes in the dietary management of diabetes, J Am Diet Assoc 81:258, 1982.

4. **Simple carbohydrates.** The small remainder of the carbohydrate kilocalories, about 5% to 15% of the total diet kilocalories, can be used as simple carbohydrates. In general, simple carbohydrates (single or double sugars found in fruits and milk, as well as sucrose-sweetened food items) should be controlled, placing greater emphasis on the complex forms. Research has indicated that small amounts of sucrose or fructose in special food items is not necessarily detrimental, but they need to be carefully controlled. Honey is a form of sugar (mainly fructose) and is *not* a sugar substitute, as some persons may believe.

5. **Sugar substitute sweeteners.** A variety of sugar substitutes are available. The most common *nonnutritive* sweetener is saccharin. Aspartame is a recently marketed *nutritive* sweetener made from two amino acids, phenylalanine and aspartic acid, and is metabolized as such. Caloric sweeteners such as fructose and sorbitol must be accounted for in the meal. A summary of dietary sweeteners is given in Table 21-2.

Protein

Normal age requirements for protein govern the amount indicated for persons with diabetes. About 15% to 20% of the total kilocalories are assigned to

Table 21-2

A Summary of Dietary Sweeteners

Sweetener	Commercial use	Comparative sweetness*	Effectiveness in carbohydrate metabolism and diabetes control	Problems
Nutritive sweeteners (provide 4 kcal/g)				
Aspartame Combination of two amino acids: aspartic acid and a methyl ester of phenylalanine	Soft drinks Chewing gum Powdered beverages Whipped toppings Puddings Gelatin Tabletop sweetener	180-200	Does not contribute significant amount of kilocalories or carbohydrates	Possibly tumerogenic† Possible source of excess phenylalanine for PKU children
Fructose Naturally occurring monosaccharide found in honey, fruits, and high-fructose corn syrup	Baked products Frosting mixes Tabletop sweetener Home food preparation	1.4 Enhanced by Use in liquids Low temperature Acidity Dilution	Absorbed more slowly than sucrose Does not require insulin for entry into cells Achieves similar level of sweetness with smaller amounts	Caloric, carbohydrate values must be considered in calculating diets and recipes Intake of more than 75 g/day increases risk of hyperglycemia

*The sweetness of sucrose is assigned the value of 1.0.
†A breakdown product of aspartame, diketopiperazine, is considered tumerogenic by some researchers.
‡Sorbitol is metabolized to fructose, then glucose.
§FDA plan to ban saccharin in 1977 failed because of saccharin's popularity.

Continued.

Table 21-2

A Summary of Dietary Sweeteners—cont'd

Sweetener	Commercial use	Comparative sweetness*	Effectiveness in carbohydrate metabolism and diabetes control	Problems
			Contributes moderate amounts of calories and carbohydrates to prevent hypoglycemia	
			Should not be used by poorly controlled, obese diabetics	
Sorbitol Sugar alcohol naturally occurring in fruits and vegetables	Baked products Sugar-free gum	0.67	Not generally recommended for diabetes control because Large amounts are needed to sweeten foods Lack of insulin results in increased conversion to glucose‡	Doses of more than 50-60 g/day result in diarrhea
Xylitol "Wood sugar" found in staw, fruits, corncobs	Banned for commercial use in the United States in 1982	1.22		Tumerogenic
L-Glucose, L-fructose: (Mirror images [isomers] of D-glucose and D-fructose)	Currently under study for possible commercial use	Same as D-glucose (0.72) and D-fructose (1.4)	Contributes no calories or carbohydrates because isomeric configuration prevents absorption	
Nonnutritive sweeteners (noncaloric)				
Saccharin	Baked products Soft drinks Tabletop sweetener	300-600	Contributes no calories or carbohydrates to the diet	Bladder cancer in test animals§
Cyclamate	Banned for commercial use in the United States in 1970			Bladder cancer in test animals

protein to meet growth and development needs in children and to maintain tissue integrity. Lean food forms are used to help control fat.

Fat

Fat should always be used in moderation with greater attention given to the control of saturated fats and cholesterol. Total fat intake is lowered to 30% or less of the day's total kilocalories, and cholesterol is limited to 300 mg/day.

These revised nutrient recommendations are summarized in Table 21-3.

Food Distribution Balance
General Rule

In general, fairly even amounts of food should be eaten throughout the day, adjusted to blood glucose self-monitoring. This will avoid excessive intakes at some points and longer fasting periods between, eliminating the "peaks and valleys" in food intake and consequent blood sugar swings. This means that a basic pattern is a regular schedule of meals at fairly consistent times through the day, with interval snacks as needed.

Daily Activity Pattern

Food distribution needs to be planned ahead and adjusted according to each day's scheduled activities. Practical consideration needs to be given to work, school, social events, and stress periods.

Exercise

For persons with insulin-dependent diabetes mellitus (IDDM), it is especially important that any exercise period or additional physical activity be accommodated in the food distribution plan. For obese adults with diabetes, regular exercise is an essential part of a successful weight management program.

Drug Therapy

The food pattern will also be influenced by any form of drug therapy required for control. As indicated, the current management goal for persons with IDDM is to maintain a normal blood glucose level as much as possible, because there is strong evidence that such tight control prevents the chronic complications of long-term uncontrolled hyperglycemia.[6] To achieve this

Table 21-3
Comparison of AHA and ADA Diet Recommendations*

	AHA Step 1 (% total kcal)	AHA Step 2 (% total kcal)	ADA/ADA (% total kcal)
Total fat	30	30	30
Monounsaturated	10-15	10-15	12-14
Saturated	10	7	10
Polyunsaturated	Up to 10	Up to 10	6-8
Carbohydrate	50-60	50-60	55-60
Protein	15-20	15-20	0.8 g/kg
Cholesterol	300 mg/day	200 mg/day	300 mg/day

*AHA, American Heart Association; ADA, American Diabetes Association and American Dietetic Association.

goal, more aggressive insulin therapy with different types of insulins now available is being used. Oral agents may be used also.

Types of Insulin

A number of insulin preparations are available for therapeutic use. According to time of action, they are rapid, intermediate, and long acting, although individual responses are highly variable.

1. **Rapid-acting insulins.** These insulins have various names, depending on the manufacturer: Actrapid, Regular, Semilente, Semitard, and Velosulin. Effect on blood glucose can be detected in about an hour, peaks at 4 to 6 hours, and lasts about 12 to 16 hours.

2. **Intermediate-acting insulins.** These insulins include Insulatard, Isophane NPH, and Protophane. Effect is detected in about 2 hours, peaks at about 11 hours, and lasts about 20 to 29 hours.

3. **Long-acting insulins.** These insulins include PZI, Ultralente, and Ultratard. Their duration is somewhat longer than the intermediate-acting insulins. They are seldom used, except for special needs, because their slow onset and extended action is more difficult to predict or control. Also, the tighter control being used today requires shorter-acting insulins with multiple injections according to self-monitoring of blood glucose levels, to meet variations in need during the day. This is especially true of the more labile or **"brittle"** forms of IDDM.

Sources of Insulin

According to commercial source, insulins may be produced from beef and pork pancreases, which had been the main U.S. source until recently. But these animal-derived insulins are immunogenic to humans, beef more so than pork, and in time they induce antiinsulin antibodies that delay or blunt their action. Now, however, human insulin is available from two sources: (1) biosynthesis by recombinant DNA technology through rapidly reproducing bacteria that have been given the human gene; and (2) chemical substitution of the terminal amino acid on the beta-chain of pork insulin. Because they carry the human insulin structure, these newer insulins are almost nonimmunogenic.

Insulin and Exercise

Exercise benefits all persons with diabetes through its action in increasing the number of insulin receptors on muscle cells, thus increasing insulin efficiency.[10] However, physical activity must be regular to be effective. A detailed history of personal activity and exercise habits provides the information needed to help a client plan a wise program of regular moderate exercise.[11] Guidelines for extra food to cover periods of heavier exercise, or athletic practice and competition, can be included. In general, exercise programs make persons feel better both physically and psychologically. Also, blood glucose self-monitoring is a simple procedure that can be a helpful means of determining the balance needed at any point in time between exercise, insulin, and food.

Oral Hypoglycemic Agents

For some persons with noninsulin-dependent diabetes mellitus (NIDDM), an oral hypoglycemic drug may be used. These drugs act to lower the elevated

"Brittle" diabetes
Form of Type I diabetes, difficult to control; sensitive to hypoglycemia and to acidosis.

blood glucose by stimulating the pancreas to produce more endogenous insulin. They belong to a group of sulfonylurea compounds and include agents such as tolbutamide and glipizide. Since their action induces increased insulin activity, their use must be balanced with food and exercise just as insulin injections would be.

Diet Management

Many of the basic diet therapy principles carry over for both types of diabetes. The nutrient ratios are approximately the same (see Table 21-1). But energy balance needs will vary widely depending on individual needs, such as growth requirements for children or weight reduction for overweight adults. A summary of the comparative diet planning needs for both types of diabetes in provided in Table 21-4.

Individual Needs

A comprehensive nutrition assessment and history will provide the necessary information to develop a personal food plan (see Chapters 10 and 17). A wide range of areas should be included, such as personal and family needs, living situation, social activities, work and school commitments, and food and exercise habits. Also, a full medical history will review the course of the person's diabetes and personal experiences with it. Then, based on this assessment of status and needs, the clinical nutritionist determines the appropriate diet prescription for the individual and calculates the nutritional needs according to the balance concept of nutritional therapy described.

Table 21-4
Dietary Strategies for the Two Main Types of Diabetes Mellitus

Dietary strategy	Type I (nonobese)	Type II (usually obese)
Decrease energy intake (kilocalories)	No	Yes
Increase frequency and number of feedings	Yes	Usually no
Have regular daily intake of kilocalories of carbohydrate, protein, and fat	Very important	Not important if average caloric intake remains in low range
Plan consistent daily ratio of protein, carbohydrate, and fat for each feeding	Desirable	Not necessary
Use extra or planned-ahead food to treat or prevent hypoglycemia	Very important	Not necessary
Plan regular times for meals/snacks	Very important	Not important
Use extra food for unusual exercise	Yes	Usually not necessary
During illness, use small, frequent feedings of carbohydrate to prevent starvation ketosis	Important	Usually not necessary because of resistance to ketosis

Diet Planning with Food Exchanges
Personal Diet Planning

Personal adaptations and approaches are important in planning nutritional therapy for any patient. But this basic principle is especially important for the person with diabetes who must eventually carry the responsibility for long-term self-care. There are numerous planning approaches used by skilled and sensitive clinical nutritionists who tailor their actions to the person's learning needs and abilities, nutritional needs, personal needs, and lifestyle. Members of the diabetes care and education practice group of the American Dietetic Association, for example, have published a helpful monograph in which they discuss no less than 11 meal planning approaches according to individual needs, such as degree of literacy, structure, complexity, and area of emphasis on weight loss and glucose control.[12] However, since the Food Exchange System is the most widely used method of meal planning, it is the approach discussed here.

The Food Exchange System

This system of diet planning is based on the concept of food equivalents and their exchange to maintain both diet control and food choice variety. It was developed jointly by the American Dietetic Association and the American Diabetes Association and has been used successfully for a number of years with periodic revisions. It is designed for use by a professional diet counselor, usually a registered dietitian (RD) with extensive clinical experience, who can adapt it to meet many needs. With such personalized initial instruction and continued counseling, the person with diabetes will find the well-written and colorfully illustrated booklet, *Exchange Lists for Meal Planning,* a helpful guide and tool for planning meals and snacks.[13] It can be a sound means of dietary regulation that is flexible enough to meet a wide variety of situations. Six food groups are used: starch/bread, meat, vegetable, fruit, milk, and fat. The revised food lists incorporate the low saturated fat modification in subgroups and highlight fiber and sodium content of foods. These revised food lists are provided in Appendix H for reference. A general description of nutrient composition and characteristics is given in Table 21-5. In using the food groups as a guide, food items in any one group may be freely exchanged within that group, since all foods in a particular group have approximately the same food value. These food groups form the basis for calculating diet needs (Table 21-6) and for helping clients learn to make wide food selections and substitutions.

Personal Meal/Snack Plan

On the basis of the individual's calculated diet prescription and food pattern, the nutritionist and the client work out a personal food plan. The client learns how to plan a menu by using the meal/snack food distribution pattern. A variety of foods from the food lists are chosen in the amounts indicated to meet the overall food plan. A sample menu based on the 2200-kcal diet as calculated in Table 21-5 is given here (see box, p. 522).

Special Concerns

In the course of daily living, a number of special concerns arise and become part of on-going diet counseling.

Table 21-5

Food Exchange Groups

Food group	Unit of exchange	Composition Carbohydrate (g)	Protein (g)	Fat (g)	Calories	Characteristic Items
Starch/bread	Varies; 1 slice bread	15	3	—	80	Variety of starch items, breads, cereals, vegetables; portions equal in carbohydrate value to 1 slice bread
Meat	28 g (1 oz)	—				Protein foods; exchange units equal to protein value of 28 g lean meal (cheese, egg, seafood)
Lean		—	7	3	55	
Medium fat		—	7	5	75	
Higher fat		—	7	8	100	
Vegetables	½ cup	5	2	—	25	Medium carbohydrate
Fruit	Varies	15	—	—	60	Portion size varies with carbohydrate value of item; all portions equaled at 10% carbohydrate
Milk	1 cup					
Skim		12	8	—	90	Equivalents to 1 cup whole milk listed; 1 cup skin + 2 fat exchanges = whole milk
Low fat		12	8	5	120	
Whole		12	8	8	150	
Fat	1 tsp					Fat food items equal to 1 tsp margarine (oil, mayonnaise, olives, avocados)
Polyunsaturated		—	—	5	45	
Monunsaturated		—	—	5	45	
Saturated		—	—	5	45	

Table 21-6

Calculation of Diabetic Diet: Short Method Using Exchange System (2200 kcal)

Food group	Total day's exchanges	Carbohydrate: 275 g (50% kcal)	Protein: 110 g (20% kcal)	Fat: 75 g (30% kcal)	Breakfast	Lunch	Dinner	Snacks PM	HS
Milk (low fat)	2	24	16	10	1				1
Vegetable	3	15	6			1	2		
Fruit	3	45 / 84			1	1	1		
Bread	13	195 / 279	39 / 61		3	3	3	2	2
Meat	7		49 / 110	35 / 45	1	2	3	1	
Fat (polyunsaturated)	6			30 / 75	1	1	2	1	1

Sample Menu Prescription:

2200 kcal—275 g carbohydrate
(50% kcal) + 110 g protein
(20% kcal) + 75 g fat (30% kcal)

Breakfast
1 medium, sliced fresh peach
Shredded Wheat cereal
1 poached egg on whole-grain toast
1 bran muffin
1 tsp margarine
1 cup low-fat milk
Coffee or tea

Lunch
Vegetable soup with wheat crackers
Tuna sandwich on whole-wheat bread
  Filling: Tuna (drained ½ cup)
          Mayonnaise (2 tsp)
          Chopped dill pickle
          Chopped celery
Fresh pear

Afternoon Snack
12 crackers with 2 tbsp peanut butter
Orange

Dinner
Pan-broiled pork chop (trimmed well)
1 cup brown rice
½-1 cup green beans
Tossed green salad
  Italian dressing (1-2 tbsp)
½ cup applesauce
1 bran muffin

Evening snack
6 cups popped, plain popcorn
1 cup low-fat milk

1. **Special diet items.** The diet of the person with diabetes is planned using regular foods. No special "dietetic" or "diabetic" food products are necessary. However, as with any consumer, label reading on processed foods is important to make wise selections.

2. **Alcohol.** Occasional use of small amounts of alcohol in the diet for persons with diabetes can be planned, but caution must be used (see Issues and Answers, p. 528). Not only must the amount, timing, frequency, and kind of drink be considered, but also the nature of the diabetes and any medications of any kind being used.

3. **Physical activity.** For any unusual physical activity, moderate or strenuous, the person with insulin-dependent diabetes mellitus (IDDM) needs to plan ahead for added food allowances to balance the exercise (see box, on facing page). This is particularly true for the young person with "brittle" diabetes engaging in strenuous athletic practice or competition. You can review the energy demands of exercise in Chapter 14.

4. **Illness.** When general illness occurs, food and insulin need to be adjusted (see box, p. 524). As needed, the texture of the food can be modified to incorporate easily digested and absorbed liquid foods with similar glucose equivalents of the usual food plan. This same procedure may be followed for

glucose equivalent replacement of meals not eaten, as shown in the box below.

5. **Travel.** When a trip is planned, the diet counselor and the client should confer to guide food choices according to what will be available. Both self-monitoring of blood glucose and insulin therapy equipment, as well as food plans, are as important on vacation or business trips as they are at home.[14] The traveler always needs to plan ahead with members of the health care team (see box, p. 525).

6. **Eating out.** Similar guidelines and suggestions can be provided for various situations when the person with diabetes eats away from home. As a general rule, the plan should be made ahead of time so that accommodations for what is eaten at home before and after the outside meal can balance with needs for the day. Practice with restaurant menus is a helpful teaching tool.

7. **Stress.** Any form of physiologic or psychosocial stress affects blood glucose levels and will be reflected in varying changes in diabetes control. These variations are caused by hormonal stress responses antagonistic to insulin. Persons with diabetes can learn useful stress-reduction and relaxation exercises and activities to help handle stress in their lives (see Chapter 16).

Goal: Person-Centered Self-Care
Changing Roles

The respective roles of patient or client and their professional therapists are changing in modern health care. In past years a traditional medical model has guided diabetes education in its methods, language, and assumed roles. The professionals viewed themselves as having major authoritative roles and assigned the passive role of "patient" to the person with diabetes. With nota-

Diabetes Education Program

Meal-Planning Guide for Active People with Type I Diabetes Mellitus

Exchange needs for	Sample menus
Moderate activity	
30 minutes	
1 bread OR	1 bran muffin OR
1 fruit	1 small orange
1 hour	
2 bread + 1 meat OR	Tuna sandwich OR
2 fruit + 1 milk	1 cup fruit salad + 1 cup milk
Strenuous activity	
30 minutes	
2 fruit OR	1 small banana OR
1 bread + 1 fat	½ bagel + 1 tsp cream cheese
1 hour	
2 bread + 1 meat +	Meat and cheese sandwich +
1 milk OR	1 cup milk OR
2 bread + 2 meat +	Hamburger +
2 fruit	1 cup orange juice

How to Modify a Diabetic Meal Plan for Sick Days

Usual food intake	Exchange	Carbohydrate (g)
½ chicken breast, roasted	3 meat	0
1 tsp margarine	1 fat	0
½ cup rice	1 bread	15
Tossed green salad, lemon wedge	Free food	0
1¼ cup strawberries	1 fruit	15
1 cup skim milk	1 milk	12
		TOTAL 42

Sick day intake*	Exchange	Carbohydrate (g)
2 cups broth	Free food	0
½ cup gelatin dessert (e.g., Jell-O)	1 fruit	15
1 cup ginger ale (regular)	2 fruit	30
2 cups herbal tea	Free food	0
		TOTAL 45

*OBJECTIVE: to provide required amounts of carbohydrate for times when the person with diabetes just doesn't feel like eating much.

ble exceptions, this model has been followed in most cases. However, because of an increasing movement toward changing roles of practitioners and consumers in the health care system (see Chapter 1), persons with diabetes are assuming a more active voice in planning and conducting their own care. Barriers in our traditional system stem from three sources: (1) our culture, (2) our health care delivery system, and (3) our professional training and habits.

Communication Needs

Essentially, much of the core problem centers on communication. For example, here is a list of words we too often use that are objectional to persons with diabetes, along with suggestions for preferred language we might use instead:

1. **"Diabetic" used as a noun.** The word "diabetic" is an adjective and should not be used alone as an impersonal noun. Use instead the phrase "person with diabetes."

2. **Compliance.** The word "compliance" raises red flags in the minds of persons with diabetes. It is purely a medical term and connotes an authoritative physician position. Instead use the word "adherence." This word has been adopted by national committees and associations working in the field of diabetes. The word "adherence" indicates that the decision-making responsibility rests with the person who has diabetes to determine courses of action in varying life situations—which is the actual fact.

3. **Patient.** In general use, the phrase "person with diabetes" is the correct reference. Persons with diabetes are patients *only* when they are in the hospital or are seeing a physician for an illness, just like anybody else.

Clinical Application

Routine meal-planning tips are all well and good. But what do you do when your "real-life" client with diabetes wants to travel or catches a cold? In both cases, the client will have too many distractions to concentrate fully on planning the most ideal menu. The fact remains, however, that in both travel and illness, diabetes management relies heavily on the food plan and, in the case of Type I diabetes, on meal/snack flexibility to meet changing demands.

Travel

Promote confidence about meal-planning skills. Review the number and type of exchanges allowed at each meal; encourage the client to practice measuring portion sizes; review tips on eating out.

Learn about the foods that will be available. For a cruise, have the client get a copy of the menu in advance. For air travel, order diabetic meals in advance. If foreign travel is involved, have the client ask the travel agent for information about foods commonly served to tourists.

Select appropriate snacks. Remind the client to meet extra carbohydrate and caloric needs during extra physical activities, such as hiking, swimming, skiing, mountain climbing.

Plan for time. Have the client avoid extended driving time and plan to include 20 g of carbohydrate for every 2 hours of travel. For emergencies and unexpected delays, the client should plan to have on hand food for two meals and two snacks, including nonperishable items and liquids.

Plan for time zone changes. The schedule may need to be changed. If so, discuss any needed meal revisions with the client for balancing the insulin-activity pattern.

Prepare companions. Companions must recognize signs and symptoms of hypoglycemia and know its treatment. Remind the client to carry quick-acting carbohydrates at all times. To support the medical regimen of insulin-dependent clients, remind them to: (1) carry an ID bracelet, pendant, or card at all times, (2) ask their physicians for a letter explaining the need for syringes, and (3) take a prescription for insulin and learn brand names used for insulin in the country to which they are traveling.

Sick-day survival

Nausea and diarrhea. Remind the client that fluid and electrolyte replacement is crucial. To replace *sodium*, the client should use salted crackers, broth or soups, as tolerated. To replace *potassium*, Coca Cola (small amounts of high-sugar foods can be tolerated as replacement for short periods of time, as during illness), tea, broth, or orange juice can be used. To replace *liquids*, the client should drink *something* at least every 2 to 3 hours.

Gastrointestinal disturbances. Insulin dosage may need to be decreased. The client should try a *clear liquid diet,* including fruit juices, fruit ices, and soups for adequate amounts of carbohydrate. *Protein supplementation* through elemental nutrition may be necessary if symptoms last longer than 72 hours. As food tolerance improves, progress to a *soft diet* that includes milk drinks, custards, and eggs. *Continued.*

Clinical Application

Colds and fever. These conditions are often treated with aspirin, which tends to lower sugar level. Remind the client of two major guidelines:

- **Do not skip meals.** If necessary, subdivide regular meals into small, frequent snacks.
- **Do not omit insulin.** If totally unable to eat, contact the physician for advice regarding insulin dosage.

In summary, the person with diabetes who is ill should (1) maintain intake of food every day, (2) replace carbohydrate solid foods with equal liquid or soft foods, (3) monitor blood frequently for sugar, and (4) contact a physician if the illness lasts more than a day or so.

---

4. **Cheating.** A particularly abusive word to many persons with diabetes, especially to parents of children and young people with diabetes, is the word "cheating." This flagrant language abuse suggests dishonesty or failure to live up to an external code. By and large, persons with diabetes do not "cheat." They may kid themselves or they may be inaccurate in their reporting, but they do not cheat. Use instead phrases such as "having difficulty" or "having a problem with."

Content: Tools for Self-Care
Necessary Skills

In recognition of the need for building self-sufficiency and responsibility with persons with diabetes and their families, a joint committee of the American Association of Diabetes Educators and the American Diabetes Association has developed an outline of learning needs.[15,16] These learning needs build on necessary skills and content areas required for good self-care:

1. Fulfillment of basic needs in relation to diabetes
2. Having a sound nutrition and meal plan
3. Understanding insulin (or oral agent) effects and how to manage them
4. Monitoring of both blood glucose and urine sugar and acetone
5. Controlling hypoglycemia
6. Dealing with illness and other special needs of daily living

These learning needs can be organized for discussion on three levels: (1) survival needs, (2) home management needs, and (3) life-style needs.

Educational Materials: Person-Centered Standards

A broad, often confusing array of diabetes education materials is available. Some are excellent, and some should be discarded. We are wisely reminded, especially by parents of some of our young adolescent clients, that whatever we use should measure up to several basic person-centered requirements. As health care providers, we should:

1. Give the client credit for having some intelligence and wanting new information.

2. Inform persons fully and completely of health care information, giving both sides of an issue when experts disagree—as surely they will on occasion.
3. Appeal to various levels of understanding, ranging from basic to sophisticated.
4. *Never* be patronizing, dehumanizing, or childish.

In the last analysis, whatever methods or materials we use, one central fact must be maintained: the person who has the diabetes is the *most* important and *fully equal* member of the diabetes care team. Approaches and strategies that involve this recognition can be developed and are the most likely ones to succeed.

To Sum Up

Diabetes mellitus is a syndrome composed of many metabolic disorders collectively characterized by hyperglycemia and other symptoms. The treatment relies heavily on a basic type of therapy—a carefully controlled diet. Diabetes is classified in two main types: insulin-dependent diabetes mellitus (IDDM) and noninsulin-dependent diabetes mellitus (NIDDM).

Blood glucose levels are controlled primarily by the pancreatic islet cell hormones: *insulin,* which facilitates passage of glucose through cell membranes via special membrane receptors; *glucagon,* which ensures adequate levels of glucose to prevent hypoglycemia; and *somatostatin,* which controls the actions of insulin and glucagon to maintain normal blood glucose levels. The diabetic state results from inadequate insulin secretion or insulin resistance from too few receptor sites. Symptoms range from polydipsia, polyuria, polyphagia, and signs of abnormal energy metabolism to fluid and electrolyte imbalances, acidosis, and coma in seriously uncontrolled conditions.

IDDM affects about 15% of all persons with diabetes. It occurs more often in children and is more severe and unstable. Its treatment involves blood glucose self-monitoring, insulin administration, and regular meals and exercise to balance insulin activity. NIDDM occurs mostly in adults, particularly those who are overweight. Acidosis is rare. Its treatment consists of weight management and exercise. The food plan for both types of diabetes should be rich in complex carbohydrates and fiber, low in simple sugars and fats, especially saturated fats and cholesterol, and moderate in protein. Moderate regular exercise increases the number of insulin receptor sites on cell membrances and aids in weight control.

Questions for Review

1. Describe the major characteristics of the two types of diabetes mellitus. Explain how these characteristics influence differences in nutritional therapy. List and describe medications used to control these conditions.
2. Identify and explain symptoms of uncontrolled diabetes mellitus.
3. Mr. Smith just found out that he has diabetes mellitus. He is a sedentary, 38-year-old man who is 5 ft, 8 in (170 cm) tall and weighs 210 lb (94 kg). No medications were prescribed. What is his desirable lean body weight? What would be an appropriate diet order in kilocalories, and how should these kilocalories be distributed among the energy nutrients? If he decides to drink, how much alcohol could be allowed and how should he fit it into his diet? Should he purchase sugar substututes or diet foods? Defend your answer. What advice would you offer Mr. Smith to help his children reduce their chances of developing diabetes?

References

1. Whitehead FW: Classification and pathogenesis of the diabetic syndrome: a historical perspective, J Am Diet Assoc 81(3):243, 1982.
2. Nestle M, et al: A case of diabetes mellitus, N Engl J Med 81:127, Oct 1982.
3. Knowler WC, et al: Diabetes incidence in Pima Indians: contribution of obesity and parental diabetes, Am J Epidemiol 113:144, 1981.
4. Berdanier CR: You are what you inherit, Nutr Today 21(5):18, Sept/Oct 1986.
5. Livingston JN: Getting the message, Diabetes Forecast 41(6):56, June 1988.
6. Dahl-Jorgensen K, et al: Effect of near normoglycaemia for two years on progression of early diabetic retinopathy, nephropathy, and neuropathy: the Oslo study, Diabetes Spectrum 1(2):98, May/June 1988.
7. Lopes-Virella MF, et al: Effect of metabolic control on lipid, lipoprotein, and apolipoprotein levels in 55 insulin-dependent diabetic patients: a longitudinal syudy, Diabetes 32:20, 1983.
8. American Diabetic Association: Nutritional recommendations and principles for individuals with diabetes mellitus: 1986, Nutr Today 22(1):29, Jan/Feb 1987.
9. Coulston AM, and Hollenbeck CB: Source and amount of dietary carbohydrate in patients with NIDDM, Top Clin Nutr 3(1):17, Jan 1988.
10. Wheeler ML, Delahanty L, and Wylie-Rosett J: Diet and exercise in noninsulin-dependent diabetes mellitus: implications for dietitians from the NIH Consensus Development Conference, J Am Diet Assoc 87(4):480, April 1987.
11. Franz MJ: Exercise and the management of diabetes mellitus, J Am Diet Assoc 87(7):872, July 1987.
12. Green J, and Holler H: Meal planning approaches in the nutrition management of the person with diabetes, Chicago, 1987, American Dietetic Association.
13. American Diabetes Association/American Dietetic Association: Exchange lists for meal planning, Chicago, 1986, ADA/ADA.
14. Jornsay DL, and Lorber DL: Diabetes and the traveler, Clin Diabetes 6(3):49, May/June 1988.
15. American Association of Diabetes Educators and American Diabetes Association: Guidelines for education of individuals with diabetes mellitus, New York, 1981, American Diabetes Association.
16. Prater B: Education guidelines for self-care living with diabetes, J Am Diet Assoc 82(3):283, March 1982.

Beebe CA (editor): Obesity management in people with diabetes, Diabetes Spectrum 1(1):17, March/April 1988.

This clinical nutrition specialist in diabetes presents a broad range of articles from contributing researchers on the difficult but vital management of obesity in diabetes, especially in NIDDM.

Beebe CA: Self blood glucose monitoring: an adjunct to dietary and insulin management of the patient with diabetes, J Am Diet Assoc 87(1):61, Jan 1987.

Wysocki T: SBGM: Has the promise been fulfilled? Diabetes Spectrum 1(2):83, May/June 1988.

These two articles provide information about the current management tool of self-monitoring of blood glucose, how it relates to diet management, and some problems in persons' use of the tool.

Berdanier CR: You are what you inherit, Nutr Today 21(5):18, Sept/Oct 1986.

This article provides an excellent discussion of the genetic factors involved in the development of disease, using the obesity-diabetes relationship as a model.

Livingston JN: Getting the message, Diabetes Forecast 41(6):57, June 1988.

This article presents the picture—literally, with an excellent illustration—of current knowledge of how insulin receptors work, which gives us a better understanding of how to treat diabetes. Written in simple style, easy to read, it would make a good teaching tool for clients and students.

Powers MA (editor): Handbook of diabetes nutritional management, Rockville, MD, 1987, Aspen Publishers, Inc.

This book provides a comprehensive source of well-organized reference material on the role of nutritional therapy in sound management of diabetes.

Topics in Clinical Nutrition: Issue topic—Diabetes Care, Top Clin Nutr 3(1): Jan 1988.

This entire issue of this popular journal presents 10 helpful articles covering a wide range of subjects involved in providing quality nutritional care for persons with diabetes.

Further Readings

Alcohol and Diabetes: Do They Mix?

Two shots of whiskey on an empty stomach can lower blood sugar dramatically. For this reason, among others, alcohol has been taboo for years for persons with diabetes. It definitely has some negative effects, since it:

- Interferes with the body's ability to regulate insulin-induced hypoglycemia. Persons in poor control are most susceptible to this effect.
- Increases serum cholesterol levels, though this effect is transient.
- Leads to hyperlipoproteinemia when used in excess by susceptible persons, including persons with diabetes.
- Leads to hyperglycemia when used in excess, though this is a transient effect usually lasting only a few hours.
- Induces a diabetic condition when used in excess by a prediabetic individual. In such persons, however, the blood sugar returns to normal following total abstinence, without having to resort to the use of insulin or other oral hypoglycemic agents.

For the person with diabetes, however, alcohol may not be quite as bad as most people think it is because it: (1) does not require insulin for its metabolism, (2) enhances the glucose-lowering effect of hypoglycemic agents, including insulin, when used in *moderate* amounts, and (3) raises HDL-cholesterol levels when used in *moderate* amounts, thus possibly providing some protection against cardiovascular disease.

In light of this information, it appears that diabetes and alcohol can mix—if shaken gently. For your clients who choose to use alcohol, you will want to suggest that they:

- Carry a personal diabetes ID at all times, in case of a hypoglycemic attack induced by alcohol
- Ask the physician if there are any contraindications to using alcohol (e.g., hypertriglycerides, gastritis, pancreatitis, some types of cardiac and renal disease) and any drug interactions (e.g., with the use of barbiturates or tranquilizers)
- Always sip alcoholic drinks slowly
- Never drink alcohol on any empty stomach
- Limit alcohol use to no more than one or two alcohol equivalents per day 2 or 3 days a week. Equivalents are:

  1½ oz (a shot glass) of distilled alcoholic beverage (whickey, Scotch, tye, vodka, brandy, cognac, rum)
  4 oz dry wine
  2 oz dry sherry
  12 oz beer (preferably Light)

- Avoid sweet drinks: liquers, sweet wines, drinks mixed with tonic, soda, fruit juice, or other liquids that have a high concentration of sugar

In addition, warn clients taking oral hypoglycemic drugs of problems that may occur when they drink alcohol—e.g., nausea, deep flushing, tachycardia, and impaired speech. The effect begins 3 to 10 minutes after taking a drink and lasts an hour or longer.

Warn clients taking insulin that they should not reduce their food intake. They should continue to eat their full diet as prescribed because of their susceptibility to hypoglycemia induced by the alcohol. Tell persons with noninsulin-dependent diabetes to consider the caloric value of the alcohol and omit two fat exchanges for each drink.

REFERENCES

Feingold KR, and Siperstein MD: Normalization of fasting blood glucose level in insulin-dependent diabetes: the role of ethonol abstention, Diab Care 6(2):186, 1983.

Franz MJ: Diabetes mellitus: considerations in the development of guidelines for the occasional use of alcohol, J Am Diet Assoc 83(2):147, 1983.

22 Renal Disease

After study of this chapter, the student should be able to:

1. Identify dietary factors that contribute to basic tissue changes in long-standing renal disease and describe the nature of these changes.

2. Compare nutritional care of patients with glomerulonephritis and nephrosis in terms of disease process, renal function, and diet modifications.

3. Describe the effects of changes in renal function that accompany chronic renal failure and the nutritional therapy for the patient on hemodialysis.

4. Relate types of renal calculi to nutritional therapy indicated in each case.

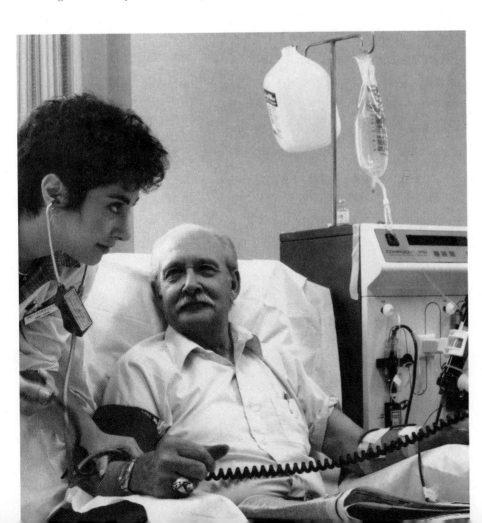

PREVIEW

Kidney diseases affect the lives of more than 8 million Americans and kill 60,000 a year. Another 3 million or more have related infections, many of which go undetected. In all, these kidney problems are a leading cause of lost work time and pay. They are the fourth leading health problem in America.

The advent of renal dialysis technology and kidney transplant techniques have prolonged the lives of the 50,000 persons in the United States today who develop kidney failure each year. But this survival is not without human and monetary cost. A scarcity of organ donors and rejection problems continue to plague successful transplant surgery. And time-consuming dialysis, although life extending, exacts an emotional and physical toll on persons with irreversible chronic renal failure. Hemodialysis costs American taxpayers some $1.4 billion each year via Medicare. Although kidney disease may not be as much a killer as heart disease or cancer, it is still a serious national and personal problem.

In this chapter in our clinical nutrition study sequence, we will examine the kidney and its functions, especially its basic functional unit, the nephron. Then on this basis we will see how disease interferes with these functions in the metabolism of nutrients and requires nutritional therapy.

Physiology of the Kidney

Nephron
The functional unit of the kidney, located in the cortex; site of the proximal tubule, descending and ascending portions of the Loop of Henle, and the distal and collecting tubules.

Renal Functions

Basic Functional Unit—The Nephron

Knowledge of the normal functions of the kidney forms the essential background for understanding therapy in renal disorders dased on the organ's impaired functioning in disease. The basic functional unit of the kidney is the **nephron.** Major advances today in treating kidney disease are based on providing maximal support for these vital nephron functions (Figure 22-1).

We are provided at birth with about 2 million of these filtering-reabsorbing nephron units, far more than we need. But we begin to lose them gradually after age 30. Each nephron is an exquisite example of a highly complex, minute tissue unit. It is adapted in fine detail to its vital function—maintaining an internal fluid environment compatible with life. These small vital units of the kidney are the master chemists of our bodies. We have the kind of body fluids and tissues that we have not merely because of what the mouth takes in but because of what the kidneys keep. Only because they work in the way they do has it become possible for us to have specific tissues of a specific nature to do specific tasks.

Specific Integrated Nephron Functions

Each kidney contains some 1 million nephrons. As the body fluid flows through these finely structured units, the nephrons perform four significant functions to support life:

1. **Filter** most constituents from the entering blood except red cells and proteins.
2. **Reabsorb** needed substances as the filtrate continues along the winding tubules.

Nephron

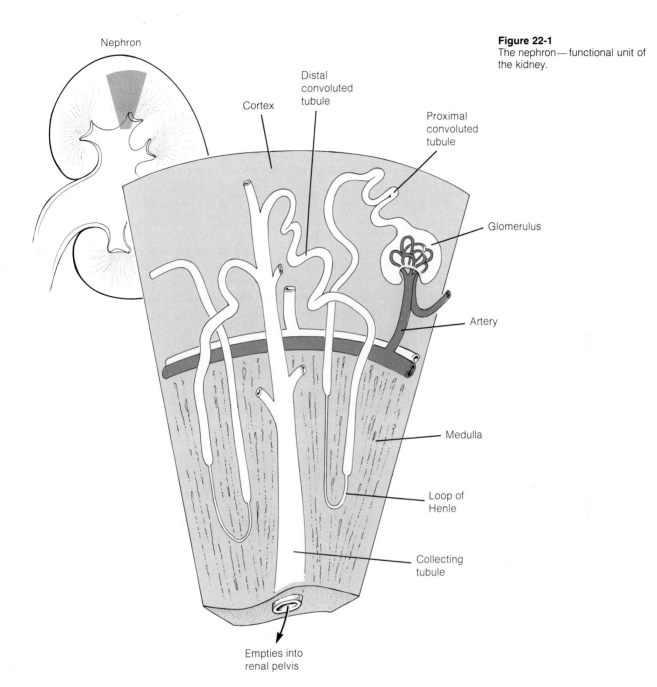

Figure 22-1
The nephron—functional unit of
the kidney.

Cortex

Distal
convoluted
tubule

Proximal
convoluted
tubule

Glomerulus

Artery

Medulla

Loop of
Henle

Collecting
tubule

Empties into
renal pelvis

3. **Secrete** additional ions to maintain acid-base balance.
4. **Excrete** unneeded materials in a concentrated urine.

Nephron Structures

Specific nephron structures, as shown in Figure 22-1, perform unique metabolic tasks to maintain body balances. These key structures include the **glomerulus** and the tubules.

Glomerulus
A convoluted cluster of blood vessels in the cortex of the kidney at the head of the nephron; site of cell-free filtrate formation.

Bowman's capsule
A cupped membrane surrounding the glomerulus; site of cell-free filtrate formation.

Medulla
Innermost portion of the kidney; site of the loop of Henle.

Glomerulus

At the head of each nephron, blood enters in a single capillary and then branches into a group of collateral capillaries. This tuft of collateral capillaries is held closely together in a cup-shaped membrane, **Bowman's capsule,** named for the young English physician, Sir William Bowman, who in 1843 first clearly established the basis of plasma filtration and consequent urine secretion based on this intimate relationship of the blood-filled glomeruli and the enveloping membrane. The filtrate formed here is cell free and virtually protein free. Otherwise it carries the same constituents as does the entering blood.

Tubules

Continuous with the base of Bowman's capsule, the nephron tubules wind in a series of convolutions toward their terminal in the renal pelvis. Specific reabsorption functions are performed by the four sections of the tubule:

1. **Proximal tubule.** In the section nearest the glomerulus, major nutrient reabsorption occurs. Essentially 100% of the glucose and amino acids and 80% to 85% of the water, sodium, potassium, chloride, and most other substances are reabsorbed. Only 15% to 30% of the filtrate remains to enter the next section.

2. **Loop of Henle.** This narrowed midsection of the renal tubule is named for the celebrated German anatomist, Friedrich Henle, who in 1845 first demonstrated its unique structure and function in creating the necessary fluid pressures for ultimately forming a concentrated urine. At this narrowed midsection, the thin loop of tubule dips into the central renal **medulla.** Here, a balanced system of water and sodium exchange through sodium pumps in the limbs of the loop creates important fluid density around the loop. This area of increased density in the central part of the kidney is important to concentrate the urine by osmotic pressure as the lower collecting tubule later passes through this same area of the kidney.

3. **Distal tubule.** This latter portion of the tubule functions primarily in providing acid-base balance through secretion of ionized hydrogen. It also conserves sodium by reabsorbing it under the influence of the adrenal hormone aldosterone, made available through the *renin-angiotensin-aldosterone mechanism.*

4. **Collecting tubule.** In the final widened section of the tubule, the filtrate is concentrated to save water and form urine for excretion. Water is absorbed under the influence of the pituitary hormone antidiuretic hormone (ADH) and the osmotic pressure of the more dense surrounding fluid in this central part of the kidney. The resulting volume of urine, now concentrated and excreted, is only 0.5% to 1% of the original water and solutes filtered at the beginning in Bowman's capsule.

General Causes of Renal Disease

A number of agents or conditions may interfere with the normal functioning of the nephrons and cause renal disease.

Inflammatory and Degenerative Disease

Inflammation of the small blood vessels and membranes in the nephrons may be short term, as in acute forms of glomerulonephritis. In other cases it may diffusely involve entire nephrons or nephron segments, disrupting normal function. Nephrotic lesions develop, leading to progressive chronic renal failure. Nutritional disturbances in the metabolism of protein, electrolytes, and water follow.

Infection and Obstruction

Bacterial infection of the urinary tract may range from occasional mild, uncomfortable bladder infection to more involved chronic recurrent disease and obstruction from kidney stones. This obstruction anywhere in the urinary tract blocks drainage, causing further infection and tissue damage.

Damage From Other Diseases

Circulatory disorders such as prolonged hypertension, often associated with the vasopressor effect of the renin-angiotensin-aldosterone mechanism, can cause degeneration of the small renal arteries and curtail efficient function. A vicious cycle ensues as the demand on the kidney in turn causes more hypertension and still more damage. Other diseases, such as diabetes mellitus and gout, may also damage kidney function. Abnormalities present from birth may lead to poor function, infection, or obstruction.

Damage From Other Agents

Environmental agents such as insecticides, solvents, and similar materials are poisons that can damage the kidneys. Some toxic drugs may also harm renal tissue.

Nutritional therapy for renal disease is based on impaired renal function and resulting clinical symptoms. In this chapter we will focus primarily on the more serious degenerative processes of glomerulonephritis, nephrotic syndrome, and renal failure. Then we briefly review the more common problems that occur in the urinary tract—obstructive kidney stones and urinary tract infection.

Disease Process

Glomerulonephritis is an inflammatory process affecting the glomeruli, the small blood vessels in the cup-shaped head of the nephron. It is most common in acute form in children 3 to 10 years of age, although 5% or more of the initial attacks occur in adults past age 50. The most common cause is a previous streptococcal infection. Glomerulonephritis has a more or less sudden onset and a brief course in its acute form, and it is usually completely cleared in a year or two. In some cases it progresses to a chronic form, involving an increased amount of renal tissue and eventually requiring dialysis and other support treatments.

Recent immunologic studies and electron microscopy have demonstrated the underlying process as an *immune complex disease*. An **antigen** or "foreign invader" in the body excites responses from the defense system to combat potentially harmful effects. In glomerular disease the antigens are usually substances attacking the body from the outside: bacteria, viruses, and chemicals, including antibiotics and other drugs. In response, **antibodies** are produced by the body to ward off or neutralize the effect of the antigen. An excess of antigen and antibodies produced leads to the the formation of *anti-*

Glomerulonephritis

Glomerulonephritis
Inflammation of the capillary glomeruli in the kidney. May result after a streptococcal infection.

Antigen
Any substance that stimulates the production of an antibody specifically designed to interact with it. Examples of antigens include toxins, bacteria, foreign proteins, etc.

Antibody
An animal protein made up of a specific sequence of amino acids that is designed to interact with a specific *antigen* during an allergic response or to prevent infection, etc.

gen-antibody complexes in the circulation, which become trapped in the glomeruli. These complexes bind components of **complement,** a series of enzymatic proteins in the blood that serve as part of the body's immune system. The activated complement in turn provides active chemical factors that attract white blood cells, whose lysosomal enzymes incite the resulting injury to the glomerulus.

These antigen-antibody complexes appear as lumpy deposits between the epithelial cells of the cupped nephron capsule and the basement membrane of the glomeruli. Lesions develop leaving scar tissue that obstructs the circulation through the glomerulus. Fatty degeneration and necrosis of the conjoined tubules follow, and ultimate destruction of the nephron results. In time, if the disease becomes progressive, the net result is a reduction in the number of functioning nephrons available in the kidneys.[1]

Clinical Symptoms

Classic symptoms include gross **hematuria** and **proteinuria.** There may be varying degrees of edema, with shortness of breath resulting from sodium and water retention and circulatory congestion. Also, there may be mild **tachycardia** and mild or marked elevation of blood pressure. The patient is generally anorexic, which contributes to feeding problems. If the disease progresses to renal insufficiency, there is **oliguria** or **anuria,** which signals development of acute renal failure.

Nutritional Therapy

The plan for nutritional care depends on the course of the disease.

General Care in Uncomplicated Disease

The general treatment is symptomatic and designed to provide optimal nutritional support. In short-term acute cases in children, pediatricians and nutritionists favor overall optimal nutrition with adequate protein, unless symptoms of oliguria or anuria develop. These complications usually last no more than 2 to 3 days and are managed by conservative treatment. Salt is usually not restricted unless complications of edema, hypertension, or oliguria become dangerous. Thus in most patients with acute uncomplicated disease, especially in children with poststreptococcal glomerulonephritis, diet modifications are not crucial. The main treatment centers on bed rest and antibiotic drug therapy. The fluid intake will be adjusted to output as a rule, including losses in vomiting and diarrhea.

Specific Therapy in Progressive Disease

If the disease process advances, however, more specific nutritional therapy measures are indicated. The nutrient factors most involved are protein, carbohydrate, sodium, potassium, and water.

1. **Protein.** If the **blood urea nitrogen (BUN)** is elevated and oliguria is present, dietary protein must be restricted. Usually the diet contains 0.5 g of protein per kilogram of ideal body weight. Some patients may use 1 g/kg as long as renal function is adequate to maintain a normal BUN level.

2. **Carbohydrate.** To provide sufficient energy from kilocalories, carbohydrate should be given liberally. This will also reduce the catabolism of tissue protein and prevent starvation ketosis.

Complement
Enzymatic protein that combines with the antigen-antibody complex, separating them when the antigen is an intact cell.

Hematuria
Presence of blood in the urine.

Proteinuria
Presence of abnormally high levels of serum protein in the urine.

Oliguria
Reduced amount of urine in comparison with fluid intake.

Anuria
Complete lack of urine secretion by the kidneys. Also known as *anuresis*.

Blood urea nitrogen (BUN)
Blood test used to identify any disorder in kidney function.

3. **Sodium.** The restriction of sodium varies with the degree of oliguria. If renal function is impaired, the sodium will be restricted to 500 to 1000 mg/day. As recovery occurs, sodium intake can be increased.

4. **Potassium.** With severe oliguria, renal clearance of potassium is impaired. Potassium intoxication may occur, requiring dialysis. Thus potassium intake is monitored carefully according to disease progression.

5. **Water.** Fluids are restricted according to the ability of the kidney to excrete urine. If restriction is not indicated, fluids can be consumed as desired.

Disease Process

The nephrotic syndrome, or **nephrosis,** is characterized by a group of symptoms resulting from kidney tissue damage and impaired nephron function. The most evident symptoms are massive **edema** and *proteinuria*. This condition may be caused by progressive glomerulonephritis. It may also be associated with other diseases, such as diabetes or connective tissue disorders—**collagen disease.** In some cases, it may result from drug reactions, especially exposure to heavy metals, or even from reaction to toxic venom following a bee sting. The primary degenerative lesion is in the capillary basement membrane of the glomerulus, permitting escape of large amounts of protein into the filtrate. The tubular changes that occur are due to the high protein concentration in the filtrate, with some protein uptake from the tubular lumen. Both filtration and reabsorption functions are disrupted.

Clinical Symptoms

The cardinal symptom is massive edema. **Ascites** is common. The abdomen becomes increasingly distended as fluid collects in the serous cavities. Often **striae** (stretch marks) appear on the stretched skin of the extremities. The massive edema is largely caused by the gross loss of protein, principally albumin, in the urine—some 4 to 10 g/day. This means that the plasma protein is greatly reduced. The albumin fraction is largely responsible for maintaining the capillary fluid shift mechanism (see Chapter 8). Thus fluid balance between tissue fluid and circulating fluid is decreased to less than 4 g/dL. Free fat, oval fat bodies, or fatty droplets are found in the urine. Protein losses are also indicated by the presence of urinary globulins and specialized binding proteins for thyroid and iron, producing signs of hypothyroidism and anemia. As serum protein loss continues, tissue proteins are broken down and general malnutrition ensues. Fatty tissue changes in the liver and general sodium retention further contribute to the edema. Severe ascites and **pedal edema** mask the gross tissue wasting.

Nutritional Therapy

Nutritional therapy is directed toward control of the major symptoms, edema and malnutrition, resulting from the massive protein losses.

Protein. Replacement of the prolonged nitrogen deficit is a fundamental and immediate need. As indicated, the plasma albumin level may have been reduced to 20% or less of its normal value. This is a major factor in the development of nephrotic ascites and edema. Daily protein needs vary according to need, from 1 g/kg/day to larger amounts in extreme cases.

Nephrotic Syndrome

Nephrosis
Inflammation of the nephron.

Edema
The presence of abnormally large amounts of fluid in the intercellular tissue spaces.

Collagen disease
Connective tissue diseases such as rheumatoid arthritis, scleroderma, lupus erythematosus, and others.

Ascites
Outflow and accumulation of fluid in the abdominal cavity. Also known as *abdominal* or *peritoneal dropsy.*

Striae
Streaks or lines on stretched skin caused by weakening of the elastic tissue by constant tension.

Pedal edema
Edema in the feet.

Kilocalories. Sufficient kilocalories must always be provided to ensure protein use for tissue synthesis. High daily intakes of 50 to 60 kcal/kg are essential. Since appetite is usually poor, much encouragement and support are needed. The food must be as appetizing as possible and in a form most easily tolerated.

Sodium. Dietary sodium must be sufficiently reduced to combat the massive edema. Usually 500 mg sodium/day (see Chapter 20) is sufficient to help initiate **diuresis.**

The general dietary management is similar to that given for hepatitis (see Chapter 19), with additional need for sodium restriction. There is no need to reduce potassium. Iron and vitamin supplements may be indicated.

Diuresis
Increased urination.

Renal Failure

The two types of renal failure, acute and chronic, are characterized by a number of symptoms reflecting interference with normal nephron functions in nutrient metabolism. Both forms have similar nutritional therapy, depending on the extent of renal tissue damage.

Acute Renal Failure
Disease Process

Renal failure may occur as an acute phase, with sudden shutdown of renal function following some metabolic insult or traumatic injury to normal kidneys. The situation is often life-threatening and is a medical emergency in which the nutritionist and nurse play important supportive roles. **Acute renal failure** may have various causes: (1) severe injury such as extensive burns or crushing injuries that cause widespread tissue destruction; (2) infectious diseases such as peritonitis; or (3) toxic agents in the environment such as carbon tetrachloride, poisonous mushrooms, or, in sensitive individuals, certain drugs such as penicillin.

Acute renal failure
Total shutdown of renal function, requiring emergency treatment.

Clinical Symptoms

The major sign of such an acute renal failure is *oliguria,* often with proteinuria or hematuria accompanying the small output. This diminished urine output results from underlying tissue problems that characterize acute renal failure. Usually blockage of the tubules is caused by cellular debris from tissue trauma or urinary failure with backup retention of filtrate materials.

Nutritional Therapy

The major challenge for nutritional therapy is the improvement of nutritional status, especially in patients with marked catabolism.[2] Depending on the patient's condition, nutrient intake may be oral or intravenous. During dialysis, total parenteral nutrition (TPN) may be used as a feeding method (see Chapter 23). Caloric demand for energy may be met by feeding a 20% to 50% glucose solution with intermittent lipid emulsions and mixtures of essential and nonessential amino acids as tolerated to prevent excessive tissue catabolism and support healing and recovery.[2,3]

Chronic Renal Failure
Disease Process

The course of renal failure may become chronic, with progressive degenerative changes in renal tissues and marked depression of all renal functions. At this stage, few functioning nephrons remain, and these gradually deteriorate (see box, p. 540). Chronic renal insufficiency may result from a variety of diseases involving the nephrons: (1) primary glomerular disease; (2) metabolic disease with renal involvement, such as insulin-dependent diabetes mellitus (IDDM); (3) exposure to toxic substances; (4) infections; (5) renal vascular disease; (6) renal tubular disease; (7) chronic pyelonephritis; or (8) congenital abnormality of both kidneys. Depending on the nature of the predisposing renal disease, there is extensive scarring of renal tissue. This distorts the kidney structure and brings vascular changes from the prolonged hypertension involved.

Clinical Symptoms

The symptom complex of advanced renal insufficiency is commonly called **uremia.** Symptoms result from the progressive loss of nephrons and the consequent decreased renal blood flow and glomerular filtration. As the nephrons are lost one by one, the remaining nephrons gradually lose their ability to maintain body water balance, concentration of solutes in body fluids (osmolality), and electrolyte and acid-base balance. This continuing loss of nephrons brings many metabolic insults.

1. **Water balance.** The increased load of solutes causes an osmotic diuresis. Increasingly the kidney cannot excrete a normal concentrated urine. Dehydration follows and may become critical. On the other hand, water intoxication may occur if there is excess fluid intake.

2. **Electrolyte balance.** A number of imbalances among electrolytes result from the decreasing nephron function:

Sodium. With osmotic diuresis, sodium loss contributes to a decreasing extracellular fluid volume. As the plasma volume decreases, renal filtration declines further, worsening the renal failure. In this state the kidney cannot respond appropriately to maintain sodium balance. Any sudden increase in sodium intake cannot be excreted readily and causes still more edema.

Potassium. The balance of potassium is usually not impaired as readily until the oliguria becomes severe or acidosis increases.

Phosphate, sulfate, and organic acids. With reduced nephron function there is reduced filtration and excretion of these materials produced by the metabolism of food nutrients. Thus these anions become concentrated in body fluids, with subsequent displacement of bicarbonate, causing metabolic acidosis.

Calcium and phosphate. Metabolism of these electrolytes is greatly disturbed as a consequence of renal tissue loss. Two metabolic functions of the kidney—activation of vitamin D hormone and parathyroid hormone control of serum calcium-phosphorus levels (see Chapter 8)—cannot proceed at normal levels. The impaired vitamin D hormone activation results in a bone disease called **osteodystrophy.** This disturbance causes bone pain, various bone deformities, awkward gait, and, in children, impaired growth. Also, there may be calcification of soft tissues, which further hinders renal function.

3. **Nitrogen retention.** Increasing loss of nephron function brings elevated amounts of nitrogenous metabolites such as urea and creatinine. The urea load results from dietary protein metabolism, the creatinine load from increasing catabolism of muscle mass.

4. **Anemia.** The normal kidney participates in the production of red blood cells, through action of a specific enzyme. The damaged kidney cannot accomplish this task, and red blood cell production is depressed. The red cells

Uremia
Presence in the blood of large amounts of byproducts of protein metabolism. Caused by impaired nephron function leading to the inability to excrete urea and other products. A toxic condition characterized by headache, nausea, vomiting, diminished vision, convulsions, or coma.

Osteodystrophy
A disease often accompanying renal failure in which calcium is lost from the bones; poor bone formation. *Renal osteodystrophy* is a result of chronic kidney disease that may begin in childhood and can result in *renal dwarfism.*

To Probe Further

The Aging Western Kidney

Renal disease typically follows a progressive downhill course. Why should this be? The work of Brenner's group at Harvard indicates that the stage may well have been set in our distant evolutionary past as the kidney adapted to meet the nitrogenous excretion needs of our hunter/scavenger, meat-eating ancestors.

Because our ancestors were carnivores, their protein intake was transient and intermittent; they could only eat after a successful hunting expedition. Thus at these times of surfeit a large number of extra nephrons had to be available to meet their needs for the prompt excretion of waste products, largely urea, and the conservation of fluid and electrolytes until the next meal became available. They achieved this metabolic task mainly by *hyperfiltration* through increased use of their many extra superficial glomeruli, largely in the outer part (**cortex**) of the kidney, which normally maintains a resting state. Only in the past 500 to 10,000 years, when population groups developed agriculture and herding, did a more continuous food intake pattern become possible. Now, in many Western countries, our adult diet averages approximately 3000 kcal and more than 100 g of protein, largely meat, *daily*.

Thus the answers to our initial questions—Why do we have far more nephrons than we seem to need? Why do we begin losing some of these nephrons through a "normal aging process" of glomerular sclerosis after age 30? Why is renal disease so inexorably progressive?—lie in a fundamental mismatch between the evolutionary design of our kidneys and the functional burden we place on them by our modern eating habits. Our sustained protein excesses, along with other solutes, impose demands for sustained increases in renal blood flow and glomeruli filtration rates. This requires that our reserve glomeruli of the outer renal cortex be in more or less continuous use and predisposes even healthy persons to the observed progressive glomerular sclerosis over time, with deterioration of normal kidney function. In health this deterioration poses no problem because we have so many extra nephrons. But when renal disease occurs, the burden is compounded. The disease accelerates the deterioration process and makes coping impossible. The downhill course inevitably ensues. The aging and vulnerable Western kidney thus seems to be related inevitably to our lifetime of large protein meals.

REFERENCES

Brenner BM, Meyer TW, and Hostetter TH: Dietary protein intake and the progressive nature of kidney disease, N Engl J Med 307(11):652, 1982.

Klahr S, Schreiner G, and Ichikawa I: The progression of renal disease, N Engl J Med 318(25):1657, June 23, 1988.

Mitch WE, Brenner BM, and Stein JM (editors): The progressive nature of renal disease, New York, 1986, Churchill Livingstone.

that are produced survive a shorter time but have a usual size and hemoglobin content.

5. **Hypertension.** When blood flow to renal tissue is increasingly impaired, the resulting *ischemia* (see Chapter 20) brings increasing hypertension through the nephrons' close relationship to the renin-angiotensin-aldosterone mechanism. In turn hypertension causes cardiovascular damage and further deterioration of the kidney.

6. **Azotemia.** The elevated blood urea nitrogen (BUN), serum creatinine, and serum uric acid levels are reflected in the characteristic laboratory finding of **azotemia.**

General Signs and Symptoms

The increasing loss of renal function brings progressive weakness, shortness of breath, general lethargy, and fatigue. There is thirst, anorexia, weight loss, and gastrointestinal irritability with diarrhea or vomiting. Increased capillary fragility brings skin, nose, oral, and gastrointestinal bleeding. Nervous system involvement brings muscular twitching, burning sensations in the extremities, or uremic convulsions. Cheyne-Stokes respiration (irregular, cyclic type of breathing) indicates acidosis. There is ulceration of the mouth, a persistent bad or metallic taste, and fetid breath. Malnutrition lowers resistance to infection. Osteodystrophy continues with aching and pain in bone and joints.

Nutritional Therapy Goals

Treatment must be individual, adjusted according to progression of the illness, type of treatment being used, and the patient's response. In general, however, basic therapy objectives are to:
- Reduce and minimize protein breakdown
- Avoid dehydration or overhydration
- Correct acidosis carefully
- Correct electrolyte depletions and avoid excesses
- Control fluid and electrolyte losses from vomiting and diarrhea
- Maintain optimal nutritional status
- Maintain appetite, general morale, and sense of well-being
- Control complications such as hypertension, bone pain, nervous system problems
- Retard progression of renal failure, postponing ultimate dialysis

These general measures of treatment involve nutritional care as a major role. The nutritionist becomes an indispensable member of the renal care team, and personal care plans for chronic renal failure include nutrient variances according to individual need.

Protein. The crucial problem is to provide sufficient protein to prevent protein breakdown, yet avoid an excess that would elevate urea levels. General limitations of protein are 0.5 g/kg/day, to help reduce azotemia and hyperkalemia and control acidosis. Protein is usually adjusted according to creatinine clearance. There is no need to restrict protein intake until the creatinine clearance falls below 40 mL/minute. Thereafter the dietary protein must be regulated according to the declining renal function (Table 22-1).

Azotemia
Term meaning nitrogen, referring to an excess of urea and other nitrogenous substances in the blood.

Creatinine
End product of the breakdown of body tissue. Found in muscles and blood; excreted in urine. High levels indicate abnormally high catabolism of body proteins, and possibly inadequate intake of carbohydrate and fat, which have a protein-sparing effect.

Table 22-1

Protein and Nitrogen
Needs in Chronic Renal
Failure

Creatinine clearance (mL/min)	Nitrogen* (g/day)	Protein (g/day)
40 and above	Unrestricted	Unrestricted
10-40	9.6	60
5-20	6.4	40†
2-10	2.5-3.0 (+1.3-2.6)	20 (+ EAA/analogs)†
8 and below	Transplantation Dialysis	
5 and below	Dialysis	

*Total protein ÷ 6.25.
†EAA, Essential amino acids; alpha-keto-, alpha-hydroxy-analogues of EAA.

If caloric requirements are liberally met, patients may be maintained in nitrogen balance for prolonged periods on as little as 35 to 40 g protein/day. However, when blood urea levels rise, protein intake must be reduced to 20 g/day. Only essential amino acids are supplied by small amounts of milk and egg protein. Thus the patient is not burdened with nonessential amino acids that make demands on the body for the disposal of their nitrogenous waste products and do little to counteract the tissue protein catabolism. In any event protein is closely controlled according to individual need, ranging in quantity from 20 to 70 g/day and having a high biologic value to supply essential amino acids.

Amino acid supplements. Promising approaches to protein replacement are being developed using mixtures of essential amino acids or of amino acid precursors. Other supplements have a relatively high proportion of nitrogen-free analogs of essential amino acids, especially *branched-chain amino acids*.[4]

Kilocalories. Adequate kilocalories are mandatory. Carbohydrate and fat must supply sufficient nonprotein kilocalories to spare dietary protein for tissue protein synthesis and energy supply. About 300 to 400 g carbohydrate is the average daily need. Sufficient fat, 75 to 90 g, is added to give the patient 2000 to 2500 total kcal daily.

Water. Total fluid intake is guarded to avoid water intoxication from overloading or dehydration from too little water. With predialysis patients, fluid intake should be sufficient to maintain adequate urine volume.

Sodium. The need for sodium intake varies. Both severe restriction and excess are to be avoided. The dietary need is closely related to the patient's handling of water. If hypertension and edema are present, the sodium intake needs to be restricted. Usually, the sodium intake will vary between 500 to 2000 mg/day.

Potassium. Serum potassium levels may be depressed or elevated. Adjustment of intake is made accordingly to maintain normal levels. If significant losses occur with severe vomiting or diarrhea, *careful* supplementation may be needed. In general the damaged kidney cannot clear potassium adequately. Thus the dietary intake is kept at about 1500 mg/day.

Phosphate and calcium. Abnormal serum levels of these electrolytes, phosphate and calcium, result from the secondary **hyperparathyroidism** caused by the damaged kidney function. Phosphate intake should be restricted early to retard or prevent this developing imbalance, which leads to the complicating bone disease osteodystrophy, before symptoms of bone pain or deformity occur.[5] Further control of phosphate levels is ensured by use of aluminum hydroxide gel to bind phosphate and prevent its intestinal absorption. A calcium supplement such as calcium lactate tablets relieves the hypocalcemia and its tetany-like effects. In some cases calcium carbonate is used because it also buffers the accompanying metabolic acidosis.

Hyperparathyroidism
Greater-than-normal levels of activity by the parathyroid glands, which regulate calcium and phosphorus. High calcium levels increase the chances of developing calcium-containing urinary calculi.

Vitamins. In more restricted protein diets, supplementary vitamins are usually advisable, since a diet of 40 g protein or less does not supply the full spectrum of vitamins needed. A multivitamin tablet or capsule is usually added to the diet of renal patients on protein restriction. To help correct the bone disease present, an activated form of vitamin D hormone may be used with caution.

Maintenance Kidney Dialysis

Since the advent of the artificial kidney machine, patients with progressive chronic renal failure have been treated both at **dialysis** centers and at home. These treatments, however, are expensive. Much of the cost is now paid under a provision of Medicare. Some 18,000 patients receive this needed artificial kidney care, usually at dialysis centers. During each treatment the patient's blood makes a number of round trips through the dialysis solution in the artificial kidney, "laundering" it to restore normal blood levels of life-sustaining substances that the patient's own kidneys can no longer accomplish. In some selected cases, an alternative form of *peritoneal dialysis* is practical for long-term ambulatory therapy at home (see box, p. 544).

Dialysis
Separating substances in solution by taking advantage of the different rates at which they pass through a semipermeable membrane.

The diet of a patient on **hemodialysis** is a very important aspect of maintaining biochemical control. Several basic objectives govern each individually tailored diet, designed to (1) maintain protein and kilocalorie balance; (2) prevent dehydration or fluid overload; (3) maintain normal serum potassium and sodium blood levels; and (4) maintain acceptable phosphate and calcium levels. Control of infection is an underlying goal. Nutritional therapy in most cases can be planned with more liberal nutrient allowances.

Hemodialysis
Removal of toxic substances from the blood by passing it through a machine that contains a semipermeable membrane and a liquid into which the substances will be diffused.

Protein. For most adult dialysis patients, a standard protein allowance of 1 g/kg lean body weight provides for nutritional needs, maintains positive nitrogen balance, does not produce excessive nitrogenous waste, and replaces the amino acids lost during each dialysis treatment. At least 75% of this daily allowance should consist of protein of high biologic value, such as eggs, meat, fish, and poultry, but little if any milk. Milk is restricted because it adds more fluid and has a high content of sodium, phosphate, and potassium.

Kilocalories. Carbohydrates and fats, depending on blood lipid levels, are supplied in generous amounts to provide the needed energy for daily activi-

Clinical Application

Nutritional Needs of Patients on Portable Dialysis Machines

Persons with end-stage renal disease used to spend up to 18 hours a week on hemodialysis machines in a hospital or dialysis center. Now approximately 2800 Americans undergo dialysis 24 hours a day, 7 days a week, without spending 1 minute in a hospital room.

These individuals use continuous ambulatory peritoneal dialysis (CAPD), a home dialysis process that introduces dialysate directly into the peritoneal cavity, where it can be exchanged for fluids that contain the metabolic waste products. This is done by attaching a disposable bag containing the dialysate to a catheter permanently inserted into the peritoneal cavity, waiting 20 to 30 minutes for the solution exchange, then lowering the bag to allow the force of gravity to cause the waste-containing fluid to drain into it. When the bag is empty, it can be folded around the waist or tucked into a pocket, allowing the user mobility.

The exchange takes place by osmosis, the rate being determined by the amount of dextrose in the solution. The most common dialysates are 1.5%, 2.5%, or 4.25% dextrose in 1.5 to 2 L of solution. Most CAPD users require three to five exchanges each day. They are not only free to move, but with good self-care they are also free from some of the extensive dietary restrictions placed on hemodialysis patients.

Protein and amino acid losses are usually minimal and easily replaced by diet. High losses were more common in early CAPD systems because of peritonitis, a common problem associated with the need to replace bags frequently.

Potassium requirements depend on the number of solution exchanges that take place each day. The fewer the number of exchanges, the greater the chance of developing high serum potassium levels. Also, patients who stop using CAPD must immediately reduce their potassium intake, since serum levels rise rapidly.

Phosphorus-binding antacids are not needed as much because of improved control of phosphorus blood levels with CAPD use.

Sodium restriction is not necessary. In patients susceptible to hypotension, high-sodium diets have been recommended.

Fluid restriction is unnecessary, since 2000 to 2200 ml of fluid may be removed with two 1.5% plus two 4.25% dextrose solutions used in 1 day. Some CAPD users even become dehydrated easily.

ties and to prevent tissue protein breakdown (see box, p. 547). The usual need is 40 kcal/kg lean body weight. Most of the carbohydrate should be supplied by simple carbohydrate foods, with control of complex carbohydrates. The complex carbohydrate food forms such as grains and legumes contribute incomplete protein and should not take up large amounts of the limited protein allowance.

CAPD does pose a few nutrition-related problems, mainly because of the amount of dextrose in the dialysate. A study of patients given three 1.5% and two 4.25% dextrose solutions in 1 day revealed an intake of more than 800 kcal above the energy value of their regular diets. In addition to posing possible weight-management problems, the extra dextrose can lead to elevated triglycerides and high-lower-density lipoprotein (LDL) levels, increasing the risk of coronary heart disease in long-term users.

Nutritionists and nurses who counsel patients being transferred from hemodialysis to the CAPD regimen are faced with a special problem: patients are often reluctant to give up their special diets. To help the individual with end-stage renal disease make the transition to CAPD as trouble free as possible, you may find it useful to explain clearly some of the possible effects of a restricted diet while on CAPD: (1) **hypotension** and dizziness from sodium depletion; (2) **potassium depletion** resulting in nausea, vomiting, muscle weakness, irregular heartbeat, or listlessness; and (3) **dehydration** caused by rapid fluid removal.

As a guide for patient counseling, you may find it helpful to use the dietary regimen followed by nutritionists at a number of clinics:

- Increase protein intake to provide 1.2 to 1.5 g/kg body weight.
- Limit phosphorus intake to 1200 mg/day by restricting phosphorus-rich foods such as nuts and legumes to one serving a week, and dairy products, including eggs, to a half-cup portion or one egg or its equivalent each day.
- Increase potassium intake by eating a wide variety of fruits and vegetables each day.
- Encourage liberal fluid intake to prevent dehydration.
- Avoid sweets and fats to control triglyceride and HDL levels.
- Maintain lean body weight by incorporating the kilocalories provided by the dialysate into the total meal plan.

Another important factor to keep in mind is that hemodialysis patients often lose their appetite. Thus the most basic aspect of your efforts to help CAPD patients adjust to this new system is to encourage them to eat.

REFERENCES

Bannister DK, et al: Nutritional effects of peritonitis in continuous ambulatory peritoneal dialysis (CAPD) patients, J Am Diet Assoc 87(1):53, Jan 1987.

Blumenkrantz MJ, et al: Metabolic balance studies and dietary protein requirements in patients undergoing continuous ambulatory peritoneal dialysis, Kidney Int 21(6):849, 1982.

Bodnar DM: Rationale for nutritional requirements for patients on continuous ambulatory peritoneal dialysis, J Am Diet Assoc 80(3):247, 1982.

Water balance. Fluid is usually limited to 400 or 500 mL/day, plus an amount equal to urinary output, if any. The total intake must account for additional fluids in the foods consumed and in water derived from metabolism of the food nutrients, as well as in fecal fluid losses. Even with this restriction there may be a mild fluid retention between dialysis treatments, with a daily weight gain in that period of about 1 lb (0.45 kg).

Sodium. To control body fluid retention and hypertension, sodium should be limited to 1000 to 2000 mg day. This restriction helps to prevent pulmonary edema or congestive heart failure from fluid overload.

Potassium. Potassium restriction is imperative to prevent hyperkalemia, which can become a problem. Potassium accumulation can easily cause cardiac arrhythmias or cardiac arrest. Thus a dietary allowance of 1500 to 2000 mg day is usually followed.

Vitamins. During the dialysis treatments, water-soluble vitamins from the blood are lost in the dialysate filtered out of the circulating blood. A daily supplement of all the water-soluble vitamins is therefore usually given. However, the fat-soluble vitamins, especially vitamins A and D, may build up. Thus multivitamin preparations used usually exclude these vitamins.

Kidney Transplant

The transplantation of kidneys from one person to another had been limited because of rejection of the foreign organ by the recipient in many cases, except when the donor and the recipient were identical twins. Now, however, the drug *cyclosporine* is providing more success with organ transplants. This drug not only helps suppress the recipient's immune system cells that attack the transplanted kidney as foreign but also helps fight off infections. Nutritional support for the surgical procedure is an important adjunct to therapy (see Chapter 23). Such successful transplantation has given new life to many persons with chronic renal failure. The quality of this extended life becomes a significant aspect of patient and family counseling (see Issues and Answers, p. 561).

Figure 22-2
Renal calculi: stones in kidney, pelvis, and ureter.

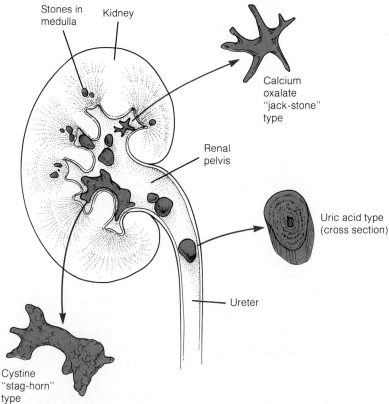

Clinical Application

Individuals on maintenance hemodialysis often have elevated triglyceride levels and depressed high-density lipoprotein (HDL) levels, a metabolic state that increases the risk of coronary heart disease. The exact mechanism causing these changes in blood lipids is unknown, although a carnitine deficiency is suspected.

Carnitine is an amino acid that carries free fatty acids into cell mitochondria, where the fatty acids can be used for energy. The body manufacturers carnitine; additional amounts are provided by the animal products in the diet.

A carnitine deficiency may occur during renal failure because of carnitine losses into the dialysate. The result is a drop in free fatty acids within muscle and other tissues, leading to an irregular heartbeat and poor function in other muscle tissues. The concurrent rise in serum free fatty acids may also trigger the production of triglycerides in the liver. These in turn are released from the liver as very-low-density lipoproteins (VLDL), thus creating another risk for heart disease.

Researchers have been able to reduce triglyceride levels in patients on maintenance hemodialysis by giving them carnitine. Side effects in one experiment affects only two out of 14 subjects, who developed weakness, a prolapsed kidney, and chewing difficulties after taking carnitine for 30 days. Symptoms disappeared after the dosage was reduced from 50 to 30 mg/kg body weight.

Carnitine: Control of Blood Lipids During Maintenance Hemodialysis

REFERENCES
Bartel LL, Hussey JL, and Shargo E: Effects of dialysis on serum carnitine, free fatty acids, and triglyceride levels in man and the rat, Metabolism 31(9):944, 1982.
Walser M: Nutritional support in renal failure: future directions, Lancet 1(8320):340, 1983.

Disease Process

Renal Calculi

The basic cause of renal calculi is unknown, but many factors contribute directly or indirectly to their formation. These factors relate to the nature of the urine itself or to the conditions of the urinary tract environment. According to the concentration of urinary constituents, the major stones formed are calcium, struvite, uric acid, and cystine stones (Figure 22-2).

Calcium Stones

By far the majority of kidney stones—about 96%—are composed of calcium compounds, usually calcium oxalate or calcium oxalate mixed with calcium phosphate.[6] In persons who form stones, which is a familial tendency, the urine produced is supersaturated with these crystalloid elements, and there is a lack of normal urine substances that prevent the crystals from forming stones. Recessive urinary calcium may result from the following:

1. **Excess calcium intake** that may come from prolonged use of large amounts of milk and alkali therapy for peptic ulcer or the use of hard water.

2. **Excess vitamin D** that may cause increased calcium absorption from the intestine as well as increased withdrawal from bone.
3. **Prolonged immobilization,** as in body casts or from extended illness or disability, that may lead to withdrawal of bone calcium and increased urinary concentration.
4. **Hyperparathyroidism** that causes excess calcium excretion. About two thirds of the persons with this endocrine disorder have renal stones, but this disorder accounts for only about 5% of total calcium stones.
5. **Renal tubular acidosis** that causes excess excretion of calcium because of defective ammonia formation.
6. **Idiopathic calciuria** that may cause some persons, even those on lower calcium diets, for unknown reasons to excrete as much as 500 mg of calcium daily.
7. **Oxalate** compounded with calcium that, because of some error in handling oxalates, accounts for about half of the calcium stones. Oxalates occur naturally only in a few food sources (see box, on the facing page).
8. **Animal protein** that has been linked to increased excretions of calcium, oxalate, and urate. A vegetarian-type diet has been recommended by some investigators as a wise choice for stone-forming persons.[7]

Struvite Stones

Struvite stones
Urinary stones made up of ammonia magnesium phosphate, a very hard crystal.

Next to calcium stones in frequency are **struvite stones,** composed of a single compound—magnesium ammonium phosphate ($MgNH_4PO_4$). These are often called "infection stones" because they are associated with urinary tract infections. The offending organism is *Proteus mirabilis.* This is a urea-splitting bacterium that contains urease, an enzyme that hydrolyzes urea to ammonia. Thus the urinary pH becomes alkaline. In the ammonia-rich environment struvite precipitates and forms large, "stag-horn" calculi. Surgical removal is usually indicated.

Uric Acid Stones

Excess uric acid excretion may be caused by an impairment in the intermediary metabolism of purine, such as occurs in gout. It may also result from a rapid tissue breakdown in wasting disease.

Cystine Stones

Cystinuria
A hereditary condition in which large amounts of cystine and other amino acids (lysine, ornithine, and arginine) are secreted in the urine. May result in the formation of urinary cystine calculi.

A hereditary metabolic defect in renal tubular reabsorption of the amino acid cystine causes this substance to accumulate in the urine. This condition is called **cystinuria.** Since this is a genetic disorder, it is characterized by early onset age and a positive family history. Cystinuria is one of the most common metabolic disorders associated with renal stones in children.

Urinary Tract Conditions

The physical changes in the urine and the organic stone matrix provide urinary tract conditions that lead to the formation of renal stones.

Physical Changes in the Urine

Susceptible persons form stones when certain changes take place in the urine. Such changes include:

1. **Urine concentration.** The concentration of the urine may result from a lower water intake or from excess water loss, as in prolonged sweating, fever, vomiting, or diarrhea.

2. **Urinary pH.** Changes in urinary pH from its mean 5.85 to 6.0 may be influenced by the diet or altered by the ingestion of acid or alkili medications.

Organic Stone Matrix

The second factor in renal stone formation is the organic matrix. This necessary core around which crystals may precipitate is a mucoprotein-carbohydrate complex. Possible sources of these organic materials include (1) bacteria masses from recurrent urinary tract infections; (2) renal epithelial tissue of the urinary tract that has sloughed off, possibly because of vitamin A deficiency; and (3) calcified plaques (Randall's plaques) formed beneath the renal epithelium in hypercalciuria. Irritation and ulceration of overlying tissue cause the plaques to slough off into the collecting tubules.

Clinical Symptoms

Severe pain and numerous urinary symptoms may result with renal stone formation, along with general weakness and sometimes fever. Laboratory examination of urine and chemical analysis of any stone passed help determine treatment.

Food Sources of Oxalates

Fruits	Vegetables	Nuts	Beverages	Other
Berries, all	Baked beans	Almonds	Chocolate	Grits
Currants	Beans, green	Cashews	Cocoa	Tofu, soy products
Concord grapes	and wax	Peanuts	Draft beer	
Figs	Beets	Peanut butter	Tea	Wheat germ
Fruit cocktail	Beet greens			
Plums	Celery			
Rhubarb	Chard, Swiss			
Tangerines	Chives			
	Collards			
	Eggplant			
	Endive			
	Kale			
	Leeks			
	Mustard greens			
	Okra			
	Peppers, green			
	Rutabagas			
	Spinach			
	Squash, summer			
	Sweet potatoes			
	Tomatoes			
	Tomato soup			
	Vegetable soup			

General Treatment

Fluid intake. A large fluid intake produces a more dilute urine and is a foundation of therapy. The dilute urine helps to prevent concentration of stone constituents.

Urinary pH. An attempt to control the solubility factor is made by changing the urinary pH to an increased acidity or alkalinity, depending on the chemical composition of the stone formed. An exception is calcium oxalate stones, since the solubility of calcium oxalate in urine is not pH dependent. Conversely, however, calcium phosphate is soluble in an acid urine.

Stone composition. When possible, dietary constituents of the stone are controlled to reduce the amount of the substance available for precipitation.

Binding agents. Materials that bind the stone elements and prevent their absorption in the intestine cause fecal excretion. For example, sodium phytate is used to bind calcium, and aluminum gels are used to bind phosphate. Glycine and calcium have a similar effect on oxalates.

Nutritional Therapy

Nutritional therapy is directly related to the stone chemistry.

Calcium Stones

A low-calcium diet of about 400 mg/day is usually given (see box on facing page). This amount is half of an average adult intake of about 800 mg/day. This lower level is achieved mainly by removal of milk and dairy products. Other calcium food sources that can be limited are leafy vegetables and whole grains. If the stone is calcium phosphate, foods containing phosphorus would also be reduced (see box, p. 552). This is also accomplished mainly by removal of milk and dairy products. Sometimes a test diet of 200 mg of calcium may be used to rule out hyperparathyroidism as a causative factor (see box, p. 553).

Since calcium stones have an alkaline chemistry, an acid ash diet may also be used to help create a urinary environment less conducive to the precipitation of the basic stone elements. The classification of food groups is based on the pH of the metabolic ash produced (see box, p. 554). An acid ash diet would increase the amount of meat, grains, eggs, and cheese (see box, p. 554). On the other hand, it would also limit the amounts of vegetables, milk, and fruits. An alkaline ash diet would outline the opposite use of foods. The use of cranberry juice has been promoted to assist in the acidification of urine. However, the commercially prepared cranberry juices on the consumer market are too dilute to be effective, since they contain only about 26% cranberry juice. Thus an inordinate volume would be required to achieve any consistent effectiveness as a urinary acidifying agent. Instead, to effect a sustained acidifying of urinary pH, most physicians rely on drugs.

Calcium oxalate stones resulting from **hyperoxaluria** would be treated by dietary avoidance of foods high in oxalates (see box, p. 549). Persons with calcium oxalate stones should avoid taking vitamin C supplements because about half the ingested ascorbate may be converted to oxalic acid.

Hyperoxaluria
Excretion of high levels of oxalate in the urine. Oxalates, found in several vegetables (e.g., spinach, tomatoes, rhubarb) combine with calcium to form urinary stones.

Low-Calcium Diet (approximately 400 mg calcium)

	Foods allowed	Foods not allowed
Beverage	Carbonated beverage, coffee, tea	Chocolate-flavored drinks, milk, milk drinks
Bread	White and light rye bread or crackers	
Cereals	Refined cereals	Oatmeal, whole-grain cereals
Desserts	Cake, cookies, gelatin desserts, pastries, pudding, sherbets, all made without chocolate, milk, or nuts; if egg yolk is used, it must be from one egg allowance.	Oatmeal, whole-grain cereals
Fat	Butter, cream (2 tbsp daily) French dressing, margarine, salad oil, shortening	Cream (except in amount allowed), mayonnaise
Fruits	Canned, cooked, or fresh fruits or juice except rhubarb	Dried fruit, rhubarb
Meat, eggs	224 g (8 oz) daily of any meat, fowl, or fish except clams, oysters, or shrimp, not more than one egg daily including those used in cooking	Clams, oysters, shrimp, cheese
Potato or substitute	Potato, hominy, macaroni, noodles, refined rice, spaghetti	Whole-grain rice
Soup	Broth, vegetable soup made from vegetables allowed	Bean or pea soup, cream or milk soup
Sweets	Honey, jam, jelly, sugar	
Vegetables	Any canned, cooked, or fresh vegetables or juice except those listed	Dried beans, broccoli, green cabbage, celery, chard, collards, endive, greens, lettuce, lentils, okra, parsley, parsnips, dried peas, rutabagas
Miscellaneous	Herbs, pickles, popcorn, relishes, salt, spices, vinegar	Chocolate, cocoa, milk gravy, nuts, olives, white sauce

*Depending on calcium content of local water supply. In instances of high calcium content, distilled water may be indicated.

Uric Acid Stones

About 4% of the total incidence of renal calculi are uric acid stones. Since uric acid is a metabolic product of *purines*, dietary control of this precursor is indicated (see box, p. 556). Purines are found in active tissue, such as glandular meat, other lean meat, and meat extractives, and in lesser amounts in plant sources such as whole grains and legumes. An effort to produce an alkaline ash to increase the urinary pH would be indicated.

Low-Phosphorus Diet (approximately 1 g phosphorus and 40 g protein)

	Foods allowed	Foods not allowed
Milk	Not more than 1 cup daily; whole, skim, or buttermilk or 3 tbsp powdered, including the amount used in cooking	
Beverages	Fruit juices, tea, coffee, carbonated drinks, Postum	Milk and milk drinks except as allowed
Bread	White only; enriched commercial, French, hard rolls, soda crackers, rush	Rye and whole-grain breads, cornbread, biscuits, muffins, waffles
Cereals	Refined cereals, such as Cream of Wheat, Cream of Rice, rice, cornmeal, dry cereals, cornflakes, spaghetti, noodles	All whole-grain cereals
Desserts	Berry or fruit-pies, cookies, cakes in average amounts; Jell-O, gelatin, angel food cake, sherbet, meringues made with egg whites, puddings if made with one egg or milk allowance	Desserts with milk and eggs, unless made with the daily allowance
Eggs	Not more than one egg daily, including those used in cooking; extra egg whites may be used	
Fats	Butter, margarine, oils, shortening	
Fruits	Fresh, frozen, canned, as desired	Dried fruits such as raisins, prunes, dates, figs, apricots
Meat	One large serving or two small servings daily of beef, lamb, veal, pork, rabbit, chicken, or turkey	Fish, shellfish (crab, oyster, shrimp, lobster, and so on), dried and cured meats (bacon, ham, chipped beef, and so on), liver, kidney, sweetbreads, brains
Cheese	None	Avoid all cheese and cheese spreads
Vegetables	Potatoes as desired; at least two servings per day of any of the following: asparagus, carrots, beets, green beans, squash, lettuce, rutabagas, tomatoes, celery, peas, onions, cucumber, corn; no more than 1 serving daily of either cabbage, spinach, broccoli, cauliflower, brussels sprouts, or artichokes	Dried vegetables such as peas, mushrooms, lima beans
Miscellaneous	Sugar, jams, jellies, syrups, salt, spices, seasonings; condiments in moderation	Chocolate, nuts, nut products such as peanut butter, cream sauces

Sample menu pattern

Breakfast	Lunch	Dinner
Fruit juice	Meat 56 g (2 oz)	Meat 56 g
Refined cereal	Potato	Potato
Egg	Vegetable	Vegetable
White toast	Salad	Salad
Butter	Bread, white	Bread, white
½ cup milk	Butter	Butter
Coffee or tea	½ cup milk	Dessert
	Dessert	Coffee or tea
	Coffee or tea	

Low-Calcium Test Diet (200 mg calcium)

	Grams	Milligrams calcium
Breakfast		
Orange juice, fresh	100	19.00
Bread (toast), white	25	19.57
Butter	15	3.00
Rice Krispies	15	3.70
Cream, 20% butterfat	35	33.95
Sugar	7	0.00
Jam	20	2.00
Distilled water, coffee, or tea*		0.00
TOTAL		81.22
Lunch		
Beef steak, cooked	100	10.00
Potato	100	11.0
Tomatoes	100	11.0
Bread	25	19.57
Butter	15	3.00
Honey	20	1.00
Applesauce	20	1.00
Distilled water, coffee, or tea		0.00
TOTAL		56.57
Dinner		
Lamb chop, cooked	90	10.00
Potato	100	11.00
Frozen green peas	80	10.32
Bread	25	19.57
Butter	15	3.00
Jam	20	2.00
Peach sauce	100	5.00
Distilled water, coffee, or tea		0.00
TOTAL		60.89
TOTAL MILLIGRAMS CALCIUM		198.68

*Use distilled water only for cooking and for beverages.

Acid and Alkaline Ash Food Groups

Acid ash	Alkaline ash	Neutral
Meat	Milk	Sugars
Whole grains	Vegetables	Fats
Eggs	Fruits (except cranberries, prunes,	Beverages (coffee, tea)
Cheese	plums)	
Cranberries		
Prunes		
Plums		

Acid Ash Diet

The purpose of this diet is to furnish a well-balanced diet in which the total acid ash is greater than the total alkaline ash each day. It lists (1) unrestricted foods, (2) restricted foods, (3) foods not allowed, and (4) sample of a day's diet.

Unrestricted foods: Eat as much a desired of the following foods.
- Bread: any, preferably whole grain; crackers, rolls
- Cereals: any, preferably whole grain
- Desserts: angel food or sunshine cake; cookies made without baking powder or soda; cornstarch pudding, cranberry desserts, custards, gelatin desserts, ice cream sherbet, plum or prune desserts; rice or tapioca pudding
- Fats: any, as in butter, margarine, salad dressings, Crisco, Spry, lard, salad oils, olive oil
- Fruits: cranberries, plums, prunes
- Meat, eggs, cheese; any meat, fish, or fowl, two servings daily; at least one egg daily
- Potato substitutes: corn, hominy, lentils, macaroni, noodles, rice, spaghetti, vermicelli
- Soup: broth as desired; other soups from foods allowed
- Sweets: cranberry or plum jelly; sugar, plain sugar candy
- Miscellaneous: cream sauce, gravy, peanut butter, peanuts, popcorn, salt, spcies, vinegar, walnuts

Restricted foods: Do not eat any more than the amount allowed each day.
- Milk: 2 cups daily (may be used in other ways than as beverage)
- Cream: ⅓ cup or less daily
- Fruits: one serving of fruit daily (in addition to prunes, plums, cranberries); certain fruits listed under "Sample menu" are not allowed at any time
- Vegetables including potato: two servings daily; certain vegetables listed under "Foods not allowed" are not allowed at any time

Foods not allowed
- Carbonated beverages, such as ginger ale, cola, root beer
- Cakes or cookies made with baking powder or soda
- Fruits: dried apricots, bananas, dates, figs, raisins, rhubarb
- Vegetables: dried beans, beet greens, dandelion greens, carrots, chard, lima beans
- Sweets: chocolate or other candies than those under "Unrestricted foods"; syrups
- Miscellaneous: other nuts, olives, pickles

Sample menu

Breakfast	Lunch	Dinner
Grapefruit	Creamed chicken	Broth
Wheatena	Steamed rice	Roast beef, gravy
Scrambled eggs	Green beans	Buttered noodles
Toast, butter, plum jam	Stewed prunes	Sliced tomato
Coffee, cream, sugar	Bread, butter	Mayonnaise
	Milk	Vanilla ice cream
		Bread, butter

Cystine Stones

About 1% of the total stones produced are cystine, since it is a relatively rare genetic disease. Cystine is a nonessential amino acid produced from the essential amino acid *methionine*. Thus a diet low in methionine is used (see box, p. 557). This diet is used with high fluid and alkali therapy.

The nutritional therapy principles in renal stone disease are outlined in Table 22-2.

Disease Process

The term *urinary tract infection (UTI)* refers to a wide variety of clinical infections in which a significant number of microorganisms are present in any portion of the urinary tract. A common form is **cystitis,** an inflammation of the bladder prevalent in young women. The condition is called recurrent UTI if three or more bouts are experienced in a year. The majority of cases are caused by aerobic members of the fecal flora, especially *Escherichia coli.* The presence of these organisms in the urine is termed **bacteriuria.** Urine produced by the normal kidney is sterile and remains so as it travels to the bladder. In UTI, however, the normal urethra has microbial flora, so that any voided urine normally contains many bacteria. Bacteriuria is present when the quantity of organisms is more than 100,000 bacteria per milliliter of urine. The female anatomy is more conducive to entry of these bacteria into the urinary tract. Recurrent cystitis occurs mostly in young and otherwise healthy women who have infections that usually correspond with sexual activity and diaphragm use. In most cases simply having the diaphragm re-

Urinary Tract Infection

Cystitis
Inflammation of the bladder. Can be caused by allergy, bacteria, gonorrhea, and other conditions. Often characterized by frequent voiding and burning. Untreated, it may lead to stone formation.

Bacteriuria
Presence of bacteria in the urine.

Stone chemistry	Nutrient modification	Diet ash

Calcium
  Phosphate
  Oxalate
	Low calcium (400 mg)
	  Low phosphorus (1000-1200 mg)
	  Low oxalate
		Acid ash

Struvite ($MgNH_4PO_4$)	Low phosphorus (1000-1200 mg) (associated with urinary infections)	Acid ash
Uric acid	Low purine	Alkaline ash
Cystine	Low methionine	Alkaline ash

Table 22-2
Summary of Diet Principles in Renal Stone Disease

Low-Purine Diet (approximately 125 mg purine)

General directions

- During acute stages use only list 1.
- After acute stage subsides and for chronic conditions, use the following schedule:
  Two days a week, not consecutive, use list 1 entirely.
  The remaining days add foods from list 2 and 3, as indicated.
  Avoid list 4 entirely.
- Keep diet moderately low in fat.

Typical meal pattern

Breakfast	Lunch	Dinner
Fruit	Egg or cheese dish	Egg or cheese dish
Refined cereal and/or egg	Vegetables, as allowed (cooked or salad)	Cream of vegetable soup, if desired
White toast	Potato or substitute	Starch (potato or substitute)
Butter, 1 tsp	White bread	Colored vegetable, as allowed
Sugar	Butter, 1 tsp	White bread, butter, 1 tsp, if desired
Coffee	Fruit or simple dessert	Salad, as allowed
Milk, if desired	Milk	Fruit or simple dessert
		Milk

Food list 1
May be used as desired; foods that contain an insignificant amount of purine bodies

Beverages
  Carbonated
  Chocolate
  Cocoa
  Coffee
  Fruit juices
  Postum
  Tea
Butter*
Bread: White and crackers, cornbread
Cereals and cereal products
  Corn
  Rice
  Tapioca
  Refined wheat
  Macaroni
  Noodles

Cheese of all kinds*
Eggs
Fats of all kinds* (moderation)
Fruits of all kinds
Gelatin, Jell-O
Milk: buttermilk, evaporated, malted, sweet
Nuts of all kinds,* peanut butter
Pies* (except mincemeat)
Sugar and sweets
Vegetables
  Artichokes
  Beets
  Beet greens
  Broccoli
  Brussels sprouts
  Cabbage
  Carrots

  Celery
  Corn
  Cucumber
  Eggplant
  Endive
  Kohlrabi
  Lettuce
  Okra
  Parsnips
  Potato, white and sweet
  Pumpkin
  Rutabagas
  Sauerkraut
  String beans
  Summer squash
  Swiss chard
  Tomato
  Turnips

*High in fat.

Food list 2
One item four times a week; foods that contain a moderate amount (up to 75 mg) of purine bodies in 100 g serving

Asparagus	Finnan haddie	Mushrooms	Salmon
Bluefish	Ham	Mutton	Shad
Bouillon	Herring	Navy beans	Spinach
Cauliflower	Kidney beans	Oatmeal	Tripe
Chicken	Lima beans	Oysters	Tuna fish
Crab	Lobster	Peas	Whitefish

Food list 3
One item once a week; foods that contain a large amount (75-150 mg) of purine bodies in 100 g serving

Bacon	Duck	Perch	Sheep
Beef	Goose	Pheasant	Shellfish
Calf tongue	Halibut	Pigeon	Squab
Carp	Lentils	Pike	Trout
Chicken soup	Liver sausage	Pork	Turkey
Codfish	Meat soups	Quail	Veal
	Partridge	Rabbit	Venison

Foods list 4
Avoid entirely; foods that contain very large amounts (150-1000 mg) of purine bodies in 100 g serving

Sweetbreads	825 mg	Kidneys (beef)	200
Anchovies	363 mg	Brains	195 mg
Sardines (in oil)	295 mg	Meat extracts	160-400 mg
Liver (calf, beef)	233 mg	Gravies	Variable

Low-Methionine Diet

	Foods allowed	Foods not allowed
Soup	Any soup made without meat stock or addition of milk	Rich meat soups, broth, canned soups made with meat broth
Meat or meat substitute	Peanut butter sandwich, spaghetti, or macaroni dish made without addition of meat, cheese, or milk; one serving per day; chicken, lamb, veal, beef, pork, crab, or bacon (3)	Fish and those not listed above
Beverages	Soy milk, tea, coffee	Milk in any form
Vegetables	Asparagus, artichoke, beans, beets, carrots, chicory, cucumber, eggplant, escarole, lettuce, onions, parsnips, potatoes, pumpkin, rhubarb, tomatoes, turnips	Those not listed as allowed

Adapted from Smith DR, Kolb FO, and Harper HA: The management of cystinuria and cystine-stone disease, J Urol 81:61, 1959.
*Optional: use in children to include protein intake. Omit if urin calcium is elevated in adults.

Continued.

Low-Methionine Diet—cont'd

	Foods allowed	Foods not allowed
Fruits	Apples, apricots, bananas, berries, cherries, fruit cocktail, grapefruit, grapes, lemon juice, nectarines, oranges, peaches, pears, pineapple, plums, tangerines, watermelon, cantaloupe	Those not listed as allowed
Salads	Raw or cooked vegetable or fruit salad	
Cereals	Macaroni, spaghetti, noodles	
Bread	Whole wheat, rye, white	
Nuts	Peanuts	
Desserts	Fresh or cooked fruit, ices, fruit pies	
Eggs		In any form
Cheese		All varieties
Concentrated sweets	Sugar, jams, jellies, syrup, honey, hard candy	
Concentrated fats	Butter, margarine, cream	
Miscellaneous	Pepper, mustard, vinegar, garlic, oil, herbs, spices	

Meal pattern

Breakfast	Lunch	Dinner
1 cup fruit juice	1 serving soup	56 g (2 oz) meat
½ cup fruit	1 serving sandwich	1 med starch
1 slice toast	1 cup fruit	½ cup vegetable
1½ pats butter	240 ml (8 oz) soy milk*	1 serving salad
2 tsp jelly	3 tsp sugar	1 tbsp dressing
1 tbsp sugar	1 tbsp cream	1 slice bread
Beverage	Beverage	1 serving dessert
1 tbsp cream		1 tbsp cream
		1 tbsp sugar
		1 tbsp cream
		1½ pats butter
		Beverage

Sample menu

Breakfast	Lunch	Dinner
Orange juice	Vegetable soup, vegetarian	Chicken, roast
Applesauce	Peanut butter sandwich	Bake potato
Whole-wheat toast	Canned peaches	Artichoke
Butter	Soy milk*	Sliced tomatoes
Jelly	Sugar	French dressing
Sugar	Cream	Whole-wheat bread
Coffee	Coffee or tea	Fruit ice
Cream		Sugar
		Cream
		Butter
		Coffee or tea

fitted to a smaller size or changing to another birth control method will solve the problem.

Clinical Symptoms

Cystitis is characterized by frequent voiding and burning on urination. Untreated, it may lead to stone formation.

Treatment

Currently antibiotic treatment has been greatly cut back. Studies show that a single dose of antibiotic is just as effective as the usual 7- to 10-day treatment in 90% of all women who have uncomplicated cystitis.[8] General nutritional measures include acidifying the urine by taking vitamin C, since cranberry juice is not effective, and drinking a large amount of fluids to produce a dilute urine. Control of UTI is an important measure, since it is a risk factor in stone formation.

Commercially prepared cranberry juice is too dilute to be effective in acidifying the urine.

To Sum Up

Through its unique functional units, the nephrons, the kidneys act as a filtration system, reabsorbing substances the body needs, secreting additional hydrogen ions to maintain a proper pH balance in the blood, and excreting unnecessary materials in a concentrated urine. Renal function can be impaired by a variety of conditions. These include inflammatory and degenerative diseases, infection and obstruction, chronic diseases such as hypertension and diabetes, environmental agents such as insecticides and solvents and other toxic substances, some medications, and trauma. Some clinical conditions affecting structure and function include glomerulonephritis, nephrotic syndrome, acute and chronic renal failure, renal calculi, and urinary tract infection. In many cases, except nephrotic syndrome, dietary protein may need to be reduced as part of the nutritional care plan. Water, electrolytes, and kilocalorie intake should also be closely monitored to match individual needs.

Chronic kidney disease at its end stage is treated by *dialysis* and *kidney transplant*. Dialysis patients must be monitored closely for protein, water, and electrolyte balance. Nutritional support of transplant patients is needed primarily as support for the surgical procedure. A normal diet is often well tolerated after surgery and convalescence.

Renal diseases have predisposing factors. For example, untreated urinary tract infections may lead to renal calculi, and progressive glomerulonephritis may lead to nephrotic syndrome. The Western diet is suspect as a predisposing factor in the development of chronic renal failure. Excess protein intake may overtax human nephrons, which were not originally designed to handle a steady diet of protein-rich foods.

Questions for Review

1. For each of the following conditions, outline the nutritional components of therapy, explaining the impact of each on kidney function: glomerulonephritis, nephrotic syndrome, and chronic renal failure.
2. Identify four clinical conditions that can impair renal function. Give an example of each, describing its effect on various structures in the kidney.
3. List the nutritional factors that must be monitored in individuals undergoing renal dialysis.

4. Outline the medical and nutritional therapy used for patients with various types of renal calculi. Describe each type of stone and explain the rationale for each aspect of therapy.
5. For what condition is a urinary tract infection a predisposing factor? What general nutritional principles are recommended in the treatment of such infections?

References

1. Klahr S, Schreiner G, and Ichikawa I: The progression of renal disease, N Engl J Med 318(25):1657, June 23, 1988.
2. Feinstein EI: Total parenteral nutritional support of patients with acute renal failure, Nutr Clin Pract 3(1):9, Feb 1988.
3. Hak LJ, and Raasch RH: Use of amino acids in patients with acute renal failure, Nutr Clin Pract 3(1):19, Feb 1988.
4. Mitch W, Abras E, and Walser M: Long-term effects of a new ketoacid-amino acid supplement in patients with chronic renal failure, Kidney Int 22(1):48, 1982.
5. Maschio G, et al: Effects of dietary protein and phosphorous restriction on the progression of early renal failure, Kidney Int 22(4):371, 1982.
6. Metheny N: Renal stones amd urinary pH, Am J Nurs 82:1372, Sept 1982.
7. Brockis JG, Levitt AJ, and Cruthers SM: The effects of vegetable and animal protein diets on calcium, urate, and oxalate excretion, Br J Urol 54:590, 1982.
8. Cystitis: less drastic solutions, Health Facts 8(51):2, 1983.

Further Readings

Bannister DK, et al: Nutritional effects of peritonitis in continuous ambulatory peritoneal dialysis (CAPD) patients, J Am Diet Assoc 87(1):53, Jan 1987.

This article describes the process of CAPD and evaluates the complication of infection of the peritoneal membrane and its effect on the nutritional status of the patient.

Feinstein EI: Total parenteral nutritional support of patients with acute renal failure, Nutr Clin Pract 3(1):9, Feb 1988.

This article discusses the causes of extensive protein catabolism seen in acute renal failure and some of the newer methods for maintaining fluid balance during TPN.

Hak LJ, and Raasch RH: Use of amino acids in patients in patients with acute renal failure, Nutr Clin Pract 3(1):19, Feb 1988.

These pharmacists present a case report of a patient with acute renal failure and discuss the types of amino acids used in TPN feedings.

Klahr S, Schreiner G, and Ichikawa I: The progression of renal disease, N Engl J Med 318(25):1657, June 23, 1988.

These authors provide an excellent review of the mechanisms underlying the progressive nature of chronic renal insufficiency to end-stage failure and the nutritional effects that accumulate.

Renal Disease: Technology vs the Quality of Life

Imagine spending up to 18 hours a week hooked up to a machine to which you literally owed your life. Imagine having a 40% chance of never being able to work outside the home again, leading a life of poverty and restricted mobility—all because of that machine. This is probably hard for most of us to imagine. Yet for approximately 55,000 Americans on maintenance dialysis, this is the reality of everyday life. And all of us on the medical-nutrition-nursing renal care team must also deal with this reality daily in our work with these persons and their families. Especially is this sensitivity needed in nutrition counseling and teaching. Food is tied up with so many personal values that when it must be drastically changed—or when choice is gone altogether—it's as if a part of the self has been diminished.

Researchers, physicians, and other renal team members, as well as clients, are becoming increasingly concerned with the *quality* of life rather than merely the *length* of life available to the person on dialysis. The only alternative currently available is kidney transplantation. On the surface, this method could be considered preferable to hemodialysis or even peritoneal dialysis because it frees the individual from any mechanical device. However, researchers are beginning to investigate the quality of life a kidney transplant provides to determine whether either method is preferable to the other.

The first issue of greatest concern is, of course, the effect of the treatment method on lifespan. Mortality rates for individuals on dialysis (8% to 15%) are in the same range as those for people recieving their first kidney transplant from a parent or a sibling (10% to 15%). However, rates among young dialysis patients with no extrarenal disease can drop as low as 2%, in contrast with rates that can soar to 30% among individuals receiving kidneys from cadavers. Still, some people feel that the benefits of increased mobility outweigh the drawbacks of a possible reduction in lifespan.

In one study, life quality measures (sleep habits, food habits, energy level, sexual activity, changes in income and/or employment, satsifaction with marriage, etc.) were examined among individuals on dialysis compared with successful transplant operations and unsuccessful operations. As expected, subjects who had had successful operations reported a near-normal quality of life—they were less tired, less inconvenienced by frequent medical treatments, and had better incomes and/or more full-time employment following renal failure than other renal patients.

Also as expected, individuals whose transplant operations were not successful indicated that the quality of their lives was the lowest of all subjects. For example, none of these subjects reported full-time employment since renal failure. They were mainly recipients of kidneys from cadavers. Thus this process is assumed to be the least desirable of all possible alternatives.

A surprising result of this study was that dialysis patients who never recieved a transplant felt that the quality of their lives was also near normal. Researchers admit that the reason for this probably includes denial or accommodation. However, they also acknowledge that human response to life experiences is an extremely complex issue, one that is difficult to assess with current "immature" research methods available for evaluating the quality of life in general.

The health care team responsible for the individual with renal failure may have its own set of parameters for determining the quality of life each mode of treatment may provide. The results of this study suggest that patients' own evaluation of their lives may involve factors much more complex than those to which the professional has been exposed. The study serves as a reminder that professionals must be open to the concerns and viewpoints of the individual faced with such major choices in treatment and relate their care planning in all areas to these personal concerns.

REFERENCES

Husbye DG, et al: Psychosocial, social, and somatic prognostic indicators in old patients undergoing long-term dialysis, Arch Int Med 147:1921, Nov 1987.

Johnson PJ, McCauley CR, and Copley JB: The quality of life of hemodialysis and transplant patients, Kidney Int 22(3):286, 1982.

23 Nutritional Care of Surgery Patients

Chapter Objectives

After study of this chapter, the student should be able to:

1. Describe the relation of malnutrition to the outcome of surgical treatment and identify means of avoiding this complicating condition.

2. Relate nutritional therapy to tissue healing.

3. Identify special nutritional problems of gastrointestinal surgery and outline an appropriate plan of care in each case.

4. Describe parenteral modes of feeding to meet unusual nutritional needs.

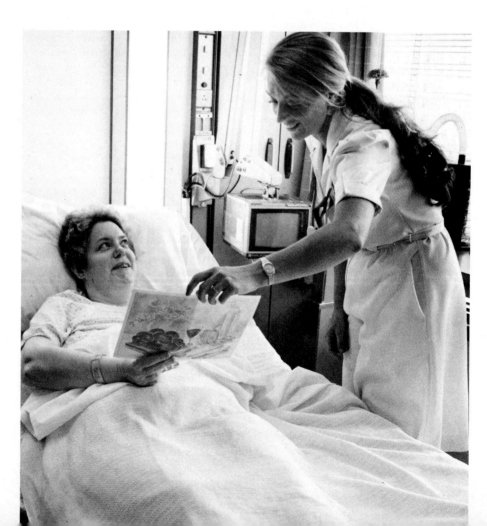

PREVIEW

A high incidence of malnutrition among hospitalized patients has been observed over the past few years. A large number of these malnourished persons are surgery patients. In numerous surveys in both American and European hospitals nearly 50% of the surgery patients have had clinical evidence of protein-energy malnutrition.

Effective nutritional support can reverse this malnutrition, markedly improve prognosis, and speed recovery. A spectrum of feeding modes, both enteral and parenteral, have helped to provide these remarkable means.

Surgery itself places physiologic and psychologic stress on patients. This state of stress brings added nutritional demands. Deficiencies can accrue easily and may lead to serious clinical problems. Careful attention to preoperative preparation, together with vigorous postoperative nutritional support, can reduce complications and provide resources for better healing and more rapid recovery.

In this chapter in our continuing clinical nutrition sequence, we will examine these nutritional demands of surgery. We will see how the type and extent of the surgical procedure, as well as the nature of any preceding injury, influence special nutritional therapy requirements and the mode of feeding needed to meet these nutritional demands.

Preoperative Nutrition

Nutrient Stores

Nutritional Needs of General Surgery Patients

Nutritional reserves fortify the patient for the demands of surgery. When time permits, nutritional preparation should correct any nutrient deficiencies. It should also provide resources for the surgery itself and for the immediate postoperative period until regular feedings can be resumed.

1. **Protein.** The most common nutritional deficiency in surgery patients is that of protein. Tissue and plasma reserves are imperative to prepare the patient for blood losses during surgery and for tissue breakdown in the immediate postoperative period of catabolism.

2. **Energy.** Sufficient kilocalories must be provided to build up any deficit. Carbohydrate is needed for glycogen stores and to spare protein for tissue synthesis.

3. **Vitamins and minerals.** Normal tissue stores of vitamins are needed for the added metabolism of carbohydrates and protein. Any deficiency state such as anemia should be corrected. Electrolytes and fluids should be in balance and correction made of any dehydration, acidosis, or alkalosis.

Persons with bleeding tendencies may be given added vitamin C before surgery.

Immediate Preoperative Period

In the usual preparation for surgery, nothing is given by mouth for at least 8 hours before surgery. This ensures that the stomach has no retained food at the time of the operation. In case of emergency surgery, if the patient has recently eaten a meal, gastric suction is used. Food in the stomach may be vomited or aspirated during surgery or recovery from anesthesia. Also, any food present may increase the possibility of postoperative gastric retention

Elemental formula
Formula whose components cannot be broken down into simpler parts.

and dilation. It may also interfere with the procedure itself, especially in abdominal surgery. Before gastrointestinal surgery, a low-residue or residue-free diet may be followed for several days to clear the operative site of any food residue. Low-residue, chemically defined formulas—**elemental formulas**—can provide a complete diet in liquid form. Such formulas, if palatable enough, can be taken orally in sufficient amounts to maintain nutritional resources. Otherwise they may be fed by tube.

Postoperative Nutrition

Healthy body tissues undergo continuous turnover, with small physiologic losses being constantly replenished by nutrients in the food eaten. In disease, however, especially surgical disease, losses are greatly increased. At the same time, replacement from food is diminished or even absent for a brief or extended period. Nutritional support, therefore, becomes all the more significant as a means of aiding recovery.

Protein

Adequate protein intake in the postoperative recovery period is of primary therapeutic concern to replace losses and supply increased demands. In addition to protein losses from tissue breakdown, added loss of plasma proteins can occur through hemorrhage, wound bleeding, and **exudates.** Increased

Exudate
Material that escapes from blood vessels and is deposited in tissues or tissue surfaces; characterized by a high content of protein, cells, or other cellular solid matter.

A negative nitrogen balance of as much as 20 g/day may occur after surgery. This represents an actual loss of tissue protein of over 1 lb/day.

metabolic losses of protein can also result from extensive tissue destruction and inflammation or from trauma and infection. If any degree of prior malnutrition or chronic infection existed, the patient's protein deficit may actually become severe and cause serious complications. There are a number of reasons for this increased protein demand:

1. **Tissue synthesis in wound healing.** Tissue proteins can be synthesized only by essential amino acids brought to the tissue by the circulating blood. The necessary essential amino acids must come either from the diet protein or by intravenous feeding. Tissue protein deficiencies are best met by oral feeding. As early as possible an intake of 100 to 150 g/day should be attempted to restore lost protein tissues and synthesize new tissue at the wound site. Although tissue protein is broken down more rapidly during stress, fortunately it is also built up more rapidly, provided sufficient amino acids are present to supply the anabolic demand. If oral feedings are possible, although appetite is poor, palatable concentrated liquid drinks or commercial formulas are useful.

2. **Avoidance of shock.** A reduction in blood volume—*hypovolemia*—from a loss of plasma proteins and a decrease in circulating red blood cell volume contribute to the potential danger of shock. When protein deficiencies exist, this danger is increased.

3. **Control of edema.** When the serum protein is low, edema develops as a result of the loss of colloidal osmotic pressure required to maintain the normal shift of fluid between the capillaries and the surrounding interstitial tissue spaces. This general edema may affect heart and lung action. Also, local edema at the surgical site delays closure of the wound and hinders normal healing.

4. **Bone healing.** In orthopedic surgery, extensive bone healing is involved. Protein is essential for proper **callus** formation and calcification. A sound protein matrix is mandatory for the anchoring of mineral matter.

Callus
Unorganized meshwork of newly grown, woven bone developed on pattern of original fibrin clot (formed after fracture) and which is normally replaced by hard adult bone.

5. **Resistance to infection.** Amino acids are necessary constituents of the proteins involved in body defense mechanisms. These defense agents include antibodies, special blood cells, hormones, and enzymes. Tissue integrity itself is a first line of defense against infections.

6. **Lipid transport.** Protein is necessary for the transport of lipids in the body's blood circulation. Special apoproteins, mostly in the liver, coat lipids to form lipoproteins, the transport form of fat. Proteins thus protect the liver, a main site of fat metabolism, from danger caused by fatty infiltration.

Multiple clinical problems may easily develop following surgery when protein deficiencies exist. There may be poor wound healing, or **dehiscence,** delayed healing of fractures, anemia, failure of gastrointestinal stomas to function, depressed lung and heart function, reduced resistance to infection, extensive weight loss, liver damage, and increased mortality risks.

Dehiscence
Splitting open, separation of the layers of a surgical wound.

Water

Water balance is a vital concern after surgery. Adequate fluid therapy is necessary to prevent dehydration. Large water losses may occur from vomiting, hemorrhage, exudates, diuresis, or fever. When drainage is involved, as is common in many surgeries, there is still more fluid loss. Intravenous therapy will supply initial needs, but oral intake should begin as soon as possible and be maintained in sufficient quantity, according to individual needs, to avoid both extremes of dehydration and water intoxication. Daily weight of the patient provides a guideline for meeting fluid requirements.

Energy

As is always the case when increased protein is demanded for tissue rebuilding, sufficient nonprotein energy kilocalories must be supplied to protect the protein for use in tissue synthesis. Adequate amounts of *carbohydrate* are essential to ensure the use of protein for building tissue and to supply the energy required for the increased metabolic demands. As protein is increased, the total kilocalories must be increased as well, since sufficient caloric intake is often crucial to the successful outcome of the surgical procedure. About 2800 kcal/day must be provided before protein can be used to tissue repair and not be diverted to help provide energy. In acute stress, as in extensive surgery or burns, when protein needs may be as high as 200 g/day, 4000 to 6000 kcal may be required. In addition to its protein-sparing action, carbohydrate also helps to avoid liver damage from depletion of glycogen reserves. *Fat* must be adequate to maintain body tissue fat reserves but it must not be excessive.

Vitamins

All of the vitamins play important roles in the healing process. Vitamin C is imperative for wound healing. It is necessary for the formation of cementing material in the ground substance of connective tissue, in capillary walls, and in the building up of new tissue. Extensive tissue regeneration, such as occurs in burns or radical surgeries, may require vitamin C supplements. As kilocalorie and protein intakes are increased, the B vitamins must also be increased. They provide essential coenzyme factors for protein and energy metabolism. Vitamin K is essential in the blood clotting mechanism.

Minerals

Replacing mineral deficiencies and ensuring continued adequacy are essential. In tissue breakdown, potassium and phosphorus are lost. Electrolyte losses, especially sodium and chloride, accompany fluid losses. Iron-deficiency anemia may develop from blood loss or malabsorption.

General Dietary Management

Oral Feeding

The majority of general surgical patients can and should progress to oral feeding as soon as possible to provide adequate nutrition. Remember that routine postoperative intravenous fluids are intended to supply hydration needs and electrolytes, not to sustain nutritional needs. Ordinary postsurgical intravenous therapy cannot supply full nutrient needs or compete with oral feedings. A rapid return to regular eating should be encouraged and maintained.

Parenteral Feeding

In cases of major tissue trauma or damage or when a patient is unable to obtain sufficient nutrients orally, parenteral feeding may be necessary. It provides crucial nutritional support from solutions containing higher percentage glucose, amino acids, electrolytes, minerals, and vitamins, with lipid emulsions fed separately about twice a week through a Y-tube connection, for needed kilocalories. Such solutions may be fed for brief periods by peripheral vein feeding or for longer periods of more severe nutritional need by central vein feeding—*total parenteral nutrition (TPN)*.

Particularly in cases of major surgery, aggressive enteral and parenteral nutrition support is often a primary factor in determining the outcome. Few clinicians, skilled and intent on their surgical task, fully realize that 50% or more of the patients awaiting or recovering from surgery are malnourished.[1] Studies repeatedly show that malnourished patients have higher postoperative morbidity and mortality than well-nourished patients do and that comprehensive nutrition assessment and vigorous therapy support a positive outcome.[2,3]

Routine Postoperative Diets

Oral intake of solid foods should be encouraged and supported as soon as possible after surgery to hasten recovery.

As rapidly as possible, as soon as intestinal peristalsis returns, water and *clear liquids* such as tea, coffee, broth, and juice may be given to help supply important fluids and some sodium and chloride. These initial liquids also help stimulate normal gastrointestinal function and early return to a full diet. Progression to *full liquids* should soon follow. Milk and milk products—including puddings, cream soups, high-protein beverages, and ice cream—supply much vital protein and carbohydrate. Each patient will progress to solid food in *soft to regular diets* according to individual tolerance.

Special Nutritional Needs for Head and Neck Surgery Patients

Head and Neck Surgery

Surgery involving mouth, throat, and neck will require modification in the manner of feeding. The patient usually cannot chew or swallow normally.

Oral Liquid Feedings

Concentrated feedings in liquid form must be planned. These feedings may consist of special enteral formulas of protein hydrolysates or amino acids with added carbohydrate, fat, vitamins, and minerals. As tolerated, milk-based beverages, soups, and fruit juices with lactose can supply frequent re-inforced oral nourishment. A milk shake–type formula supplemented with skim milk powder or other protein concentrate can supply 20 g of protein and 400 kcal (see Chapter 19).

Tube Feedings

Patients who are comatose or severely debilitated or who have undergone radical neck or facial surgery may require tube feeding. New developments in small-bore feeding tubes have made this method of feeding easier. In cases of long-term need, rapid development of sophisticated delivery systems and standardized formulas has made continued home enteral nutrition possible for many patients.[4]

A wide variety of feeding tubes for enteral nutrition are available. Usually a nasogastric tube is used (see Chapter 24). In cases of esophageal obstruction, surgical insertion of a special tube may be made through the abdominal wall, a procedure called a *gastrostomy*. In other cases a special Moss tube may be placed during surgery for short-term postsurgical feeding to allow early intake of an elemental formula and avoid postoperative **paralytic** or **adynamic ileus.** The tube may be removed 2 days after surgery and can be followed by oral elemental formula and a full low-residue diet soon thereafter. In general the tube feeding formula will be prescribed according to the patient's need and tolerance. Small amounts of formula are used at first and gradually increased. Usually 2 L of formula is sufficient for a 24-hour period. The feeding should not exceed 240 to 360 ml (8 to 12 oz) in each 3- to 4-hour interval. Two general types of formula may be used:

1. **Commercial formulas.** A number of commercial formulas of different types are available for selection and use according to individual need. These products may be made from **intact nutrient** sources for use with an intact bowel able to digest and absorb them. Others may use predigested or **elemental nutrients,** which are readily absorbed with only minimal residue. Still others may be formulas designed for special problems, or single-nutrient modules of protein, carbohydrate, and fat, which may be mixed to meet the patient's specific needs.

2. **Blended food mixtures.** Sometimes blended food mixtures are preferred by some persons, especially older patients at home who feel comforted by "regular food." Any food that will liquefy in a high-speed blender can be used, or strained baby food may be added to simplify the mixing process. Ingredients may include a milk base, with added egg, strained meat, vegetable, fruit, fruit juices, nonfat dry milk, cream, vitamins, or minerals as needed (Table 23-1). Some patients may wish to use blended food mixtures because of the cost factor involved in long-term use of commercial formula products. Close nutritional monitoring of such blended formulas is necessary, however. Sometimes when they are diluted to go through the tube, the nutrient density may not compare with that of a commercial formula. With both commercial and blended home formulas, diarrhea may be a problem from bacterial contamination caused by poor handling of formula and equipment or by intolerance of an ingredient such as lactose.[5] However, these problems can be evaluated and prevented.

Although long-term tube feeding may well meet physiologic needs, it also carries psychologic burdens. Support for the quality of life must also be a part of patient care planning.

Paralytic or adynamic ileus
Obstruction of the intestines, resulting from inhibition of bowel motility.

Commercial formulas provide the advantages of convenience, formulation to meet special needs, and sanitation. They have disadvantages of cost (especially with long-term use) and osmolality problems with concentration of materials in solution.

Intact nutrient
A nutrient in its natureal undigested form, such as protein.

Elemental nutrient
A single nutrient component as rendered normally by digestion, such as an amino acid.

Blended food formulas provide the advantages of lower cost, calculation to meet personal tolerances, usually less problems with osmolality, and the psychologic advantage of being "real food." They have the disadvantage of problems with sanitation in mixing and storing.

Table 23-1

Sample Tube Feeding Formula (2500 ml, 3000 kilocalories)

Ingredients	Amount	Protein	Fat	Carbohydrate
Homogenized milk	1 L	32	40	48
Eggs	3	21	16	
Apple juice	400 ml			55
Vegetable oil	30 ml		30	
Strained baby food (112 g [4 oz] jars)				
Beef liver	4 jars	56	12	14
Beets	2 jars	3		20
Peaches	2 jars	1	1	59
Sustagen	1½ cups (225 g)	52	7	150
(Water as needed to total 2500 ml)				
TOTALS		165	106	346
TOTAL CALORIES			2998	

Special Nutritional Needs for Gastrointestinal Surgery Patients

Vagotomy
Interruption of the impulses carried by the vagus nerve(s), resulting in prevention of increased flow or acidity of gastric secretions.

Gastric Resection

Nutrition Problems

A number of nutrition problems may develop following gastric surgery, depending on the type of surgical procedure (Figure 23-1) and the patient's response. A partial gastrectomy may create little postoperative difficulty. A total gastrectomy is another matter, however, since there is complete excision of the stomach and the remaining portion of the esophagus is joined to the jejunum—*anastomosis*. This resectioning may produce serious nutritional deficits and requires careful individual assessment and diet planning. When a **vagotomy** is also performed, there is increased gastric fullness and distention. The stomach portion remaining becomes atonic and empties poorly, so that food fermentation follows, producing flatus and diarrhea. After gastric surgery about 50% of the patients fail to regain weight to optimal levels. The nutritional care of patients who have had gastric surgery primarily falls into two phases: the immediate postoperative period and a later "dumping syndrome."

Immediate Postoperative Period

Generally, after surgery, frequent small oral feedings are resumed according to the patient's tolerance. A typical pattern of simple dietary progression may cover about a 2-week period. The basic principles of such a general diet therapy for this immediate postoperative period involve (1) *size* of meals—small frequent and (2) *type* of food—simple, easily digested, mild, low in bulk. Increasingly, however, surgeons are using a needle-catheter jejunostomy procedure to provide earlier nutritional support with an elemental formula.

Later "Dumping Syndrome"

After patients have recovered from surgery and begin to eat food in greater volume and variety, they may experience increasing discomfort following

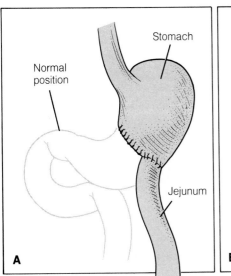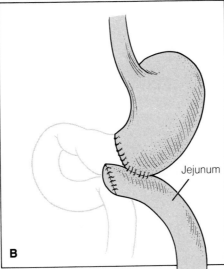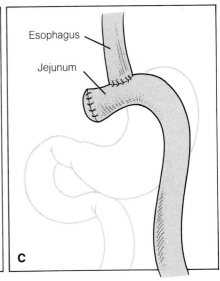

Figure 23-1
Gastric surgery. **A,** Partial gastrectomy, Billroth I. **B,** Partial gastrectomy, Billroth II. **C,** Total gastrectomy.

meals. About 10 to 15 minutes after eating, there is a cramping, full feeling. The pulse is rapid, and there is a wave of weakness, cold sweating, and dizziness; frequently nausea and vomiting follow. Such distressing reactions to food intake increase anxiety, so the person eats less and less. This postgastrectomy complex of symptoms is commonly called *dumping syndrome*. A more precise term used by some clinicians is *jejunal hyperosmolar syndrome*. This difficulty is more likely to occur in patients who have had total gastrectomy. The symptoms of shock result when a meal containing a high proportion of readily soluble carbohydrate rapidly enters the jejunum, which has been attached to the esophagus. This entering food mass is a concentrated hyperosmolar solution in relation to the surrounding extracellular fluid. To achieve osmotic balance, water is drawn from the blood into the intestine, causing a rapid decrease in the circulating blood volume (see Chapter 8). As a result, the blood pressure drops, and signs of cardiac insufficiency appear: rapid pulse, sweating, weakness, and tremors. In about 2 hours a second sequence of events follows. The concentrated solution of simple carbohydrate is rapidly absorbed, causing a **postprandial** rise in blood glucose. In response, an overproduction of insulin is stimulated, which in turn leads to an eventual drop in the blood sugar below normal fasting levels. Symptoms of mild hypoglycemia result. Dramatic relief of these distressing symptoms and gradual regaining of lost weight follow careful control of the diet with the pattern given here (see box, p. 570).

Gallbladder Surgery
Nutrition Problems

For patients suffering from acute **cholecystitis** or **cholelithiasis** (Figure 23-2), the treatment is usually surgical removal of the gallbladder—*cholecystectomy*. Following surgery, control of fat in the diet aids wound healing and comfort. The presence of fat in the duodenum continues to stimulate the **cholecystokinin mechanism** (see Chapter 19), which causes contraction and

Postprandial
Occurring after dinner, or after a meal.

Cholecystitis
Inflammation of the gallbladder.

Cholelithiasis
Formation of gallstones.

Cholicystokinin mechanism
Hormone secreted by mucosa of upper intestine, which stimulates contraction of the gallbladder.

Diet for Postoperative Dumping Syndrome

General description

- Five or six small meals daily.
- Relative high fat content to retard passage of food and help maintain weight.
- High protein content (meat, egg, cheese) to rebuild tissue and maintain weight.
- Relatively low carbohydrate content to prevent rapid passage of quickly utilized foods.
- No milk; no sugar, sweets, or desserts; no alcohol or sweet carbonated beverages.
- Liquids between meals only; avoid fluids for at least 1 hour before and after meals.
- Relatively low-roughage foods; raw foods as tolerated.

Meal pattern

Breakfast
   2 scrambled eggs with 1 to 2 tbsp butter or margarine
   ½ to 1 slice bread or small serving cereal with butter or margarine
   2 crisp bacon strips
   1 serving solid fruit*

Midmorning sandwich of:
   1 slice bread
   Butter or margarine
   56 g (2oz) lean meat

Lunch
   112 g (4 oz) lean meat with 1 or 2 tbsp butter or margarine
   ½ to 1 slice bread with butter or margarine
   ½ banana or other solid fruit*

Midafternoon
   Same snack as midmorning

Dinner
   112 g lean meat with 1 or 2 tbsp butter or margarine
   Green or colored vegetable† with butter or margarine
   ½ to 1 slice bread with butter or margarine (or small serving starchy vegetable substitute)
   1 serving solid fruit*

Bedtime
   56 g meat or 2 eggs or 56 g cheese or cottage cheese
   1 slice bread or 5 crackers
   Butter or margarine

*Fruit choice: applesauce, baked apple, canned fruit (drained), banana, orange or grapefruit sections.
†Vegetable choice: asparagus, spinach, green beans, squash, beets, carrots, green peas.

pain in the surgical area. There is also a period of readjustment to the more aqueous supply of liver bile available to assist fat digestion and absorption.

Dietary Management

Depending on individual tolerance and response, a relatively low-fat diet may need to be followed for a brief time with moderate fat use thereafter, as

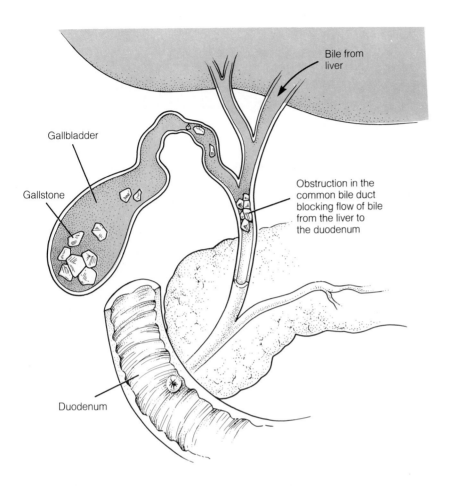

Figure 23-2
Gallbladder with stones (chole-lithiasis).

Bile from liver

Gallbladder

Gallstone

Obstruction in the common bile duct blocking flow of bile from the liver to the duodenum

Duodenum

recommended in the U.S. Dietary Guidelines for all healthy Americans. The low-fat regimen outlined for gallbladder disease (see Chapter 19) may serve as a guide.

Ileostomy and Colostomy

In cases of intestinal lesion or obstruction or when inflammatory bowel disease (see Chapter 19) involves the entire colon, the treatment of choice is usually resection of the intestine to remove the diseased portion. An *ileostomy*, usually permanent but sometimes temporary, may also be established. In this procedure the end of the remaining small intestine, the ileum, is attached to an opening in the abdominal wall, and a **stoma** is formed to provide for discharge of the intestinal contents (Figure 23-3). In other cases, a temporary or permanent *colostomy* may be indicated with resection of only the final left side of the colon, and a stoma is made with the remaining descending colon.

Nutrition Problems

An ileostomy and a colostomy produce different problems in management. With an ileostomy, the intestinal contents at the point of the ileus are unformed, irritating, and even erosive to the skin. The ileostomy drains freely, almost continuously, and should not be irrigated. Thus establishment of controlled functioning is difficult. Many patients, however, do develop a reasonable degree of regularity in regard to meals. Some sort of ap-

Stoma

From Greek *stoma,* mouth. A temporary or permanent opening, surgically established, in the abdominal wall as part of the ileostomy or colostomy procedure.

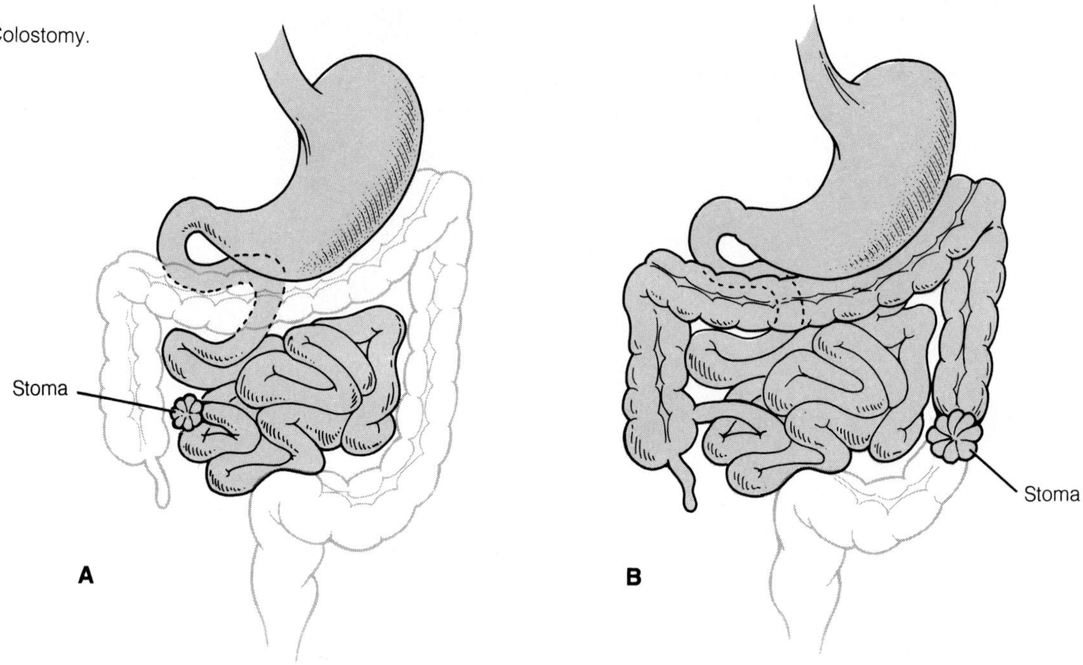

Figure 23-3
A, Ileostomy. **B,** Colostomy.

pliance is necessary to hold the discharge. A modified, alternative procedure called the *continent ileostomy* is sometimes done. Here the surgeon forms a reservoir inside the abdominal cavity out of intestinal tissue, and a one-way valve holds the collection until the patient periodically inserts a cathether to empty it.[6] This method eliminates the need for the usual exterior plastic appliance.

A colostomy is more manageable. The normal contents of the intestine at this point in the colon are solid or semisolid, since more water and electrolytes have been absorbed by the proximal colon. The consistency of the discharge and its less irritating nature create fewer control problems. Often a sigmoid colostomy can be adequately controlled by simple dietary measures and periodic irrigation, so that in many cases no protective appliance is needed. Coping with any ostomy is difficult at best, however, and patients need much support and practical help and resources in learning good self-care.[7,8]

Dietary Management

A relatively low-residue diet (see Chapter 19) is usually used in the immediate postoperative period. But as soon as possible the diet should be advanced to a regular pattern of food to provide (1) optimal nutrition and physical rehabilitation and (2) an additional means of psychologic support. Diet counseling with the patient and family will help establish the most successful pattern of meals and avoid those foods that cause individual discomfort. In general, persons with ostomies should eat regular diets of food that agrees with them, sufficient in quantity and nutrient value to maintain proper weight and energy. A low-residue diet may be used occasionally when diarrhea occurs.

Rectal Surgery
Nutrition Problems

For a brief period following rectal surgery, a *hemorrhoidectomy*, there is pain on elimination. Thus bowel movements should be delayed until initial healing is begun.

Dietary Management

A clear fluid or nonresidue diet is indicated for initial use. The basic foods used are almost completely digested and nutrients absorbed in the small intestine, leaving minimal residue for elimination by the colon. In some cases a nonresidue commercial formula may be used during the initial postoperative period.

Nutritional Support Base

A major concern of therapy for the patient with extensive burns is rigorous nutritional support. The clinical nutritionist on the burn team is in a most strategic position to assess, plan, implement, and monitor the nutritional care for these patients.[9,10] Strong assistance is needed in nursing care. Three important factors guide this vital nutritional therapy: (1) large catabolic losses, (2) essential anabolic healing demands, and (3) deep personal support needs.

Treatment and Prognosis

The plan of care and its outcome depend on several factors:
1. *Age*—elderly persons and very young children are most vulnerable
2. *Health condition*—the presence of any preexisting condition, such as diabetes, heart or renal disease, or any other associated injuries, complicates care
3. *Burn severity*—the location and severity of the burn wounds and the time elapsed before treatment are significant

Degree and Extent of Burns

The depth of the burn wound affects its healing process: (1) *first-degree* burns—**erythema**— involve cell necrosis above the basal layer of the epidermis; (2) *second-degree* burns involve erythema and blistering, and necrosis within the dermis; and (3) *third-degree* burns result in a full-thickness skin loss, including the fat layer. Second- and third-degree burns covering 15% to 20% or more of the total body surface, or even 10% in children and elderly persons, usually cause extensive fluid loss and require intravenous fluid and electrolyte replacement therapy. Burns of severe depth covering more than 50% of the body surface area are often fatal, especially in infants and older persons. Patients with major burn injuries are usually transferred for care to a specialized burn care facility.

Stages of Nutritional Care

The nutritional care of the patient with massive burns is constantly adjusted to individual responses and needs. At all times attention to amino acid needs is vital, in addition to critical fluid-electrolyte balance and energy (kilocalories) support.[9,10] Generally three stages of care can be identified: (1) immediate "ebb" or shock period and following "flow" or recovery response; (2)

Special Nutritional Needs for Patients with Burns

Erythema
Redness of the skin produced by congestion of the capillaries, resulting from a variety of causes, one of which can be radiant heat, i.e., burns.

secondary critical period of vigorous feeding; and (3) the follow-up period of reconstructive surgery and rehabilitation.

Stage 1: Immediate Shock Period

Massive flooding edema occurs at the burn site during the first hours after injury to about the second day. Loss of enveloping skin surface and exposure of tissue fluids lead to immediate loss of water and electrolytes, mainly sodium, and large protein depletion. In an effort to balance this loss, water shifts from the surrounding tissue spaces in the body, only adding to the continuous loss at the burn site. As a result water circulating in the blood is withdrawn, thus decreasing the overall blood volume (**hypovolemia**) and blood pressure. Blood concentration and diminished urine output occur as a result. Cell dehydration follows as cell water is drawn out to balance the tissue fluid losses. Cell potassium is also withdrawn and circulating serum potassium levels rise.

Immediate intravenous fluid therapy replaces water and electrolytes by use of a salt solution such as **lactated Ringer's solution,** helping to prevent shock. Acute renal failure is a rare occurrence when resuscitation is started early. During the first part of this initial shock period, the first 12 to 14 hours after the injury, **colloid** solutions such as albumin or plasma are not effective since most of such solutions are lost in fluids at the burn site. Usually vascular endothelial permeability returns to normal after the first day, however, and colloid solutions can then be used to help restore plasma volume. During this initial period, no attempt is made to meet nutritional requirements in protein and kilocalories because (1) glucose-free balanced electrolyte solutions are the need, since infusion of glucose at this time may result in hyperglycemia; and (2) an *adynamic ileus* develops after the injury and precludes any use of the gastrointestinal tract at this time.

Stage 1: Recovery Period

After about 48 to 72 hours, tissue fluids and electrolytes are gradually reabsorbed into the general circulation, balance is established, and the pattern of massive tissue loss is reversed. At this point a sudden **diuresis** occurs, indicating successful therapy. The patient returns to preinjury weight by about the end of the first week. A careful check of fluid intake and output is essential, with constant checks for signs of dehydration or overhydration.

Stage 2: Secondary Feeding Period

Toward the end of the first postburn week, adequate bowel function returns, and a vigorous feeding period must begin. At this point, despite the patient's depression and anorexia, life may well depend on rigorous nutritional therapy. Several factors necessitate this increased intake:

1. **Tissue destruction.** The massive burn injury has brought large losses of protein and electrolytes that must be replaced.

2. **Tissue catabolism.** Tissue protein breakdown has followed the injury, with consequent loss of lean body mass and nitrogen.

3. **Increased metabolism.** Increased metabolic demands arise from additional needs. **Sepsis** or fever make extra kilocalories necessary for energy needs. Extra carbohydrate and B vitamins are needed for energy as the body resources mobilize to meet heightened basal metabolic require-

Hypovolemia
An abnormally low volume of circulating blood plasma.

Lactated Ringer's solution
Sterile solution of calcium chloride, potassium chloride, sodium chloride, and sodium lactate in water given to replenish fluid and electrolytes.

Colloid
Glutinous, gluelike; a dispersion of matter throughout a medium.

Diuresis
Increased urine excretion.

Sepsis
Presence in the blood or other tissues of pathogenic microorganisms or their toxins—the condition associated with such presence.

ments. Tissue regeneration requires extra protein and key vitamins such as ascorbic acid. The success of follow-up skin grafting requires optimal tissue health.

Stage 2: Nutritional Therapy

Successful nutritional therapy during this critical period is based on vigorous energy and protein therapy:

1. **High energy.** From 3500 to 5000 kcal, with a high percentage of carbohydrate, is necessary to spare protein for tissue regeneration and to supply the greatly increased metabolic demands for energy.

2. **High protein.** Depending on the extent of the burn injury, individual needs will vary from 150 g to as high as 400 g. Children will require 2 to 4 times the normal protein needs for age. In general most adults require an increased amount of protein, 2 to 3 g/kg body weight, to achieve nitrogen balance.

3. **High vitamins.** From 1 to 2 g of vitamin C may be needed for tissue regeneration. Increased thiamin, riboflavin, and niacin are necessary to metabolize the extra carbohydrate and protein.

Stage 2: Dietary Management

To meet these crucial nutrient demands, either enteral or parenteral modes of feeding may be used.

1. **Enteral feeding.** To achieve the necessary intake of increased nutrient density indicated, a careful intake record must be maintained. Oral feedings are desirable if tolerated by the patient. Concentrated oral liquids must be given using protein hydrolysates or amino acids to ensure adequate intake. Commercial formulas are usually used to supply large amounts of nourishment. Solid foods according to individual food preferences are added by about the second week. Tube feeding may be required by some patients in the beginning. In this case low-bulk defined formula solutions may be given through small-bore feeding tubes. In either case, continuous support and encouragement are necessary. Food should be made as attractive and appetizing as possible, supplying items particularly liked and respecting disliked foods.

2. **Parenteral feeding.** For some patients, oral intake and tube feedings may be inadequate to meet the accelerated demands, or they may be impossible because of associated injuries or complications. In these cases parenteral feeding through a large central vein or peripheral vein is needed to provide the essential nutritional support.

Stage 3: Follow-up Reconstruction

Continuous vigorous nutrition is essential to maintain tissue integrity for successful skin grafting or plastic reconstructive surgery. The patient will need not only physical rebuilding of body resources but also much personal support to rebuild the human will and spirit, since there may be disfigurement and disability. Health team members can do much to help instill the courage and confidence the person must have to face the future again. Whatever the future demands, however, optimal physical stamina gained through persistent, supportive care—medical, nutritional, and nursing—will help each patient rebuild the personal resources needed to cope.

Total Parenteral Nutrition: Care of the Malnourished or Hypermetabolic Patient

TPN Development

In nutritional therapy, the term *parenteral* means any feeding method other than by the normal gastrointestinal route. In current usage it refers to special feeding of concentrated nutrient solutions through central and peripheral veins to achieve necessary nutritional support when the gastrointestinal tract cannot be used. The development of this basic surgical technique, it has provided a major advance in critical patient care.

The complete sustaining of increased nutritional requirements through a large central vein has been termed *total parenteral nutrition (TPN)*. The similar feeding method through a somewhat smaller peripheral vein, called *peripheral parenteral nutrition (PPN)*, can be used in many cases as a viable alternative.[11] It may also be used in conjunction with enteral feeding, such as oral intake or tube feeding, as is frequently the case in transition feeding.[12] On the special nutrition support team, a clinical nutritionist with special advanced training designs and calculates these special feedings according to individual needs, and the pharmacist mixes the indicated solutions. Presently the clinical nutrition specialist and the physician have available a wide spectrum of formulas and delivery systems from which to plan individual nutritional therapy according to the clinical problems presented.

Indications for TPN Use

Several basic factors govern decisions concerning the use of TPN. Since there are risks involved, careful assessment of each of these factors is necessary.

Availability of Gastrointestinal Tract

If major abdominal injury renders the gut totally unavailable for use, an alternative means of sustaining nutrition is an obvious necessity. In other cases the gut may be unavailable because of obstruction, **fistulas,** or malignant disease. Or the patient may be unable to eat because of coma, severe anorexia, or mental disturbance.

Degree of Malnutrition

If a patient is malnourished, any medical treatment attempted will have less chance of success. Studies indicate that there is far more general malnutrition among hospitalized patients than was previously assumed. Also, it is clear that disease imposes an even greater threat to positive nutritional status. Thus the assessment of nutritional status becomes an important part of overall care, especially for hospitalized patients (see Chapter 17). For the more severely malnourished patient, more serious consideration of TPN is indicated.

Degree of Hypermetabolism or Catabolism

If a patient is suffering from major trauma or severe sepsis or malignant disease, the rate of catabolism takes a devastating toll on the body resources. This toll may be measured in nitrogen balance studies, with a loss ranging up to 15 g of nitrogen over 24 hours. Catabolic periods follow surgery, with more extensive surgery bringing the greatest losses of body resources. Malignant disease and its radiation treatment and chemotherapy (see Chapter 24), or any critical illness, place additional demands on the body's metabolism.

Fistula
Abnormal passage, usually between two internal organs, or leading from an internal organ to the surface of the body.

Patient with limited or impossible use of gut	Metabolic rate, degree of catabolism (nitrogen loss per 24 hr)	Degree of malnutrition*
Situation 1	Normal (0-8 g)	Severe
Situation 2	Moderate (8-15 g)	Moderate
Situation 3	Severe (15 g)	Normal

Table 23-2
Patient Situations
Imposing Need for TPN

*In terms of percent of normal standards of nutritional assessment.

Basic Rules for Use of TPN

Using the three basic factors above, most clinicians have formed general rules to guide the choice of TPN as a preferred means of therapy. Combinations of these factors indicating need for TPN are given in Table 23-2. Two basic rules have evolved in practice:

1. **The "rule of five."** If a patient has been unable to eat for 5 days and is highly likely to be unable to eat for at least another week, TPN should be considered *then* rather than waiting until malnutrition exists.
2. **Weight loss rule.** Any patient who has lost 7% of the usual body weight over 2 months or who has been deprived of oral nourishment for 5 to 7 days or longer is a candidate for TPN.

Patient Candidates for TPN

Based on these considerations, candidates for vigorous nutritional therapy through TPN can be identified. These candidates include: (1) *severely malnourished patients being prepared for surgery,* such as those with cancer of the esophagus or stomach; (2) *patients with postoperative complications,* such as those with fistulas or short bowel syndrome; (3) *patients with inflammatory bowel disease,* such as those with acute Crohn's disease, radiation enteritis, or ulcerative colitis; and (4) *patients with malabsorption or inadequate oral intake,* such as those with chronic malnutrition, major trauma as in burns, malignant neoplasms, or acute and chronic relapsing pancreatitis.

Nutrition Assessment

General Assessment

Initial individual assessment provides the necessary basis for (1) identifying patients requiring special therapy, (2) calculating their nutritional requirements, and (3) determining the specific nutrient formulation to meet these requirements. This is the task of the clinical nutritionist on the TPN team. This initial assessment is done by standard methods: anthropometric measures, biochemical laboratory data, clinical observations, and dietary evaluations, together with a detailed history. These general methods are described in Chapter 17 and can be reviewed there.

Specific TPN Procedures

Specific TPN nutritional assessment is done according to individual patient and clinical situations and includes the following:

1. **Degree of weight loss.** Interpret measures of current body weight and height in terms of desirable lean body weight for height, usual body weight,

Table 23-3

Indications of Severe
Protein-Calorie Malnutri-
tion According to
Percentage of Recent
Weight Loss

% Body weight loss	Time period
2%	1 week
5%	1 month
7.5%	3 months
10%	6 months

and amount of recent weight change. Compare patient's amount of recent weight change with the values indicating malnutrition given in Table 23-3.

2. **Body fat stores and skeletal muscle mass.** Using caliper measures of triceps skinfold (TSF) and standard reference tables for TSF data, estimate the patient's body fat stores. Using the upper midarm circumference (MAC) measure, calculate the midarm muscle circumference (MAMC) and compare with standard reference tables:

$$MAMC(cm) = MAC(cm) - [0.314 \times TSF(mm)].$$

3. **Lean body mass.** Using amount of creatinine output in a 24-hour urine collection, determine the creatinine-height index using standard tables.

4. **Degree of catabolism.** Using amount of urea nitrogen output in a 24-hour urine collection and the nitrogen value of the diet during the same 24-hour period, calculate the overall nitrogen balance for the period:

$$N \text{ balance} = N \text{ intake (protein intake} \div 6.25) - N \text{ loss (urinary urea } N + 4).$$

5. **Immune function.** Use total lymphocyte count or percentage of lymphocytes in total white blood cell count to determine general immune system function. Skin testing for sensitivity to common recall antigens can also give immune function data.

6. **Plasma protein compartment.** Use the serum albumin level as a measure of the body's visceral protein mass. Also, using laboratory data for total iron-binding capacity (TIBC), calculate the value for transferrin, the body's iron transport compound: transferrin (mg/dL) = [TIBC(μg/dL) × 0.8] − 43. Reference standards for these measures are given in Table 23-4. Monitoring of these nutritional assessment data continues throughout therapy.

Nutritional Requirements: TPN Prescription

The TPN prescription and plan of nutritional care are based on calculation of the basic nutritional requirements plus additional needs resulting from the patient's degree of catabolism, malnutrition, and any activity (see box, p. 581). This same principle guides nutritional therapy in any feeding mode. Nutritional needs are fundamental: energy, protein, electrolytes, vitamins, and minerals.

Energy Requirements

The kilocalorie needs of the critically ill patient will range from 2000 to 5000 kcal/day in major trauma or sepsis. The great difference is seen in comparing health and illness needs. This large energy input is necessary to meet the increased basal metabolic demands and the large energy cost of catabolism, fever, malnutrition, and any physical activity.

In health about 35 kcal/kg body weight are required for maintenance, whereas in catabolic illness it is about 50 to 60 kcal/kg.

$$\text{Nitrogen} = \frac{\text{Total protein}}{6.25}$$

Laboratory data	Normal values	Degree of malnutrition	
		Moderate	Severe
Serum albumin (g/dL)	3.5	2.1-3.0	<2.1
Serum transferrin (mg/dL)	180-260	100-150	<100
Total lymphocyte count			
Per mm³	1500-4000	800-1200	<800
% of WBC	20%-53%		

Table 23-4
Determination of Protein-Calorie Malnutrition by Plasma Values

Protein Requirements

Protein is needed to maintain nitrogen balance and provide essential amino acids. In addition, an adequate ratio of nitrogen to nonnitrogen kilocalories is necessary to protect the nitrogen sources for use in tissue protein synthesis. For meeting the metabolic stress of illness, the ratio should be 150 to 200 kcal/g of nitrogen. In terms of protein intake, the patient needs a minimum of 1.2 to 1.5 g protein/kg body weight. Compare this increased requirement with the usual maintenance adult requirements in health: 0.8 to 1.0 g protein/kg.

Electrolyte Requirements

Individual monitoring data are used to determine electrolyte balances and needs. An example of the electrolyte composition of a basic TPN formula is given in Table 23-5.

Vitamin and Mineral Requirements

Added vitamin and mineral needs are created by hypermetabolic effects and depleted states. An evaluation of the extent of these needs is based on individual assessment data. Particular attention is paid to trace elements. These needs are reflected in Table 23-5.

Preparation of TPN Solutions

With the development of the TPN technique, products for use in TPN nutrient solutions have also been developing. They are used by the TPN team in formulating nutritional needs for each patient, based on the nutritional requirements for protein, energy, electrolytes, vitamins, and minerals.

Protein-Nitrogen Source

Remember that 6.25 g protein, amino acids, equals 1 g nitrogen. Currently the nitrogen source of choice is crystalline amino acids, both essential and nonessential. A number of commercial products are available in a variety of compositions and dilutions. After the individual patient prescription is determined by the TPN physician and clinical nutritionist, the team pharmacist mixes accurate solutions for each patient as indicated. However, all team members should know about these solutions and keep up with the various commercial product changes. For example, the usual amino acid need is supplied by a 3.5% or 4.25% dilution. This dilution is achieved by mixing 1 L of a standard 7% or 8.5% amino acid solution with 1 L of dextrose solution.

6.25 g protein = 1 g nitrogen

Table 23-5

Example of Basic TPN Formula Components

Components	Amounts
Basic solution	
Crystalline amino acids	2.75%
Dextrose	25%
Additives	
Electrolytes	
Na	50 mEq/L
Cl	50 mEq/L
K	40 mEq/l
HPO_4	25 mEq/L
Ca	5 mEq/L
Mg	8 mEq/L
Vitamins	
Multiple (MVI)	1.7 mlconc/L
Vitamin C (day)	500 mg
Trace elements solution (day)	
Zn	3 mg
Cu	1.6 mg
Cr	2 μg
Se	120 μg
Mn	2 μg
I	120 μg
Fe	1.5 μg
Other additives (as needed)	
Regular insulin	0-25 units/L
Heparin	1000 units/L

Nonprotein Energy Source—Kilocalories

Nonprotein kilocalories to meet energy demands and protect protein for tissue synthesis are supplied by glucose solutions and fat emulsions.

1. **Glucose (dextrose).** Dextrose solutions range from the 5% solution, used traditionally in peripheral intravenous support of fluid and electrolytes postsurgically, to the hypertonic 70% solution available for TPN formulations. The usual solution used for TPN is 50% dextrose. When this solution is mixed with amino acid solution, it renders a 25% dextrose solution in the formula. Dextrose solutions given intravenously do not deliver the classic 4 kcal/g. In the *anhydrous* form, these solutions are 91% calorigenic, providing 3.75 kcal/g. Thus a final solution of 25% dextrose solution would provide 850 kcal. For example, a liter solution of 25% glucose and 2.75% amino acid (Travasol), as shown in Table 23-5, would provide 4.63 g nitrogen and a kilocalorie/nitrogen ratio of 183:1. This ratio will vary with different solutions. In common TPN dextrose solutions using the *monohydrate* form, the energy value of the dextrose is a little less—3.4 kcal/g instead of the usual fuel factor for carbohydrate of 4 kcal/g.

2. **Fat.** Emulsions of fat provide a concentrated source of nonprotein kilo-

Clinical Application

The percentage of a substance in a solution indicates how many grams of that substance are present in 100 mL (2 dL). For example:

5% dextrose (D) solution = 5 g dextrose/100 mL

This is written as D_5W and read as "5% dextrose in water." The subscript after *D* indicates the percentage of dextrose present. Other nutrient designations are similar. For example:

3.5% amino acid (AA) solution = 3.5 g AA/100 mL
0.9% normal saline (NaCl) solution = 0.9 g NaCl/100 mL

Suppose your patient is on a typical TPN solution. Her formula prescription reads: 25% dextrose, 3.5% amino acids, 3 L/day. This solution and volume would be achieved by mixing 1500 ml $D_{50}W$ plus 1500 mL 7% AA solution. How much carbohydrate (dextrose) and protein (amino acids) and how many kilocalories would she be receiving? You can calculate this easily by simple ratio and proportion:

Carbohydrate (dextrose)

$$\frac{50 \text{ g dextrose}}{100 \text{ mL}} \text{ as } \frac{\textbf{x} \text{ g dextrose}}{1500 \text{ mL}}$$

Read this mathematic statement as "50 g of dextrose is to 100 mL of solution as x g dextrose is to 1500 mL of solution." Now cross multiply and divide by 100 mL.

$$100\textbf{ x} = 50 \times 1500 \text{ (75,000)}$$
$$\textbf{x} = 75,000 \div 100$$
$$\textbf{x} = 750 \text{ g dextrose}$$

Protein (amino acids)

$$\frac{7 \text{ g AA}}{100 \text{ mL}} \text{ as } \frac{\textbf{x} \text{ g AA}}{1500 \text{ mL}}$$
$$100\textbf{ x} = 7 \times 1500 \text{ (10,500)}$$
$$\textbf{x} = 10,500 \div 100$$
$$\textbf{x} = 105 \text{ g amino acids}$$

Kilocalories (kcal)

You can now calculate the total kilocalories in this solution simply by multiplying kilocalorie value per grams of dextrose (**D**) (monohydrate) in the solution (3.4 kcal/g) and of protein (AA) (4 kcal/g):

750 g D × 3.4 kcal/g = 2550 kcal
105 g AA × 4.0 kcal/g = 420 kcal
TOTAL = 2970 kcal

Additional kilocalories from a supplement of fat emulsion (500 mL twice a week) would be added to this total.

Calculating Nutrient Composition of Intravenous Solutions

calories and ensure a necessary supply of the main essential fatty acid, linoleic acid (see Chapter 4). Commercial products include Intralipid and Lyposyn, for example. Both come in 10% (1.1 kcal/ml) and 20% (2.0 kcal/ml) concentrations. They are fat emulsions derived from soy oil (Intralipid) and safflower oil (Liposyn). Both contain neutral triglycerides of predominantly unsaturated fatty acids. They are usually used a supplement to the main TPN solution, provided separately according to need, usually one to two bottles a week for adults. They are administered separately through a Y-connector tube. They are never mixed with the main dextrose–amino acid solution because the emulsion would break down.

Electrolytes. The formulation of electrolytes is based on the usual requirements for normal electrolyte balance with adjustments according to individual patient monitoring. A general ratio of electrolytes is shown in Table 23-5.

Vitamins. Multivitamin formulas are available for use in TPN solutions, as are individual vitamins for formulating the solution according to special patient needs. Multiple formulas such as MVI (multiple vitamin injection) supply water-soluble B vitamins and vitamin C, as well as water-soluble forms of vitamins A, D, and E. Since vitamins B_{12}, folate, and K may alter their form when added to the rest of the vitamin formula, they are added separately and not on a daily basis, as indicated in Table 23-5.

Minerals. Caution is needed in adding minerals to the TPN solution. Incompatibilities of certain electrolytes and other components may result in the formation of an insoluble **precipitate,** depending on factors such as ion concentration and solution pH. More attention has been given recently to the need for added trace elements, as well as the need for close monitoring of calcium balance.

Precipitate
To cause a substance in solution to settle down in solid particles.

Mixing the Formula

The pharmacist on the TPN team mixes the components of the specific solution for the patient's prescription according to a rigid protocol. A laminar flow hood provides an aseptic environment in which the solutions, open medication vials, and other materials can be handled safely. To ensure stability, the individual solutions are ordered and mixed daily, following prescription adjustments made on the basis of constant TPN monitoring protocol.

Administration of TPN
TPN Team

The insertion of the central vein TPN line is a surgical procedure done by the physician (Figure 23-4). It is usually performed at the bedside following strict aseptic procedures. The nurse on the TPN team has special training in care of the patient on TPN and is responsible for administering the formula (see box on facing page), and for maintaining the rigid protocols developed to avoid infection or other complications. The clinical nutrition specialist on the TPN team, a clinical dietitian with advanced academic degree and special TPN training, is responsible for constant nutrition assessment and monitoring, interpretation of data, and calculating formula needs in close collaboration with the physician. The team pharmacist is responsible for mixing the formulas according to individual prescription worked out by the physician and clinical nutritionist. In the hands of a well-trained TPN team, risks have been minimized and complications controlled by team effort.

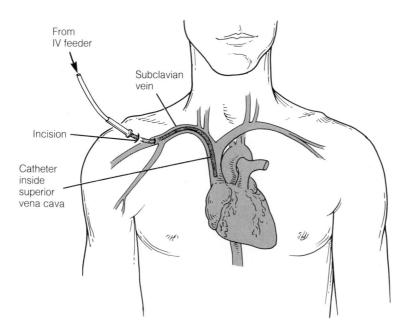

From
IV feeder

Subclavian
vein

Incision

Catheter
inside
superior
vena cava

Figure 23-4
Catheter placement for total parenteral nutrition (TPN) made by feeding via subclavian vein to superior vena cava.

Clinical Application

Careful administration of TPN formulas is essential. Specific protocols will vary somewhat. Usually, however, they include the following points:

- **Start slowly.** Give time to adapt to the increased glucose concentration and osmolality of the solution.
- **Schedule carefully.** During the first 24 hours, 1 to 2 L is given by continuous drip, the slow rate regulated usually by an infusion pump.
- **Monitor closely.** Note metabolic effects of glucose (not to exceed 200 mg/dL) and electrolytes.
- **Increase volume cautiously.** Watch the effect of all changes and proceed slowly.
- **Maintain a constant rate.** Keep the correct hourly infusion rate, with no "catch up" or "slow down" effort to meet original volume order.
- **Discontinue slowly.** Take patient off of TPN feeding gradually, reducing rate and daily volume about 1 L/day.

Administration of TPN Formula

Home TPN for Long-Term Use

Experience from home use of other long-term medical equipment, such as that used for renal dialysis, has led to the practice of self-infusion of parenteral nutrients at home in special cases of long-term need (see Issues and Answers, p. 586). Home TPN can greatly reduce the cost of such treatment. In the hands of selected, well-trained patients and families it allows mobility and travel. It offers special promise in long-term management of such conditions as severe abdominal injury or chronic severe inflammatory bowel disease. Special equipment, solutions, and guidelines for training selected patients and families have been developed and are successfully being used in many cases.

To Sum Up

The nutritional demands of surgery begin before the patient reaches the operating table. Preoperatively the task is to correct any existing deficiencies and build nutrient reserves to meet surgical demands. Postoperatively it is to replace losses and support recovery. The additional task of encouraging eating is often required during this period.

Pre- and postsurgical feedings are given in a variety of ways. The oral route is always preferred, but damage to the intestinal tract or a poor appetite may require other enteral or parenteral feedings. Diets are modified according to the surgical procedure performed. For the depleted surgical patient, nutritional support relies heavily on biomedical technology to facilitate enteral and parenteral feedings administer by specially trained TPN team members.

Questions for Review

1. Describe the general impact of imbalances of the following nutritional factors during the preoperative, immediate postoperative, and postoperative periods: protein, kilocalories, vitamins, minerals, and fluids.
2. Describe the major surgical effects for which nutrition therapy must be planned following these procedures: mouth, throat, and neck surgery; gastric resection; cholescystectomy; and rectal surgery.
3. Write a 1-day meal plan for a person experiencing the postgastrectomy "dumping syndrome." What general dietary guidelines are used? Why?
4. Describe the difference in care between an ileostomy and a colostomy. What are the dietary implications of each?
5. Outline the nutritional care of a burn patient from treatment for immediate shock through recovery and tissue reconstruction.
6. What is TPN? For whom is it usually recommended? Why? Describe the operation of the TPN team.

References

1. Mughal MM, and Meguid MM: The effect of nutritional status on the morbidity after elective surgery for benign gastrointestinal disease, J Parenteral Enteral Nutr 11(2):140, Mar/Apr 1987.
2. Church JM, and Hill GL: Assessing the efficacy of intravenous nutrition in general surgical patients: dynamic nutritional assessment with plasma proteins, J Parenteral Enteral Nutr 11(2):135, Mar/Apr 1987.
3. Glassman RG: Nutrition assessment: a critical review, Top Clin Nutr 1(4):16, Oct 1986.
4. Nelson JK, Palumbo PJ, and O'Brien PC: Home enteral nutrition: observations of a newly established program, Nutr Clin Prac 1(4):193, Aug 1986.
5. Kohn CL, and Kiethley JK: Techniques for evaluating and managing diarrhea in the tube-fed patient, Nutr Clin Prac 2(6):250, Dec 1987.

6. Rathgeber MG: Nutrition and osto-mies, ADA practice group: Dietitians in Nutrition Support Newsletter 8(6):5, May 1987.
7. Mullen BD, and McGinn KA: The ostomy book, Palo Alto, CA, 1980, Bull Publishing Co.
8. Knebel F: Diet for smooth digestion, Am Health 2(4):72, 1983.
9. Del Savio N: Nutritional support for thermally injured patients: the role of the dietitian, Nutr Supp Serv 4(10):10, Oct 1984.
10. Luterman A, Adams M, and Curreri W: Nutritional management of the burn patient, Crit Care Q 7:34, 1984.
11. Kelly SF: Peripheral vein TPN: a viable alternative to the central venous approach, Clin Consultations 1(2):1, 1981.
12. Wade JE: Transitional enteral feeding, Clin Consultations 1(2):10, 1981.

Further Readings

ASPEN: Guidelines for use of total parenteral nutrition in the hospitalized adult patient, J Parenteral Enteral Nutr 10(5):441, Sept/Oct 1986.

This is the guiding statement from the American Society for Parenteral and Enteral Nutrition (ASPEN) concerning the use of TPN as a special feeding mode in highly stressed cases.

Beck SL, Rose NR, and Zagoren A: Home total parenteral nutrition utilizing implanted infusion ports, Nutr Clin Prac 2(1):26, Feb 1987.

Burch K, et al: Development of an assist device for a blind home total parenteral nutrition patient, Nutr Clin Prac 3(1):23, Feb 1988.

Gelman D: Staying home, feeling better, Newsweek CVIII(1):48, July 1986.

Marein C, et al: Home parenteral nutrition, Nutr Clin Prac 1(4):179, Aug 1986.

This group of articles describes programs for home use of special nutrition support feeding, developed to meet both medical and personal needs with the advances in technology for formulas and delivery systems.

Cunningham JJ, Harris LJ, and Briggs SE: Nutritional support of the severely burned infant, Nutr Clin Prac 3(2):69, Apr 1988.

Del Savio N: Nutritional support for the thermally injured patient: the role of the dietitian, Nutr Supp Serv 4(10):10, Oct 1984.

These two articles present a case report of an injured infant and a description of nutritional responsibilities in the care of burn patients.

Kohn CL, and Keithley JK: Techniques for evaluating and managing diarrhea in the tube-fed patient, Nutr Clin Pract 2(6):250, Dec 1987.

Nelson JK, Palumbo PJ, and O'Brien PC: Home enteral nutrition: observations of a newly established program, Nutr Clin Pract 1(4):193, Aug 1986.

These two articles provide guidance for mamaging successful tube feeding for persons in need of special nutrition support.

Mamel JJ: Percutaneous endoscopic gastrostomy, Nutr Clin Pract 2(2):65, Apr 1987.

This is an excellent review with illustrations of the gastrostomy method of feeding through a special tube surgically placed through the abdominal wall into the stomach, which has successfully maintained nutritional status of children and adults during periods of feeding problems.

The Challenge of Long-Term TPN Therapy

The purpose of any nonoral feeding method is to restore the patient to the oral feeding state, if possible. How long this will take varies according to the original nutritional and health status of the patient, as well as the extent of the illness. Persons with inflammatory bowel syndrome (see Chapter 19) have been known to require 2 to 3 months to reap the clinical benefits of "bowel rest" afforded by TPN. At least one individual with "no bowel" syndrome has done very well on TPN for more than a decade. Although this makes TPN's potential for long-term use seem tremendous, it is not without its drawbacks.

First of all, the intestinal effects of TPN suggest potential hazards with long-term use. The lack of food in the alimentary canal results in:

- Reduced secretion of hormones and enzymes into the gastrointestinal tract
- **Cholestasis,** caused by an increased viscosity of bile that is *not* secreted into the gastrointestinal tract
- Mucosal atrophy and *hypoplasia,* possibly resulting from reduced levels of cholecystokinin
- Less insulin secreted in response to the same amount of glucose obtained orally

These difficulties do not interfere with the ability to digest foods for 2 to 3 months. But what if the patient graduates to oral or tube feedings after that? Will there be difficulties with (1) undigested foods, (2) a higher risk for gallstones, (3) impaired nutrient absorption across an atrophied mucosa, or (4) a risk of hyperglycemia?

These questions may indicate the need for *very* careful monitoring and *gradual* refeeding for such patients; however, such concerns still must be verified and/or measured.

Other problems regarding long-term TPN *have* been verified and measured. These problems have more to do with the nature of the formula solution rather than the bowel. Their potential for malnutrition warrants careful control and prevention methods on the part of the health care professional.

The TPN process uses solutions of glucose, fats, and amino acids, as well as vitamin and mineral supplements. The nature of the glucose and fat solutions is discussed in the text. During use of these solutions, glucose levels must be carefully monitored, since excessive amounts may result in:

- Hyperglycemia
- Respiratory distress, especially in critically ill patients—excessive glucose intake raises the respiratory quotient (CO_2/O_2) by increasing CO_2 production
- Lipogenesis

These problems may not be desirable in individual patients. The best defense against them is a solution that derives half of its nonprotein energy from fats and half from glucose.

Amino acid solutions have been associated with several nutritional imbalances, including deficiencies in the following:

Carnitine. Carnitine is an amino acid that helps incorporate fatty acids into the cell for energy use (see Chapter 6). Patients on long-term TPN have developed muscle weakness, high bilirubin levels, and hypoglycemia, and plasma carnitine levels have been found to be low. Symptoms subside after carnitine supplementation.

Cholestasis
Suppression or stoppage of the bile flow.

Calcium. Amino acid solutions provide extra sulfur such as in methionine and cysteine, which binds with calcium and promotes its excretion. As a result premature infants on TPN have been known to develop a painful bone disease characterized by osteomalacia and associated with the resulting calcium deficiency.

Amino acid solutions have also been known to induce *metabolic alkalosis,* a condition that may be symptomless or marked by irritability, hypoxia, neuromuscular hyperexcitability, impaired gastrointestinal motility, polyuria, tetany, and other symptoms. It is associated with a loss of endogenous acids such as gastric hydrochloric acid (HCl), which occurs in several conditions in which TPN is indicated for (e.g., chronic vomiting and fistulas). Ironically, this loss can be aggravated by TPN, specifically by the lactate or acetate that is added to amino acid solutions to *prevent* this condition's counterpart, *metabolic acidosis.* Since acetate is added to all commercial solutions, the health care professional must be prepared to correct its pH by adding water or HCl. Arginine HCl and ammonium chloride can also be used, although with caution if renal or hepatic insufficiency is suspected. Sodium chloride and potassium chloride have also been used, but they are not as effective as HCl.

Vitamin and mineral supplements may create a problem because of the difficulty that is connected with their release from solution or because of the variability in requirements among patients, as in the examples that follow:

Iron. Iron dextran, the supplement frequently used in TPN solutions, does not release iron as easily as desired. Ferrous citrate is recommended by at least one study, which found that 74% to 81% of its iron was readily available for binding with ferritin in the blood.

Biotin. One patient, who developed delirium, dermatitis, severe depression, anorexia, and nausea and vomiting, was relieved of his symptoms after 1 week of biotin supplementation at 300 μg/day.

Thus for maximal promotion of the nutritional status of patients requiring long-term TPN, the health care professional should do the following:

- Carefully monitor a *gradual* refeeding program to avoid problems created by reduced gastrointestinal secretions and mucosal atrophy.
- Provide sufficient fats (i.e., half of the nonprotein kilocalories) to prevent respiratory distress in very ill patients and spare protein for tissue repair and development.
- Be aware of deficiency symptoms and potential effects of "undesirable" additives (sulfur, ammonia) found in amino acid solutions, and be prepared to adjust the solution appropriately.
- Adjust vitamin and mineral levels to suit individual needs.
- Select solutions from which nutrients are readily available.

REFERENCES

Borum PR: Carnitine—who needs it? Nutr Today 21(6):4, Nov/Dec 1986.

Cole D, and Zlotkin S: Increased sulfate as an etiological factor in the hypercalciuria associated with total parenteral nutrition, Am J Clin Nutr 37:108, Jan 1983.

Levenson JL: Biotin-responsive depression hyperalimentation, J Parenteral Enteral Nutr 7:181, Mar/Apr 1983.

Marshall MW: The nutritional importance of biotin—an update, Nutr Today 22(6):26, Nov/Dec 1987.

Sayers MH, et al: Supplementation of total parenteral nutrition solutions with ferrous citrate, J Parenteral Enteral Nutr 7:117, Mar/Apr 1983.

24 Nutrition and Cancer

Chapter Objectives

After study of this chapter, the student should be able to:

1. Relate nutrition to development of the cancer cell and to the body's defense system.
2. Identify nutritional effects of the various medical therapies for cancer and describe ways of handling eating problems.
3. List ways cancer affects nutritional requirements and outline dietary management to meet these needs.

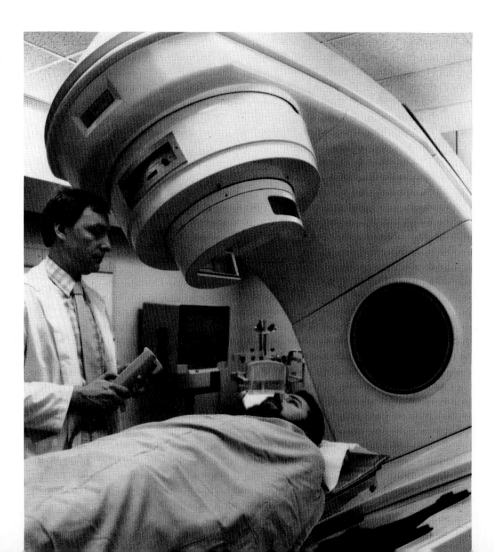

PREVIEW

The American Cancer Society estimates that approximately 440,000 Americans die of cancer each year, with about 25% dying of lung cancer. In its multiple forms cancer has become one of our major public health problems. It is second only to heart disease and accounts for about 20% of the total deaths in the United States each year.

In current study and practice, important nutritional relationships exist in two basic areas: (1) *prevention*, related to the environment and the body's defense system; and (2) *therapy*, related to nutritional support for medical treatments and rehabilitation. To understand these nutritional relationships, we must clarify them in terms of cancer's physiologic basis in the structure and function of cells, and the body's defense systems, both in immunity and the healing process.

In this chapter in our continuing study sequence on clinical nutrition, we will examine these issues relating nutrition to the cancer process in its varying forms. We will look at the significance of nutritional support in cancer therapy and explore many practical means of managing dietary problems.

Multiple Forms of Cancers

Difficulties in the study of cancer have arisen from its varying nature and multiple forms. The word **cancer** is a general term used to designate any one of many malignant tumors or **neoplasms** (new growth). There are many different forms of cancer, varying worldwide and changing with population migrations. There are multiple causes and often conflicting research results because of the large number of variables involved. Thus it is clear that we are dealing with a wide range of malignant tumors collectively known as cancer. We would be more correct, then, to use the plural term "cancers" in discussing this great variety of neoplasms.

To better understand cancer development, therefore, we should view it as a growth process that has its physiologic basis in the structure and function of cells. Since nutrition is fundamental to all tissue growth, we need to look briefly at the cancer cell to understand the relationship of nutritional factors to cancer. This misguided cell and its tumor tissue represent normal cell growth that has "gone wild."

The Cancer Cell

The marvel of human life is that the process of cell growth and reproduction goes on almost flawlessly over and over again, guided by the cell's genes. In adult humans some 3 to 4 million cells complete the normal life-sustaining process of cell division every second, largely without mistake, guided by the genetic code. The central question in cell biology has been: How are the process and rate of cell reproduction maintained so precisely in normal cells? The question in cancer research, based on increased knowledge of normal cell physiology, then follows: How and why is this normal, precise regulation of cell reproduction and function lost in cancer cells, and why do cancer cells

The Process of Cancer Development

Cancer
Celullar tumor whose natural course is fatal; unlike benign tumor cells, cancer growths are invasive and spread easily.

Neoplasm
Any new or abnormal growth; uncontrolled or progressive growth. Also called a tumor.

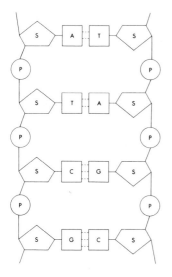

Figure 24-1
Diagram of a portion of DNA structure. Note the components. The sugar deoxyribose and phosphate form the parallel bars of the ladderlike structure (a double helix); the connecting nitrogenous bases (the pyrimidines, thymine and cytosine, and the purines, adenine and guanine) form the rungs (*A*, adenine; *T*, thymine; *C*, cytosine; *G*, guanine; *S*, sugar—deoxyribose; *P*, phosphate). The dotted lines represent the hydrogen bonding between the nitrogenous bases.

then remain mutant and malformed, functionally immature and imperfect, incapable of normal cell life?

The first part of the answer lies in the nature of the cell's genetic material and its regulating components. The specific genetic material in the cell's nucleus is arranged as chromosomes and genes, which hold the controlling agent, *deoxyribonucleic acid (DNA)*. Specific sites along the chromosome threads are called genes. Each gene carries specific information that controls synthesis of specific proteins and transmits genetic heritage. A single chromosome thread is made up of hundreds of genes arranged end to end, and each gene of DNA is made up of some 600 to several thousand smaller subunits called nucleotides. The nucleic acids, DNA and its companion *ribonucleic acid (RNA)*, compose the controlling system by which both the cell and thus the organism sustain life.

The structure of DNA is that of a very large polynucleotide made up of many individual mononucleotides, each one of which has three parts: (1) a sugar (deoxyribose); (2) a phosphate; and (3) a specific nitrogenous base—adenine, cytosine, guanine, or thymine. It is the pairing of these nitrogenous bases, as shown in Figure 24-1, that incorporates the "genetic code" and enables the DNA to transmit messages to guide protein structure. The DNA appears as a twisted ladder or spiral staircase in structure and is thus called a "helix," the Greek word meaning "coil."

Gene Control of Cell Reproduction and Function
The Normal Cell

Cells arise only from preexisting cells by division and carry the preexisting cell's genetic pattern. Normally the various cell structures and functions operate in an orderly manner under gene control, directing the cell's specific processes of protein synthesis. Gene action, however, can be switched on and off, depending on the position of a cell in the body, the stage of body development, and the external environment. Specific regulator genes control such function by producing a repressor substance as needed to regulate operator genes and structural genes. This orderly regulation of induction and repression in cell activity, however, can be lost with mutation of these regulatory genes. Control is also lost when a specific gene for some reason moves from its position to another location on the chromosome.

The Cancer Cell

A cell may become malignant when one of these potentially cancer-causing genes is translocated and reinserted into a highly active part of the DNA. This has been shown to occur, for example, in patients with Burkitt's lymphoma and the blood cancer, acute nonlymphocytic leukemia. Now apparently these root causes of damaged DNA and the cell's impaired ability to repair it are joined by the recently discovered cellular genes called *protooncogenes,* which in their developed form of oncogenes can cause neoplastic growth.[1] This search for genetic damage and the explanation of how that damage affects biochemical function in the cell are key lines of current research promising further unfolding the mysteries of cancer.

Cancer Cell Derivation. The source of the cancer cell is now clear. It is derived from a normal cell that has lost control over cell reproduction and is thereby transformed from a normal cell (Figure 24-2) into a cancer cell.

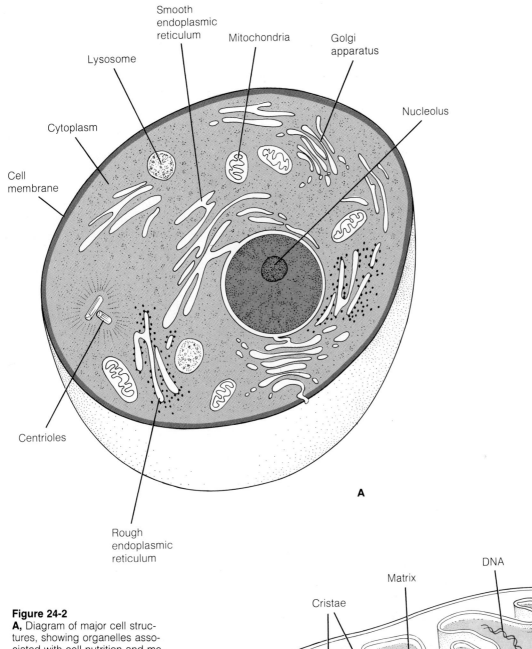

Figure 24-2
A, Diagram of major cell structures, showing organelles associated with cell nutrition and metabolism. **B,** Structure of a mitochondrion, the "powerhouse" of the cell.

Sarcoma
Tumor, usually malignant, arising from connective tissue.

Carcinoma
Tumor, usually malignant, arising from epithelial tissue.

Cancer Tumor Types

On this basis of cell nature and differentiation, it is possible to classify cancer tumor types according to (1) the type of *originating tissue,* with tumors arising from connective tissues called **sarcomas** and those from epithelial tissues called **carcinomas;** and (2) the *degree of cell tissue change,* with tumor stages defined in relation to rate of growth, degree of autonomy, and invasiveness.

Relation to Aging Process

Since the incidence of cancer increases with age, a relationship exists between cancer development and the aging process in cells, tissues, and organ systems.

Causes of Cancer Cell Development

The underlying cause of cancer, as indicated, is the fundamental loss of control over normal cell reproduction. Researchers have discovered several interrelated causes contributing to this loss of cell control.

Mutations

Gene mutations result from loss of one or more regulatory genes in the cell nucleus. Such a mutant gene may be inherited, although some environmental agent may contribute to its expression.

Chemical Carcinogens

A number of chemical carcinogens (hydrocarbons) can interfere with the structure or function of regulatory genes. Exposure to such agents may be by individual choice, as in cigarette smoking, or by exposure to general environmental substances, such as pesticide residues, water and air pollutants, food additives and contaminants, and occupational hazards.[2,3] However, many of our natural environmental agents can carry more hazard (for example, excessive sunshine causes skin cancer *melanoma*) than do manmade agents.[2] Possible cancer-causing actions of these agents may be mutation, effect on regulation of gene function, or activation of a dormant virus.

Radiation

In some instances radiation may be sufficient to cause chromosome breakage and incorrect rejoining. Such radiation damage may come from x-rays, radioactive materials, atomic exhausts or wastes, or sunlight. Our pursuit of the bronzed look has taken a large toll: sun-related skin cancer has risen rapidly in the United States and Europe, afflicting younger and younger persons. The common forms on the head and neck are usually basal cell carcinoma and are easily cured by surgical removal. However, a far more lethal form, *malignant melanoma,* strikes more than 15,000 Americans a year, killing some 45% of them.

Oncogenic Viruses

Oncogenic, or tumor-producing, viruses that interfere with the function of the regulatory genes have been identified in animals and are the focus of much current research.[1] Although oncogenes were first found in viruses, their evolutionary history indicates that they are also present and functioning in normal vertebrate cells. It is their abnormal expression that can lead to cancerous growth. A virus is little more than a packet of genetic information encased in a protein coat. It contains a small chromosome, DNA or RNA, with a relatively small number of genes, usually fewer than five and never more than several hundred. In contrast, cells of complex organisms have tens of thousands of genes. Generally, when viruses produce disease, they act as parasites, taking over the cell machinery to replicate themselves.

Epidemiologic Factors

Studies of cancer distribution and occurrence in relation to such factors as race, diet, region, sex, age, heredity, and occupation show variable and conflicting results. The specific role of diet in cancer etiology is still unclear (see Issues and Answers, p. 608). However, the incidence of cancer does vary a great deal from country to country, and that of specific cancer types varies from 6- to 300-fold. Although our cancer rates have not changed markedly over the past few decades, cancer is *endemic* in our population. The U.S. incidence rates are appreciably greater than those in many other countries. Also, racial incidence of cancer seems to change as population groups migrate and aquire the different cancer characteristics of the new population. Although specific dietary factors have been hard to pinpoint in the cause of cancer, worldwide studies do show significant correlation of mortality from breast cancer, for example, with the consumption of fat in the diet.

Stress Factors

The idea that emotions may play a part in malignancy is not new. Galen, a second century Greek physician, wrote of such relationships, as have many different kinds of "healers" since that time. However, these relationships are difficult to measure. Even with great technologic and scientific advances, Western medicine holds fast to its basic tenet that a thing must be measurable under controlled conditions to be said to exist.

Nonetheless, increasing observations are being made of relationships between cancer and less measurable factors of stress. Clinicians and researchers have reported that psychic trauma, especially the loss of a central relationship, does seem to carry with it a strong cancer correlation. The cause of a possible relationship between such trauma and cancer may lie in two physiologic areas: (1) damage to the thymus gland and the immune system, and (2) neuroendocrine effects mediated through the hypothalamus, pituitary, and adrenal cortex. This automatic cascade of physiologic events triggered by stress (see Chapter 16) may well provide the neurologic currency that converts anxiety to malignancy. Such a stressful state may also make a person more vulnerable to other factors present, influencing the integrity of the immune system, food behaviors, and nutritional status. It may also act as an environmental agent whose physiologic impact stimulates the expression of an underlying mutant or damaged gene.

Components of the Immune System

The human body's defense system is remarkably efficient and complex. Several components of special type cells protect not only against external invaders such as bacteria and viruses but also against internal "aliens" such as malignant tumor cells.

Two major populations of cells provide the immune system's primary line of defense for detecting and destroying malignant cells that arise daily in the body. These cells mediate specific **cellular immunity** and **humoral immu-**

The Body's Defense System

Cellular immunity
Specific, acquired immunity in which the role of the T-lymphocytes predominates.

Humoral immunity
Acquired immunity in which the role of antibodies (produced by B-lymphocytes and plasma cells) predominates.

nity, as well as providing supportive backup biologic systems. These two populations of lymphoid cells, or *lymphocytes* (a type of white cell), develop early in life from a common stem cell in fetal liver and bone marrow (Figure 24-3). They then differentiate and populate the peripheral lymphoid organs during the latter stages of gestation. One type are called *T cells,* traced from the thymus-derived cells, and the other *B cells,* traced from bursa-derived cells. Both T and B lymphocytes are derived from precursor cells in the bone marrow.

T Cells

After precursor cells migrate to the thymus, the T cell population is differentiated in this small gland, which lies posterior to the sternum and anterior to the great vessels partly covering the trachea. The majority of the circulating small lymphocytes in blood, lymph, and certain areas of the lymph nodes and spleen are T cells. When these cells meet an antigen, an alien substance, they proliferate and initiate specific cellular immune responses: (1) they activate the *phagocytes,* special cells that have intracellular killing and degrading mechanisms for destroying invaders; and (2) they cause an inflammatory response through chemical mediators released by the antigen-stimulated T cells. Scientists have now discovered that some T lymphocytes can do even

The thymus is a small organ, weighing about 14 g (½ oz) at birth. It reaches its largest size of 37 g (1⅓ oz) at puberty and reduces in older age to 7 g (¼ oz).

Figure 24-3
Development of the T and B cells, lymphocyte components of the body's immune system.

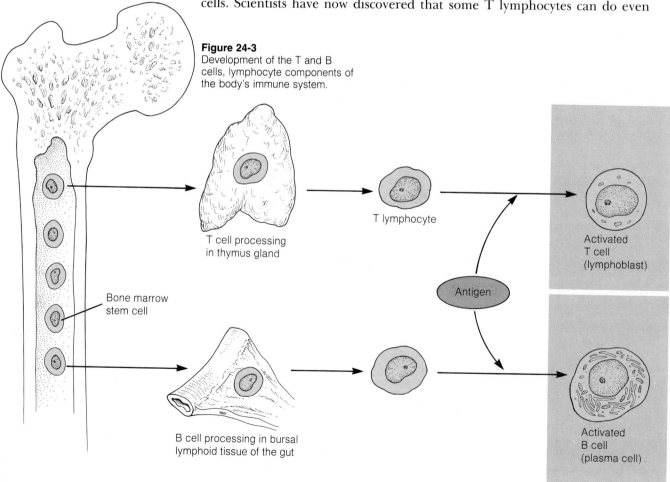

Bone marrow stem cell

T cell processing in thymus gland

T lymphocyte

Antigen

Activated T cell (lymphoblast)

B cell processing in bursal lymphoid tissue of the gut

Activated B cell (plasma cell)

more, not only proliferating in response to an antigen but also attacking it. These special T cells are called "helper cell-independent cytotoxic T lymphocytes," abbreviated more graphically to the name *HIT cells.*

B Cells

The B cell population matures first in the bone marrow and then, following migration, in the solid peripheral lymphoid tissues of the body—the lymph nodes, spleen, and gut. These cells are responsible for synthesis and secretion of specialized protein known as *antibodies.* When the B cells contact an antigen, they increase and initiate specific humoral immune responses: (1) they produce specific antibodies in the blood; and (2) they produce a particular antibody secretion in the bowel and upper respiratory mucosa. This combination of antigen and antibody then attracts phagocytes and initiates the inflammatory response for healing. Teams of researchers and clinicians have been able to develop specially tailored proteins called *monoclonal antibodies* and use them to diagnose and treat a number of diseases, including cancer.[4] As their name implies, these special antibodies are produced by identical descendents, or clones, of a single cell through specific techniques involving injection and development in laboratory mice. These controlled products are specific antibodies for specific targets.

Relation to Nutrition

Immune System

Nutritional support is necessary to maintain the integrity of this efficient human immune system. Several malnourished populations have displayed changes in the structure and function of the immune system because of atrophy of the basic tissues involved: liver, bowel wall, bone marrow, spleen, and lymphoid tissue. The role of nutrition in maintaining normal immunity and in combating sustained attacks in malignancy is fundamental.

The Healing Process

Tissue integrity, essential for the healing process, is maintained through protein synthesis. Such strength of tissue is a front line of the body's defense system. This process of healing requires optimal nutritional intake to support (1) cell function and structure of all its parts involving DNA, RNA, amino acids, and proteins, and (2) the integrity of all the immune system components. Wise and early use of vigorous nutritional support for cancer patients has been shown to provide recovery of normal nutritional status, including **immunocompetence,** thereby improving their response to therapy and prognosis.

Surgery

Operable Tumors

Early diagnosis of operable tumors has led to successful surgical treatment of a large number of cancer patients. The success of any surgery depends in large measure on the sound nutritional status of the patient (see Chapter 23). But this is especially true of cancer patients because their general condition may be weakened. Optimal nutritional status preoperatively and maximal nutritional support postoperatively are fundamental to the healing process.

Immunocompetence
The ability or capacity to develop an immune response, such as antibody production or cell-mediated immunity, following exposure to antigen.

Nutritional Support for Cancer Therapy

Nutrition Relationships

Nutrition has both general and specific relationships: (1) support of the general healing process and overall body metabolism, and (2) specific modifications of nutrient factors, texture, or feeding method according to the surgical site and organ function involved. Prevention of problems through early detection and surgical treatment has significantly increased cancer cure rates. Surgical treatment may also be used with other forms of therapy for removal of single metastases or for prevention and alleviation of symptoms.

Radiation

Treatment Role

Radiation
Electromagnetic phenomenon that has properties combining both wave and particle functions. Spans the entire spectrum from low-frequency radio waves, through white light, to high-frequency gamma rays.

Following the discovery of **radiation** in the nineteenth century, scientists found that it could damage body tissue. Continued study of its use and control revealed that normal tissue could largely withstand an amount of radiation that would damage and destroy cancer tissue. The subsequent role of radiation in cancer treatment has developed around controlled use with two types of tumor: (1) those responsive to therapy within a dose level tolerable to health of normal tissue, and (2) those that can be targeted without damage to overlying vital organ tissue.

Forms

Radiation used in cancer therapy is produced from three main sources: (1) *x-rays,* the oldest form of cancer treatment, or electromagnetic waves similar to heat and light rays, with varying penetration according to the speed at which the electrons strike the target; and (2) *radioactive isotopes,* such as cobalt 60, and (3) *atomic particles,* derived from radioactive materials.

Effects

Palliative care
Care that gives relief but no cure.

Radiotherapy may be used alone or in conjunction with other therapies both for curative and **palliative care** for some 50% of all cancer patients at some time during the course of their disease. Radiation effects will influence nutritional status and therapy a great deal, depending on the site and intensity of treatment:

1. *Head and neck* radiation will affect the oral mucosa and salivary secretions, as well as the esophagus, influencing taste sensations and sensitivity to food temperature and texture
2. *Abdomen* radiation may produce denuded bowel mucosa, loss of villi and absorbing surface area, vascular changes from intimal thickening, thrombosis, ulcer formation, or inflammation. Obstruction, fistula formation, or strictures may further contribute to general malabsorption, compounded by curtailment of food intake due to anorexia and nausea.

Chemotherapy

Drug Development

Although chemotherapy has been recognized as a valid cancer therapy over the past few decades, the most effective agents currently in use have largely been developed only within the past few years. Intensive research has resulted in the development of a large number of effective *antineoplastic drugs.* Their therapeutic use is based on two general principles related to rate and mode of action.

Rate of Action

The so-called cell or log (logarithm)-kill hypothesis of the action of chemotherapeutic agents on tumors indicates that a single dose can only be as much as 99.9% effective in killing the tumor cells. Thus if as large a tumor as is compatible with life can be treated with a drug tolerable at a toxicity level that is 99.9% effective, the tumor is gradually reduced with successive doses that cause "fractional killing" with each dose. This process finally brings the tumor within the capability of the body's own immune system to take over and make the final kill and cure. The smaller the tumor, either because of early detection or initial treatment by surgery or radiation, the greater the possible effectiveness of the chemotherapeutic agents. Two other principles of dosage rate for greater effectiveness are also important: (1) aggressive use of maximal tolerable dosages in repeated series, and (2) use of several drugs together for a *synergistic* effect.

Mode of Action

Chemotherapeutic agents are effective because they disrupt the normal processes in the cell responsible for cell growth and reproduction. Some agents interfere with DNA synthesis. Others disrupt DNA structure and RNA replication. Others prevent prevent cell division by mitosis, or cause hormonal imbalances, or make unavailable the specific amino acids necessary for protein synthesis. It is this diversity in mode of action that provides a basis for grouping drugs into certain classes of chemotherapeutic agents: (1) alkaloids, (2) alkylating agents, (3) antibiotics, (4) antimetabolites, (5) enzymes, and (6) hormones. They are usually used in combined therapy or as adjuvant therapy in conjunction with surgery or radiation.

Toxic Effects

Chemotherapeutic agents have the same effects on rapidly reproducing normal cells as they do on the rapidly reproducing cancer cells. Interference with normal function is most apparent in normal cells of the bone marrow, the gastrointestinal tract, and the hair follicles, accounting for a number of the toxic side effects and problems in nutritional management:

1. **Bone marrow effects** include interference with production of red blood cells (anemia), white cells (infections), and platelets (bleeding).

2. **Gastrointestinal effects** include nausea and vomiting, **stomatitis,** anorexia, ulcers, and diarrhea.

3. **Hair follicle effects** include alopecia (baldness) and general hair loss.

Stomatitis
Inflammation of the oral mucosa.

Therapeutic Problems and Goals

Numerous problems present needs for nutritional therapy and care of patients with cancer. In general, nutritional therapy deals with problems (1) related to the disease process itself and (2) related to medical treatment of the disease. Thus the basic objectives of nutritional therapy in cancer are to (1) meet the increased metabolic demands of the disease and prevent catabolism as much as possible, and (2) alleviate symptoms of the disease and its treatment through adaptations of food and the feeding process.

Nutritional Therapy

Problems Related to the Disease Process

General feeding problems pose a great challenge to the nutritionist who is planning care and to the nurse who is providing supportive assistance. These problems relate to the overall systemic effects of the neoplastic disease process itself and to the specific individual responses to the type of cancer involved.

General Systemic Reactions

Anorexia
Lack or loss of appetite.

The disease process causes three basic systemic effects: (1) **anorexia,** (2) a hypermetabolic state, and (3) a negative nitrogen balance. These effects are often accompanied by a continuing weight loss. These effects may vary widely with individual patients, according to type and stage of the disease, from mild, scarcely discernible responses to the extreme forms of debilitating **cachexia** seen in advanced disease.[5] This extreme weight loss and weakness is caused by abnormalities in glucose metabolism, in which cancer patients cannot produce glucose efficiently from carbohydrates and instead "feed" off their own tissue protein and convert it to glucose. The "new-old" drug, hydrazine sulfate, seems to correct this metabolic error, allowing patients to conserve more energy.[6]

Cachexia
Profound and marked state of bodily dysfunction; general ill health and malnutrition.

The anorexia is frequently accompanied by depression or discomfort during normal eating.[7] This contributes further to a limited nutrient intake at the very time the disease process causes an increased metabolic rate and nutrient demand. Often this imbalance of decreased intake and increased demand creates a negative nitrogen balance, an indication of body-tissue wasting. Sometimes a true tissue loss of protein is masked by outward nitrogen equilibrium as the growing tumor retains nitrogen at the expense of the host, further compounding the problem.

Specific Responses Related to Type of Cancer

Interrelated functional and metabolic problems stem from specific types of cancer and their effects on the body. All of these factors contribute to nutritional depletion. In addition to the primary nutritional deficiencies induced by the disease process itself, secondary difficulties in ingestion and use of nutrients relate to specific tumors that cause obstructions or lesions in the gastrointestinal tract or adjacent tissue. Thus these conditions curtail intake or absorption of adequate nutrients.

Problems Related to Cancer Treatment

Each of the medical treatments for cancer entails physiologic stress, toxic tissue effects, or changes in normal body function. Thus the benefit achieved is not without attendant problems. Nutritional support seeks to alleviate these problems.

Surgery

Beyond the regular nutritional needs surrounding any surgical procedure and its healing process, gastrointestinal surgery poses special problems for normal eating and digesting and absorbing of food nutrients. In head and neck surgery, or resections in the oropharyngeal area, sometimes necessitated by cancer, food intake is greatly affected. A creative variety of food forms and semiliquid textures as well as modes of feeding must be devised. Often the mechanical problems of food ingestion make long-term tube feeding necessary.[8]

Gastrectomy may cause numerous postgastrectomy "dumping" problems

Clinical Application

Chemotherapy creates an almost "catch-22" situation in terms of the nutritional management of patients with cancer. On the one hand, it works best in the patient who is well nourished. On the other hand, it often triggers nausea and vomiting to such a degree that the patient cannot consume enough food to be well nourished. The resulting course of malnutrition may be further aggravated by alterations in taste acuity. To help prevent this problem of malnutrition, there are several things you may do:

- **Obtain a detailed history of emesis** Include data about onset, duration, and severity. Estimate the severity by degree of weight loss, electrolyte depletion, and retching. Also record factors aggravating or relieving emesis.
- **Limit food intake** Do this selectively and carefully to avoid taste aversions to foods previously enjoyed by the patient.
- **Evaluate emetic effect of antiemetic drugs** Note drugs used in patient's medical chemotherapy, anticipating possible emetic effects, as well as effectiveness of any antiemetic drugs being used to control the nausea (Table 24-1). Relate personal food plan and support counseling with patient and family about these effects.
- **Identify potential psychogenic causes** These are suspected when emesis occurs before the drug is administerd, or just as it is administered. Anticipatory nausea and vomiting have also been associated with the office or clinic visit itself, a person (e.g., the physician or nurse), or an event associated with treatment. This is most often seen in patients on chemotherapy for more than 6 months.
- **Identify other illnesses** Congestive heart failure, influenza, bowel obstruction may also be responsible for nausea and vomiting.
- **Identify other drugs, treatments** Use of other emetic drugs (e.g., antibiotics, digitalis, narcotics) or radiation therapy may aggravate nausea and vomiting during chemotherapy.

The nausea itself occurs when an area in the medulla of the brain—the vomiting center (VC)—is stimulated directly or indirectly by messages sent from the gastrointestinal tract or the cerebral cortex. The chemoreceptor trigger zone (CTZ), located near the VC, can also transmit stimuli induced by chemotherapy drugs. These three stimulatory routes suggest that the control of nausea and vomiting lies in a careful evaluation of three factors: (1) ingested food items, (2) psychologic influences, and (3) the emetic effects of any and all drugs, treatments, or illnesses occurring simultaneously.

Controlling Nausea and Vomiting in Patients Receiving Chemotherapy

REFERENCE
Huber SL, and Ballentine R: Therapeutic trends in the management of chemotherapy-induced nausea and vomiting, Nutr Support Serv 2(10):30, 1982.

Stenosis
Narrowing or contraction of a
duct or opening.

Endarteritis
Inflammation of the inner lining
of an artery.

requiring frequent, small, low-carbohydrate feedings (see Chapter 19). *Vagotomy* contributes to gastric stasis. Various intestinal resections or tumor excisions may cause steatorrhea due to general malabsorption, fistulas, or **stenosis.** Pancreatectomy causes loss of digestive enzymes, induced insulin-dependent diabetes mellitus, and general weight loss.

Radiation

Radiation to the oropharyngeal area often produces a loss of taste sensation, with increasing anorexia and nausea.[9,10] Other means of tempting appetite through food appearance and aroma, as well as texture, must be developed. Abdominal radiation may cause intestinal damage, with tissue edema and congestion, decreased peristalsis, or **endarteritis** in small blood vessels. In the intestinal wall there may be fibrosis, stenosis, necrosis, or ulceration. General malabsorption or fistulas may develop, as well as hemorrhage, obstruction, and diarrhea, all contributing to nutritional problems. The liver is somewhat more resistant to damage from radiation in adults, but children are more vulnerable.

Chemotherapy

The major nutritional problems during chemotherapy relate to (1) the gastrointestinal symptoms caused by the effect of the toxic drugs on the rapidly developing mucosal cells; (2) the anemia associated with bone marrow effects; and (3) the general systemic toxicity effect on appetite. Stomatitis, nausea, diarrhea, and malabsorption contribute to many food intolerances. Antiemetic drugs such as prochlorperazine (Compazine) may be used (Table 24-1). Such drugs act on the vomiting center in the brain to prevent the nausea response. Prolonged vomiting seriously affects fluid and electrolyte balance. Certain chemotherapeutic drugs also have special effects. For example, monoaminoxidase (MAO) inhibitors may be used for pretreatment relief of mental and emotional depression or for palliative therapy. These antidepressant drugs cause well-known pressor effects when used with tyramine-rich foods. Thus these foods should be avoided when using such drugs (see Chapter 18).

Principles of Nutritional Therapy

Two important principles of nutritional therapy, vital in any sound nutrition practice but especially essential in care of patients with cancer, provide the basis for planning nutritional care of each patient: (1) personal nutritional assessment, and (2) vigorous nutrition therapy to maintain good nutritional status and support medical treatment.

Nutrition Assessment

It is far more difficult to replenish a nutritionally depleted patient than to maintain a good nutritional status from the outset of the disease process. Therefore a primary goal in nutritional therapy is to prevent a depleted state. Both initial assessment for baseline data and regular monitoring thereafter during treatment are necessary. A detailed personal history is essential to determine individual needs, desires, and tolerances. All of these procedures are found in Chapter 17.

Table 24-1

Medications Used to Control Nausea and Vomiting in Patients Receiving Chemotherapy*

Antiemetic drug/action	Cancer chemotherapeutic drug counteracted	Dosage used	Side effects	Comments
Phenothiazines Action: blocks CTZ stimulation by dopamine	Moderate emetic-potential drugs			
Examples Compazine (prochlorperazine) Torecan (thiethylperazine) Phenergan (promethazine)		5-10 mg, orally or parenterally before chemotherapy; every 4-6 hr after, for 24-48 hr	Sedation Orthostatic hypertension	Less effective when given on an "as needed" basis
Droperidol (inapsine) Action: sedative and antiemetic	Cisplatin	0.5 mg intravenously 1 hr before chemotherapy; every 4 hr after	Somnolence	Some patients given up to 1.5 mg intravenously developed a tolerance for the drug
Corticosteroids Dexamethasone (Hexadrol, Decadron)	Cyclophosphamide Doxorubicin	10 mg intramuscularly before chemotherapy	Perianal stinging if given too rapidly	Moderate to high relief in 70% of the patients
Methylprednisolone (SoluMedrol)	Nitrogen mustard Mitomycin Methyl-CCNU	250 mg intravenously every 6 hr for 4 doses beginning 2 hr	Swelling Facial rash Weakness, lethargy	Effects of methylprednisolone considered disappointing
Tetrahydrocannabinol (THC, marijuana)	Variety of agents studied Methotrexate 5-FU Methyl-CCNU Cyclophosphamide Doxorubicin Nitrosoureas Mechlorethamine Cisplatin	10 mg/m²	Somnolence Visual hallucinations	Patients (usually older) not used to THC refused to continue it because of CNS effects. Response associated with extent of THC-induced "high". Most effective with fluorouracil, cyclophosphamide, methotrexate, doxorubicin
Metoclopramide (Reglan)	Cisplatin	Single 20 mg dose, given orally halfway through a 6 hr infusion of cisplatin (100 mg/m²); higher doses might be possible intravenously (1-3 mg/kg/dose)	Sedation	Works well for patients who do not respond to other antiemetic drugs

*Data modified from studies reported by Huber, S.L., and Ballentine, R.: Nutr. Support Serv. 2(10):30, 1982.

Nutritional Therapy and Plan of Care

The nutritionist, in consultation with the physician, develops an individual plan of nutritional care based on interpretation of the nutrition assessment data. This nutritional therapy outline is then incorporated into the nursing care plan as the nutritionist works with the nursing staff to carry it out. Primary care provided by the experienced clinical nutritionist on a regular basis is a necessary part of the oncology team practice. This vigorous care often makes the difference in the success rate of medical therapy. Thus the clinical nutritionist can assess individual patient needs, plan and manage nutritional care, monitor progress and responses to therapy, and make adjustments in care according to status and tolerances.

Nutritional Needs

Although individual needs will vary, of course, guidelines for nutritional therapy must meet increased nutrient needs.

1. **Energy.** Great energy demands are placed on the cancer patient. These demands result from the hypermetabolic state of the disease process and the tissue-healing requirements. Of this total dietary kilocaloric value, there must be sufficient carbohydrate to spare protein for vital tissue symthesis. For the adult patient with good nutritional status, about 2000 kcal/day will provide for maintenance needs. A more malnourished patient may require 3000 to 4000 kcal, depending on the degree of malnutrition and body trauma.

2. **Protein.** Tissue protein synthesis, a necessary component of healing and rehabilitation, requires essential amino acids and nitrogen. Efficient protein use, which depends on an optimum protein/kilocalorie ratio, promotes tissue building, prevents tissue wastage (catabolism), and helps make up tissue deficits. An adult patient with good nutritional status will need about 80 to 100 g/day of protein to meet maintenance needs and assure anabolism. A malnourished patient will need more, 100 to 200 g/day to replenish tissue and restore positive nitrogen balance.

3. **Vitamins and minerals.** Key vitamins and minerals control protein and energy metabolism through their roles in cell enzyme systems. They also play a necessary part in structural development and tissue integrity. Hence an optimum intake of vitamins and minerals, at least to the recommended dietary allowances (RDA) levels but frequently to the higher potency therapeutic levels, is indicated. Depending on individual nutritional status, supplements to dietary sources may be needed.

4. **Fluids.** Adequate fluid intake is important for two reasons: (1) to replace gastrointestinal losses or losses caused by infection and fever, and (2) to help the kidneys dispose of the metabolic breakdown products from the destroyed cancer cells as well as from the toxic drugs used in treatment. For example, some toxic drugs such as cyclophosphamide (Cytoxan) require as much as 2 to 3 L of forced fluids daily to prevent hemorrhagic cystitis.

Nutritional Management

The specific feeding method used depends on the individual patient's condition. However, the classic dictum of nutritional management should prevail: "If the gut works, use it." The spectrum of management approaches includes four feeding methods—two enteral forms and two parenteral forms.

Enteral Feeding: Oral Diet and Nutrient Supplementation

An oral diet with supplementation is the most desired form of feeding, of course, whenever it is possible. A carefully designed personal plan of care based on nutrition assessment data and including adjustments in texture, temperature, food choices, and tolerances, as well as family food patterns, can often meet needs.[11] The hospitalized patient's diet can be supplemented with familiar foods from home as the clinical nutritionist plans with the family. Personal food tolerances will vary according to the current treatment and nature of the disease. A number of adjustments in food texture, temperature, amount, timing, taste, appearance, and form can be made to help alleviate symptoms of common problems in successive parts of the gastrointestinal tract. Difficulties in eating may be caused by loss of appetite, problems in the mouth or with swallowing, or various gastrointestinal problems.

Loss of Appetite

Anorexia is a major problem and curtails food intake when it is needed most. It is a general systemic effect of the cancer disease process itself. It is further induced by the cancer treatment and progressively enhanced by personal anxiety, depression, and stress of the illness. Such a vicious cycle, if not countered by much effort, can lead to more malnutrition and the well-recognized starvation "cancer cachexia," a syndrome of emaciation, debilitation, and malnutrition. A vigorous program of eating, *not dependent on appetite for stimulus,* must be planned with patient and family. The overall goal is to provide food with as much *nutrient density* as possible so that "every bite will count."

Mouth Problems

Eating difficulties may stem from sore mouth, stomatitis, or taste changes. Sore mouth often results from chemotherapy or from radiation to the head and neck area. It is increased by any state of malnutrition or from infections such as **candidiasis** (thrush), with numerous ulcerations of the oral and throat mucosa. Frequent small meals and snacks, soft in texture, bland in nature, and cool or cold in temperature, are often better tolerated. There may also be alterations in the tongue's taste buds, causing taste distortion ("taste blindness") and inability to distinguish the basic tastes of salt, sweet, sour, or bitter, with consequent food aversions. Since the aversion is often toward basic protein foods, a high protein/energy liquid drink supplement may be needed. *Dental problems* may also contribute to mouth difficulties and should be corrected. *Salivary secretions* are also affected by cancer treatment, so foods with a high liquid content should be used. Solid foods may be swallowed more easily with use of sauces, gravies, broth, yogurt, or salad dressings. A food processor or blender can render foods in semisolid or liquid forms and make them easier to swallow. If the swallowing problem is especially severe because of tumor growth or therapy, guides for a special swallowing training program, including progressive food textures, exercises, and positions, can be followed.[12]

Candidiasis
Superficial fungous infection (genus: *Candida*) of moist parts of the body (infection of oral mucous membranes is called *thrush*).

Gastrointestinal Problems

Eating difficulties may include nausea and vomiting (see box, p. 599). There may be general indigestion, bloating, or specific surgery responses such as the postgastrectomy "dumping" syndrome. Nausea is often enhanced by foods that are hot, sweet, fatty, or spicy, so these can be avoided according to individual tolerance. Frequent small feedings of cold foods, soft to liquid in texture, may have more appeal. These can be eaten slowly with rests in between. Antinausea drugs may be prescribed to help with food tolerance (Table 24-1). Other food problems may include general diarrhea, constipation, flatuence, or specific lactose intolerance or surgery responses, such as occur with intestinal resections and various ostomies.[13] The effect of chemotherapy or radiation treatment on the mucosal cells secreting lactase contributes to lactose intolerance. In such cases a nutrient supplement formula with a non-milk protein base may be needed.

A number of commercial nutrient supplement products are available. A comparative review of these products will provide the basis for developing a formulary in the hospital setting for a limited number of such products. A food processor or blender can be used at home to produce creative solid and liquid food combinations from regular foods for interval liquid supplementation.

Figure 24-4
Types of tube feeding. **A,** Common nasogastric feeding tube; **B,** gastrostomy-jejunal enteral feeding tube.

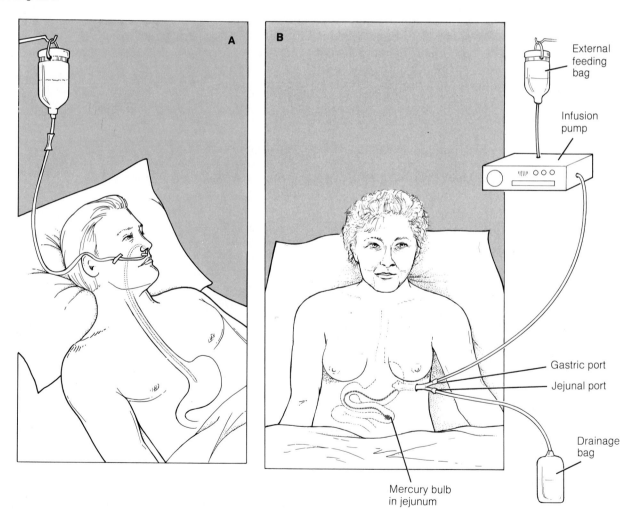

Enteral Feeding: Tube

When the patient is unable to eat but the gastrointestinal tract can still be used, tube feedings may be needed to provide the necessary nutritional support (Figure 24-4). The route of entry may vary from the traditional nasogastric tube to alternate surgical placements of esophagostomy, gastrostomy, or jejunostomy tubes. Individual problems surrounding the use of tube feedings may result from personal needs or from concentration of the formula.

Personal Problems

Many patients have negative attitudes toward nasogastric tubes (Table 24-2). Such an unnatural feeding method carries with it emotional problems for the patient. However, there is better acceptance with the small-caliber feeding tubes. Some highly motivated patients have even learned to pass their tubes themselves. Patients can be fed in some instances by pump-monitored slow drip during the night and freed from the tube during the day. The development of sophisticated enteral formulas and delivery systems has also made home enteral nutrition both feasible and practical.[14]

Table 24-2

Problem-Solving Tips for Patients Receiving Enteral Nutrition

Problem	Suggested solutions
Thirst, oral dryness	Lubricate lips Chew sugarless gum Brush teeth Rinse mouth frequently CAUTION: use lemon drops sparingly because of carcinogenic effects
Tube discomfort	Gargle with a mixture of warm water and mouth wash Gently blow nose Clean tube regularly with water or water-soluble lubricant If persistent, pull tube out gently, clean it, and reinsert Request smaller tube
Tension, fullness	Relax, breathe deeply after each feeding
Loud stomach noises	Take feedings in private
Limited mobility	Change positions in bed or chair Walk around the house or hospital corridor
Gustatory distress General dissatisfaction with feeding	Warm or chill feedings CAUTION: feedings that are too cold may cause diarrhea Serve favorite foods that have been liquefied
Persistent hunger	Chew a favorite food, then spit it out Chew gum Suck lemon drops (sparingly)
Inability to drink	Rinse mouth frequently with water and other liquids

Osmolality Problems

The concentration of the formula, it *osmolality,* as well as its specific composition of nutrients, are important considerations in selecting a product in order to avoid imbalances in the gastrointestinal fluid and electrolyte circulation. It must be of proper dilution and administered at an appropriate rate. Jejunostomy feedings given by **gavage** must be administered very slowly to prevent dumping symptoms. Blended formulas are rarely used by hospitals because there are too many uncontrolled factors. For example, hospital use of raw egg for patient fare is banned by most state health regulations; powdered egg white is a substitute.

Parenteral Feeding

When the gastrointestinal system cannot be used and nutritional support is vital, two additional modes of parenteral feeding may be needed. First, *peripheral parenteral nutrition (PPN)* can be used for brief periods to administer solutions of dextrose, amino acids, vitamins, and minerals, with intermittent fat emulsions. Second, to meet greater nutritional support requirements over a longer period of time, *total parenteral nutrition (TPN)* through a larger central vein may be used for feeding a more concentrated formula of these ingredients.[15] The TPN process requires surgical placement and careful assessment and administration. These procedures are found in Chapter 23. The use of TPN with cancer patients has been questioned by some practitioners. In many cases, however, it has been a significant means of turning metabolic status from catabolism to anabolism, often avoiding the serious development of cancer cachexia.[16]

To Sum Up

Cancer is a term applied to abnormal, malignant growths in various body tissue sites. The cancerous cell is derived from a normal cell that loses control over cell reproduction. Cancer cell development occurs via mutation, carcinogens, radiation, and oncogenic viruses. It is also influenced by many epidemiologic factors such as diet, alcohol, and smoking, as well as physical and psychologic stress factors. Cell development is mediated by the body's immune system, primarily its T cells, a type of white cell found in blood, lymph, and certain parts of the lymph nodes and spleen, and B cells, which manufacture and secrete antibodies.

Cancer therapy consists primarily of surgery, radiation, and chemotherapy. Supportive nutritional therapy for the cancer patient should be highly individualized and depends on the response of each body system to the disease and to the treatment itself. It is based on a thorough nutritional assessment and provided by a number of routes—oral, tube feeding, peripheral vein, TPN. The oral route is preferred if at all possible. Nutrient requirements and feeding mode must be designed for specific physical and psychologic needs of individual patients.

Questions for Review

1. What is cancer? Identify and describe several major causes of cancer cell formation.
2. How does your body attempt to defend itself against cancer? What nutritional factors may diminish this ability?
3. List and describe the rationale and mode of action of the types of therapies used to treat cancer.

4. Differentiate those factors challenging cancer recovery that are associated with the disease versus the type of therapy used.
5. Outline the general procedure for the nutritional management of a cancer patient.

References

1. Bishop JM: The molecular genetics of cancer, Science 235:305, Jan 1987.
2. Ames BN, Magaw R, and Gold LS: Ranking possible carcinogen hazards, Science 236:271, Apr 17, 1987.
3. Newberne PM, and Connor MW: Food additives and cancer and contaminants: an update, Cancer 58(suppl):1851, Oct 15, 1986.
4. Langone J: Monoclonals: the super antibodies, Discover 4(6):68, 1983.
5. Trant AS: Taste and anorexia in cancer patients: a review, Top Clin Nutr 1(2):17, Apr 1986.
6. Seligmann J, and Witherspoon D: A new, old cancer drug, Newsweek, June 6, 1983, p. 95.
7. Little LV, and Aljadir LP: Nutrition and quality of life of cancer patients, Top Clin Nutr 1(2):61, Apr 1986.
8. Krey SH, et al: Prolonged use of modular enteral hyperalimentation, Nutr Clin Pract 1(3):140, June 1986.
9. Donaldson SS: Nutritional support as an adjunct to radiation therapy, J Parenteral Enteral Nutr 8:302, 1984.
10. Hearne BE, et al: Enteral nutrition support in head and neck cancer: tube vs oral feeding during radiation therapy, J Am Diet Assoc 85:669, 1985.
11. Coulston AM, and Darbinian JA: Nutrition management in patients with cancer, Top Clin Nutr 1(2):26, Apr 1986.
12. Rosenbaum, EH, et al: Nutrition for the cancer patient, Palo Alto, CA, 1980, Bull Publishing Co.
13. Mullen BD, and McGinn KA: The ostomy book, Palo Alto, CA, 1980, Bull Publishing Co.
14. Nelson JK, Palumbo PJ, and O'Brien PC: Home enteral nutrition in cancer patients, Top Clin Nutr 1(2):37, Apr 1986.
15. Bell SJ, Coffey LM, and Blackburn GL: Use of total parenteral nutrition in cancer patients, Top Clin Nutr 1(2):37, Apr 1986.
16. Brennan MF, and Ekman L: Metabolic consequences of nutritional support of the cancer patient, Cancer 54:2627, 1984.

Further Readings

Cancer 58(suppl), Oct 15, 1986.
This entire supplemental issue of this journal is devoted to issues involved in diet and cancer, including such topics as etiology, pathophysiology of malnutrition, modes of therapy, risk reduction, medical treatment effects, and family nutrition education.
Lingard CD, et al: Planning and implementing a nutrition program for children with cancer, Top Clin Nutr 1(2):71, Apr 1986.
Rickard KA, et al: Advances in nutritional care of children with neoplastic diseases: a review of treatment, research, and application, J Am Diet Assoc 86(12):1666, Dec 1986.
These two excellent articles from the clinical team at James Whitcomb Riley Hospital for Children provide a comprehensive background in medical treatment and nutritional support for children with cancer.
Radman M, and Wagner R: The high fidelity of DNA duplication, Sci Am 259(2):40, Aug 1988.
For those fascinated by the nature of DNA and its vast human control system, which lies at the genetic heart of diseases such as cancer, this is a gem! Its very readable text and fine illustrations clarify our marvelous "high-fidelity" system of some 3 billion nucleotide letters to spell "human being" that goes on and on, generation after generation, with exceedingly few mistakes.

Dietary Guidelines for Cancer Prevention

The American public is always searching for a means of preventing devastating diseases before they start. At the turn of this century they sought relief from killer infections that have become virtually nonexistent. Today the battle is being waged against heart disease, cancer, and cerebrovascular accident (CVA, stroke). The medical community responded, first establishing guidelines to reduce the risk of hypertension and coronary heart disease, both of which may lead to CVA. Then the lay community anxiously awaited guidelines for cancer prevention as well.

Following study by a group of experts, such public guidelines were reported. A National Research Council (NRC) panel of nutrition scientists, including clinicians, researchers, and educators, issued guidelines, based on current knowledge and expert opinion, in their report *Diet, Nutrition, and Cancer*. The recommendations were a set of six "interim" dietary guidelines intended to reduce the risk of developing a variety of cancers:

1. Reduce fat intake to 30% of total kilocalories in the diet.
2. Include fruit, especially citrus; vegetables, especially carotene-rich ones; and whole grains in the diet daily.
3. Avoid foods preserved by pickling or smoking.
4. Avoid food contamination with carcinogens of any source (intentional additives, unintended contaminants, naturally occurring compounds).
5. Continue efforts to identify mutagens in foods, test their carcinogenic properties and, if it can be done without reducing the nutritive value of the food, remove them or limit their content in that food.
6. Avoid excessive alcohol intake.

If these diet and cancer guidelines sound familiar, it is because most of them are. They have already been included in the U.S. dietary goals issued earlier by the Department of Agriculture. These initial dietary goals were developed primarily to reduce the risk of heart disease, diabetes mellitus, hypertension, and other interrelated chronic disease. The two new statements added by the NRC cancer panel are common sense issues: (1) avoiding carcinogen-contaminated foods and (2) identifying, testing, and limiting the use of carcinogenic mutagens. However in this case these two added guidelines are directed at the food industry, rather than the public.

This NRC report and its recommended interim guidelines have been criticized by some persons in the scientific community. Also, some ask, since these guidelines have been presented before and today are considered common sense nutrition, why were they redeveloped by such a prestigious body as the NRC? Some critics suspect that the NRC's Committee on Diet, Nutrition, and Cancer felt "pressured" into providing information that would meet the public's demand for preventive measures against chronic disease. These critics do not take issue with the guidelines per se. However, they believe that the suggestion is made that the guidelines *will*, without complete certainty, prevent cancer, when in most cases this is not entirely known. However, the executive summary of the NRC committee's findings states clearly that evidence regarding the effect of many of their recommendations is inconclusive, and so they used the word "interim" in their title.

Fats are strongly associated with cancer of the breast, prostate, and bowel, in per capita, as well as case-control, studies; an increase of 10% to 40% of total kilocalories as fat increases tumor incidence. No one yet knows *how* fats contribute to tumor formation.

Citrus fruits are recommended sources of vitamin C, which is associated with a lower risk for cancer in the stomach and esophagus. Vitamin C has inhibited the in vivo and in vitro formation of carcinogenic N-nitroso compounds in laboratory tests. However, it has not been shown to have any effect on **preformed** tumors.

Carotene-rich vegetables are recommended for vitamin A, which in epidemiologic studies shows an inverse relationship with cancer of the lung, bladder, and larynx. Unfortunately no one yet knows whether this effect is caused by vitamin A itself, the carotenoids (vitamin A precursors) or other factors in food, or retinoids (synthetic analogs of vitamin A that lack its toxic effects but also inhibit neoplasms). Despite its anticancer effect, vitamin A supplement cannot be recommended because (1) it is highly toxic in large amounts, and (2) it may not be effective if carotene (found only in food) is the primary preventive agent.

Whole grains are recommended for the anticancer properties of the fiber they contain. Specific components, bran and cellulose, of fiber have been associated with inhibiting cancer formation or growth, especially in the colon. The NRC committee admits there is no conclusive evidence associating total fiber intake to cancer prevention.

Pickled and smoked foods are associated with cancer of the stomach and esophagus in China, Japan, Iceland, and elsewhere. Some preparation methods produce high levels of such compounds as polycycline aromatic and N-nitroso hydrocarbons, which can become mutagens and change the genetic material in cells in bacteria and animals. Thus they are suspected of being carcinogenic in humans.

Contamination with carcinogens occurs when a large amount of an additive is purposefully used, environmental additives such as pesticides and industrial chemicals enter the food supply, or naturally occurring toxins develop from molds such as aflatoxin or from bacterial action such as nitrosamine formation. Control over such contamination is primarily the responsibility of the food industry and government enforcement of the Delaney Clause (see Chapter 9), designed to prohibit the addition of any substance demonstrating carcinogenic properties in any amounts of foods. This recommendation is beyond the control of the general public, other than by political action such as boycotting against offending food companies and lobbying to encourage representatives to enforce the Delaney Clause.

Mutagens are substances that change part of the genetic material in cells; the change is almost always suspected of being carcinogenic. Some mutagens occur naturally in foods, such as mutagenic flavonoids (quercetin, kaemopterol). Others occur during the cooking process, especially in high-heat processes such as charcoal broiling. However, even the committee believes that no one can determine how these mutagens actually contribute to the incidence of cancer in the United States.

It is recommended that **alcohol** use be moderate, based on limited evidence associating heavy beer drinking with colorectal cancer and alcohol-induced cirrhosis with liver cancer. In combination with cigarette smoking, alcohol has certainly contributed to the risk of cancer of the mouth, larynx, esophagus, and respiratory tract. However, the key question to alcohol limitation remains: How much is *too* much?

Some critics also state that they suspect the NRC Committee of being somewhat selective in its formation of guidelines. For instance, even though an inverse relationship was found between stomach cancer and milk consumption, no recommendation was made to increase milk intake.

The irony of this situation is that no critic can take issue with any of the recommendations made, based on the general principle of health promotion. On the one hand they are all reasonable statements, given the extent of our knowledge and experiences. On the other hand, however, the NRC may have come close to "telling the public what it wants to know" without the possession of firm evidence. Whether or not the advice is harmful, and this certainly does *not* seem to be the case, it might be misleading to some persons who constantly seek dietary cures and preventions.

REFERENCES

Harper AE: A matter of opinion: firm recommendations, infirm basis, Nutr Today 17(4):16, 1982.

Kline K: Breast cancer: the diet-cancer connection, Nutr Today 21(3):11, May/June 1986.

National Research Council, executive summary: Diet, nutrition, and cancer, Nutr Today 17(4):20, 1982.

Watson RR, and Leonard TK: Selenium and vitamins A, E, and C: nutrients with cancer prevention properties, J Am Diet Assoc 86(4):505, Apr 1986.

25 Nutrition Support in Disabling Disease

Chapter Objectives

After study of this chapter, the student should be able to:

1. Describe the multidisciplinary team approach to long-term care and rehabilitation in disabling disease, why it is imperative, and the interrelated roles of each team member.
2. Plan practical means of helping persons with disabling disease or injury achieve as much independence in eating as possible.
3. Identify special needs of older disabled persons and how they may be met.
4. Describe a nutritional support program and its rationale for each of the following disabling diseases: rheumatoid arthritis, COPD, and AIDS.

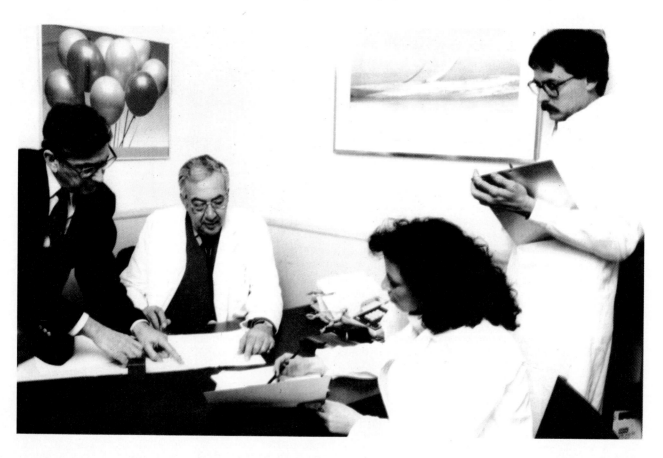

PREVIEW

In addition to primary care clinical problems, persons with severe or disabling illness or injury often require long-term specialized care, which carries added physical, mental, and social burdens. Such situations often require tremendous coping resources from the patient and family.

As a fundamental part of the specialized team care, personal nutrition support plays a vital role in the healing and restoring process. Patients undergoing severe physical difficulties require basic and specialized nutritional and emotional support. The practical necessity of handling the daily activity of eating, as well as meeting nutritional needs, requires patience and planning.

A positive approach to health within personal capacity in each case seeks to build personal strengths and resources. Nutritional care focuses on this integral relationship of nutrition to overall health promotion, as well as on the treatment of specific disease.

In this final chapter in our study of clinical nutrition, we will look at long-term care and rehabilitation needs of persons with disabling conditions. We will apply these principles of nutritional support to three examples of such health problems that bring malnutrition and sometimes devasting consequences—rheumatoid arthritis, progressive pulmonary failure, and AIDS.

Goals of Supportive Care

Positive goals guide care for disabling disease or injury. Successful support is rooted in a positive philosophy, based on the optimal potential of each person affected. This approach requires a specialized team working together with the patient and family to meet individual needs. It is built on clearly defined preventive and restorative personal care objectives. To the greatest degree possible within each situation, two goals are fundamental in planning care: (1) to prevent further **disability,** and (2) to restore potential function. Health workers and clients alike have developed many creative techniques of care to meet these twin goals. Both of these key principles also apply to nutritional support.

Methods: The Team Approach

How can these goals be met? How can the health care system draw on its various resources and levels of care to meet these tremendous needs? In some devastating cases obstacles may seem almost insurmountable. In others, when the underlying disease may as yet lack a cure, the prognosis is poor. Nonetheless, these support goals remain valid. Everyone involved persists toward them. Often the patient's initial reaction is one of defeat and resignation or withdrawal. Certainly the patient and family cannot carry the overwhelming burden alone. They cannot accomplish the necessary care alone. Such a complex and complicated process requires a strong *team approach.* A number of sensitive and skilled specialists lend their particular expertise. They bring their unique training and insights and resources to identify specific personal needs.

Nutrition Support and Rehabilitation

Disability
Mental or physical impairment that prevents the individual from performing one or more gainful activities; not synonymous with *handicap*, which implies serious disadvantage.

At all times, however, these health care specialists remember that the most important member of the team is the patient. They always work *with* the patient and family to help develop some solutions. Goal setting is always personal. These three partners—professional specialists, patient, and family— form a greater health team. The undertaking is always shared and supportive, whatever the nature of the condition (see box, p. 615), its individual limitations, or its outcome.

In our discussion here, we will look first at some of the general needs of disabled persons such as socioeconomic and psychologic problems, some special needs of older disabled persons, and daily eating problems. Then we will consider several specific disabling diseases as examples of current health problems that require special nutrition support. In each case we will focus on the particular nutrition principles that help meet these support needs.

Socioeconomic and Psychologic Factors in Rehabilitation

The general attitudes of society toward disabled persons varies between extremes of overprotection and avoidance. These social attitudes result mainly from years of negative conditioning and are not easily changed. Some people are repelled by deformities or severe illness, perhaps because they sense their own vulnerability and mortality. Others completely ignore them. Neither extreme is helpful. But at the same time overprotection robs persons of their selfhood and smothers the *will* to fight against surrounding odds and develop self-acceptance. However, disabled persons do have varying special needs, and social avoidance of these needs creates additional problems in everyday living. There are doorways not made for wheelchairs, unmanageable stairs and curbings, lack of access to public transportation, and many other daily barriers.

Economic Problems and Living Situations

Care for disabling injury or severe illness is a long and costly process. A major area of exploration for the health care team is one of financial resources and assistance needed. Also, continuing long-term economic problems may revolve around employment capabilities or earning capacities or the means for providing care.

Disabled persons face many practical problems of everyday living. Whether a person needs long-term hospital care or can maintain independent living, perhaps with an attendant, depends on a number of physical and situational factors. If the person can maintain a home with help, then the necessary special equipment for maximal self-care and added care by the attendant must be provided.

Psychologic Barriers

Positive resolution of many practical and emotional problems requires tremendous psychologic adjustment. Each person struggles with self-image and physical body trauma. It is small wonder that they often withdraw in defeat and exhaustion. Personality changes occur during rehabilitation processes that test both inner strength and physical stamina. Depending on personal resources and strengths, the person may or may not be able to function. Much of the health team's keen insight and concern are directed toward supporting each person's efforts to meet individual needs. That many disabled persons do reach self-care goals in some measure is evident in the remarkable achievements some attain, despite or perhaps because of their difficulties.[1]

America is aging. Population projections indicate that 50 years from now approximately one person in six will be over 65. And with older age comes an increased number of disabled elderly persons. The U.S. Rehabilitation Services Administration, using a baseline of one disabled American in 10, estimates that the odds of being disabled increase to one in three after age 65. Increased services, including rehabilitation services, will be needed. But rehabilitation needs of older persons differ, of course, from those of younger people. Three life-changing events of aging determine these needs—retirement, chronic illnesses, and general physical decline.

Vocational Rehabilitation

Without adequate planning ahead, many older persons experience stressful disorientation with retirement. They have had a lifetime of active involvement in a familiar working environment, and now that sense of stability and identity is no longer there. Supportive activities focus on vocational planning and effective use of leisure time. At this point, many persons have not been accustomed to viewing leisure activities in a positive manner. They need help in making this adjustment. In addition, vocational programs following retirement can help persons find gainful employment. Or they can help retired healthy Americans find ways of contributing their wisdom and skills to others now working in the same field. In turn, such activity can enhance the health and social assets of the older person.

Residual Disabilities from Illnesses

In the age group of 60 to 75, the so-called "young-old," rehabilitation must focus on problems resulting from chronic diseases of aging—heart disease, hypertension, strokes, or cancer. Chronic illnesses may also be related to damaging health behaviors such as alcoholism, smoking, excessive eating of foods high in fat and salt, and a sedentary life. Survival after heart attack or stroke, which now occurs more frequently with modern medical care, may leave an older person with chronic disabilities. However, early efforts at rehabilitation help prevent disability, avoid complications, and restore reasonable function.

Physical Decline in Aging

In the age group of 75 to 85 and older, the so-called "old-old," there is a marked increase in disability. Much of this increase comes from falls and resulting fractures, chronic brain failure, disorders in locomotion, impaired senses of perception, and increased problems with drug reactions and interactions. Older persons may have several different diseases and take a number of different drugs or receive a variety of medical treatments. In this age group minor disabilities often result in major handicaps. Mental and physical dependency may require supportive care in the home or long-term care facility. Common health problems in both the young-old and old-old groups involve nutritional care as well. These problems include arthritis, cardiorespiratory and cardiovascular insufficiency, depression, sensory deprivation, infections, skin and foot disorders, and nutritional deficiencies from poor dentition and fad diets.

Special Needs of Older Disabled Persons

Rehabilitation of the elderly person focuses on those needs unique to the aging process.

In general, however, disease and disability do not affect only the young-old and old-old, nor are all of these groups disabled. Many of the disabled are young people,[1,2] and many older adults continue to be fit and healthy. But the increasing age of the general population inevitably brings with it an increasing number of older adults with chronic disease and various disabilities of aging. Even minor disabilities may cause major **handicaps** in everyday living. Minor injuries can bring major debilitating results. In any case, the twin goals of rehabilitation care continue to be prevention of further disability and restoration of the maximal function available.

Prevention of Malnutrition

Kilocalories

The rehabilitative process of physical therapy involves hard work. The patient tires easily, and the energy intake must be sufficient to meet the energy output demands. Excess kilocalories must be avoided to prevent obesity. But sufficient energy for tissue metabolism is essential.

Protein

General protein needs are based on maintaining strength of tissue structure and function. Tissue and organ integrity protect against catabolism, **decubitus ulcers,** infections, and negative nitrogen balance. Dietary protein in optimal quantity and quality ensures the necessary supply of all essential amino acids required for tissue synthesis. In addition to these general needs, severe trauma such as that involved in **spinal cord injury** brings special needs to meet the catabolic response.[2,3] In the early period following injury, the metabolic process usually follows three stages:

1. **Early catabolic period.** This initial stage peaks about 2 weeks after the injury and may remain for several more weeks. Nitrogen replacement needs may require plasma transfusion or special feedings.

2. **Late catabolic period.** In this latter stage nitrogen excretion lessens. This condition may remain for some weeks or months, especially if it is compounded by infections or decubitus ulcers.

3. **Positive nitrogen balance.** This resolution of the metabolic problem is finally reached after protein therapy by dietary means and the clearing of any infection or ulcers. Sometimes as much as 150 g of protein per day or more is needed, with supplementation according to individual requirements.

Carbohydrate

General energy needs are great. They are met by optimal dietary carbohydrate as the body's major fuel source (see Chapters 5 and 14). Severe trauma requires maximal carbohydrate, especially in the early stages following injury. More breakdown of tissue protein and fat occurs to provide needed energy. But this only adds to the negative nitrogen balance. Thus sufficient carbohydrate foods are important to provide the needed energy and spare protein for its essential tissue rebuilding function.

Fat

At any point in rehabilitation care the diet must supply linoleic acid, the essential fatty acid, and a moderate amount of fat for the body's general metabolic activities and tissue integrity. The general dietary recommendation that fat supply about 30% of the total kilocalories is sufficient. Some fat for food

General Basic Principles of Supportive Nutritional Care

Handicap
Mental or physical defect that may or may not be congenital that prevents the individual from participating in normal life activities; implies disadvantage.

Decubitus ulcer
Bed sore.

Spinal cord injury
Partial or complete severing of the spinal cord caused by trauma. Partial severance results in general muscle weakness and sensory motor loss. Complete severance results in total paralysis of muscles that are controlled by nerves leaving the spinal cord *below* the level of injury, especially in *paraplegia* or *quadriplegia*.

To Probe Further

Invisible Disability

Persons with obvious disabling conditions receive cues from others that help them adapt to their disabilities. Anyone with a disability undergoes some revision of self-concept, a disruption in familiar role patterns, and a period of adjustment to the limitations. This adjustment often involves stages of the classic mode of the "sick role": (1) exemption from normal responsibility, (2) wanting to get well, and (3) cooperation with health professionals.

The person with an invisible disability such as kidney failure, some types of cancer, cardiovascular disease, or diabetes is often denied these supportive cues and feedback in the difficult task of adjustment. These conditions are not apparent or easily observed by casual acquaintances. Often this reinforces the use of denial of the actual limitations, and thus more damage through poor self-care results. The person often avoids the sick role and ignores the limitations of the condition. Yet these persons need rehabilitative support and training as much as those with more obvious disabilities.

These psychologic aspects of invisible disability carry implications for all members of the health team. Because the loss is not tangible, the patient or client often lacks the support for grieving, which hinders adjustment. Health professionals must be aware of the psychodynamics of the adaptive process, anticipate needs, offer guidance, and assist the client in mourning outwardly. Then the healing process can begin.

REFERENCE
Falvo DR, Allen H, and Maki DR: Psychosocial aspects of invisible disability, Rehab Lit 43:2, Jan/Feb 1982.

---

palatability also aids appetite, which tends to be poor in the course of long-confining illness.

Vitamins and Minerals

Optimal intake of vitamins and minerals for metabolic activity and maintenance of tissue reserves is needed. The normal RDA standards for age and sex are adequate in most cases. However, a deficiency state such as anemia indicates need for supplementation. In some rehabilitation centers multivitamin preparations are given routinely to ensure adequate amounts.

Restoration of Eating Ability
Normal Development of the Eating Process

In the normal growth and development of a child, the feeding and eating process develops through an overlapping and interdependent series of physical and physiologic stages. The usual activities of eating—swallowing, chewing, hand and utensil use—gradually develop with motor ability. The learning comes with much practice and patience. In a sense, the injured person must "start over" and relearn these basic skills.

Thus, with an understanding of these normal patterns, the disabled person works with the professional team of occupational and physical therapists, nutritionists, and nurses to find adaptive procedures to restore basic eating ability. For each client four aspects of the eating process will require individual attention: (1) the nature and degree of motor control; (2) eating position; (3) use of adapted utensils; and (4) supportive individual needs. For example, blind persons will need a description of the food served, its placement on the plate named generally in a clockwise direction to help remember it, and a follow-up training course in preparing food with a number of assistive tools and techniques.

Personal Food Plan

As indicated, the personal food plan must fulfill basic nutritional needs, in increased amounts to meet additional metabolic demands. In addition, appetite and motivation must be supported to accomplish the task. Sensory stimuli such as variety in food texture, color, and flavor can enhance appetite and help motivate the learning of new adapted modes of eating. Also, "comfort foods" or familiar ethic dishes and well-liked foods can encourage the sometimes frustrating and difficult process of relearning how to eat.

Independence in Daily Living

With each disabled person the goal is to achieve as much independence in daily living as possible (see Issues and Answers, p. 624). Maximum use is made of individual neuromotor resources and emotional reserves. These personal resources are aided by self-help devices as needed. A large number of these creative devices are available, many of them due to the inventive mind of a concerned occupational therapist.[4]

Special Disabling Conditions Requiring Supportive Nutritional Care

Several representative disabling conditions can illustrate various areas of need for supportive nutritional care. Here we will briefly review as examples three such conditions, each attacking primarily a special body system—skeletal, respiratory, defense. Each in turn relates to malnutrition and nutritional support needs: (1) *rheumatoid arthritis,* in which distorted small joints in the arms and hands make eating difficult and a general underlying inflammatory process can compromise nutritional status; (2) *chronic obstructive pulmonary disease (COPD),* in which attendant malnutrition increases risk of respiratory system failure; and (3) *acquired immune deficiency syndrome (AIDS),* in which a virus attacks cells vital to the body's defense system, bringing gross malnutrition and devastating consequences.

Rheumatoid Arthritis
Clinical Characteristics

The general term "arthritis" comes from the Greek word *arthron,* meaning "joint." Its underlying chronic, systemic, inflammatory disease process attacks the joints and brings swelling, heat, and pain.[5,6] Its cause is as yet unclear, but possible contributory factors include trauma, infection, genetic influences, immunologic components, and stress.[5] The joint damage involves tissue changes in the synosheaths. The disease primarily affects the small joints of the upper extremities. But more severe effects may occur, especially in juvenile forms involving other joints and sometimes internal organs such as liver and heart, depending on the type of the disease. There is progressive joint deformity and destruction.

This disability dramatically affects activities of daily living, especially the fundamental necessity of obtaining and eating food. There is hand and wrist involvement, including destruction of wrist ligaments and tendons, with weakened finger and hand grip strength, and limited finger movement (Figure 25-1). All of these changes limit ability to self-feed, shop for food, or prepare it. Also, elbow and shoulder involvement hinder bringing food to the mouth. Further tissue damage in the *temporomandibular joint (TMJ)* of the jaws limits normal opening and closing of the mouth and alters chewing ability. Other nonjoint problems such as anemia of chronic disease, decrease in salivary secretions, dysphagia, and bone disease, further complicate nutrition problems leading to overall malnutrition. In its juvenile form in children and adolescents, this resulting malnutrition can cause serious growth retardation.

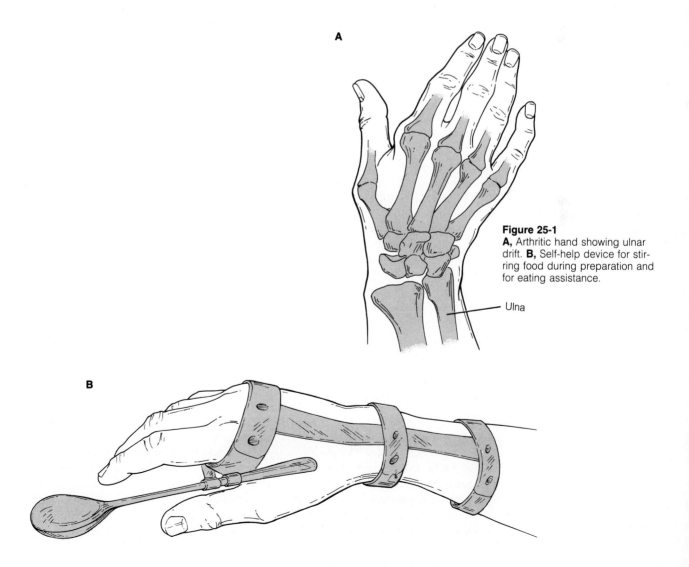

A

Figure 25-1
A, Arthritic hand showing ulnar drift. **B,** Self-help device for stirring food during preparation and for eating assistance.

Ulna

B

Nutritional Therapy

Appropriate nutrition support must begin with early screening and continuing assessment of individual needs. Medical treatment, which may involve a number of drugs for control of the inflammatory process, has implications for nutritional therapy. These drug groups include: (1) salicylates (aspirin); (2) nonsteroidal antiinflammatory agents such as gold salts or D-penicillamine; and (3) corticosteroids. Steroid therapy is usually restricted to more severe disease or lack of response to other drugs. These corticosteroids do control symptoms, but at the price of serious side effects such as growth retardation in children and metabolic imbalances. Thus initial history must assess potential drug-nutrient-food interactions (see Chapter 18) and their nutritional effects.[5-7] Also, the history should include any of the numerous unproven regimens for arthritis that the patient may be using.[8] Special functional assessment of eating ability is needed, including any swallowing problem from lack of salivary secretions and dysphagia (see box on facing page).

Standard nutritional assessment is essential (see Chapter 17). On the basis of these data, nutritional needs can be determined and monitored:

1. **Energy.** Energy needs, especially for children, vary widely and must be determined on an individual basis. In general, needs will involve basal energy expenditure plus added multiples for increased metabolic factors, such as stress of disease activity, sepsis, fever, skeletal injury, or surgery (see Chapter 23). If the client is receiving physical therapy, an additional physical activity factor is used. Total kilocalories are increased as needed to achieve desirable weight gain during growth, or decreased if indicated for obese adults. Follow-up monitoring will determine any needed adjustments in energy estimates.

2. **Protein.** Protein needs vary with protein status, surgical therapy, proteinuria, and nitrogen balance. The RDA standards for age and sex can guide protein needs for children to meet basic growth needs. States of malnutrition will require more. A well-nourished adult patient will need about 0.5 to 1.0 g of protein/kg/day during quiet disease periods. Increases may be needed during active inflammatory disease periods.

3. **Vitamins and minerals.** Standard recommendations for vitamins and minerals are used. Specific supplementation may be used if needed, such as calcium and vitamin D if bone disease is involved.

The course of rheumatoid arthritis is unpredictable. The disease is usually progressive and some degree of permanent disability may result. But after years of disease many persons are capable of self-care with rehabilitation training and are fully employable. There is no "special" diet for rheumatoid arthritis. No diet will cure the disease or decrease its symptoms. But certainly continuing optimum nutritional support is important maintenance therapy.

Osteoarthritis

This milder form of arthritis in older adults is more appropriately called *degenerative joint disease* because there is minimal inflammation involved. It is also chronic and may progress, limiting movement of affected joints, mostly in the hands. Marked disability is uncommon. There is no cure, but appropriate pain-controlling medication and nutritional support for general health promotion may help relieve symptoms. Depending on degree of hand joint involvement, self-feeding devices may assist eating.

Clinical Application

The swallowing reflex is frequently diminished or absent in disabled persons. The reflex may be enhanced, however, by the use of an ice collar or by brushing the neck with a small brush such as a paint brush just before eating. The liquid or semisolid food should be placed behind the front teeth, and the patient should slowly tilt the head back and swallow. This routine can be learned as the helper uses the repeated statement, "Tilt and swallow . . . tilt and swallow . . . ."

Tilt and Swallow

Conditions of Muscular Weakness or Incoordination

Similar eating problems may stem from conditions involving muscular weakness and incoordination. Weakness in muscle action may come from disuse following an injury or from underlying neuromuscular disease. As long as the tissue has adequate blood and nerve supply, muscles weakened by injury can be strengthened by appropriate exercises as the healing process ensues. However, certain neuromuscular disorders cause wasting of the muscle or denervation of muscle action by brain or spinal injury. These conditions cause more serious problems. They include neuromuscular disorders such as **amyotrophic lateral sclerosis (ALS)**,[9] *myasthenia gravis, spinal cord injury*, and **cerebrovascular accident (CVA),** or stroke.

Muscular incoordination may result from brain damage that brings uncontrolled muscular movements. The nature of the problem depends on the site of the brain lesion. A number of clinical problems may be associated with incoordination and resulting feeding disabilities. These conditions include *cerebral palsy*, which may require early nasogastric tube feeding in young children to support growth, then extensive continuing efforts to develop some degree of oral self-feeding.[10] Other conditions resulting in feeding problems and requiring nutritional support are *multiple sclerosis, Huntington's disease*, and *Parkinson's disease*.

Amyotrophic lateral sclerosis
Muscular weakness and atrophy in the arm and hands caused by damage to motor neurons. Deterioration continues without remission.

Cerebrovascular accident (CVA)
Stroke; brain tissue damage caused by reduced blood flow from arterial blockage or breakage; may result in *hemiplegia, hemiparesis*, or *hemianopsia*.

Chronic Obstructive Pulmonary Disease (COPD)
Clinical Characteristics

Malnutrition is common with the debilitating condition of *chronic obstructive pulmonary disease (COPD)*. This term describes a group of disorders in which the airflow in the lungs is limited and respiratory system failure develops. The two main interrelated COPD conditions are chronic bronchitis and emphysema. Malnutrition usually accompanies COPD, and its presence increases the illness and death rates associated with the disease process. Anorexia and significant weight loss reflect a growing inability to maintain adequate nutritional status, which in turn severely compromises pulmonary function.[11,12] Progression of the disease process with its increasing shortness of breath prevents the person from living a normal life. Eventually, in progressive respiratory failure, the patient becomes dependent on a mechanical respirator and controlled oxygen supply.

Nutritional Therapy

Respiratory failure is actually a failure of the pulmonary gas exchange of oxygen and carbon dioxide. Its common manifestations are *hypoxemia,* deficient oxygenation of the blood, and *hypercapnia* (from Greek word *kapnos,* meaning "smoke"), excess carbon dioxide in the blood. Thus nutritional therapy is guided by the *respiratory quotient (RQ),* the ratio of carbon dioxide produced in comparison to oxygen consumed, per unit of time, by each of the fuel nutrients. This becomes apparent in the special diet ratios used[11]:

1. **Fat.** Contrary to generally recommended diets, fat is the favored fuel source in COPD because of its lower oxidative RQ value (0.7 compared to 1.0 for carbohydrate). Also, fat is a concentrated source of needed kilocalories. It is lower in osmolality than carbohydrate, and it does not contribute to the hyperglycemia often seen in critically ill patients fed formulas largely composed of dextrose and amino acids. Fat should provide about 30% to 50% of the nonprotein kilocalories in the diet.

2. **Carbohydrate.** Conversely, a lower-than-usual amount of carbohydrate is recommended because of its less favorable RQ value. The metabolic effect of larger amounts of carbohydrate is to increase oxygen consumption and carbon dioxide production and retention. This is a critical imbalance for a patient with failing respiratory function. Carbohydrate should provide no more than about 50% of the nonprotein kilocalories in the diet.

3. **Protein.** The need for protein in ill persons' diets to counteract the catabolic stress on body tissue protein is well understood. The recommended amount for this purpose ranges from 1.0 to 2.5 g protein/kg/day. This amount is adjusted according to degree of malnutrition and stress. However, in respiratory failure more is not better, and protein allowances must be carefully prescribed. In a prudent diet for failing pulmonary function, protein should provide about 15% of the total kilocalories.

4. **Energy.** Adequate energy intake is based on extent of protein-calorie malnutrition and loss of lean body mass. Individual needs are calculated to cover basal energy expenditure, with added amounts for metabolic activity factors according to the degree of disease activity and its physiologic stress. Based on body weight, energy needs are about 25 to 35 kcal/kg/day for maintenance and 45 kcal/kg/day for anabolic needs to restore lean body mass.[12,13]

Special Enteral/Parenteral Feeding

Enteral feeding is the preferred mode, orally for dietary supplementation if possible, but by nasogastric tube if needed. Appropriate commercial formula, based on the recommended nutrient ratio given here, is available.[14]

General guidelines for dietary modifications in COPD for professional use, based on these nutrition support principles, are available.[14] Suggestions for use in counseling COPD patients in menu planning and food preparation are included.

Acquired Immune Deficiency Syndrome (AIDS)
Clinical Characteristics

The devastating disease of AIDS has become our modern-day "Black Plague," the epidemic that exterminated a third of the population of Europe in the Middle Ages.[15] Since it was initially described in 1981, AIDS has become a prevalent, infectious, fatal disease of alarming proportions. The infectious agent is believed by most researchers in the field to be *human immu-*

nodeficiency virus (HIV). It is spread by sexual contact, inoculation with contaminated blood, and perinatal transmission to babies.[16] It is not known how many persons with HIV infection will progress to *AIDS-related complex (ARC)* and to AIDS. However, the U.S. Surgeon General projects 270,000 cases of AIDS, with 179,000 deaths, by the year 1991.[17]

The AIDS virus attacks the T cells of the body's defense system (see Figure 24-3 and discussion in chapter 24) leaving it defenseless against infections normally killed by our immune systems. The disease runs an erratic course with unpredictable periods of remission. But it is always relentlessly fatal. The underlying disease process brings gross malnutrition. Symptoms include anorexia, fever, weight loss, diarrhea, malabsorption, and opportunistic infections with swelling of the glands, especially the lymph nodes.

Nutritional Therapy

Nutritional care of persons with AIDS focuses on maximum nutrition support to (1) help counteract the generalized catabolic effects of the disease and its severe malnutrition, and (2) provide specific intervention for individual complications present at various stages of the disease. These stages vary from the asymptomatic period of HIV infection through periods of "constitutional disease" that vary in severity and duration.[18,19] A host of available disease agents—parasitic, bacterial, viral—common to our environment may invade the body, now defenseless, without an active immune system. Resulting infections and malignancy can affect the entire gastrointestinal tract.[20] Review of the nutritional care for cancer patients with similar gastrointestinal problems as described in Chapter 24 will reinforce many approaches for relieving these symptoms. In any case, in care of AIDS patients, three basic nutritional support principles guide therapy:

1. **Energy.** A high-calorie diet is needed to combat the potential and progressive weight loss, a major evidence of the developing malnutrition and metabolic stress of severe illness. Regular nutrition assessment and monitoring provide a basis for estimating nutritional needs.

2. **Protein.** Increased protein is needed to combat the catabolic effect of the disease with extensive loss of lean body mass. A goal for kilocalorie-to-nitrogen ratio is at least 150:1 (see Chapter 23).

3. **Vitamins and minerals.** Needs vary at different stages of the disease. Dietary supplementation, if needed, should be guided and monitored by the clinical nutritionist on the care team, since overuse may even depress immune function, and single-item use can upset the overall nutrient balance and cause deficiencies of other competing nutrients.

Enteral/Parenteral Therapy

Oral high-calorie, high-protein supplement formulas may be used as the disease progresses, according to gastrointestinal tolerance. Or they may be given as a tube feeding if indicated. If esophagitis becomes severe, gastrostomy tube feeding may be used. Nutritional support in advanced disease may require TPN.

The ARIS Project in Santa Clara County, California, has produced an excellent booklet for patients with AIDS and their families.[21] It provides simple, clear, supportive guidance for dealing with a variety of eating problems and boosting the energy and protein intake. The AIDS team clinical dietitian at your health care center can supply other helpful resources.

To Sum Up

Individuals facing disabling illness and injury confront many interacting challenges, including social attitudes and financial, physical, and psychologic barriers. The team approach, involving family, friends, and health professionals, becomes an essential basis of care.

The basic principles of nutrition care involve *prevention* of malnutrition and *restoration* of eating ability. To avoid malnutrition, the nutritionist must assess individual nutritional needs to meet fundamental energy requirements. There must be sufficient nutrient intake to meet a variety of needs: protein and fat (linoleic acid) to promote tissue and organ integrity; carbohydrate demands to counteract impaired postinjury metabolism; and vitamins and minerals, sometimes supplemented to prevent deficiencies. A frequent goal is to restore eating ability, often with assistive devices.

Special disabling conditions that require special nutrition support include: (1) rheumatoid arthritis and other diseases affecting muscle weakness and coordination; (2) COPD with progressive respiratory failure and malnutrition; and (3) AIDS with progressive loss of lean body weight, malnutrition, and fatal consequences.

Questions for Review

1. What are the two goals of rehabilitative therapy for disabling conditions? How do the basic principles of nutritional support help meet these goals?
2. Describe the functions of major nutrients in preventing or retarding the catabolic process in long-term disabling illness or injury.
3. Identify several disease processes or injuries that result in eating disabilities. Give examples of the therapy used in each case.
4. Describe the clinical characteristics and special nutritional therapy for rheumatoid arthritis, COPD, and AIDS.

References

1. Odgers S: Suddenly disabled: how I learned to live a full life from a wheelchair, Med Self-Care 19:26, Winter 1982.
2. Ainsley BM, and Blackburn GL: Nutritional needs of a paraplegic patient, JAMA 248:2180, Nov 1982.
3. Gines DJ: Long-term nutritional care for the client with spinal cord injury, Top Clin Nutr 3(3):61, July 1988.
4. Cassell JA: Interview: Fred Sammons, OTR, Top Clin Nutr 3(3):71, July 1988.
5. Garceau AO, Dwyer JT, and Holland M: A practical approach to nutrition in the patient with juvenile rheumatoid arthritis, Clin Nutr 8(2):55, Mar/Apr 1989.
6. Tonger-Decker R: Nutritional considerations in rheumatoid arthritis, J Am Diet Assoc 88(3):327, Mar 1985.
7. Bigaoutte J, Timchalk MA, and Kremer J: Nutritional adequacy of diet and supplements in patients with rheumatoid arthritis who take medications, J Am Diet Assoc 87(12):1687, Dec 1987.
8. Wolman PG: Management of patients using unproven regimens for arthritis, J Am Diet Assoc 87(9):1211, Sept 1987.
9. Slowie LA, Paige MS, and Antel JP: Nutritional considerations in the management of patients with amyotropic lateral sclerosis (ALS), J Am Diet Assoc 83(1):44, Jan 1983.
10. Gisel EG, and Patrick J: Identification of children with cerebral palsy unable to maintain a normal nutritional state, Lancet 1:283, Feb 6, 1988.
11. Miller MA: A practical approach to eating and breathing in respiratory failure, Top Clin Nutr 1(4):61, 1986.

12. Armstrong JN: Nutrition and the respiratory patient, Nutr Support Serv 6(3):8, Mar 1986.
13. Pingleton Sk, and Harmon GS: Nutritional management in acute respiratory failure, JAMA 257:3094, June 12, 1987.
14. Monograph: Dietary modification in chronic pulmonary disease, Columbus, OH, 1986, Ross Laboratories, Inc.
15. Clarke M: Plagues, man, and history, Newsweek CXI(19):85, May 9, 1988.
16. Bentler M, and Standish M: Nutrition support of the pediatric patient with AIDS, J Am Diet Assoc 87(4):488, Apr 1987.
17. Surgeon General's report on acquired immune deficiency syndrome, US Department of Health and Human Services, Washington, DC, 1987, US Government Printing Office.
18. Collins CL: Nutrition care in AIDS, Dietetic Currents 15(3):11, 1988.
19. Garcia ME, Collins CL, and Mansell PWA: The acquired immune deficiency syndrome, Nutr Clin Pract 2(3):108, June 1987.
20. Gelt A, and Miller S: AIDS and gastroenterology, Am J Gastroenterol 81:619, 1986
21. Taber-Pike J, et al: Nutrition and AIDS: guidelines for PWAs/PWARCs, Campbell, CA, 1987, ARIS Project. (Address inquiries: Bill Horn, Nutrition Services, The ARIS Project, 595 Millich Drive, Suite 104, Campbell, CA 95008)

Further Readings

Bentler M, and Standish M: Nutrition support of the pediatric patient with AIDS, J Am Diet Assoc 87(4):488, Apr 1987.

Collins CL: Nutrition care in AIDS, Dietetic Currents 15(3):11, 1988.

Dwyer JT, et al: Unproven nutrition therapies for AIDS: what is the evidence? Nutr Today 23(2):25, Mar/Apr 1988.

Garcia ME, Collins CL, and Mansell PWA: The acquired immune deficiency syndrome: nutritional complications and assessment of body weight status, Nutr Clin Pract 2(3):108, June 1987.

These four articles provide helpful background in different areas of nutrition support for persons with AIDS.

Garceau AO, Dwyer JT, and Holland M: A practical approach to nutrition in the patient with juvenile rheumatoid arthritis, Clin Nutr 8(2):55, Mar/Apr 1989.

Tonger-Decker R: Nutritional considerations in rheumatoid arthritis, J Am Diet Assoc 88(3):327, Mar 1988.

These two articles provide excellent background information with many practical considerations for nutritional support of children and adults with rheumatoid arthritis.

Keim NL, et al: Dietary evaluation of outpatients with chronic obstructive pulmonary disease, J Am Diet Assoc 86(7):902, July 1986.

Pingleton SK, and Harmon GS: Nutritional management in acute respiratory failure, JAMA 257:3094, June 12, 1987.

These two articles provide discussions about nutrient support for persons with COPD in progressive respiratory failure.

Independent Living vs The Kindness of Strangers

"I have always relied on the kindness of strangers." If this author's famous line for his lead character Blanche conjures up images of a blithe Southern belle, you're right—you're right—but think again. In today's reality, you may well think of a once-independent career woman now confined to her wheelchair, much of her financial resources gone to pay for lengthy and highly specialized care. Before 1978 she would have relied on the "kindness of strangers" to meet most of her basic needs, including transportation to keep medical appointments and purchase food and help in meal preparation and personal care.

In 1978 the Rehabilitation Act of 1973 was amended to allocate federal funds to establish independent living centers for disabled persons. As an example, the number of Americans who cannot perform even simple activities of daily living because of a major illness, disabling injury, or chronic health condition rose dramatically by 83.2% in the one decade between 1966 and 1976 and has been gradually rising during the 1980s. In 1980 about 15% of the free living population was disabled. This rise is caused primarily by new technologies that have virtually wiped out the infectious diseases that used to kill the disabled, as well as those that, together with nutrition, have extended the general life span. The causes of disability have changed, too, with rheumatoid arthritis and diabetes replacing heart disease and other causes.

Disabled persons have traditionally been barred from many activities because of limited mobility. Jobs, education, and recreational facilities have often been denied to them because of inadequate physical access or facilities and even fear and prejudice. Promotion of access, as well as independent living, has been a strong civil rights issue in many parts of the United States with many positive results.

The passage of legislation establishing independent living centers across the United States enabled disabled persons to meet their basic needs. It also promoted political awareness among local communities. This legislation has opened the door to disabled persons who can and want to be self-reliant individuals capable of enriching their lives and contributing to their communities. Unfortunately, this support and any future assistance are in jeopardy. Since 1980 the federal administration has been reluctant to enforce new regulations regarding the needs of disabled persons. Also, there have been cutbacks in programs providing income support through the Social Security Administration. Public support for these programs is also lessening, since the proportion of the public being served is relatively small and their needs are highly specialized.

Will the disabled person once again find it necessary to rely on "the kindness of strangers?" How will the loss of contributed income from working disabled persons affect the economy? And will the "kind strangers" be capable of filling the gap?

REFERENCE
DeJong G, and Lifchez R: Physical disability and public policy, Sci Am 248(6):40, 1983.

Appendixes

A

Nutritive Values of the Edible Part of Foods

Foods, Approximate Measures, Units, and Weight		(g)	Water (%)	Food Energy (cal)	Protein (g)	Fat (g)	Saturated (total) (g)	Oleic (g)	Linoleic (g)
							Fatty Acids		
								Unsaturated	
Dairy Products (Cheese, Cream, Imitation Cream, Milk; Related Products)									
Cheese:									
Natural:									
Blue	1 oz	28	42	100	6	8	5.3	1.9	.2
Camembert (3 wedges per 4 oz container)	1 wedge	38	52	115	8	9	5.8	2.2	.2
Cheddar:									
Cut pieces	1 oz	28	37	115	7	9	6.1	2.1	.2
	1 cu in	17.2	37	70	4	6	3.7	1.3	.1
Shredded	1 cup	113	37	455	28	37	24.2	8.5	.7
Cottage (curd not pressed down):									
Creamed (cottage cheese, 4% fat):									
Large curd	1 cup	225	79	235	28	10	6.4	2.4	.2
Small curd	1 cup	210	79	220	26	9	6.0	2.2	.2
Low fat (2%)	1 cup	226	79	205	31	4	2.8	1.0	.1
Low fat (1%)	1 cup	226	82	165	28	2	1.5	.5	.1
Uncreamed (cottage cheese dry curd, less than ½% fat)	1 cup	145	80	125	25	1	.4	.1	Tr
Cream	1 oz	28	54	100	2	10	6.2	2.4	.2
Mozzarella, made with—									
Whole milk	1 oz	28	48	90	6	7	4.4	1.7	.2
Part skim milk	1 oz	28	49	80	8	5	3.1	1.2	.1
Parmesan, grated:									
Cup, not pressed down	1 cup	100	18	455	42	30	19.1	7.7	.3
Tablespoon	1 tbsp	5	18	25	2	2	1.0	.4	Tr
Ounce	1 oz	28	18	130	12	9	5.4	2.2	.1
Provolone	1 oz	28	41	100	7	8	4.8	1.7	.1
Ricotta, made with—									
Whole milk	1 cup	246	72	430	28	32	20.4	7.1	.7
Part skim milk	1 cup	246	74	340	28	19	12.1	4.7	.5
Romano	1 oz	28	31	110	9	8	—	—	—
Swiss	1 oz	28	37	105	8	8	5.0	1.7	.2
Pasteurized process cheese:									
American	1 oz	28	39	105	6	9	5.6	2.1	.2
Swiss	1 oz	28	42	95	7	7	4.5	1.7	.1
Pasteurized process cheese food, American	1 oz	28	43	95	6	7	4.4	1.7	.1
Pasteurized process cheese spread, American	1 oz	28	48	80	5	6	3.8	1.5	.1
Cream, sweet:									
Half-and-half (cream and milk)	1 cup	242	81	315	7	28	17.3	7.0	.6
	1 tbsp	15	81	20	Tr	2	1.1	.4	Tr
Light, coffee, or table	1 cup	240	74	470	6	46	28.8	11.7	1.0
	1 tbsp	15	74	30	Tr	3	1.8	.7	.1
Whipping, unwhipped (volume about double when whipped):									
Light	1 cup	239	64	700	5	74	46.2	18.3	1.5
	1 tbsp	15	64	45	Tr	5	2.9	1.1	.1
Heavy	1 cup	238	58	820	5	88	54.8	22.2	2.0
	1 tbsp	15	58	80	Tr	6	3.5	1.4	.1
Whipped topping (pressurized)	1 cup	60	61	155	2	13	8.3	3.4	.3
	1 tbsp	3	61	10	Tr	1	.4	.2	Tr
Cream, sour	1 cup	230	71	495	7	48	30.0	12.1	1.1
	1 tbsp	12	71	25	Tr	3	1.6	.6	.1

From Adams, C.F., and Richardson, M.: Nutritive value of foods, Home and Garden Bulletin No. 72, U.S. Department of Agriculture, Washington, D.C., 1981, U.S. Government Printing Office.
Blanks indicate no data available.
Tr, Trace.
For notes, see end of table.

Nutrients in Indicated Quantity

Carbohydrate (g)	Calcium (mg)	Phosphorus (mg)	Iron (mg)	Potassium (mg)	Vitamin A Value (IU)	Thiamin (mg)	Riboflavin (mg)	Niacin (mg)	Ascorbic Acid (mg)
1	150	110	.1	73	200	.01	.11	.3	0
Tr	147	132	.1	71	350	.01	.19	.2	0
Tr	204	145	.2	28	300	.01	.11	Tr	0
Tr	124	88	.1	17	180	Tr	.06	Tr	0
1	815	579	.8	111	1200	.03	.42	.1	0
6	135	297	.3	190	370	.05	.37	.3	Tr
6	126	277	.3	177	340	.04	.34	.3	Tr
8	155	340	.4	217	160	.05	.42	.3	Tr
6	138	302	.3	193	80	.05	.37	.3	Tr
3	46	151	.3	47	40	.04	.21	.2	0
1	23	30	.3	34	400	Tr	.06	Tr	0
1	163	117	.1	21	260	Tr	.08	Tr	0
1	207	149	.1	27	180	.01	.10	Tr	0
4	1376	807	1.0	107	700	.05	.39	.3	0
Tr	69	40	Tr	5	40	Tr	.02	Tr	0
1	390	229	.3	30	200	.01	.11	.1	0
1	214	141	.1	39	230	.01	.09	Tr	0
7	509	389	.9	257	1210	.03	.48	.3	0
13	669	449	1.1	308	1060	.05	.46	.2	0
1	302	215	—	—	160	—	.11	Tr	0
1	272	171	Tr	31	240	.01	.10	Tr	0
Tr	174	211	.1	46	340	.01	.10	Tr	0
1	219	216	.2	61	230	Tr	.08	Tr	0
2	163	130	.2	79	260	.01	.13	Tr	0
2	159	202	.1	69	220	.01	.12	Tr	0
10	254	230	.2	314	260	.08	.36	.2	2
1	16	14	Tr	19	20	.01	.02	Tr	Tr
9	231	192	.1	292	1730	.08	.36	.1	2
1	14	12	Tr	18	110	Tr	.02	Tr	Tr
7	166	146	.1	231	2690	.06	.30	.1	1
Tr	10	9	Tr	15	170	Tr	.02	Tr	Tr
7	154	149	.1	179	3500	.05	.26	.1	1
Tr	10	9	Tr	11	220	Tr	.02	Tr	Tr
7	61	54	Tr	88	550	.02	.04	Tr	0
Tr	3	3	Tr	4	30	Tr	Tr	Tr	0
10	268	195	.1	331	1820	.08	.34	.2	2
1	14	10	Tr	17	90	Tr	.02	Tr	Tr

Foods, Approximate Measures, Units, and Weight		(g)	Water (%)	Food Energy (cal)	Protein (g)	Fat (g)	Saturated (total) (g)	Oleic (g)	Linoleic (g)
							Fatty Acids		
								Unsaturated	
Cream products, imitation (made with vegetable fat):									
Sweet:									
Creamers:									
Liquid (frozen)	1 cup	245	77	335	2	24	22.8	.3	Tr
	1 tbsp	15	77	20	Tr	1	1.4	Tr	0
Powdered	1 cup	94	2	515	5	33	30.6	.9	Tr
	1 tsp	2	2	10	Tr	1	.7	Tr	0
Whipped topping:									
Frozen	1 cup	75	50	240	1	19	16.3	1.0	.2
	1 tbsp	4	50	15	Tr	1	.9	.1	Tr
Powdered, made with whole milk	1 cup	80	67	150	3	10	8.5	.6	.1
	1 tbsp	4	67	10	Tr	Tr	.4	Tr	Tr
Pressurized	1 tbsp	4	60	10	Tr	1	.8	.1	Tr
Sour dressing (imitation sour cream) made with	1 cup	235	75	415	8	39	31.2	4.4	1.1
nonfat dry milk	1 tbsp	12	75	20	Tr	2	1.6	.2	.1
Milk:									
Fluid:									
Whole (3.3% fat)	1 cup	244	88	150	8	8	5.1	2.1	.2
Lowfat (2%):									
No milk solids added	1 cup	244	89	120	8	5	2.9	1.2	.1
Lowfat (1%)									
No milk solids added	1 cup	244	90	100	8	3	1.6	.7	.1
Nonfat (skim):									
No milk solids added	1 cup	245	91	85	8	Tr	.3	.1	Tr
Buttermilk	1 cup	245	90	100	8	2	1.3	.5	Tr
Canned:									
Evaporated, unsweetened:									
Whole milk	1 cup	252	74	340	17	19	11.6	5.3	0.4
Skim milk	1 cup	255	79	200	19	1	.3	.1	Tr
Sweetened, condensed	1 cup	306	27	980	24	27	16.8	6.7	.7
Dried:									
Buttermilk	1 cup	120	3	465	41	7	4.3	1.7	.2
Nonfat instant:									
Envelope, net wt, 3.2 oz[5]	1 envelope	91	4	325	32	1	.4	.1	Tr
Cup[7]	1 cup	68	4	245	24	Tr	.3	.1	Tr
Milk beverages:									
Chocolate milk (commercial):									
Regular	1 cup	250	82	210	8	8	5.3	2.2	.2
Lowfat (2%)	1 cup	250	84	180	8	5	3.1	1.3	.1
Lowfat (1%)	1 cup	250	85	160	8	3	1.5	.7	.1
Eggnog (commercial)	1 cup	254	74	340	10	19	11.3	5.0	.6
Malted milk, home-prepared with 1 cup of whole milk and 2 to 3 heaping tsp of malted milk powder (about ¾ oz):									
Chocolate	1 cup of milk plus ¾ oz of powder	265	81	235	9	9	5.5	—	—
Natural	1 cup of milk plus ¾ oz of powder	265	81	235	11	10	6.0	—	—
Shakes, thick:[8]									
Chocolate, container, net wt, 10.6 oz	1 container	300	72	355	9	8	5.0	2.0	.2
Vanilla, container, net wt, 11 oz	1 container	313	74	350	12	9	5.9	2.4	.2
Milk desserts, frozen:									
Ice cream:									
Regular (about 11% fat):									
Hardened	½ gal	1064	61	2155	38	115	71.3	28.8	2.6
	1 cup	133	61	270	5	14	8.9	3.6	.3
	3 fl oz container	50	61	100	2	5	3.4	1.4	.1
Soft serve (frozen custard)	1 cup	173	60	375	7	23	13.5	5.9	.6
Rich (about 16% fat), hardened	½ gal	1188	59	2805	33	190	118.3	47.8	4.3
	1 cup	148	59	350	4	24	14.7	6.0	.5
Ice milk:									
Hardened (about 4.3% fat)	½ gal	1048	69	1470	41	45	28.1	11.3	1.0
	1 cup	131	69	185	5	6	3.5	1.4	.1
Soft serve (about 2.6% fat)	1 cup	175	70	225	8	5	2.9	1.2	0.1
Sherbet (about 2% fat)	½ gal	1542	66	2160	17	31	19.0	7.7	.7
	1 cup	193	66	270	2	4	2.4	1.0	.1

For notes, see end of table.

Nutrients in Indicated Quantity

Carbohydrate (g)	Calcium (mg)	Phosphorus (mg)	Iron (mg)	Potassium (mg)	Vitamin A Value (IU)	Thiamin (mg)	Riboflavin (mg)	Niacin (mg)	Ascorbic Acid (mg)
28	23	157	.1	467	220[1]	0	0	0	0
2	1	10	Tr	29	10[1]	0	0	0	0
52	21	397	.1	763	190[1]	0	.16[1]	0	0
1	Tr	8	Tr	16	Tr[1]	0	Tr[1]	0	0
17	5	6	.1	14	650[1]	0	0	0	0
1	Tr	Tr	Tr	1	30[1]	0	0	0	0
13	72	69	Tr	121	290[1]	.02	.09	Tr	1
1	4	3	Tr	6	10[1]	Tr	Tr	Tr	Tr
1	Tr	1	Tr	1	20[1]	0	0	0	0
11	266	205	.1	380	20[1]	.09	.38	.2	2
1	14	10	Tr	19	Tr	.01	.02	Tr	Tr
11	291	228	.1	370	310[2]	.09	.40	.2	2
12	297	232	.1	377	500	.10	.40	.2	2
12	300	235	.1	381	500	.10	.41	.2	2
12	302	247	.1	406	500	.09	.34	.2	2
12	285	219	.1	371	80[3]	.08	.38	.1	2
25	657	510	.5	764	610[3]	.12	.80	.5	5
29	738	497	.7	845	1000[4]	.11	.79	.4	3
166	868	775	.6	1136	1000[3]	.28	1.27	.6	8
59	1421	1119	.4	1910	260[3]	.47	1.90	1.1	7
47	1120	896	.3	1552	2160[6]	.38	1.59	.8	5
35	837	670	.2	1160	1610[6]	.28	1.19	.6	4
26	280	251	.6	417	300[3]	.09	.41	.3	2
26	284	254	.6	422	500	.10	.42	.3	2
26	287	257	.6	426	500	.10	.40	.2	2
34	330	278	.5	420	890	.09	.48	.3	4
29	304	265	.5	500	330	.14	.43	.7	2
27	347	307	.3	529	380	.20	.54	1.3	2
63	396	378	.9	672	260	.14	.67	.4	0
56	457	361	.3	572	360	.09	.61	.5	0
254	1406	1075	1.0	2052	4340	.42	2.63	1.1	6
32	176	134	.1	257	540	.05	.33	.1	1
12	66	51	Tr	96	200	.02	.12	.1	Tr
38	236	199	.4	338	790	.08	.45	.2	1
256	1213	927	.8	1771	7200	.36	2.27	.9	5
32	151	115	.1	221	900	.04	.28	.1	1
232	1409	1035	1.5	2117	1710	.61	2.78	.9	6
29	176	129	.1	265	210	.08	.35	.1	1
38	274	202	.3	412	180	.12	.54	.2	1
469	827	594	2.5	1585	1480	.26	.71	1.0	31
59	103	74	.3	198	190	.03	.09	.1	4

Foods, Approximate Measures, Units, and Weight		(g)	Water (%)	Food Energy (cal)	Protein (g)	Fat (g)	Saturated (total) (g)	Oleic (g)	Linoleic (g)
Milk desserts, other:									
Custard, baked	1 cup	265	77	305	14	15	6.8	5.4	.7
Puddings:									
From home recipe:									
Starch base:									
Chocolate	1 cup	260	66	385	8	12	7.6	3.3	.3
Vanilla (blancmange)	1 cup	255	76	285	9	10	6.2	2.5	.2
Tapioca cream	1 cup	165	72	220	8	8	4.1	2.5	.5
From mix (chocolate) and milk:									
Regular (cooked)	1 cup	260	70	320	9	8	4.3	2.6	.2
Instant	1 cup	260	69	325	8	7	3.6	2.2	.3
Yogurt:									
With added milk solids:									
Made with lowfat milk:									
Fruit-flavored[9]	1 container, net wt 8 oz	227	75	230	10	3	1.8	.6	.1
Plain	1 container, net wt 8 oz	227	85	145	12	4	2.3	.8	.1
Made with nonfat milk	1 container, net wt 8 oz	227	85	125	13	Tr	.3	.1	Tr
Without added milk solids:									
Made with whole milk	1 container, net wt 8 oz	227	88	140	8	7	4.8	1.7	.1
Eggs									
Eggs, large (24 oz per dozen):									
Raw:									
Whole, without shell	1 egg	50	75	80	6	6	1.7	2.0	.6
White	1 white	33	88	15	3	Tr	0	0	0
Yolk	1 yolk	17	49	65	3	6	1.7	2.1	.6
Cooked:									
Fried in butter	1 egg	46	72	85	5	6	2.4	2.2	.6
Hard-cooked, shell removed	1 egg	50	75	80	6	6	1.7	2.0	.6
Poached	1 egg	50	74	80	6	6	1.7	2.0	.6
Scrambled (milk added) in butter; also omelet	1 egg	64	76	95	6	7	2.8	2.3	.6
Fats, Oils; Related Products									
Butter:									
Regular (1 brick or 4 sticks per lb):									
Stick (½ cup)	1 stick	113	16	815	1	92	57.3	23.1	2.1
Tablespoon (about ⅛ stick)	1 tbsp	14	16	100	Tr	12	7.2	2.9	.3
Pat (1-in square, ⅓ in high; 90 per lb)	1 pat	5	16	35	Tr	4	2.5	1.0	.1
Whipped (6 sticks or two 8 oz containers per lb)									
Stick (½ cup)	1 stick	76	16	540	1	61	38.2	15.4	1.4
Tablespoon (about ⅛ stick)	1 tbsp	9	16	65	Tr	8	4.7	1.9	.2
Pat (1¼ in square, ⅓ in high; 120 per lb)	1 pat	4	16	25	Tr	3	1.9	.8	.1
Fats, cooking (vegetable shortenings)	1 cup	200	0	1770	0	200	48.8	88.2	48.4
	1 tbsp	13	0	110	0	13	3.2	5.7	3.1
Lard	1 tbsp	13	0	115	0	13	5.1	5.3	1.3
Margarine:									
Regular (1 brick or 4 sticks per lb):									
Stick (½ cup)	1 stick	113	16	815	1	92	16.7	42.9	24.9
Tablespoon (about ⅛ stick)	1 tbsp	14	16	100	Tr	12	2.1	5.3	3.1
Pat (1-in square, ⅓ in high; 90 per lb)	1 pat	5	16	35	Tr	4	.7	1.9	1.1
Soft, two 8 oz containers per lb	1 container	227	16	1635	1	184	32.5	71.5	65.4
	1 tbsp	14	16	100	Tr	12	2.0	4.5	4.1
Whipped (6 sticks per lb):									
Stick (½ cup)	1 stick	76	16	545	Tr	61	11.2	28.7	16.7
Tablespoon (about ⅛ stick)	1 tbsp	9	16	70	Tr	8	1.4	3.6	2.1
Oils, salad or cooking:									
Corn	1 cup	218	0	1925	0	218	27.7	53.6	125.1
	1 tbsp	14	0	120	0	14	1.7	3.3	7.8
Olive	1 cup	216	0	1910	0	216	30.7	154.4	17.7
	1 tbsp	14	0	120	0	14	1.9	9.7	1.1
Peanut	1 cup	216	0	1910	0	216	37.4	98.5	67.0
	1 tbsp	14	0	120	0	14	2.3	6.2	4.2
Safflower	1 cup	218	0	1925	0	218	20.5	25.9	159.8
	1 tbsp	14	0	120	0	14	1.3	1.6	10.0
Soybean oil, hydrogenated	1 cup	218	0	1925	0	218	31.8	93.1	75.6
(partially hardened)	1 tbsp	14	0	120	0	14	2.0	5.8	4.7

For notes, see end of table.

Nutrients In Indicated Quantity

Carbohydrate (g)	Calcium (mg)	Phosphorus (mg)	Iron (mg)	Potassium (mg)	Vitamin A Value (IU)	Thiamin (mg)	Riboflavin (mg)	Niacin (mg)	Ascorbic Acid (mg)
29	297	310	1.1	387	930	.11	.50	.3	1
67	250	255	1.3	445	390	.05	.36	.3	1
41	298	232	Tr	352	410	.08	.41	.3	2
28	173	180	.7	223	480	.07	.30	.2	2
59	265	247	.8	354	340	.05	.39	.3	2
63	374	237	1.3	335	340	.08	.39	.3	2
42	343	269	.2	439	120[10]	.08	.40	.2	1
16	415	326	.2	531	150[10]	.10	.49	.3	2
17	452	355	.2	579	20[10]	.11	.53	.3	2
11	274	215	.1	351	280	.07	.32	.2	1
1	28	90	1.0	65	260	.04	.15	Tr	0
Tr	4	4	Tr	45	0	Tr	.09	Tr	0
Tr	26	86	.9	15	310	.04	.07	Tr	0
1	26	80	.9	58	290	.03	.13	Tr	0
1	28	90	1.0	65	260	.04	.14	Tr	0
1	28	90	1.0	65	260	.04	.13	Tr	0
1	47	97	.9	85	310	.04	.16	Tr	0
Tr	27	26	.2	29	3470[11]	.01	.04	Tr	0
Tr	3	3	Tr	4	430[11]	Tr	Tr	Tr	0
Tr	1	1	Tr	1	150[11]	Tr	Tr	Tr	0
Tr	18	17	.1	20	2310[11]	Tr	.03	Tr	0
Tr	2	2	Tr	2	290[11]	Tr	Tr	Tr	0
Tr	1	1	Tr	1	120[11]	0	Tr	Tr	0
0	0	0	0	0	—	0	0	0	0
0	0	0	0	0	—	0	0	0	0
0	0	0	0	0	0	0	0	0	0
Tr	27	26	.2	29	3750[12]	.01	.04	Tr	0
Tr	3	3	Tr	4	470[12]	Tr	Tr	Tr	0
Tr	1	1	Tr	1	170[12]	Tr	Tr	Tr	0
Tr	53	53	.4	59	7500[12]	.01	.08	.1	0
Tr	3	3	Tr	4	470[12]	Tr	Tr	Tr	0
Tr	18	17	.1	20	2500[12]	Tr	.03	Tr	0
Tr	2	2	Tr	2	310[12]	Tr	Tr	Tr	0
0	0	0	0	0	—	0	0	0	0
0	0	0	0	0	—	0	0	0	0
0	0	0	0	0	—	0	0	0	0
0	0	0	0	0	—	0	0	0	0
0	0	0	0	0	—	0	0	0	0
0	0	0	0	0	—	0	0	0	0
0	0	0	0	0	—	0	0	0	0
0	0	0	0	0	—	0	0	0	0
0	0	0	0	0	—	0	0	0	0
0	0	0	0	0	—	0	0	0	0

Foods, Approximate Measures, Units, and Weight		(g)	Water (%)	Food Energy (cal)	Protein (g)	Fat (g)	Fatty Acids		
							Saturated (total) (g)	Unsaturated	
								Oleic (g)	Linoleic (g)
Soybean-cottonseed oil blend,	1 cup	218	0	1925	0	218	38.2	63.0	99.6
hydrogenated	1 tbsp	14	0	120	0	14	2.4	3.9	6.2
Salad dressings:									
Commercial:									
Blue cheese:									
Regular	1 tbsp	15	32	75	1	8	1.6	1.7	3.8
Low calorie (5 cal per tsp)	1 tbsp	16	84	10	Tr	1	.5	.3	Tr
French:									
Regular	1 tbsp	16	39	65	Tr	6	1.1	1.3	3.2
Low calorie (5 cal per tsp)	1 tbsp	16	77	15	Tr	1	.1	.1	.4
Italian:									
Regular	1 tbsp	15	28	85	Tr	9	1.6	1.9	4.7
Low calorie (2 cal per tsp)	1 tbsp	15	90	10	Tr	1	.1	.1	.4
Mayonnaise	1 tbsp	14	15	100	Tr	11	2.0	2.4	5.6
Mayonnaise type:									
Regular	1 tbsp	15	41	65	Tr	6	1.1	1.4	3.2
Low calorie (8 cal per tsp)	1 tbsp	16	81	20	Tr	2	.4	.4	1.0
Tartar sauce, regular	1 tbsp	14	34	75	Tr	8	1.5	1.8	4.1
Thousand Island:									
Regular	1 tbsp	16	32	80	Tr	8	1.4	1.7	4.0
Low calorie (10 cal per tsp)	1 tbsp	15	68	25	Tr	2	.4	.4	1.0
From home recipe:									
Cooked type[13]	1 tbsp	16	68	25	1	2	.5	.6	.3
Fish, Shellfish, Meat, Poultry, Related Products									
Fish and shellfish:									
Bluefish, baked with butter or margarine	3 oz	85	68	135	22	4	—	—	—
Clams:									
Raw, meat only	3 oz	85	82	65	11	1	—	—	—
Canned, solids and liquid	3 oz	85	86	45	7	1	.2	Tr	Tr
Crabmeat (white or king), canned, not pressed down	1 cup	135	77	135	24	3	.6	0.4	0.1
Fish sticks, breaded, cooked, frozen (stick, 4 × 1 × ½ in)	1 fish stick or 1 oz	28	66	50	5	3	—	—	—
Haddock, breaded, fried[14]	3 oz	85	66	140	17	5	1.4	2.2	1.2
Ocean perch, breaded, fried[14]	1 fillet	85	59	195	16	11	2.7	4.4	2.3
Oysters, raw, meat only (13-19 medium Selects)	1 cup	240	85	160	20	4	1.3	.2	.1
Salmon, pink, canned, solids and liquid	3 oz	85	71	120	17	5	.9	.8	.1
Sardines, Atlantic, canned in oil, drained solids	3 oz	85	62	175	20	9	3.0	2.5	.5
Scallops, frozen, breaded, fried, reheated	6 scallops	90	60	175	16	8	—	—	—
Shad, baked with butter or margarine, bacon	3 oz	85	64	170	20	10	—	—	—
Shrimp:									
Canned meat	3 oz	85	70	100	21	1	.1	.1	Tr
French fried[16]	3 oz	85	57	190	17	9	2.3	3.7	2.0
Tuna, canned in oil, drained solids	3 oz	85	61	170	24	7	1.7	1.7	.7
Tuna salad[17]	1 cup	205	70	350	30	22	4.3	6.3	6.7
Meat and meat products:									
Bacon (20 slices per lb, raw), broiled or fried, crisp	2 slices	15	8	85	4	8	2.5	3.7	.7
Beef, cooked:[18]									
Cuts braised, simmered, or pot roasted:									
Lean and fat (piece, 2½ × 2½ × ¾ in)	3 oz	85	53	245	23	16	6.8	6.5	.4
Lean only from item directly above	2.5 oz	72	62	140	22	5	2.1	1.8	.2
Ground beef, broiled:									
Lean with 10% fat	3 oz or patty 3 × ⅝ in	85	60	185	23	10	4.0	3.9	.3
Lean with 21% fat	2.9 oz or patty 3 × ⅝ in	82	54	235	20	17	7.0	6.7	.4
Roast, oven cooked, no liquid added:									
Relatively fat, such as rib:									
Lean and fat (2 pieces, 4⅛ × 2¼ × ¼ in)	3 oz	85	40	375	17	33	14.0	13.6	.8
Lean only	1.8 oz	51	57	125	14	7	3.0	2.5	.3
Relatively lean, such as heel of round:									
Lean and fat (2 pieces, 4⅛ × 2¼ × ¼ in)	3 oz	85	62	165	25	7	2.8	2.7	.2
Lean only	2.8 oz	78	65	125	24	3	1.2	1.0	0.1

For notes, see end of table.

Nutrients in Indicated Quantity

Carbohydrate (g)	Calcium (mg)	Phosphorus (mg)	Iron (mg)	Potassium (mg)	Vitamin A Value (IU)	Thiamin (mg)	Riboflavin (mg)	Niacin (mg)	Ascorbic Acid (mg)
0	0	0	0	0	—	0	0	0	0
0	0	0	0	0	—	0	0	0	0
1	12	11	Tr	6	30	Tr	.02	Tr	Tr
1	10	8	Tr	5	30	Tr	.01	Tr	Tr
3	2	2	.1	13	—	—	—	—	—
2	2	2	.1	13	—	—	—	—	—
1	2	1	Tr	2	Tr	Tr	Tr	Tr	—
Tr	Tr	1	Tr	2	Tr	Tr	Tr	Tr	—
Tr	3	4	.1	5	40	Tr	.01	Tr	—
2	2	4	Tr	1	30	Tr	Tr	Tr	—
2	3	4	Tr	1	40	Tr	Tr	Tr	—
1	3	4	.1	11	30	Tr	Tr	Tr	Tr
2	2	3	.1	18	50	Tr	Tr	Tr	Tr
2	2	3	.1	17	50	Tr	Tr	Tr	Tr
2	14	15	.1	19	80	.01	.03	Tr	Tr
0	25	244	.6	—	40	.09	.08	1.6	—
2	59	138	5.2	154	90	.08	.15	1.1	8
2	47	116	3.5	119	—	.01	.09	.9	—
1	61	246	1.1	149	—	.11	.11	2.6	—
2	3	47	.1	—	0	.01	.02	.5	—
5	34	210	1.0	296	—	.03	.06	2.7	2
6	28	192	1.1	242	—	.10	.10	1.6	—
8	226	343	13.2	290	740	.34	.43	6.0	—
0	167[15]	243	.7	307	60	.03	.16	6.8	—
0	372	424	2.5	502	190	.02	.17	4.6	—
9	—	—	—	—	—	—	—	—	—
0	20	266	.5	320	30	.11	.22	7.3	—
1	98	224	2.6	104	50	.01	.03	1.5	—
9	61	162	1.7	195	—	.03	.07	2.3	—
0	7	199	1.6	—	70	.04	.10	10.1	—
7	41	291	2.7	—	590	.08	.23	10.3	2
Tr	2	34	.5	35	0	.08	.05	.8	—
0	10	114	2.9	184	30	.04	.18	3.6	—
0	10	108	2.7	176	10	.04	.17	3.3	—
0	10	196	3.0	261	20	.08	.20	5.1	—
0	9	159	2.6	221	30	.07	.17	4.4	—
0	8	158	2.2	189	70	.05	.13	3.1	—
0	6	131	1.8	161	10	.04	.11	2.6	—
0	11	208	3.2	279	10	.06	.19	4.5	—
0	10	199	3.0	268	Tr	.06	.18	4.3	—

Foods, Approximate Measures, Units, and Weight		(g)	Water (%)	Food Energy (cal)	Protein (g)	Fat (g)	Saturated (total) (g)	Oleic (g)	Linoleic (g)
							Fatty Acids		
							Saturated (total) (g)	**Unsaturated**	
								Oleic (g)	Linoleic (g)
Steak:									
Relatively fat-sirloin, broiled:									
Lean and fat (piece, 2½ × 2½ × ¾ in)	3 oz	85	44	330	20	27	11.3	11.1	.6
Lean only	2.0 oz	56	59	115	18	4	1.8	1.6	.2
Relatively lean-round, braised:									
Lean and fat (piece, 4⅛ × 2¼ × ½ in)	3 oz	85	55	220	24	13	5.5	5.2	.4
Lean only	2.4 oz	68	61	130	21	4	1.7	1.5	.2
Beef, canned:									
Corned beef	3 oz	85	59	185	22	10	4.9	4.5	.2
Corned beef hash	1 cup	220	67	400	19	25	11.9	10.9	.5
Beef, dried, chipped	2½ oz jar	71	48	145	24	4	2.1	2.0	.1
Beef and vegetable stew	1 cup	245	82	220	16	11	4.9	4.5	.2
Beef potpie (home recipe), baked (piece, ⅓ of 9-in diameter pie)[19]	1 piece	210	55	515	21	30	7.9	12.8	6.7
Chili con carne with beans, canned	1 cup	255	72	340	19	16	7.5	6.8	.3
Chop suey with beef and pork (home recipe)	1 cup	250	75	300	26	17	8.5	6.2	.7
Heart, beef, lean, braised	3 oz	85	61	160	27	5	1.5	1.1	.6
Lamb, cooked:									
Chop, rib (cut 3 per lb with bone), broiled:									
Lean and fat	3.1 oz	89	43	360	18	32	14.8	12.1	1.2
Lean only	2 oz	57	60	120	16	6	2.5	2.1	.2
Leg, roasted:									
Lean and fat (2 pieces, 4⅛ × 2¼ × ¼ in)	3 oz	85	54	235	22	16	7.3	6.0	.6
Lean only	2.5 oz	71	62	130	20	5	2.1	1.8	.2
Shoulder, roasted:									
Lean and fat (3 pieces, 2½ × 2½ × ¼ in)	3 oz	85	50	285	18	23	10.8	8.8	.9
Lean only	2.3 oz	64	61	130	17	6	3.6	2.3	.2
Liver, beef, fried (slice, 6½ × 2⅜ × ⅜ in)[20]	3 oz	85	56	195	22	9	2.5	3.5	.9
Pork, cured, cooked:									
Ham, light cure, lean and fat, roasted (2 pieces, 4⅛ × 2¼ × ¼ in)[22]	3 oz	85	54	245	18	19	6.8	7.9	1.7
Luncheon meat:									
Boiled ham, slice (8 per 8 oz pkg)	1 oz	28	59	65	5	5	1.7	2.0	.4
Canned, spiced or unspiced:									
Slice, approx. 3 × 2 × ½ in	1 slice	60	55	175	9	15	5.4	6.7	1.0
Pork, fresh, cooked:[18]									
Chop, loin (cut 3 per lb with bone), broiled:									
Lean and fat	2.7 oz	78	42	305	19	25	8.9	10.4	2.2
Lean only	2 oz	56	53	150	17	9	3.1	3.6	.8
Roast, oven cooked, no liquid added:									
Lean and fat (piece, 2½ × 2½ × ¾ in)	3 oz	85	46	310	21	24	8.7	10.2	2.2
Lean only	2.4 oz	68	55	175	20	10	3.5	4.1	.8
Shoulder cut, simmered:									
Lean and fat (3 pieces, 2½ × 2½ × ¼ in)	3 oz	85	46	320	20	26	9.3	10.9	2.3
Lean only	2.2 oz	63	60	135	18	6	2.2	2.6	.6
Sausages (see also Luncheon meat):									
Bologna, slice (8 per 8 oz pkg)	1 slice	28	56	85	3	8	3.0	3.4	.5
Braunschweiger, slice (6 per 6 oz pkg)	1 slice	28	53	90	4	8	2.6	3.4	.8
Brown and serve (10-11 per 8 oz pkg), browned	1 link	17	40	70	3	6	2.3	2.8	.7
Deviled ham, canned	1 tbsp	13	51	45	2	4	1.5	1.8	.4
Frankfurter (8 per 1 lb pkg), cooked (reheated)	1 frankfurter	56	57	170	7	15	5.6	6.5	1.2
Meat, potted (beef, chicken, turkey), canned	1 tbsp	13	61	30	2	2	—	—	—
Pork link (16 per 1 lb pkg), cooked	1 link	13	35	60	2	6	2.1	2.4	.5
Salami:									
Dry type, slice (12 per 4 oz pkg)	1 slice	10	30	45	2	4	1.6	1.6	.1
Cooked type, slice (8 per 8 oz pkg)	1 slice	28	51	90	5	7	3.1	3.0	.2
Vienna sausage (7 per 4 oz can)	1 sausage	16	63	40	2	3	1.2	1.4	.2
Veal, medium fat, cooked, bone removed:									
Cutlet (4⅛ × 2¼ × ½ in), braised or broiled	3 oz	85	60	185	23	9	4.0	3.4	.4
Rib (2 pieces, 4⅛ × 2¼ × ¼ in), roasted	3 oz	85	55	230	23	14	6.1	5.1	.6
Poultry and poultry products:									
Chicken, cooked:									
Breast, fried, bones removed, ½ breast (3.3 oz with bones)[23]	2.8 oz	79	58	160	26	5	1.4	1.8	1.1
Drumstick, fried, bones removed (2 oz with bones)[23]	1.3 oz	38	55	90	12	4	1.1	1.3	.9
Half broiler, broiled, bones removed (10.4 oz with bones)	6.2 oz	176	71	240	42	7	2.2	2.5	1.3

For notes, see end of table.

Nutrients in Indicated Quantity

Carbohydrate (g)	Calcium (mg)	Phosphorus (mg)	Iron (mg)	Potassium (mg)	Vitamin A Value (IU)	Thiamin (mg)	Riboflavin (mg)	Niacin (mg)	Ascorbic Acid (mg)
0	9	162	2.5	220	50	.05	.15	4.0	—
0	7	146	2.2	202	10	.05	.14	3.6	—
0	10	213	3.0	272	20	.07	.19	4.8	—
0	9	182	2.5	238	10	.05	.16	4.1	—
0	17	90	3.7	—	—	.01	.20	2.9	—
24	29	147	4.4	440	—	.02	.20	4.6	—
0	14	287	3.6	142	—	.05	.23	2.7	0
15	29	184	2.9	613	2400	.15	.17	4.7	17
39	29	149	3.8	334	1720	.30	.30	5.5	6
31	82	321	4.3	594	150	.08	.18	3.3	—
13	60	248	4.8	425	600	.28	.38	5.0	33
1	5	154	5.0	197	20	.21	1.04	6.5	1
0	8	139	1.0	200	—	.11	.19	4.1	—
0	6	121	1.1	174	—	.09	.15	3.4	—
0	9	177	1.4	241	—	.13	.23	4.7	—
0	9	169	1.4	227	—	.12	.21	4.4	—
0	9	146	1.0	206	—	.11	.20	4.0	—
0	8	140	1.0	193	—	.10	.18	3.7	—
5	9	405	7.5	323	45,390[21]	.22	3.56	14.0	23
0	8	146	2.2	199	0	.40	.15	3.1	—
0	3	47	.8	—	0	.12	.04	.7	—
1	5	65	1.3	133	0	.19	.13	1.8	—
0	9	209	2.7	216	0	.75	.22	4.5	—
0	7	181	2.2	192	0	.63	.18	3.8	—
0	9	218	2.7	233	0	.78	.22	4.8	—
0	9	211	2.6	224	0	.73	.21	4.4	—
0	9	118	2.6	158	0	.46	.21	4.1	—
0	8	111	2.3	146	0	.42	.19	3.7	—
Tr	2	36	.5	65	—	.05	.06	.7	—
1	3	69	1.7	—	1850	.05	.41	2.3	—
Tr	—	—	—	—	—	—	—	—	—
0	1	12	.3	—	0	.02	.01	.2	—
1	3	57	.8	—	—	.08	.11	1.4	—
0	—	—	—	—	—	Tr	.03	.2	—
Tr	1	21	.3	35	0	.10	.04	.5	—
Tr	1	28	.4	—	—	.04	.03	.5	—
Tr	3	57	.7	—	—	.07	.07	1.2	—
Tr	1	24	.3	—	—	.01	.02	.4	—
0	9	196	2.7	258	—	.06	.21	4.6	—
0	10	211	2.9	259	—	.11	.26	6.6	—
1	9	218	1.3	—	70	.04	.17	11.6	—
Tr	6	89	.9	—	50	.03	.15	2.7	—
0	16	355	3.0	483	160	.09	.34	15.5	—

Foods, Approximate Measures, Units, and Weight		(g)	Water (%)	Food Energy (cal)	Protein (g)	Fat (g)	Saturated (total) (g)	Oleic (g)	Linoleic (g)
							Nutrients in Indicated Quantity		
								Fatty Acids	
							Saturated (total) (g)	**Unsaturated**	
Chicken, canned, boneless	3 oz	85	65	170	18	10	3.2	3.8	2.0
Chicken a la king, cooked (home recipe)	1 cup	245	68	470	27	34	12.7	14.3	3.3
Chicken and noodles, cooked (home recipe)	1 cup	240	71	365	22	18	5.9	7.1	3.5
Chicken chow mein:									
Canned	1 cup	250	89	95	7	Tr	—	—	—
From home recipe	1 cup	250	78	255	31	10	2.4	3.4	3.1
Chicken potpie (home recipe), baked, piece (⅓ of 9-in diameter pie)[19]	1 piece	232	57	545	23	31	11.3	10.9	5.6
Turkey, roasted, flesh without skin:									
Dark meat, piece, 2½ × 1⅝ × ¼ in	4 pieces	85	61	175	26	7	2.1	1.5	1.5
Light meat, piece, 4 × 2 × ¼ in	2 pieces	85	62	150	28	3	.9	.6	.7
Light and dark meat:									
Chopped or diced	1 cup	140	61	265	44	9	2.5	1.7	1.8
Pieces (1 slice white meat, 4 × 2 × ¼ in with 2 slices dark meat, 2½ × 1⅝ × ¼ in)	3 pieces	85	61	160	27	5	1.5	1.0	1.1
Fruits and Fruit Products									
Apples, raw, unpeeled, without cores:									
2¾-in diameter (about 3 per lb with cores)	1 apple	138	84	80	Tr	1	—	—	—
3¼-in diameter (about 2 per lb with cores)	1 apple	212	84	125	Tr	1	—	—	—
Apple juice, bottled or canned[24]	1 cup	248	88	120	Tr	Tr	—	—	—
Applesauce, canned:									
Sweetened	1 cup	255	76	230	1	Tr	—	—	—
Unsweetened	1 cup	244	89	100	Tr	Tr	—	—	—
Apricots:									
Raw, without pits (about 12 per lb with pits)	3 apricots	107	85	55	1	Tr	—	—	—
Canned in heavy syrup (halves and syrup)	1 cup	258	77	220	2	Tr	—	—	—
Dried:									
Uncooked (28 large or 37 medium halves per cup)	1 cup	130	25	340	7	1	—	—	—
Cooked, unsweetened, fruit and liquid	1 cup	250	76	215	4	1	—	—	—
Apricot nectar, canned	1 cup	251	85	145	1	Tr	—	—	—
Avocados, raw, whole, without skins and seeds:									
California, mid- and late-winter (with skin and seed, 3⅛-in diameter; wt 10 oz)	1 avocado	216	74	370	5	37	5.5	22.0	3.7
Florida, late summer and fall (with skin and seed, 3⅝-in diameter; wt 1 lb)	1 avocado	304	78	390	4	33	6.7	15.7	5.3
Banana without peel (about 2.6 per lb with peel)	1 banana	119	76	100	1	Tr	—	—	—
Banana flakes	1 tbsp	6	3	20	Tr	Tr	—	—	—
Blackberries, raw	1 cup	144	85	85	2	1	—	—	—
Blueberries, raw	1 cup	145	83	90	1	1	—	—	—
Cantaloupe; see muskmelons									
Cherries:									
Sour (tart), red, pitted, canned, water pack	1 cup	244	88	105	2	Tr	—	—	—
Sweet, raw, without pits and stems	10 cherries	68	80	45	1	Tr	—	—	—
Cranberry juice cocktail, bottled, sweetened	1 cup	253	83	165	Tr	Tr	—	—	—
Cranberry sauce, sweetened, canned, strained	1 cup	277	62	405	Tr	1	—	—	—
Dates:									
Whole, without pits	10 dates	80	23	220	2	Tr	—	—	—
Chopped	1 cup	178	23	490	4	1	—	—	—
Fruit cocktail, canned, in heavy syrup	1 cup	255	80	195	1	Tr	—	—	—
Grapefruit:									
Raw, medium, 3¾-in diameter (about 1 lb 1 oz):									
Pink or red	½ grapefruit with peel[28]	241	89	50	1	Tr	—	—	—
White	½ grapefruit with peel[28]	241	89	45	1	Tr	—	—	—
Canned, sections with syrup	1 cup	254	81	180	2	Tr	—	—	—
Grapefruit juice:									
Raw, pink, red, or white	1 cup	246	90	95	1	Tr	—	—	—
Canned, white:									
Unsweetened	1 cup	247	89	100	1	Tr	—	—	—
Sweetened	1 cup	250	86	135	1	Tr	—	—	—
Frozen, concentrate, unsweetened:									
Undiluted, 6 fl oz can	1 can	207	62	300	4	1	—	—	—
Diluted with 3 parts water by volume	1 cup	247	89	100	1	Tr	—	—	—
Dehydrated crystals, prepared with water (1 lb yields about 1 gal)	1 cup	247	90	100	1	Tr	—	—	—

For notes, see end of table.

Nutrients in Indicated Quantity

Carbohydrate (g)	Calcium (mg)	Phosphorus (mg)	Iron (mg)	Potassium (mg)	Vitamin A Value (IU)	Thiamin (mg)	Riboflavin (mg)	Niacin (mg)	Ascorbic Acid (mg)
0	18	210	1.3	117	200	.03	.11	3.7	3
12	127	358	2.5	404	1130	.10	.42	5.4	12
26	26	247	2.2	149	430	.05	.17	4.3	Tr
18	45	85	1.3	418	150	.05	.10	1.0	13
10	58	293	2.5	473	280	.08	.23	4.3	10
42	70	232	3.0	343	3090	.34	.31	5.5	5
0	—	—	2.0	338	—	.03	.20	3.6	—
0	—	—	1.0	349	—	.04	.12	9.4	—
0	11	351	2.5	514	—	.07	.25	10.8	—
0	7	213	1.5	312	—	.04	.15	6.5	—
20	10	14	.4	152	120	.04	.03	.1	6
31	15	21	.6	233	190	.06	.04	.2	8
30	15	22	1.5	250	—	.02	.05	.2	2[25]
61	10	13	1.3	166	100	.05	.03	.1	3[25]
26	10	12	1.2	190	100	.05	.02	.1	2[25]
14	18	25	.5	301	2890	.03	.04	.6	11
57	28	39	.8	604	4490	.05	.05	1.0	10
86	87	140	7.2	1273	14,170	.01	.21	4.3	16
54	55	88	4.5	795	7500	.01	.13	2.5	8
37	23	30	.5	379	2380	.03	.03	.5	36[26]
13	22	91	1.3	1303	630	.24	.43	3.5	30
27	30	128	1.8	1836	880	.33	.61	4.9	43
26	10	31	.8	440	230	.06	.07	.8	12
5	2	6	.2	92	50	.01	.01	.2	Tr
19	46	27	1.3	245	290	.04	.06	.6	30
22	22	19	1.5	117	150	.04	.09	.7	20
26	37	32	.7	317	1660	.07	.05	.5	12
12	15	13	.3	129	70	.03	.04	.3	7
42	13	8	.8	25	Tr	.03	.03	.1	81
104	17	11	.6	83	60	.03	.03	.1	6
58	47	50	2.4	518	40	.07	.08	1.8	0
130	105	112	5.3	1153	90	.16	.18	3.9	0
50	23	31	1.0	411	360	.05	.03	1.0	5
13	20	20	.5	166	540	.05	.02	.2	44
12	19	19	.5	159	10	.05	.02	.2	44
45	33	36	.8	343	30	.08	.05	.5	76
23	22	37	.5	399	([29])	.10	.05	.5	93
24	20	35	1.0	400	20	.07	.05	.5	84
32	20	35	1.0	405	30	.08	.05	.5	78
72	70	124	.8	1250	60	.29	.12	1.4	286
24	25	42	.2	420	20	.10	.04	.5	96
24	22	40	.2	412	20	.10	.05	.5	91

Foods, Approximate Measures, Units, and Weight		(g)	Nutrients in Indicated Quantity						
			Water (%)	Food Energy (cal)	Protein (g)	Fat (g)	Fatty Acids		
							Saturated (total) (g)	Unsaturated	
								Oleic (g)	Linoleic (g)
Grapes, European type (adherent skin), raw:									
Thompson seedless	10 grapes	50	81	35	Tr	Tr	—	—	—
Tokay and Emperor, seeded types	10 grapes[30]	60	81	40	Tr	Tr	—	—	—
Grapejuice:									
Canned or bottled	1 cup	253	83	165	1	Tr	—	—	—
Frozen concentrate, sweetened:									
Undiluted, 6 fl oz can	1 can	216	53	395	1	Tr	—	—	—
Diluted with 3 parts water by volume	1 cup	250	86	135	1	Tr	—	—	—
Grape drink, canned	1 cup	250	86	135	Tr	Tr	—	—	—
Lemon, raw, size 165, without peel and seeds (about 4 per lb with peels and seeds)	1 lemon	74	90	20	1	Tr	—	—	—
Lemon juice:									
Raw	1 cup	244	91	60	1	Tr	—	—	—
Canned, or bottled, unsweetened	1 cup	244	92	55	1	Tr	—	—	—
Frozen, single strength, unsweetened, 6 fl oz can	1 can	183	92	40	1	Tr	—	—	—
Lemonade concentrate, frozen:									
Undiluted, 6 fl oz can	1 can	219	49	425	Tr	Tr	—	—	—
Diluted with 4⅓ parts water by volume	1 cup	248	89	105	Tr	Tr	—	—	—
Limeade concentrate, frozen:									
Undiluted, 6 fl oz can	1 can	218	50	410	Tr	Tr	—	—	—
Diluted with 4⅓ parts water by volume	1 cup	247	89	100	Tr	Tr	—	—	—
Limejuice:									
Raw	1 cup	246	90	65	1	Tr	—	—	—
Canned, unsweetened	1 cup	246	90	65	1	Tr	—	—	—
Muskmelons, raw, with rind, without seed cavity:									
Cantaloupe, orange-fleshed (with rind and seed cavity, 5-in diameter, 2⅓ lb)	½ melon with rind[33]	477	91	80	2	Tr	—	—	—
Honeydew (with rind and seed cavity, 6½-in diameter, 5¼ lb)	⅒ melon with rind[33]	226	91	50	1	Tr	—	—	—
Oranges, all commercial varieties, raw:									
Whole, 2⅝-in diameter, without peel and seeds (about 2½ per lb with peel and seeds)	1 orange	131	86	65	1	Tr	—	—	—
Sections without membranes	1 cup	180	86	90	2	Tr	—	—	—
Orange juice:									
Raw, all varieties	1 cup	248	88	110	2	Tr	—	—	—
Canned, unsweetened	1 cup	249	87	120	2	Tr	—	—	—
Frozen concentrate:									
Undiluted, 6 fl oz can	1 can	213	55	360	5	Tr	—	—	—
Diluted with 3 parts water by volume	1 cup	249	87	120	2	Tr	—	—	—
Dehydrated crystals, prepared with water (1 lb yields about 1 gal)	1 cup	248	88	115	1	Tr	—	—	—
Orange and grapefruit juice:									
Frozen concentrate:									
Undiluted, 6 fl oz can	1 can	210	59	330	4	1	—	—	—
Diluted with 3 parts water by volume	1 cup	248	88	110	1	Tr	—	—	—
Papayas, raw, ½-in cubes	1 cup	140	89	55	1	Tr	—	—	—
Peaches:									
Raw:									
Whole, 2½-in diameter, peeled, pitted (about 4 per lb with peels and pits)	1 peach	100	89	40	1	Tr	—	—	—
Sliced	1 cup	170	89	65	1	Tr	—	—	—
Canned, yellow-fleshed, solids and liquid (halves or slices):									
Syrup pack	1 cup	256	79	200	1	Tr	—	—	—
Water pack	1 cup	244	91	75	1	Tr	—	—	—
Dried:									
Uncooked	1 cup	160	25	420	5	1	—	—	—
Cooked, unsweetened, halves and juice	1 cup	250	77	205	3	1	—	—	—
Frozen, sliced, sweetened:									
10-oz container	1 container	284	77	250	1	Tr	—	—	—
Cup	1 cup	250	77	220	1	Tr	—	—	—
Pears:									
Raw, with skin, cored:									
Bartlett, 2½-in diameter (about 2½ per lb with cores and stems)	1 pear	164	83	100	1	1	—	—	—
Bosc, 2½-in diameter (about 3 per lb with cores and stems)	1 pear	141	83	85	1	1	—	—	—

For notes, see end of table.

Nutrients in Indicated Quantity

Carbohydrate (g)	Calcium (mg)	Phosphorus (mg)	Iron (mg)	Potassium (mg)	Vitamin A Value (IU)	Thiamin (mg)	Riboflavin (mg)	Niacin (mg)	Ascorbic Acid (mg)
9	6	10	.2	87	50	.03	.02	.2	2
10	7	11	.2	99	60	.03	.02	.2	2
42	28	30	.8	293	—	.10	.05	.5	Tr[25]
100	22	32	.9	255	40	.13	.22	1.5	32[31]
33	8	10	.3	85	10	.05	.08	.5	10[31]
35	8	10	.3	88	—	.03[32]	.03[32]	.3	([32])
6	19	12	.4	102	10	.03	.01	.1	39
20	17	24	.5	344	50	.07	.02	.2	112
19	17	24	.5	344	50	.07	.02	.2	102
13	13	16	.5	258	40	.05	.02	.2	81
112	9	13	.4	153	40	.05	.06	.7	66
28	2	3	.1	40	10	.01	.02	.2	17
108	11	13	.2	129	Tr	.02	.02	.2	26
27	3	3	Tr	32	Tr	Tr	Tr	Tr	6
22	22	27	.5	256	20	.05	.02	.2	79
22	22	27	.5	256	20	.05	.02	.2	52
20	38	44	1.1	682	9240	.11	.08	1.6	90
11	21	24	.6	374	60	.06	.04	.9	34
16	54	26	.5	263	260	.13	.05	.5	66
22	74	36	.7	360	360	.18	.07	.7	90
26	27	42	.5	496	500	.22	.07	1.0	124
28	25	45	1.0	496	500	.17	.05	.7	100
87	75	126	.9	1500	1620	.68	.11	2.8	360
29	25	42	.2	503	540	.23	.03	.9	120
27	25	40	.5	518	500	.20	.07	1.0	109
78	61	99	.8	1308	800	.48	.06	2.3	302
26	20	32	.2	439	270	.15	.02	.7	102
14	28	22	.4	328	2450	.06	.06	.4	78
10	9	19	.5	202	1330[34]	.02	.05	1.0	7
16	15	32	.9	343	2260[34]	.03	.09	1.7	12
51	10	31	.8	333	1100	.03	.05	1.5	8
20	10	32	.7	334	1100	.02	.07	1.5	7
109	77	187	9.6	1520	6240	.02	.30	8.5	29
54	38	93	4.8	743	3050	.01	.15	3.8	5
64	11	37	1.4	352	1850	.03	.11	2.0	116[35]
57	10	33	1.3	310	1630	.03	.10	1.8	103[35]
25	13	18	.5	213	30	.03	.07	.2	7
22	11	16	.4	83	30	.03	.06	.1	6

Foods, Approximate Measures, Units, and Weight		(g)	Water (%)	Food Energy (cal)	Protein (g)	Fat (g)	Saturated (total) (g)	Oleic (g)	Linoleic (g)
							Fatty Acids		
								Unsaturated	
D'Anjou, 3-in diameter (about 2 per lb with cores and stems)	1 pear	200	83	120	1	1	—	—	—
Canned, solids and liquid, syrup pack, heavy (halves or slices)	1 cup	255	80	195	1	1	—	—	—
Pineapple:									
Raw, diced	1 cup	155	85	80	1	Tr	—	—	—
Canned, heavy syrup pack, solids and liquid:									
Crushed, chunks, tidbits	1 cup	255	80	190	1	Tr	—	—	—
Slices and liquid:									
Large	1 slice; 2¼ tbsp liquid	105	80	80	Tr	Tr	—	—	—
Medium	1 slice; 1¼ tbsp liquid	58	80	45	Tr	Tr	—	—	—
Pineapple juice, unsweetened, canned	1 cup	250	86	140	1	Tr	—	—	—
Plums:									
Raw, without pits:									
Japanese and hybrid (2⅛-in diameter, about 6½ per lb with pits)	1 plum	66	87	30	Tr	Tr	—	—	—
Prune-type (1½-in diameter, about 15 per lb with pits)	1 plum	28	79	20	Tr	Tr	—	—	—
Canned, heavy syrup pack (Italian prunes), with pits and liquid:									
Cup	1 cup[36]	272	77	215	1	Tr	—	—	—
Portion	3 plums; 2¾ tbsp liquid[36]	140	77	110	1	Tr	—	—	—
Prunes, dried, "softenized," with pits:									
Uncooked	4 extra large or 5 large prunes[36]	49	28	110	1	Tr	—	—	—
Cooked, unsweetened, all sizes, fruit and liquid	1 cup[36]	250	66	255	2	1	—	—	—
Prune juice, canned or bottled	1 cup	256	80	195	1	Tr	—	—	—
Raisins, seedless:									
Cup, not pressed down	1 cup	145	18	420	4	Tr	—	—	—
Packet, ½ oz (1½ tbsp)	1 packet	14	18	40	Tr	Tr	—	—	—
Raspberries, red:									
Raw, capped, whole	1 cup	123	84	70	1	1	—	—	—
Frozen, sweetened, 10 oz container	1 container	284	74	280	2	1	—	—	—
Rhubarb, cooked, added sugar:									
From raw	1 cup	270	63	380	1	Tr	—	—	—
From frozen, sweetened	1 cup	270	63	385	1	1	—	—	—
Strawberries:									
Raw, whole berries, capped	1 cup	149	90	55	1	1	—	—	—
Frozen, sweetened:									
Sliced, 10 oz container	1 container	284	71	310	1	1	—	—	—
Whole, 1 lb container (about 1¾ cups)	1 container	454	76	415	2	1	—	—	—
Tangerine, raw, 2⅜-in diameter, size 176, without peel (about 4 per lb with peels and seeds)	1 tangerine	86	87	40	1	Tr	—	—	—
Tangerine juice, canned, sweetened	1 cup	249	87	125	1	Tr	—	—	—
Watermelon, raw, 4 × 8 in wedge with rind and seeds (1/16 of 32⅔ lb melon, 10 × 16 in)	1 wedge with rind and seeds	926	93	110	2	1	—	—	—
Grain Products									
Bagel, 3-in diameter:									
Egg	1 bagel	55	32	165	6	2	.5	.9	.8
Water	1 bagel	55	29	165	6	1	.2	.4	.6
Barley, pearled, light, uncooked	1 cup	200	11	700	16	2	.3	.2	.8
Biscuits, baking powder, 2-in diameter (enriched flour, vegetable shortening):									
From home recipe	1 biscuit	28	27	105	2	5	1.2	2.0	1.2
From mix	1 biscuit	28	29	90	2	3	.6	1.1	.7
Breadcrumbs (enriched)[38]:									
Dry, grated	1 cup	100	7	390	13	5	1.0	1.6	1.4
Soft; see White bread									
Breads:									
Boston brown bread, canned, slice, 3¼ × ½ in[38]	1 slice	45	45	95	2	1	.1	.2	.2
Cracked-wheat bread (¾ enriched wheat flour, ¼ cracked wheat)[38]:									
Slice (18 per loaf)	1 slice	25	35	65	2	1	.1	.2	.2
French or Vienna bread, enriched[38]									
Slice:									
French (5 × 2½ × 1 in)	1 slice	35	31	100	3	1	.2	.4	.4

For notes, see end of table.

Nutrients in Indicated Quantity

Carbohydrate (g)	Calcium (mg)	Phosphorus (mg)	Iron (mg)	Potassium (mg)	Vitamin A Value (IU)	Thiamin (mg)	Riboflavin (mg)	Niacin (mg)	Ascorbic Acid (mg)
31	16	22	.6	260	40	.04	.08	.2	8
50	13	18	.5	214	10	.03	.05	.3	3
21	26	12	.8	226	110	.14	.05	.3	26
49	28	13	.8	245	130	.20	.05	.5	18
20	12	5	.3	101	50	.08	.02	.2	7
11	6	3	.2	56	30	.05	.01	.1	4
34	38	23	.8	373	130	.13	.05	.5	80[27]
8	8	12	.3	112	160	.02	.02	.3	4
6	3	5	.1	48	80	.01	.01	.1	1
56	23	26	2.3	367	3130	.05	.05	1.0	5
29	12	13	1.2	189	1610	.03	.03	.5	3
29	22	34	1.7	298	690	.04	.07	.7	1
67	51	79	3.8	695	1590	.07	.15	1.5	2
49	36	51	1.8	602	—	.03	.03	1.0	5
112	90	146	5.1	1106	30	.16	.12	.7	1
11	9	14	.5	107	Tr	.02	.01	.1	Tr
17	27	27	1.1	207	160	.04	.11	1.1	31
70	37	48	1.7	284	200	.06	.17	1.7	60
97	211	41	1.6	548	220	.05	.14	.8	16
98	211	32	1.9	475	190	.05	.11	.5	16
13	31	31	1.5	244	90	.04	.10	.9	88
79	40	48	2.0	318	90	.06	.17	1.4	151
107	59	73	2.7	472	140	.09	.27	2.3	249
10	34	15	.3	108	360	.05	.02	.1	27
30	44	35	.5	440	1040	.15	.05	.2	54
27	30	43	2.1	426	2510	.13	.13	.9	30
28	9	43	1.2	41	30	.14	.10	1.2	0
30	8	41	1.2	42	0	.15	.11	1.4	0
158	32	378	4.0	320	0	.24	.10	6.2	0
13	34	49	.4	33	Tr	.08	.08	.7	Tr
15	19	65	.6	32	Tr	.09	.08	.8	Tr
73	122	141	3.6	152	Tr	.35	.35	4.8	Tr
21	41	72	.9	131	0[39]	.06	.04	.7	0
13	22	32	.5	34	Tr	.08	.06	.8	Tr
19	15	30	.8	32	Tr	.14	.08	1.2	Tr

Foods, Approximate Measures, Units, and Weight		(g)	Water (%)	Food Energy (cal)	Protein (g)	Fat (g)	Saturated (total) (g)	Oleic (g)	Linoleic (g)
							Fatty Acids		
							Saturated (total) (g)	**Unsaturated**	
								Oleic (g)	Linoleic (g)
Vienna (4¾ × 4 × ½ in)	1 slice	25	31	75	2	1	.2	.3	.3
Italian bread enriched:									
Slice, 4½ × 3¼ × ¾ in	1 slice	30	32	85	3	Tr	Tr	Tr	.1
Raisin bread, enriched[38]:									
Slice (18 per loaf)	1 slice	25	35	65	2	1	.2	.3	.2
Rye bread:									
American, light (⅔ enriched wheat flour, ⅓ rye flour):									
Slice (4¾ × 3¾ × 7/16 in)	1 slice	25	36	60	2	Tr	Tr	Tr	.1
Pumpernickel (⅔ rye flour, ⅓ enriched wheat flour):									
Slice (5 × 4 × ⅜ in)	1 slice	32	34	80	3	Tr	.1	Tr	.2
White bread, enriched[38]:									
Soft-crumb type[38]:									
Slice (18 per loaf)	1 slice	25	36	70	2	1	.2	.3	.3
Slice, toasted	1 slice	22	25	70	2	1	.2	.3	.3
Slice (22 per loaf)	1 slice	20	36	55	2	1	.2	.2	.2
Slice, toasted	1 slice	17	25	55	2	1	.2	.2	.2
Slice (24 per loaf)	1 slice	28	36	75	2	1	.2	.3	.3
Slice, toasted	1 slice	24	25	75	2	1	.2	.3	.3
Slice (28 per loaf)	1 slice	24	36	65	2	1	.2	.3	.2
Slice, toasted	1 slice	21	25	65	2	1	.2	.3	.2
Cubes	1 cup	30	36	80	3	1	.2	.3	.3
Crumbs	1 cup	45	36	120	4	1	.3	.5	.5
Firm-crumb type[38]:									
Slice (20 per loaf)	1 slice	23	35	65	2	1	.2	.3	.3
Slice, toasted	1 slice	20	24	65	2	1	.2	.3	.3
Slice (34 per loaf)	1 slice	27	35	75	2	1	.2	.3	.3
Slice, toasted	1 slice	23	24	75	2	1	.2	.3	.3
Whole-wheat bread:									
Soft-crumb type:									
Slice (16 per loaf)	1 slice	28	36	65	3	1	.1	.2	.2
Slice, toasted	1 slice	24	24	65	3	1	.1	.2	.2
Firm-crumb type:									
Slice (18 per loaf)	1 slice	25	36	60	3	1	.1	.2	.3
Slice, toasted	1 slice	21	24	60	3	1	.1	.2	.3
Breakfast cereals:									
Hot type, cooked:									
Corn (hominy) grits, degermed:									
Enriched	1 cup	245	87	125	3	Tr	Tr	Tr	.1
Unenriched	1 cup	245	87	125	3	Tr	Tr	Tr	.1
Farina, quick-cooking, enriched	1 cup	245	89	105	3	Tr	Tr	Tr	.1
Oatmeal or rolled oats	1 cup	240	87	130	5	2	.4	.8	.9
Wheat, rolled	1 cup	240	80	180	5	1	—	—	—
Wheat, whole-meal	1 cup	245	88	110	4	1	—	—	—
Ready-to-eat:									
Bran flakes (40% bran), added sugar, salt, iron, vitamins	1 cup	35	3	105	4	1	—	—	—
Bran flakes with raisins, added sugar, salt, iron, vitamins	1 cup	50	7	145	4	1	—	—	—
Corn flakes:									
Plain, added sugar, salt, iron, vitamins	1 cup	25	4	95	2	Tr	—	—	—
Sugar-coated, added salt, iron, vitamins	1 cup	40	2	155	2	Tr	—	—	—
Corn, oat flour, puffed, added sugar, salt, iron, vitamins	1 cup	20	4	80	2	1	—	—	—
Corn, shredded, added sugar, salt, iron, thiamin, niacin	1 cup	25	3	95	2	Tr	—	—	—
Oats, puffed, added sugar, salt, minerals, vitamins	1 cup	25	3	100	3	1	—	—	—
Rice, puffed:									
Plain, added iron, thiamin, niacin	1 cup	15	4	60	1	Tr	—	—	—
Presweetened, added salt, iron, vitamins	1 cup	28	3	115	1	0	—	—	—
Wheat flakes, added sugar, salt, iron, vitamins	1 cup	30	4	105	3	Tr	—	—	—
Wheat, puffed:									
Plain, added iron, thiamin, niacin	1 cup	15	3	55	2	Tr	—	—	—
Presweetened, added salt, iron, vitamins	1 cup	38	3	140	3	Tr	—	—	—

For notes, see end of table.

Nutrients in Indicated Quantity

Carbohydrate (g)	Calcium (mg)	Phosphorus (mg)	Iron (mg)	Potassium (mg)	Vitamin A Value (IU)	Thiamin (mg)	Riboflavin (mg)	Niacin (mg)	Ascorbic Acid (mg)
14	11	21	.6	23	Tr	.10	.06	.8	Tr
17	5	23	.7	22	0	.12	.07	1.0	0
13	18	22	.6	58	Tr	.09	.06	.6	Tr
13	19	37	.5	36	0	.07	.05	.7	0
17	27	73	.8	145	0	.09	.07	.6	0
13	21	24	.6	26	Tr	.10	.06	.8	Tr
13	21	24	.6	26	Tr	.08	.06	.8	Tr
10	17	19	.5	21	Tr	.08	.05	.7	Tr
10	17	19	.5	21	Tr	.06	.05	.7	Tr
14	24	27	.7	29	Tr	.11	.07	.9	Tr
14	24	27	.7	29	Tr	.09	.07	.9	Tr
12	20	23	.6	25	Tr	.10	.06	.8	Tr
12	20	23	.6	25	Tr	.08	.06	.8	Tr
15	25	29	.8	32	Tr	.12	.07	1.0	Tr
23	38	44	1.1	47	Tr	.18	.11	1.5	Tr
12	22	23	.6	28	Tr	.09	.06	.8	Tr
12	22	23	.6	28	Tr	.07	.06	.8	Tr
14	26	28	.7	33	Tr	.11	.06	.9	Tr
14	26	28	.7	33	Tr	.09	.06	.9	Tr
14	24	71	.8	72	Tr	.09	.03	.8	Tr
14	24	71	.8	72	Tr	.07	.03	.8	Tr
12	25	57	.8	68	Tr	.06	.03	.7	Tr
12	25	27	.8	68	Tr	.05	.03	.7	Tr
27	2	25	.7	27	Tr[40]	.10	.07	1.0	0
27	2	25	.2	27	Tr[40]	.05	.02	.5	0
22	147	113[41]	([42])	25	0	.12	.07	1.0	0
23	22	137	1.4	146	0	.19	.05	.2	0
41	19	182	1.7	202	0	.17	.07	2.2	0
23	17	127	1.2	118	0	.15	.05	1.5	0
28	19	125	5.6	137	1540	.46	.52	6.2	0
40	28	146	7.9	154	2200[43]	([44])	([44])	([44])	0
21	([44])	9	([44])	30	([44])	([44])	([44])	([44])	13[45]
37	1	10	([44])	27	1760	.53	.60	7.1	21[45]
16	4	18	5.7	—	880	.26	.30	3.5	11
22	1	10	.6	—	0	.33	.05	4.4	13
19	44	102	4.0	—	1100	.33	.38	4.4	13
13	3	14	.3	15	0	.07	.01	.7	0
26	3	14	([44])	43	1240[45]	([44])	([44])	([44])	15[45]
24	12	83	4.8	81	1320	.40	.45	5.3	16
12	4	48	.6	51	0	.08	.03	1.2	0
33	7	52	([44])	63	1680	.50	.57	6.7	20[45]

Foods, Approximate Measures, Units, and Weight		(g)	Water (%)	Food Energy (cal)	Protein (g)	Fat (g)	Fatty Acids		
							Saturated (total) (g)	Unsaturated Oleic (g)	Linoleic (g)
Wheat, shredded, plain	1 oblong biscuit or ½ cup spoon-size biscuits	25	7	90	2	1	—	—	—
Wheat germ, without salt and sugar, toasted	1 tbsp	6	4	25	2	1	—	—	—
Buckwheat flour, light, sifted	1 cup	98	12	340	6	1	.2	.4	.4
Bulgur, canned, seasoned	1 cup	135	56	245	8	4	—	—	—
Cake icings; see Sugars and sweets									
Cakes made from cake mixes with enriched flour[46]:									
Angelfood:									
Piece, 1/12 of cake	1 piece	53	34	135	3	Tr	—	—	—
Coffeecake:									
Piece, 1/6 of cake	1 piece	72	30	230	5	7	2.0	2.7	1.5
Cupcakes, made with egg, milk, 2½-in diameter:									
Without icing	1 cupcake	25	26	90	1	3	.8	1.2	.7
With chocolate icing	1 cupcake	36	22	130	2	5	2.0	1.6	.6
Devil's food with chocolate icing:									
Piece, 1/16 of cake	1 piece	69	24	235	3	8	3.1	2.8	1.1
Cupcake, 2½-in diameter	1 cupcake	35	24	120	2	4	1.6	1.4	.5
Gingerbread:									
Piece, 1/9 of cake	1 piece	63	37	175	2	4	1.1	1.8	1.1
White, 2 layer with chocolate icing:									
Piece, 1/16 of cake	1 piece	71	21	250	3	8	2.0	2.9	1.2
Yellow, 2 layer with chocolate icing:									
Piece, 1/16 of cake	1 piece	69	26	235	3	8	3.0	3.0	1.3
Cakes made from home recipes using enriched flour[47]:									
Boston cream pie with custard filling:									
Whole cake (8-in diameter)	1 cake	825	35	2490	41	78	23.0	30.1	15.2
Piece, 1/12 of cake	1 piece	69	35	210	3	6	1.9	2.5	1.3
Fruitcake, dark:									
Slice, 1/30 of loaf	1 slice	15	18	55	1	2	.5	1.1	.5
Plain, sheet cake:									
Without icing:									
Whole cake (9-in sq)	1 cake	777	25	2830	35	108	29.5	44.4	23.9
Piece, 1/9 of cake	1 piece	86	25	315	4	12	3.3	4.9	2.6
With uncooked white icing:									
Piece, 1/9 of cake	1 piece	121	21	445	4	14	4.7	5.5	2.7
Pound[49]:									
Loaf, 8½ × 3½ × 3¼ in	1 loaf	565	16	2725	31	170	42.9	73.1	39.6
Slice, 1/17 of loaf	1 slice	33	16	160	2	10	2.5	4.3	2.3
Spongecake:									
Whole cake (9¾-in diameter tube cake)	1 cake	790	32	2345	60	45	13.1	15.8	5.7
Piece, 1/12 of cake	1 piece	66	32	195	5	4	1.1	1.3	.5
Cookies made with enriched flour[50,51]:									
Brownies with nuts:									
Home-prepared, 1¾ × 1¾ × 7/8 in:									
From home recipe	1 brownie	20	10	95	1	6	1.5	3.0	1.2
From commercial recipe	1 brownie	20	11	85	1	4	.9	1.4	1.3
Frozen, with chocolate icing, 1½ × 1¾ × 7/8 in[52]	1 brownie	25	13	105	1	5	2.0	2.2	.7
Chocolate chip:									
Commercial, 2¼-in diameter, 3/8 in thick	4 cookies	42	3	200	2	9	2.8	2.9	2.2
From home recipe, 2 1/3-in diameter	4 cookies	40	3	205	2	12	3.5	4.5	2.9
Fig bars, square (1 5/8 × 1 5/8 × 3/8 in) or rectangular (1½ × 1¾ × ½ in)	4 cookies	56	14	200	2	3	.8	1.2	.7
Gingersnaps, 2-in diameter, ¼ in thick	4 cookies	28	3	90	2	2	.7	1.0	.6
Macaroons, 2¾-in diameter, ¼ in thick	2 cookies	38	4	180	2	9	—	—	—
Oatmeal with raisins, 2 5/8-in diameter, ¼ in thick	4 cookies	52	3	235	3	8	2.0	3.3	2.0
Plain, prepared from commercial chilled dough, 2½-in diameter, ¼ in thick	4 cookies	48	5	240	2	12	3.0	5.2	2.9
Sandwich type (chocolate or vanilla), 1¾-in diameter, 3/8 in thick	4 cookies	40	2	200	2	9	2.2	3.9	2.2
Vanilla wafers, 1¾-in diameter, ¼ in thick	10 cookies	40	3	185	2	6	—	—	—

For notes, see end of table.

Nutrients in Indicated Quantity

Carbohydrate (g)	Calcium (mg)	Phosphorus (mg)	Iron (mg)	Potassium (mg)	Vitamin A Value (IU)	Thiamin (mg)	Riboflavin (mg)	Niacin (mg)	Ascorbic Acid (mg)
20	11	97	.9	87	0	.06	.03	1.1	0
3	3	70	.5	57	10	.11	.05	.3	1
78	11	86	1.0	314	0	.08	.04	.4	0
44	27	263	1.9	151	0	.08	.05	4.1	0
32	50	63	.2	32	0	.03	.08	.3	0
38	44	125	1.2	78	120	.14	.15	1.3	Tr
14	40	59	.3	21	40	.05	.05	.4	Tr
21	47	71	.4	42	60	.05	.06	.4	Tr
40	41	72	1.0	90	100	.07	.10	.6	Tr
20	21	37	.5	46	50	.03	.05	.3	Tr
32	57	63	.9	173	Tr	.09	.11	.8	Tr
45	70	127	.7	82	40	.09	.11	.8	Tr
40	63	126	.8	75	100	.08	.10	.7	Tr
412	553	833	8.2	734[48]	1730	1.04	1.27	9.6	2
34	46	70	.7	61[48]	140	.09	.11	.8	Tr
9	11	17	.4	74	20	.02	.02	.2	Tr
434	497	793	8.5	614[48]	1320	1.21	1.40	10.2	2
48	55	88	.9	68[48]	150	.13	.15	1.1	Tr
77	61	91	.8	74	240	.14	.16	1.1	Tr
273	107	418	7.9	345	1410	.90	.99	7.3	0
16	6	24	.5	20	80	.05	.06	.4	0
427	237	885	13.4	687	3560	1.10	1.64	7.4	0
36	20	74	1.1	57	300	.09	.14	.6	Tr
10	8	30	.4	38	40	.04	.03	.2	Tr
13	9	27	.4	34	20	.03	.02	.2	Tr
15	10	31	.4	44	50	.03	.03	.2	Tr
29	16	48	1.0	56	50	.10	.17	.9	Tr
24	14	40	.8	47	40	.06	.06	.5	Tr
42	44	34	1.0	111	60	.04	.14	.9	Tr
22	20	13	.7	129	20	.08	.06	.7	0
25	10	32	.3	176	0	.02	.06	.2	0
38	11	53	1.4	192	30	.15	.10	1.0	Tr
31	17	35	.6	23	30	.10	.08	.9	0
28	10	96	.7	15	0	.06	.10	.7	0
30	16	25	.6	29	50	.10	.09	.8	0

Foods, Approximate Measures, Units, and Weight		(g)	Water (%)	Food Energy (cal)	Protein (g)	Fat (g)	Saturated (total) (g)	Oleic (g)	Linoleic (g)
Cornmeal									
Whole-ground, unbolted, dry form	1 cup	122	12	435	11	5	.5	1.0	2.5
Bolted (nearly whole-grain), dry form	1 cup	122	12	440	11	4	.5	.9	2.1
Degermed, enriched:									
Dry form	1 cup	138	12	500	11	2	.2	.4	.9
Cooked	1 cup	240	88	120	3	Tr	Tr	.1	.2
Degermed, unenriched:									
Dry form	1 cup	138	12	500	11	2	.2	.4	.9
Cooked	1 cup	240	88	120	3	Tr	Tr	.1	.2
Crackers[38]:									
Graham, plain, 2½-in square	2 crackers	14	6	55	1	1	.3	.5	.3
Rye wafers, whole-grain, 1⅞ × 3½ in	2 wafers	13	6	45	2	Tr	—	—	—
Saltines, made with enriched flour	4 crackers or 1 packet	11	4	50	1	1	.3	.5	.4
Danish pastry (enriched flour), plain without fruit or nuts[54]:									
Round piece, about 4¼-in diameter × 1 in	1 pastry	65	22	275	5	15	4.7	6.1	3.2
Ounce	1 oz	28	22	120	2	7	2.0	2.7	1.4
Doughnuts, made with enriched flour[38]:									
Cake type, plain, 2½-in diameter, 1 in high	1 doughnut	25	24	100	1	5	1.2	2.0	1.1
Yeast-leavened, glazed, 3¾-in diameter, 1¼ in high	1 doughnut	50	26	205	3	11	3.3	5.8	3.3
Macaroni, enriched, cooked (cut lengths, elbows, shells):									
Firm stage (hot)	1 cup	130	64	190	7	1	—	—	—
Tender stage:									
Cold macaroni	1 cup	105	73	115	4	Tr	—	—	—
Hot macaroni	1 cup	140	73	155	5	1	—	—	—
Macaroni (enriched) and cheese[55]:									
Canned	1 cup	240	80	230	9	10	4.2	3.1	1.4
From home recipe (served hot)[56]	1 cup	200	58	430	17	22	8.9	8.8	2.9
Muffins made with enriched flour[38]:									
From home recipe:									
Blueberry, 2⅜-in diameter, 1½ in high	1 muffin	40	39	110	3	4	1.1	1.4	.7
Bran	1 muffin	40	35	105	3	4	1.2	1.4	.8
Corn (enriched degermed cornmeal and flour), 2⅜-in diameter, 1½ in high	1 muffin	40	33	125	3	4	1.2	1.6	.9
Plain, 3-in diameter, 1½ in high	1 muffin	40	38	120	3	4	1.0	1.7	1.0
From mix, egg, milk:									
Corn, 2⅜-in diameter, 1½ in high[58]	1 muffin	40	30	130	3	4	1.2	1.7	.9
Noodles (egg noodles), enriched, cooked	1 cup	160	71	200	7	2	—	—	—
Noodles, chow mein, canned	1 cup	45	1	220	6	11	—	—	—
Pancakes (4-in diameter)[38]:									
Buckwheat, made from mix (with buckwheat and enriched flour), egg and milk added	1 cake	27	58	55	2	2	.8	.9	.4
Plain									
Made from home recipe using enriched flour	1 cake	27	50	60	2	2	.5	.8	.5
Made from mix with enriched flour, egg and milk added	1 cake	27	51	60	2	2	.7	.7	.3
Pies, piecrust made with enriched flour, vegetable shortening (9-in diameter):									
Apple:									
Sector, ⅐ of pie	1 sector	135	48	345	3	15	3.9	6.4	3.6
Banana cream:									
Sector, ⅐ of pie	1 sector	130	54	285	6	12	3.8	4.7	2.3
Blueberry:									
Sector, ⅐ of pie	1 sector	135	51	325	3	15	3.5	6.2	3.6
Cherry:									
Sector, ⅐ of pie	1 sector	135	47	350	4	15	4.0	6.4	3.6
Custard:									
Sector, ⅐ of pie	1 sector	130	58	285	8	14	4.8	5.5	2.5
Lemon meringue:									
Sector, ⅐ of pie	1 sector	120	47	305	4	12	3.7	4.8	2.3
Mince:									
Sector, ⅐ of pie	1 sector	135	43	365	3	16	4.0	6.6	3.6
Peach:									
Sector, ⅐ of pie	1 sector	135	48	345	3	14	3.5	6.2	3.6
Pecan:									
Sector, ⅐ of pie	1 sector	118	20	495	6	27	4.0	14.4	6.3
Pumpkin:									
Sector, ⅐ of pie	1 sector	130	59	275	5	15	5.4	5.4	2.4

For notes, see end of table.

Nutrients in Indicated Quantity

Carbohydrate (g)	Calcium (mg)	Phosphorus (mg)	Iron (mg)	Potassium (mg)	Vitamin A Value (IU)	Thiamin (mg)	Riboflavin (mg)	Niacin (mg)	Ascorbic Acid (mg)
90	24	312	2.9	346	620[53]	.46	.13	2.4	0
91	21	272	2.2	303	590[53]	.37	.10	2.3	0
108	8	137	4.0	166	610[53]	.61	.36	4.8	0
26	2	34	1.0	38	140[53]	.14	.10	1.2	0
108	8	137	1.5	166	610[53]	.19	.07	1.4	0
26	2	34	.5	38	140[53]	.05	.02	.2	0
10	6	21	.5	55	0	.02	.08	.5	0
10	7	50	.5	78	0	.04	.03	.2	0
8	2	10	.5	13	0	.05	.05	.4	0
30	33	71	1.2	73	200	.18	.19	1.7	Tr
13	14	31	.5	32	90	.08	.08	.7	Tr
13	10	48	.4	23	20	.05	.05	.4	Tr
22	16	33	.6	34	25	.10	.10	.8	0
39	14	85	1.4	103	0	.23	.13	1.8	0
24	8	53	.9	64	0	.15	.08	1.2	0
32	11	70	1.3	85	0	.20	.11	1.5	0
26	199	182	1.0	139	260	.12	.24	1.0	Tr
40	362	322	1.8	240	860	.20	.40	1.8	Tr
17	34	53	.6	46	90	.09	.10	.7	Tr
17	57	162	1.5	172	90	.07	.10	1.7	Tr
19	42	68	.7	54	120[57]	.10	.10	.7	Tr
17	42	60	.6	50	40	.09	.12	.9	Tr
20	96	152	.6	44	100[57]	.08	.09	.7	Tr
37	16	94	1.4	70	110	.22	.13	1.9	0
26	—	—	—	—	—	—	—	—	—
6	59	91	.4	66	60	.04	.05	.2	Tr
9	27	38	.4	33	30	.06	.07	.5	Tr
9	58	70	.3	42	70	.04	.06	.2	Tr
51	11	30	.9	108	40	.15	.11	1.3	2
40	86	107	1.0	264	330	.11	.22	1.0	1
47	15	31	1.4	88	40	.15	.11	1.4	4
52	19	34	.9	142	590	.16	.12	1.4	Tr
30	125	147	1.2	178	300	.11	.27	.8	0
45	17	59	1.0	60	200	.09	.12	.7	4
56	38	51	1.9	240	Tr	.14	.12	1.4	1
52	14	39	1.2	201	990	.15	.14	2.0	4
61	55	122	3.7	145	190	.26	.14	1.0	Tr
32	66	90	1.0	208	3210	.11	.18	1.0	Tr

Foods, Approximate Measures, Units, and Weight		(g)	Water (%)	Food Energy (cal)	Protein (g)	Fat (g)	Saturated (total) (g)	Oleic (g)	Linoleic (g)
							Fatty Acids		
								Unsaturated	
Piecrust (home recipe) made with enriched flour and vegetable shortening, baked	1 pie shell, 9-in diameter	180	15	900	11	60	14.8	26.1	14.9
Pizza (cheese) baked, 4¾-in sector; ⅛ of 12-in diameter pie[19]	1 sector	60	45	145	6	4	1.7	1.5	0.6
Popcorn, popped:									
Plain, large kernel	1 cup	6	4	25	1	Tr	Tr	.1	.2
With oil (coconut) and salt added, large kernel	1 cup	9	3	40	1	2	1.5	.2	.2
Sugar coated	1 cup	35	4	135	2	1	.5	.2	.4
Pretzels, made with enriched flour:									
Dutch, twisted, 2¾ × 2⅝ in	1 pretzel	16	5	60	2	1	—	—	—
Thin, twisted, 3¼ × 2¼ × ¼ in	10 pretzels	60	5	235	6	3	—	—	—
Stick, 2¼ in long	10 pretzels	3	5	10	Tr	Tr	—	—	—
Rice, white, enriched:									
Instant, ready-to-serve, hot	1 cup	165	73	180	4	Tr	Tr	Tr	Tr
Long grain:									
Raw	1 cup	185	12	670	12	1	.2	.2	.2
Cooked, served hot	1 cup	205	73	225	4	Tr	.1	.1	.1
Parboiled:									
Raw	1 cup	185	10	685	14	1	.2	.1	.2
Cooked, served hot	1 cup	175	73	185	4	Tr	.1	.1	.1
Rolls, enriched:									
Commercial:									
Brown-and-serve (12 per 12-oz pkg), browned	1 roll	26	27	85	2	2	.4	.7	.5
Cloverleaf or pan, 2½-in diameter, 2 in high	1 roll	28	31	85	2	2	.4	.6	.4
Frankfurter and hamburger (8 per 11½-oz pkg)	1 roll	40	31	120	3	2	.5	.8	.6
Hard, 3¾-in diameter, 2 in high	1 roll	50	25	155	5	2	.4	.6	.5
Hoagie or submarine, 11½ × 3 × 2½ in	1 roll	135	31	390	12	4	.9	1.4	1.4
From home recipe:									
Cloverleaf, 2½-in diameter, 2 in high	1 roll	35	26	120	3	3	.8	1.1	.7
Spaghetti, enriched, cooked:									
Firm stage, "al dente," served hot	1 cup	130	64	190	7	1	—	—	—
Tender stage, served hot	1 cup	140	73	155	5	1	—	—	—
Spaghetti (enriched) in tomato sauce with cheese:									
From home recipe	1 cup	250	77	260	9	9	2.0	5.4	.7
Canned	1 cup	250	80	190	6	2	.5	.3	.4
Spaghetti (enriched) with meat balls and tomato sauce:									
From home recipe	1 cup	248	70	330	19	12	3.3	6.3	.9
Canned	1 cup	250	78	260	12	10	2.2	3.3	3.9
Toaster pastries	1 pastry	50	12	200	3	6	—	—	—
Waffles, made with enriched flour, 7-in diameter[38]:									
From home recipe	1 waffle	75	41	210	7	7	2.3	2.8	1.4
From mix, egg and milk added	1 waffle	75	42	205	7	8	2.8	2.9	1.2
Wheat flours:									
All-purpose or family flour, enriched:									
Sifted, spooned	1 cup	115	12	420	12	1	.2	.1	0.5
Unsifted, spooned	1 cup	125	12	455	13	1	.2	.1	.5
Cake or pastry flour, enriched, sifted, spooned	1 cup	96	12	350	7	1	.1	.1	.3
Self-rising, enriched, unsifted, spooned	1 cup	125	12	440	12	1	.2	.1	.5
Whole-wheat, from hard wheats, stirred	1 cup	120	12	400	16	2	.4	.2	1.0
Legumes (Dry), Nuts, Seeds; Related Products									
Almonds, shelled:									
Chopped (about 130 almonds)	1 cup	130	5	775	24	70	5.6	47.7	12.8
Slivered, not pressed down (about 115 almonds)	1 cup	115	5	690	21	62	5.0	42.2	11.3
Beans, dry:									
Common varieties as Great Northern, navy, and others:									
Cooked, drained:									
Great Northern	1 cup	180	69	210	14	1	—	—	—
Pea (navy)	1 cup	190	69	225	15	1	—	—	—
Canned, solids and liquid:									
White with:									
Frankfurters (sliced)	1 cup	255	71	365	19	18	—	—	—
Pork and tomato sauce	1 cup	255	71	310	16	7	2.4	2.8	.6
Pork and sweet sauce	1 cup	255	66	385	16	12	4.3	5.0	1.1
Red kidney	1 cup	255	76	230	15	1	—	—	—

For notes, see end of table.

Nutrients in Indicated Quantity

Carbohydrate (g)	Calcium (mg)	Phosphorus (mg)	Iron (mg)	Potassium (mg)	Vitamin A Value (IU)	Thiamin (mg)	Riboflavin (mg)	Niacin (mg)	Ascorbic Acid (mg)
79	25	90	3.1	89	0	.47	.40	5.0	0
22	86	89	1.1	67	230	.16	.18	1.6	4
5	1	17	.2	—	—	—	.01	.1	0
5	1	19	.2	—	—	—	.01	.2	0
30	2	47	.5	—	—	—	.02	.4	0
12	4	21	.2	21	0	.05	.04	.7	0
46	13	79	.9	78	0	.20	.15	2.5	0
2	1	4	Tr	4	0	.01	.01	.1	0
40	5	31	1.3	—	0	.21	([59])	1.7	0
149	44	174	5.4	170	0	.81	.06	6.5	0
50	21	57	1.8	57	0	.23	.02	2.1	0
150	111	370	5.4	278	0	.81	.07	6.5	0
41	33	100	1.4	75	0	.19	.02	2.1	0
14	20	23	.5	25	Tr	.10	.06	.9	Tr
15	21	24	.5	27	Tr	.11	.07	.9	Tr
21	30	34	.8	38	Tr	.16	.10	1.3	Tr
30	24	46	1.2	49	Tr	.20	.12	1.7	Tr
75	58	115	3.0	122	Tr	.54	.32	4.5	Tr
20	16	36	.7	41	30	.12	.12	1.2	Tr
39	14	85	1.4	103	0	.23	.13	1.8	0
32	11	70	1.3	85	0	.20	.11	1.5	0
37	80	135	2.3	408	1080	.25	.18	2.3	13
39	40	88	2.8	303	930	.35	.28	4.5	10
39	124	236	3.7	665	1590	.25	.30	4.0	22
29	53	113	3.3	245	1000	.15	.18	2.3	5
36	54[60]	67[60]	1.9	74[60]	500	.16	.17	2.1	([60])
28	85	130	1.3	109	250	.17	.23	1.4	Tr
27	179	257	1.0	146	170	.14	.22	.9	Tr
88	18	100	3.3	109	0	0.74	0.46	6.1	0
95	20	109	3.6	119	0	.80	.50	6.6	0
76	16	70	2.8	91	0	.61	.38	5.1	0
93	331	583	3.6	—	0	.80	.50	6.6	0
85	49	446	4.0	444	0	.66	.14	5.2	0
25	304	655	6.1	1005	0	.31	1.20	4.6	Tr
22	269	580	5.4	889	0	.28	1.06	4.0	Tr
38	90	266	4.9	749	0	.25	.13	1.3	0
40	95	281	5.1	790	0	.27	.13	1.3	0
32	94	303	4.8	668	330	.18	.15	3.3	Tr
48	138	235	4.6	536	330	.20	.08	1.5	5
54	161	291	5.9	—	—	.15	.10	1.3	—
42	74	278	4.6	673	10	.13	.10	1.5	—

Foods, Approximate Measures, Units, and Weight		(g)	Water (%)	Food Energy (cal)	Protein (g)	Fat (g)	Saturated (total) (g)	Oleic (g)	Linoleic (g)
								Nutrients in Indicated Quantity → Fatty Acids → Unsaturated		
Lima, cooked, drained	1 cup	190	64	260	16	1	—	—	—
Blackeye peas, dry, cooked (with residual cooking liquid)	1 cup	250	80	190	13	1	—	—	—
Brazil nuts, shelled (6-8 large kernels)	1 oz	28	5	185	4	19	4.8	6.2	7.1
Cashew nuts, roasted in oil	1 cup	140	5	785	24	64	12.9	36.8	10.2
Coconut meat, fresh:									
Piece, about 2 × 2 × ½ in	1 piece	45	51	155	2	16	14.0	.9	.3
Shredded or grated, not pressed down	1 cup	80	51	275	3	28	24.8	1.6	.5
Filberts (hazelnuts), chopped (about 60 kernels)	1 cup	115	6	730	14	72	5.1	55.2	7.3
Lentils, whole, cooked	1 cup	200	72	210	16	Tr	—	—	—
Peanuts, roasted in oil, salted (whole, halves, chopped)	1 cup	144	2	840	37	72	13.7	33.0	20.7
Peanut butter	1 tbsp	16	2	95	4	8	1.5	3.7	2.3
Peas, split, dry, cooked	1 cup	200	70	230	16	1	—	—	—
Pecans, chopped or pieces (about 120 large halves)	1 cup	118	3	810	11	84	7.2	50.5	20.0
Pumpkin and squash kernels, dry, hulled	1 cup	140	4	775	41	65	11.8	23.5	27.5
Sunflower seeds, dry, hulled	1 cup	145	5	810	35	69	8.2	13.7	43.2
Walnuts:									
Black:									
Chopped or broken kernels	1 cup	125	3	785	26	74	6.3	13.3	45.7
Ground (finely)	1 cup	80	3	500	16	47	4.0	8.5	29.2
Persian or English, chopped (about 60 halves)	1 cup	120	4	780	18	77	8.4	11.8	42.2
Sugars and Sweets									
Cake icings:									
Boiled, white:									
Plain	1 cup	94	18	295	1	0	0	0	—
With coconut	1 cup	166	15	605	3	13	11.0	.9	Tr
Uncooked:									
Chocolate made with milk and butter	1 cup	275	14	1035	9	38	23.4	11.7	1.0
Creamy fudge from mix and water	1 cup	245	15	830	7	16	5.1	6.7	3.1
White	1 cup	319	11	1200	2	21	12.7	5.1	.5
Candy:									
Caramels, plain or chocolate	1 oz	28	8	115	1	3	1.6	1.1	.1
Chocolate:									
Milk, plain	1 oz	28	1	145	2	9	5.5	3.0	.3
Semisweet, small pieces (60 per oz)	1 cup or 6-oz pkg	170	1	860	7	61	36.2	19.8	1.7
Chocolate-coated peanuts	1 oz	28	1	160	5	12	4.0	4.7	2.1
Fondant, uncoated (mints, candy corn, other)	1 oz	28	8	105	Tr	1	.1	.3	.1
Fudge, chocolate, plain	1 oz	28	8	115	1	3	1.3	1.4	.6
Gum drops	1 oz	28	12	100	Tr	Tr	—	—	—
Hard	1 oz	28	1	110	0	Tr	—	—	—
Marshmallows	1 oz	28	17	90	1	Tr	—	—	—
Chocolate-flavored beverage powders (about 4 heaping tsp per oz):									
With nonfat dry milk	1 oz	28	2	100	5	1	.5	.3	Tr
Without milk	1 oz	28	1	100	1	1	.4	.2	Tr
Honey, strained or extracted	1 tbsp	21	17	65	Tr	0	0	0	0
Jams and preserves	1 tbsp	20	29	55	Tr	Tr	—	—	—
	1 packet	14	29	40	Tr	Tr	—	—	—
Jellies	1 tbsp	18	29	50	Tr	Tr	—	—	—
	1 packet	14	29	40	Tr	Tr	—	—	—
Syrups:									
Chocolate-flavored syrup or topping:									
Thin type	1 fl oz or 2 tbsp	38	32	90	1	1	.5	.3	Tr
Fudge type	1 fl oz or 2 tbsp	38	25	125	2	5	3.1	1.6	.1
Molasses, cane:									
Light (first extraction)	1 tbsp	20	24	50	—	—	—	—	—
Blackstrap (third extraction)	1 tbsp	20	24	45	—	—	—	—	—
Sorghum	1 tbsp	21	23	55	—	—	—	—	—
Table blends, chiefly corn, light and dark	1 tbsp	21	24	60	0	0	0	0	0
Sugars:									
Brown, pressed down	1 cup	220	2	820	0	0	0	0	0
White:									
Granulated	1 cup	200	1	770	0	0	0	0	0
	1 tbsp	12	1	45	0	0	0	0	0
	1 packet	6	1	23	0	0	0	0	0
Powdered, sifted, spooned into cup	1 cup	100	1	385	0	0	0	0	0

For notes, see end of table.

Nutrients in Indicated Quantity

Carbohydrate (g)	Calcium (mg)	Phosphorus (mg)	Iron (mg)	Potassium (mg)	Vitamin A Value (IU)	Thiamin (mg)	Riboflavin (mg)	Niacin (mg)	Ascorbic Acid (mg)
49	55	293	5.9	1163	—	.25	.11	1.3	—
35	43	238	3.3	573	30	.40	.10	1.0	—
3	53	196	1.0	203	Tr	.27	.03	.5	—
41	53	522	5.3	650	140	.60	.35	2.5	—
4	6	43	.8	115	0	.02	.01	.2	1
8	10	76	1.4	205	0	.04	.02	.4	2
19	240	388	3.9	810	—	.53	—	1.0	Tr
39	50	238	4.2	498	40	.14	.12	1.2	0
27	107	577	3.0	971	—	.46	.19	24.8	0
3	9	61	.3	100	—	.02	.02	2.4	0
42	22	178	3.4	592	80	.30	.18	1.8	—
17	86	341	2.8	712	150	1.01	.15	1.1	2
21	71	1602	15.7	1386	100	.34	.27	3.4	—
29	174	1214	10.3	1334	70	2.84	.33	7.8	—
19	Tr	713	7.5	575	380	.28	.14	.9	—
12	Tr	456	4.8	368	240	.18	.09	.6	—
19	119	456	3.7	540	40	.40	.16	1.1	2
75	2	2	Tr	17	0	Tr	0.03	Tr	0
124	10	50	.8	277	0	.02	.07	.3	0
185	165	305	3.3	536	580	.06	.28	.6	1
183	96	218	2.7	238	Tr	.05	.20	.7	Tr
260	48	38	Tr	57	860	Tr	.06	Tr	Tr
22	42	35	.4	54	Tr	.01	.05	.1	Tr
16	65	65	.3	109	80	.02	.10	.1	Tr
97	51	255	4.4	553	30	.02	.14	.9	0
11	33	84	.4	143	Tr	.10	.05	2.1	Tr
25	4	2	.3	1	0	Tr	Tr	Tr	0
21	22	24	.3	42	Tr	.01	.03	.1	Tr
25	2	Tr	.1	1	0	0	Tr	Tr	0
28	6	2	.5	1	0	0	0	0	0
23	5	2	.5	2	0	0	Tr	Tr	0
20	167	155	.5	227	10	.04	.21	.2	1
25	9	48	.6	142	—	.01	.03	.1	0
17	1	1	.1	11	0	Tr	.01	.1	Tr
14	4	2	.2	18	Tr	Tr	.01	Tr	Tr
10	3	1	.1	12	Tr	Tr	Tr	Tr	Tr
13	4	1	.3	14	Tr	Tr	.01	Tr	1
10	3	1	.2	11	Tr	Tr	Tr	Tr	1
24	6	35	.6	106	Tr	.01	.03	.2	0
20	48	60	.5	107	60	.02	.08	.2	Tr
13	33	9	.9	183	—	.01	.01	Tr	—
11	137	17	3.2	585	—	.02	.04	.4	—
14	35	5	2.6	—	—	—	.02	Tr	—
15	9	3	.8	1	0	0	0	0	0
212	187	42	7.5	757	0	.02	.7	.4	0
199	0	0	.2	6	0	0	0	0	0
12	0	0	Tr	Tr	0	0	0	0	0
6	0	0	Tr	Tr	0	0	0	0	0
100	0	0	.1	3	0	0	0	0	0

				Nutrients in Indicated Quantity					
							Fatty Acids		
								Unsaturated	
							Saturated (total) (g)	Oleic (g)	Linoleic (g)
Foods, Approximate Measures, Units, and Weight		(g)	Water (%)	Food Energy (cal)	Protein (g)	Fat (g)			

Vegetable and Vegetable Products

Asparagus, green:									
Cooked, drained:									
Cuts and tips, 1½- to 2-in lengths:									
From raw	1 cup	145	94	30	3	Tr	—	—	—
From frozen	1 cup	180	93	40	6	Tr	—	—	—
Spears, ½-in diameter at base:									
From raw	4 spears	60	94	10	1	Tr	—	—	—
From frozen	4 spears	60	92	15	2	Tr	—	—	—
Canned, spears, ½-in diameter at base	4 spears	80	93	15	2	Tr	—	—	—
Beans:									
Lima, immature seeds, frozen, cooked, drained:									
Thick-seeded types (Fordhooks)	1 cup	170	74	170	10	Tr	—	—	—
Thin-seeded types (baby limas)	1 cup	180	69	210	13	Tr	—	—	—
Snap:									
Green:									
Cooked, drained:									
From raw (cuts and French style)	1 cup	125	92	30	2	Tr	—	—	—
From frozen:									
Cuts	1 cup	135	92	35	2	Tr	—	—	—
French style	1 cup	130	92	35	2	Tr	—	—	—
Canned, drained solids (cuts)	1 cup	135	92	30	2	Tr	—	—	—
Yellow or wax:									
Cooked, drained:									
From raw (cuts and French style)	1 cup	125	93	30	2	Tr	—	—	—
From frozen (cuts)	1 cup	135	92	35	2	Tr	—	—	—
Canned, drained solids (cuts)	1 cup	135	92	30	2	Tr	—	—	—
Beans, mature. See Beans, dry and Blackeye peas, dry.									
Bean sprouts (mung):									
Raw	1 cup	105	89	35	4	Tr	—	—	—
Cooked, drained	1 cup	125	91	35	4	Tr	—	—	—
Beets:									
Cooked, drained, peeled:									
Whole beets, 2-in diameter	2 beets	100	91	30	1	Tr	—	—	—
Diced or sliced	1 cup	170	91	55	2	Tr	—	—	—
Canned, drained solids:									
Whole beets, small	1 cup	160	89	60	2	Tr	—	—	—
Diced or sliced	1 cup	170	89	65	2	Tr	—	—	—
Beet greens, leaves and stems, cooked, drained	1 cup	145	94	25	2	Tr	—	—	—
Blackeye peas, immature seeds, cooked and drained:									
From raw	1 cup	165	72	180	13	1	—	—	—
From frozen	1 cup	170	66	220	15	1	—	—	—
Broccoli, cooked, drained:									
From raw:									
Stalk, medium size	1 stalk	180	91	45	6	1	—	—	—
Stalks cut into ½-in pieces	1 cup	155	91	40	5	Tr	—	—	—
From frozen:									
Stalk, 4½ to 5 in long	1 stalk	30	91	10	1	Tr	—	—	—
Chopped	1 cup	185	92	50	5	1	—	—	—
Brussels sprouts, cooked, drained:									
From raw, 7-8 sprouts (1¼- to 1½-in diameter)	1 cup	155	88	55	7	1	—	—	—
From frozen	1 cup	155	89	50	5	Tr	—	—	—
Cabbage:									
Common varieties:									
Raw:									
Coarsely shredded or sliced	1 cup	70	92	15	1	Tr	—	—	—
Finely shredded or chopped	1 cup	90	92	20	1	Tr	—	—	—
Cooked, drained	1 cup	145	94	30	2	Tr	—	—	—
Red, raw, coarsely shredded or sliced	1 cup	70	90	20	1	Tr	—	—	—
Savoy, raw, coarsely shredded or sliced	1 cup	70	92	15	2	Tr	—	—	—
Cabbage, celery (also called pe-tsai or wongbok), raw, 1-in pieces	1 cup	75	95	10	1	Tr	—	—	—
Cabbage, white mustard (also called bokchoy or pakchoy), cooked, drained	1 cup	170	95	25	2	Tr	—	—	—
Carrots:									
Raw, without crowns and tips, scraped:									
Whole, 7½ × 1⅛ in, or strips, 2½ to 3 in long	1 carrot or 18 strips	72	88	30	1	Tr	—	—	—

For notes, see end of table.

Nutrients in Indicated Quantity

Carbohydrate (g)	Calcium (mg)	Phosphorus (mg)	Iron (mg)	Potassium (mg)	Vitamin A Value (IU)	Thiamin (mg)	Riboflavin (mg)	Niacin (mg)	Ascorbic Acid (mg)
5	30	73	.9	265	1310	.23	.26	2.0	38
6	40	115	2.2	396	1530	.25	.23	1.8	41
2	13	30	.4	110	540	.10	.11	.8	16
2	13	40	.7	143	470	.10	.08	.7	16
3	15	42	1.5	133	640	.05	.08	.6	12
32	34	153	2.9	724	390	.12	.09	1.7	29
40	63	227	4.7	709	400	.16	.09	2.2	22
7	63	45	.8	189	680	.09	.11	.6	15
8	54	43	.9	205	780	.09	.12	.5	7
8	49	39	1.2	177	690	.08	.10	.4	9
7	61	34	2.0	128	630	.04	.07	.4	5
6	63	46	.8	189	290	.09	.11	.6	16
8	47	42	.9	221	140	.09	.11	.5	8
7	61	34	2.0	128	140	.04	.07	.4	7
7	20	67	1.4	234	20	.14	.14	.8	20
7	21	60	1.1	195	30	.11	.13	.9	8
7	14	23	.5	208	20	.03	.04	.3	6
12	24	39	.9	354	30	.05	.07	.5	10
14	30	29	1.1	267	30	.02	.05	.2	5
15	32	31	1.2	284	30	.02	.05	.2	5
5	144	36	2.8	481	7400	.10	.22	.4	22
30	40	241	3.5	625	580	.50	.18	2.3	28
40	43	286	4.8	573	290	.68	.19	2.4	15
8	158	112	1.4	481	4500	.16	.36	1.4	162
7	136	96	1.2	414	3880	.14	.31	1.2	140
1	12	17	.2	66	570	.02	.03	.2	22
9	100	104	1.3	392	4810	.11	.22	.9	105
10	50	112	1.7	423	810	.12	.22	1.2	135
10	33	95	1.2	457	880	.12	.16	.9	126
4	34	20	.3	163	90	.04	.04	.2	33
5	44	26	.4	210	120	.05	.05	.3	42
6	64	29	.4	236	190	.06	.06	.4	48
5	29	25	.6	188	30	.06	.04	.3	43
3	47	38	.6	188	140	.04	.06	.2	39
2	32	30	.5	190	110	.04	.03	.5	19
4	252	56	1.0	364	5270	.07	.14	1.2	26
7	27	26	.5	246	7930	.04	.04	.4	6

Foods, Approximate Measures, Units, and Weight		(g)	Water (%)	Food Energy (cal)	Protein (g)	Fat (g)	Nutrients in Indicated Quantity		
							Fatty Acids		
							Saturated (total) (g)	Unsaturated	
								Oleic (g)	Linoleic (g)
Grated	1 cup	110	88	45	1	Tr	—	—	—
Cooked (crosswise cuts), drained	1 cup	155	91	50	1	Tr	—	—	—
Canned:									
Sliced, drained solids	1 cup	155	91	45	1	Tr	—	—	—
Strained or junior (baby food)	1 oz (1¾ to 2 tbsp)	28	92	10	Tr	Tr	—	—	—
Cauliflower:									
Raw, chopped	1 cup	115	91	31	3	Tr	—	—	—
Cooked, drained:									
From raw (flower buds)	1 cup	125	93	30	3	Tr	—	—	—
From frozen (flowerets)	1 cup	180	94	30	3	Tr	—	—	—
Celery, Pascal type, raw:									
Stalk, large outer, 8 × 1½ in, at rood end	1 stalk	40	94	5	Tr	Tr	—	—	—
Pieces, diced	1 cup	120	94	20	1	Tr	—	—	—
Collards, cooked, drained:									
From raw (leaves without stems)	1 cup	190	90	65	7	1	—	—	—
From frozen (chopped)	1 cup	170	90	50	5	1	—	—	—
Corn, sweet:									
Cooked, drained:									
From raw, ear 5 × 1¾ in	1 ear[61]	140	74	70	2	1	—	—	—
From frozen:									
Ear, 5 in long	1 ear[61]	229	73	120	4	1	—	—	—
Kernels	1 cup	165	77	130	5	1	—	—	—
Canned:									
Cream style	1 cup	256	76	210	5	2	—	—	—
Whole kernel:									
Vacuum pack	1 cup	210	76	175	5	1	—	—	—
Wet pack, drained solids	1 cup	165	76	140	4	1	—	—	—
Cowpeas; see Blackeye peas									
Cucumber slices, ⅛ in thick (large, 2⅛-in diameter; small, 1¾-in diameter):									
With peel	6 large or 8 small slices	28	95	5	Tr	Tr	—	—	—
Without peel	6½ large or 9 small pieces	28	96	5	Tr	Tr	—	—	—
Dandelion greens, cooked, drained	1 cup	105	90	35	2	1	—	—	—
Endive, curly (including escarole), raw, small pieces	1 cup	50	93	10	1	Tr	—	—	—
Kale, cooked, drained:									
From raw (leaves without stems and midribs)	1 cup	110	88	45	5	1	—	—	—
From frozen (leaf style)	1 cup	130	91	40	4	1	—	—	—
Lettuce, raw:									
Butterhead, as Boston types:									
Head, 5-in diameter	1 head[63]	220	95	25	2	Tr	—	—	—
Leaves	1 outer or 2 inner or 3 heart leaves	15	95	Tr	Tr	Tr	—	—	—
Crisphead, as Iceberg:									
Head, 6-in diameter	1 head[64]	567	96	70	5	1	—	—	—
Wedge, ¼ of head	1 wedge	135	96	20	1	Tr	—	—	—
Pieces, chopped or shredded	1 cup	55	96	5	Tr	Tr	—	—	—
Looseleaf (bunching varieties including romaine or cos), chopped or shredded pieces	1 cup	55	94	10	1	Tr	—	—	—
Mushrooms, raw, sliced or chopped	1 cup	70	90	20	2	Tr	—	—	—
Mustard greens, without stems and midribs, cooked, drained	1 cup	140	93	30	3	1	—	—	—
Okra pods, 3 × ⅝ in, cooked	10 pods	106	91	30	2	Tr	—	—	—
Onions:									
Mature:									
Raw:									
Chopped	1 cup	170	89	65	3	Tr	—	—	—
Sliced	1 cup	115	89	45	2	Tr	—	—	—
Cooked (whole or sliced), drained	1 cup	210	92	60	3	Tr	—	—	—
Young green, bulb (⅜-in diameter) and white portion of top	6 onions	30	88	15	Tr	Tr	—	—	—
Parsley, raw, chopped	1 tbsp	4	85	Tr	Tr	Tr	—	—	—
Parsnips, cooked (diced or 2-in lengths)	1 cup	155	82	100	2	1	—	—	—
Peas, green:									
Canned:									
Whole, drained solids	1 cup	170	77	150	8	1	—	—	—
Strained (baby food)	1 oz (1¾ to 2 tbsp)	28	86	15	1	Tr	—	—	—
Frozen, cooked, drained	1 cup	160	82	110	8	Tr	—	—	—

For notes, see end of table.

Nutrients in Indicated Quantity

Carbohydrate (g)	Calcium (mg)	Phosphorus (mg)	Iron (mg)	Potassium (mg)	Vitamin A Value (IU)	Thiamin (mg)	Riboflavin (mg)	Niacin (mg)	Ascorbic Acid (mg)
11	41	40	.8	375	12,100	.07	.06	.7	9
11	51	48	.9	344	16,280	.08	.08	.8	9
10	47	34	1.1	186	23,250	.03	.05	.6	3
2	7	6	.1	51	3690	.01	.01	.1	1
6	29	64	1.3	339	70	.13	.12	.8	90
5	26	53	.9	258	80	.11	.10	.8	69
6	31	68	.9	373	50	.07	.09	.7	74
2	16	11	.1	136	110	.01	.01	.1	4
5	47	34	.4	409	320	.04	.04	.4	11
10	357	99	1.5	498	14,820	.21	.38	2.3	144
10	299	87	1.7	401	11,560	.10	.24	1.0	56
16	2	69	.5	151	310[62]	.09	.08	1.1	7
27	4	121	1.0	291	440[62]	.18	.10	2.1	9
31	5	120	1.3	304	580[62]	.15	.10	2.5	8
51	8	143	1.5	248	840[62]	.08	.13	2.6	13
43	6	153	1.1	204	740[62]	.06	.13	2.3	11
33	8	81	.8	160	580[62]	.05	.08	1.5	7
1	7	8	.3	45	70	.01	.01	.1	3
1	5	5	.1	45	Tr	.01	.01	.1	3
7	147	44	1.9	244	12,290	.14	.17	—	19
2	41	27	.9	147	1650	.04	.07	.3	5
7	206	64	1.8	243	9130	.11	.20	1.8	102
7	157	62	1.3	251	10,660	.08	.20	.9	49
4	57	42	3.3	430	1580	.10	.10	.5	13
Tr	5	4	.3	40	150	.01	.01	Tr	1
16	108	118	2.7	943	1780	.32	.32	1.6	32
4	27	30	.7	236	450	.08	.08	.4	8
2	11	12	.3	96	180	.03	.03	.2	3
2	37	14	.8	145	1050	.03	.04	.2	10
3	4	81	.6	290	Tr	.07	.32	2.9	2
6	193	45	2.5	308	8120	.11	.20	.8	67
6	98	43	.5	184	520	.14	.19	1.0	21
15	46	61	.9	267	Tr[65]	.05	.07	.3	17
10	31	41	.6	181	Tr[65]	.03	.05	.2	12
14	50	61	.8	231	Tr[65]	.06	.06	.4	15
3	12	12	.2	69	Tr[65]	.02	.01	.1	8
Tr	7	2	.2	25	300	Tr	.01	Tr	6
23	70	96	.9	587	50	.11	.12	.2	16
29	44	129	3.2	163	1170	.15	.10	1.4	14
3	3	18	.3	28	140	.02	.03	.3	3
19	30	138	3.0	216	960	.43	.14	2.7	21

Foods, Approximate Measures, Units, and Weight		(g)	Water (%)	Food Energy (cal)	Protein (g)	Fat (g)	Saturated (total) (g)	Oleic (g)	Linoleic (g)
							Fatty Acids		
							Saturated	**Unsaturated**	
							(total) (g)	Oleic (g)	Linoleic (g)
Peppers, hot, red, without seeds, dried (ground chili powder, added seasonings)	1 tsp	2	9	5	Tr	Tr	—	—	—
Peppers, sweet (about 5 per lb, whole), stem and seeds removed:									
Raw	1 pod	74	93	15	1	Tr	—	—	—
Cooked, boiled, drained	1 pod	73	95	15	1	Tr	—	—	—
Potatoes, cooked:									
Baked, peeled after baking (about 2 per lb, raw)	1 potato	156	75	145	4	Tr	—	—	—
Boiled (about 3 per lb, raw):									
Peeled after boiling	1 potato	137	80	105	3	Tr	—	—	—
Peeled before boiling	1 potato	135	83	90	3	Tr	—	—	—
French-fried, strip, 2 to 3½ in long:									
Prepared from raw	10 strips	50	45	135	2	7	1.7	1.2	3.3
Frozen, oven heated	10 strips	50	53	110	2	4	1.1	.8	2.1
Hashed brown, prepared from frozen	1 cup	155	56	345	3	18	4.6	3.2	9.0
Mashed, prepared from:									
Raw:									
Milk added	1 cup	210	83	135	4	2	.7	.4	Tr
Milk and butter added	1 cup	210	80	195	4	9	5.6	2.3	0.2
Dehydrated flakes (without milk), water, milk, butter, and salt added	1 cup	210	79	195	4	7	3.6	2.1	.2
Potato chips, 1¾ × 2½-in oval cross section	10 chips	20	2	115	1	8	2.1	1.4	4.0
Potato salad, made with cooked salad dressing	1 cup	250	76	250	7	7	2.0	2.7	1.3
Pumpkin, canned	1 cup	245	90	80	2	1	—	—	—
Radishes, raw (prepackaged) stem ends, rootlets cut off	4 radishes	18	95	5	Tr	Tr	—	—	—
Sauerkraut, canned, solids and liquid	1 cup	235	93	40	2	Tr	—	—	—
Southern peas; see Blackeye peas									
Spinach:									
Raw, chopped	1 cup	55	91	15	2	Tr	—	—	—
Cooked, drained:									
From raw	1 cup	180	92	40	5	1	—	—	—
From frozen:									
Chopped	1 cup	205	92	45	6	1	—	—	—
Leaf	1 cup	190	92	45	6	1	—	—	—
Canned, drained solids	1 cup	205	91	50	6	1	—	—	—
Squash, cooked:									
Summer (all varieties), diced, drained	1 cup	210	96	30	2	Tr	—	—	—
Winter (all varieties), baked, mashed	1 cup	205	81	130	4	1	—	—	—
Sweet potatoes:									
Cooked (raw, 5 × 2 in; about 2½ per lb):									
Baked in skin, peeled	1 potato	114	64	160	2	1	—	—	—
Broiled in skin, peeled	1 potato	151	71	170	3	1	—	—	—
Candied, 2½ × 2-in piece	1 piece	105	60	175	1	3	2.0	.8	.1
Canned:									
Solid pack (mashed)	1 cup	255	72	275	5	1	—	—	—
Vacuum pack, piece 2¾ × 1 in	1 piece	40	72	45	1	Tr	—	—	—
Tomatoes:									
Raw, 2⅗-in diameter (3 per 12 oz pkg)	1 tomato[66]	135	94	25	1	Tr	—	—	—
Canned, solids and liquid	1 cup	241	94	50	2	Tr	—	—	—
Tomato catsup	1 cup	273	69	290	5	1	—	—	—
	1 tbsp	15	69	15	Tr	Tr	—	—	—
Tomato juice, canned:									
Cup	1 cup	243	94	45	2	Tr	—	—	—
Glass (6 fl oz)	1 glass	182	94	35	2	Tr	—	—	—
Turnips, cooked, diced	1 cup	155	35	35	1	Tr	—	—	—
Turnip greens, cooked, drained:									
From raw (leaves and stems)	1 cup	145	94	30	3	Tr	—	—	—
From frozen (chopped)	1 cup	165	93	40	4	Tr	—	—	—
Vegetables, mixed, frozen, cooked	1 cup	182	83	115	6	1	—	—	—
Miscellaneous Items									
Baking powders for home use:									
Sodium aluminum sulfate:									
With monocalcium phosphate monohydrate	1 tsp	3.0	2	5	Tr	Tr	0	0	0
With monocalcium phosphate monohydrate, calcium sulfate	1 tsp	2.9	1	5	Tr	Tr	0	0	0
Straight phosphate	1 tsp	3.8	2	5	Tr	Tr	0	0	0
Low sodium	1 tsp	4.3	2	5	Tr	Tr	0	0	0
Barbecue sauce	1 cup	250	81	230	4	17	2.2	4.3	10.0

For notes, see end of table.

Nutrients in Indicated Quantity

Carbohydrate (g)	Calcium (mg)	Phosphorus (mg)	Iron (mg)	Potassium (mg)	Vitamin A Value (IU)	Thiamin (mg)	Riboflavin (mg)	Niacin (mg)	Ascorbic Acid (mg)
1	5	4	.3	20	1300	Tr	.02	.2	Tr
4	7	16	.5	157	310	.06	.06	.4	94
3	7	12	.4	109	310	.05	.05	.4	70
33	14	101	1.1	782	Tr	.15	.07	2.7	31
23	10	72	.8	556	Tr	.12	.05	2.0	22
20	8	57	.7	385	Tr	.12	.05	1.6	22
18	8	56	.7	427	Tr	.07	.04	1.6	11
17	5	43	.9	326	Tr	.07	.01	1.3	11
45	28	78	1.9	439	Tr	.11	.03	1.6	12
27	50	103	.8	548	40	.17	.11	2.1	21
26	50	101	.8	525	360	.17	.11	2.1	19
30	65	99	.6	601	270	.08	.08	1.9	11
10	8	28	.4	226	Tr	.04	.01	1.0	3
41	80	160	1.5	798	350	.20	.18	2.8	28
19	61	64	1.0	588	15,680	.07	.12	1.5	12
1	5	6	.2	58	Tr	.01	.01	.1	5
9	85	42	1.2	329	120	.07	.09	.5	33
2	51	28	1.7	259	4460	.06	.11	.3	28
6	167	68	4.0	583	14,580	.13	.25	.9	50
8	232	90	4.3	683	16,200	.14	.31	.8	39
7	200	84	4.8	688	15,390	.15	.27	1.0	53
7	242	53	5.3	513	16,400	.04	.25	.6	29
7	53	53	.8	296	820	.11	.17	1.7	21
32	57	98	1.6	945	8610	.10	.27	1.4	27
37	46	66	1.0	342	9230	.10	.08	.8	25
40	48	71	1.1	367	11,940	.14	.09	.9	26
36	39	45	.9	200	6620	.06	.04	.4	11
63	64	105	2.0	510	19,890	.13	.10	1.5	36
10	10	16	.3	80	3120	.02	.02	.2	6
6	16	33	.6	300	1110	.07	.05	.9	28[67]
10	14[68]	46	1.2	523	2170	.12	.07	1.7	41
69	60	137	2.2	991	3820	.25	.19	4.4	41
4	3	8	.1	54	210	.01	.01	.2	2
10	17	44	2.2	552	1940	.12	.07	1.9	39
8	13	33	1.6	413	1460	.09	.05	1.5	29
8	54	34	.6	291	Tr	.06	.08	.5	34
5	252	49	1.5	—	8270	.15	.33	.7	68
6	195	64	2.6	246	11,390	.08	.15	.7	31
24	46	115	2.4	348	9010	.22	.13	2.0	15
1	58	87	—	5	0	0	0	0	0
1	183	45	—	—	0	0	0	0	0
1	239	359	—	6	0	0	0	0	0
2	207	314	—	471	0	0	0	0	0
20	53	50	2.0	435	900	.03	.03	.8	13

Foods, Approximate Measures, Units, and Weight		(g)	Water (%)	Food Energy (cal)	Protein (g)	Fat (g)	Saturated (total) (g)	Oleic (g)	Linoleic (g)
							Fatty Acids	**Unsaturated**	
Beverages, alcoholic:									
Beer	12 fl oz	360	92	150	1	0	0	0	0
Gin, rum, vodka, whisky:									
80 proof	1½ fl oz jigger	42	67	95	—	—	0	0	0
86 proof	1½ fl oz jigger	42	64	105	—	—	0	0	0
90 proof	1½ fl oz jigger	42	62	110	—	—	0	0	0
Wines:									
Dessert	3½ fl oz glass	103	77	140	Tr	0	0	0	0
Table	3½ fl oz glass	102	86	85	Tr	0	0	0	0
Beverages, carbonated, sweetened, nonalcoholic:									
Carbonated water	12 fl oz	366	92	115	0	0	0	0	0
Cola type	12 fl oz	369	90	145	0	0	0	0	0
Fruit-flavored sodas and Tom Collins mixer	12 fl oz	372	88	170	0	0	0	0	0
Ginger ale	12 fl oz	366	92	115	0	0	0	0	0
Root beer	12 fl oz	370	90	150	0	0	0	0	0
Chili powder; see Peppers, hot, red									
Chocolate:									
Bitter or baking	1 oz	28	2	145	3	15	8.9	4.9	.4
Semisweet; see Candy, chocolate									
Gelatin, dry	1 7 g envelope	7	13	25	6	Tr	0	0	0
Gelatin dessert prepared with gelatin dessert powder and water	1 cup	240	84	140	4	0	0	0	0
Mustard, prepared, yellow	1 tsp or individual serving pouch or cup	5	80	5	Tr	Tr	—	—	—
Olives, pickled, canned:									
Green	4 medium or 3 extra large or 2 giant[69]	16	78	15	Tr	2	.2	1.2	.1
Ripe, Mission	3 small or 2 large[69]	10	73	15	Tr	2	.2	1.2	.1
Pickles, cucumber:									
Dill, medium, whole, 3¾ in long, 1¼-in diameter	1 pickle	65	93	5	Tr	Tr	—	—	—
Fresh-pack, slices 1½-in diameter, ¼ in thick	2 slices	15	79	10	Tr	Tr	—	—	—
Sweet gherkin, small, whole, about 2½ in long, ¾-in diameter	1 pickle	15	61	20	Tr	Tr	—	—	—
Relish, finely chopped, sweet	1 tbsp	15	63	20	Tr	Tr	—	—	—
Popsicle, 3 fl oz size	1 popsicle	95	80	70	0	0	0	0	0
Soups:									
Canned, condensed:									
Prepared with equal volume of milk:									
Cream of chicken	1 cup	245	85	180	7	10	4.2	3.6	1.3
Cream of mushroom	1 cup	245	83	215	7	14	5.4	2.9	4.6
Tomato	1 cup	250	84	175	7	7	3.4	1.7	1.0
Prepared with equal volume of water:									
Bean with pork	1 cup	250	84	170	8	6	1.2	1.8	2.4
Beef broth, bouillon, consomme	1 cup	240	96	30	5	0	0	0	0
Beef noodle	1 cup	240	93	65	4	3	.6	.7	.8
Clam chowder, Manhattan type (with tomatoes, without milk)	1 cup	245	92	80	2	3	.5	.4	1.3
Cream of chicken	1 cup	240	92	95	3	6	1.6	2.3	1.1
Cream of mushroom	1 cup	240	90	135	2	10	2.6	1.7	4.5
Minestrone	1 cup	245	90	105	5	3	.7	.9	1.3
Split pea	1 cup	245	85	145	9	3	1.1	1.2	.4
Tomato	1 cup	245	91	90	2	3	.5	.5	1.0
Vegetable beef	1 cup	245	92	80	5	2	—	—	—
Vegetarian	1 cup	245	92	80	2	2	—	—	—
Dehydrated:									
Bouillon cube, ½ in	1 cube	4	4	5	1	Tr	—	—	—
Mixes:									
Unprepared:									
Onion	1½ oz pkg	43	3	150	6	5	1.1	2.3	1.0
Prepared with water:									
Chicken noodle	1 cup	240	95	55	2	1	—	—	—
Onion	1 cup	240	96	35	1	1	—	—	—
Tomato vegetable with noodles	1 cup	240	93	65	1	1	—	—	—
Vinegar, cider	1 tbsp	15	94	Tr	Tr	0	0	0	0
White sauce, medium, with enriched flour	1 cup	250	73	405	10	31	19.3	7.8	.8
Yeast:									
Baker's dry, active	1 pkg	7	5	20	3	Tr	—	—	—
Brewer's, dry	1 tbsp	8	5	25	3	Tr	—	—	—

For notes, see end of table.

Nutrients in Indicated Quantity

Carbohydrate (g)	Calcium (mg)	Phosphorus (mg)	Iron (mg)	Potassium (mg)	Vitamin A Value (IU)	Thiamin (mg)	Riboflavin (mg)	Niacin (mg)	Ascorbic Acid (mg)
14	18	108	Tr	90	—	.01	.11	2.2	—
Tr	—	—	—	1	—	—	—	—	—
Tr	—	—	—	1	—	—	—	—	—
Tr	—	—	—	1	—	—	—	—	—
8	8	—	—	77	—	.01	.02	.2	—
4	9	10	.4	94	—	Tr	.01	.1	—
29	—	—	—	—	0	0	0	0	0
37	—	—	—	—	0	0	0	0	0
45	—	—	—	—	0	0	0	0	0
29	—	—	—	0	0	0	0	0	0
39	—	—	—	0	0	0	0	0	0
8	22	109	1.9	235	20	.01	.07	.4	0
0	—	—	—	—	—	—	—	—	—
34	—	—	—	—	—	—	—	—	—
Tr	4	4	.1	7	—	—	—	—	—
Tr	8	2	.2	7	40	—	—	—	—
Tr	9	1	.1	2	10	Tr	Tr	—	—
1	17	14	.7	130	70	Tr	.01	Tr	4
3	5	4	.3	—	20	Tr	Tr	Tr	1
5	2	2	.2	—	10	Tr	Tr	Tr	1
5	3	2	.1	—	—	—	—	—	—
18	0	—	Tr	—	0	0	0	0	0
15	172	152	0.5	260	610	0.05	0.27	0.7	2
16	191	169	.5	279	250	.05	.34	.7	1
23	168	155	.8	418	1200	.10	.25	1.3	15
22	63	128	2.3	395	650	.13	.08	1.0	3
3	Tr	31	.5	130	Tr	Tr	.02	1.2	—
7	7	48	1.0	77	50	.05	.07	1.0	Tr
12	34	47	1.0	184	880	.02	.02	1.0	—
8	24	34	.5	79	410	.02	.05	.5	Tr
10	41	50	.5	98	70	.02	.12	.7	Tr
14	37	59	1.0	314	2350	.07	.05	1.0	—
21	29	149	1.5	270	440	.25	.15	1.5	1
16	15	34	.7	230	1000	.05	.05	1.2	12
10	12	49	.7	162	2700	.05	.05	1.0	—
13	20	39	1.0	172	2940	.05	.05	1.0	—
Tr	—	—	—	4	—	—	—	—	—
23	42	49	.6	238	30	.05	.03	.3	6
8	7	19	.2	19	50	.07	.05	.5	Tr
6	10	12	.2	58	Tr	Tr	Tr	Tr	2
12	7	19	.2	29	480	.05	.02	.5	5
1	1	1	.1	15	—	—	—	—	—
22	288	233	.5	348	1150	.12	.43	.7	2
3	3	90	1.1	140	Tr	.16	.38	2.6	Tr
3	17[70]	140	1.4	152	Tr	1.25	.34	3.0	Tr

Footnotes to accompany pp. A-1 to A-35.

[1] Vitamin A value is largely from beta-carotene used for coloring. Riboflavin value for powdered sweet creamers applies to products with added riboflavin.

[2] Applies to product without added vitamin A. With added vitamin A, value is 500 IU.

[3] Applies to product without vitamin A added.

[4] Applies to product with added vitamin A. Without added vitamin A, value is 20 IU.

[5] Yields 1 qt of fluid milk when reconstituted according to package directions.

[6] Applies to product with added vitamin A.

[7] Weight applies to product with label claim of 1⅓ cups equal 3.2 oz.

[8] Applies to products made from thick shake mixes and that do not contain added ice cream. Products made from milk shake mixes are higher in fat and usually contain added ice cream.

[9] Content of fat, vitamin A, and carbohydrate varies. Consult the label when precise values are needed for special diets.

[10] Applies to product made with milk containing no added vitamin A.

[11] Based on year-round average.

[12] Based on average vitamin A content of fortified margarine. Federal specifications for fortified margarine require a minimum of 15,000 IU of vitamin A per pound.

[13] Fatty acid values apply to product made with regular-type margarine.

[14] Dipped in egg, milk or water, and breadcrumbs; fried in vegetable shortening.

[15] If bones are discarded, value for calcium will be greatly reduced.

[16] Dipped in egg, breadcrumbs, and flour or batter.

[17] Prepared with tuna, celery, salad dressing (mayonnaise type), pickle, onion, and egg.

[18] Outer layer of fat on the cut was removed to within approximately ½ in of the lean. Deposits of fat within the cut were not removed.

[19] Crust made with vegetable shortening and enriched flour.

[20] Regular-type margarine used.

[21] Value varies widely.

[22] About one fourth of the outer layer of fat on the cut was removed. Deposits of fat within the cut were not removed.

[23] Vegetable shortening used.

[24] Also applies to pasteurized apple cider.

[25] Applies to product without added ascorbic acid. For value of product with added ascorbic acid, refer to label.

[26] Based on product with label claim of 45% of U.S. RDA in 6 fl oz.

[27] Based on product with label claim of 100% of U.S. RDA in 6 fl oz.

[28] Weight includes peel and membranes between sections. Without these parts, the weight of the edible portion is 123 g for ½ pink or red grapefruit and 118 g for ½ white grapefruit.

[29] For white-fleshed varieties, value is about 20 IU per cup; for red-fleshed varieties, 1080 IU.

[30] Weight includes seeds. Without seeds, weight of the edible portion is 57 g.

[31] Applies to product without added ascorbic acid. With added ascorbic acid, based on claim that 6 fl oz of reconstituted juice contains 45% or 50% of the U.S. RDA, value in milligrams is 108 or 120 for a 6 fl oz can (undiluted, frozen concentrate grape juice), 36 or 40 for 1 cup of diluted juice (diluted frozen concentrate grape juice).

[32] For products with added thiamin and riboflavin but without added ascorbic acid, values in milligrams would be .60 for thiamin, .80 for riboflavin, and Tr for ascorbic acid. For products with only ascorbic acid added, value varies with the brand. Consult the label.

[33] Weight includes rind. Without rind, the weight of the edible portion is 272 g for cantaloup and 149 g for honeydew melon.

[34] Represents yellow-fleshed varieties. For white-fleshed varieties, value is 50 IU for 1 peach, 90 IU for 1 cup of slices.

[35] Value represents products with added ascorbic acid. For products without added ascorbic acid, value in milligrams is 116 for a 10 oz container, 103 for 1 cup.

[36]Weight includes pits. After removal of the pits, the weight of the edible portion is 258 g for 1 cup plums in heavy syrup, 133 g for 3 plums in heavy syrup, 43 g for 4 dried prunes, and 213 g for 1 cup cooked, unsweetened prunes.

[37]Weight includes rind and seeds. Without rind and seeds, weight of the edible portion is 426 g.

[38]Made with vegetable shortening.

[39]Applies to product made with white cornmeal. With yellow cornmeal, value is 30 IU.

[40]Applies to white varieties. For yellow varieties, value is 150 IU.

[41]Applies to products that do not contain disodium phosphate. If disodium phosphate is an ingredient, value is 162 mg.

[42]Value may range from less than 1 mg to about 8 mg, depending on the brand. Consult the label.

[43]Applies to product with added nutrient. Without added nutrient, value is trace.

[44]Value varies with the brand. Consult the label.

[45]Applies to product with added nutrient. Without added nutrient, value is trace.

[46]Excepting angelfood cake, cakes were made from mixes containing vegetable shortening; icings, with butter.

[47]Excepting spongecake, vegetable shortening used for cake portion; butter, for icing. If butter or margarine used for cake portion, vitamin A values would be higher.

[48]Applies to product made with a sodium aluminum-sulfate type of baking power. With a low-sodium type of baking powder containing potassium, value would be about twice the amount shown.

[49]Equal weights of flour, sugar, eggs, and vegetable shortening.

[50]Products are commercial unless otherwise specified.

[51]Made with enriched flour and vegetable shortening except for macaroons, which do not contain flour or shortening.

[52]Icing made with butter.

[53]Applies to yellow varieties; white varieties contain only a trace.

[54]Contains vegetable shortening and butter.

[55]Made with corn oil.

[56]Made with regular margarine.

[57]Applies to product made with yellow cornmeal.

[58]Made with enriched degermed cornmeal and enriched flour.

[59]Product may or may not be enriched with riboflavin. Consult the label.

[60]Value varies with the brand. Consult the label.

[61]Weight includes cob. Without cob, weight is 77 g for 1 ear cooked, drained sweet corn, 126 g for 1 frozen 5-in ear.

[62]Based on yellow varieties. For white varieties, value is trace.

[63]Weight includes refuse of outer leaves and core. Without these parts, weight is 163 g.

[64]Weight includes core. Without core, weight is 539 g.

[65]Value based on white-fleshed varieties. For yellow-fleshed varieties, value in IU is 70 for 1 cup chopped raw onions, 50 for 1 cup sliced raw onions, and 80 for 1 cup cooked onions.

[66]Weight inclues cores and stem ends. Without these parts, weight is 123 g.

[67]Based on year-round average. For tomatoes marketed from November through May, value is about 12 mg; from June through October, 32 mg.

[68]Applies to product without calcium salts added. Value for products with calcium salts added may be as much as 63 mg for whole tomatoes, 241 mg for cut forms.

[69]Weight includes pits. Without pits, weight is 13 g for 4 medium (or 3 extra large or 2 giant) green pickled olives, 9 g for 3 small (or 2 large) ripe pickled olives.

[70]Value may vary from 6 to 60 mg.

B

Cholesterol Content of Foods

Item	Amount of Cholesterol in		Refuse from Item as Purchased (%)
	100 g Edible Portion[1] (mg)	Edible Portion of 450 g (1 lb) as Purchased (mg)	
Beef, raw			
With bone[2]	70	270	15
Without bone[2]	70	320	0
Brains, raw	>2000	>9000	0
Butter	250	1135	0
Cavier or fish roe	>300	>1300	0
Cheese			
Cheddar	100	455	0
Cottage, creamed	15	70	0
Cream	120	545	0
Other (25%-30% fat)	85	385	0
Cheese spread	65	295	0
Chicken, flesh only, raw	60	—	0
Crab			
In shell[2]	125	270	52
Meat only[2]	125	565	0
Egg, whole	550	2200	12
Egg white	0	0	0
Egg yolk			
Fresh	1500	6800	0
Frozen	1280	5800	0
Dried	2950	13,380	0
Fish			
Steak[2]	70	265	16
Fillet[2]	70	320	0
Heart, raw	150	680	0
Ice cream	45	205	0
Kidney, raw	375	1700	0
Lamb, raw			
With bone[2]	70	265	16
Without bone[2]	70	320	0
Lard and other animal fat	95	430	0
Liver, raw	300	1360	0
Lobster			
Whole[2]	200	235	74
Meat only[2]	200	900	0
Margarine			
All vegetable fat	0	0	0
Two-thirds animal fat, one-third vegetable fat	65	295	0
Milk			
Fluid, whole	11	50	0

From Watt, B.K., and Merrill, A.L.: Composition of foods—raw, processed, prepared, U.S. Department of Agriculture, Agriculture Handbook No. 8, Dec. 1963.

[1]Data apply to 100 g of edible portion of the item, although it may be purchased with the refuse indicated and described or implied in the first column.

[2]Items that have the same chemical composition for the edible portion but differ in the amount of refuse.

| Item | Amount of Cholesterol in | | Refuse from Item as Purchased (%) |
	100 g Edible Portion[1] (mg)	Edible Portion of 450 g (1 lb) as Purchased (mg)	
Dried, whole	85	385	0
Fluid, skim	3	15	0
Mutton			
With bone[2]	65	250	16
Without bone[2]	65	295	0
Oysters			
In shell[2]	>200	>90	90
Meat only[2]	>200	>900	0
Pork			
With bone[2]	70	260	18
Without bone[2]	70	320	0
Shrimp			
In shell[2]	125	390	31
Flesh only[2]	125	565	0
Sweetbreads (thymus)	250	1135	0
Veal			
With bone[2]	90	320	21
Without bone[2]	90	410	0

C

Dietary Fiber in Selected Plant Foods

Food	Amount	Weight (g)	Total Dietary Fiber (g)	Noncellulose Polysaccharides (g)	Cellulose (g)	Lignin (g)
Apple	1 med					
Flesh		138	1.96	1.29	0.66	0.01
Skin		100	3.71	2.21	1.01	0.49
Banana	1 small	119	2.08	1.33	0.44	0.31
Beans						
Baked	1 cup	255	18.53	14.45	3.59	0.48
Green, cooked	1 cup	125	4.19	2.31	1.61	0.26
Bread						
White	1 slice	25	0.68	0.50	0.18	Trace
Whole meal	1 slice	25	2.13	1.49	0.33	0.31
Broccoli, cooked	1 cup	155	6.36	4.53	1.78	0.05
Brussels sprouts, cooked	1 cup	155	4.43	3.08	1.24	0.11
Cabbage, cooked	1 cup	145	4.10	2.55	1.00	0.55
Carrots, cooked	1 cup	155	5.74	3.44	2.29	Trace
Cauliflower, cooked	1 cup	125	2.25	0.84	1.41	Trace
Cereals						
All-Bran	1 oz	30	8.01	5.35	1.80	0.86

Adapted from Southgate, D.A.T., and others: A guide to calculating intakes of dietary fiber, J. Hum. Nutr. **30:**303, 1976.

Food	Amount	Weight (g)	Total Dietary Fiber (g)	Noncellulose Polysaccharides (g)	Cellulose (g)	Lignin (g)
Corn Flakes	1 cup	25	2.75	1.82	0.61	0.33
Grapenuts	¼ cup	30	2.10	1.54	0.38	0.17
Puffed Wheat	1 cup	15	2.31	1.55	0.39	0.37
Rice Krispies	1 cup	30	1.34	1.04	0.23	0.07
Shredded Wheat	1 biscuit	25	3.07	2.20	0.66	0.21
Special K	1 cup	30	1.64	1.10	0.22	0.32
Cherries	10 cherries	68	0.84	0.63	0.17	0.05
Cookies						
Ginger	4 snaps	28	0.56	0.41	0.08	0.07
Oatmeal	4 cookies	52	2.08	1.64	0.21	0.22
Plain	4 cookies	48	0.80	0.68	0.05	0.06
Corn	1 cup	165	7.82	7.11	0.51	0.20
Canned	1 cup	165	9.39	8.20	1.06	0.13
Flour						
Bran	1 cup	100	44.00	32.70	8.05	3.23
White	1 cup	115	3.62	2.90	0.69	0.03
Whole meal	1 cup	120	11.41	7.50	2.95	0.96
Grapefruit	½ cup	100	0.44	0.34	0.04	0.06
Jam, strawberry	1 tbsp	20	0.22	0.17	0.02	0.03
Lettuce	⅙ head	100	1.53	0.47	1.06	Trace
Marmalade, orange	1 tbsp	20	0.14	0.13	0.01	Trace
Onions, raw, sliced	1 cup	100	2.10	1.55	0.55	Trace
Orange	1 cup	200	0.58	0.44	0.08	0.06
Parsnips, raw, diced	1 cup	100	4.90	3.77	1.13	Trace
Peanuts	1 oz	30	2.79	1.92	0.51	0.36
Peanut butter	1 tbsp	16	1.21	0.90	0.31	Trace
Peach, flesh and skin	1 med	100	2.28	1.46	0.20	0.62
Pear	1 med					
Flesh		164	4.00	2.16	1.10	0.74
Skin		100	8.59	3.72	2.18	2.67
Peas, canned	1 cup	170	13.35	8.84	3.91	0.60
Peas, raw or frozen	1 cup	100	7.75	5.48	2.09	0.18
Plums	1 plum	66	1.00	0.65	0.15	0.20
Potato, raw	1 med	135	4.73	3.36	1.38	Trace
Raisins	1 oz	30	1.32	0.72	0.25	0.35
Strawberries	1 cup	149	2.65	1.39	1.04	0.22
Tomato						
Raw	1 med	135	1.89	0.88	0.61	0.41
Canned, drained	1 cup	240	2.04	1.08	0.89	0.07
Turnips, raw	1 med	100	2.20	1.50	0.70	Trace

D

Sodium and Potassium Content of Foods, 100 g, Edible Portion

Food and Description	Sodium (mg)	Potassium (mg)
Almonds		
Dried	4	773
Roasted and salted	198	773
Apples		
Raw, pared	1	110
Frozen, sliced, sweetened	14	68
Apple juice, canned or bottled	1	101
Applesauce, canned, sweetened	2	65
Apricots		
Raw	1	281
Canned, syrup pack, light	1	239
Dried, sulfured, cooked, fruit, and liquid	8	318
Asparagus		
Cooked spears, boiled, drained	1	183
Canned spears, green		
Regular pack, solids and liquid	236[1]	166
Special dietary pack (low sodium), solids and liquid	3	166
Frozen		
Cuts and tips, cooked, boiled, drained	1	220
Spears, cooked, boiled, drained	1	238
Avocados, raw, all commercial varieties	4	604
Bacon, cured, cooked, broiled or fried, drained	1021	236
Bacon, Canadian, cooked, broiled or fried, drained	2555	432
Bananas, raw, common	1	370
Bass, black sea, raw	68	256
Beans, common, mature seeds, dry		
White		
Cooked	7	416
Canned, solids and liquid, with pork and tomato sauce	463	210
Red, cooked	3	340
Beans, lima		
Immature seeds		
Cooked, boiled, drained	1	422
Canned		
Regular pack, solids and liquid	236[1]	222
Special dietary pack (low sodium), solids and liquid	4	222
Frozen, thin-seeded types, commonly called baby limas, cooked, boiled, drained	129	394
Mature seeds, dry, cooked	2	612
Beans, mung, sprouted seeds, cooked, boiled, drained	4	156
Beans, snap		
Green		
Cooked, boiled, drained	4	151
Canned		
Regular pack, solids and liquid	236[1]	95

Numbers in parentheses denote values inputed, usually from another form of the food or from a similar food. Dashes denote lack of reliable data for a constituent believed to be present in measurable amount. Values are selected from Watt, B.K., and Merrill, A.L.: Composition of foods—raw, processed, prepared, U.S. Department of Agriculture, Agriculture Handbook No. 8, Dec. 1963.
For notes, see end of table.

Food and Description	Sodium (mg)	Potassium (mg)
Special dietary pack (low sodium), solids and liquid	2	95
Frozen, cut, cooked, boiled, drained	1	152
Yellow or wax		
Cooked, boiled, drained	3	151
Canned		
Regular pack, solids and liquid	236[1]	95
Special dietary pack (low sodium), solids and liquid	2	95
Frozen, cut, cooked, boiled, drained	1	164
Beef		
Retail cuts, trimmed to retail level		
Round	60	370
Rump	60	370
Hamburger, regular ground, cooked	47	450
Beef, corned, boneless		
Cooked, medium fat	1740	150
Canned corned-beef hash (with potato)	540	200
Beef, dried, cooked, creamed	716	153
Beef potpie, commercial, frozen, unheated	366	93
Beets, common, red		
Canned		
Regular pack, solids and liquid	236[1]	167
Special dietary pack (low sodium), solids and liquid	46	167
Beet greens, common, cooked, boiled, drained	76	332
Biscuits, baking powder, made with enriched flour	626	117
Blackberries, including dewberries, boysenberries, and young-berries, raw	1	170
Blueberries		
Raw	1	81
Frozen, not thawed, sweetened	1	66
Bouillon cubes or powder	24,000	100
Bran, added sugar and malt extract	1060	1070
Bran flakes (40% bran), added thiamine	925	—
Bran flakes with raisins, added thiamine	800	—
Breads		
Cracked wheat	529	134
French or Vienna, enriched	580	90
Italian, enriched	585	74
Raisin	365	233
Rye, American (⅓ rye, ⅔ clear flour)	557	145
White, enriched, made with 3%-4% nonfat dry milk	507	105
Whole wheat, made with 2% nonfat dry milk	527	273
Bread stuffing mix and stuffings prepared from mix, dry form	1331	172
Broccoli		
Cooked spears, boiled, drained	10	267
Frozen, spears, cooked, boiled, drained	12	220
Brussels sprouts, frozen, cooked, boiled, drained	14	295
Buffalo fish, raw	52	293
Bulgur (parboiled wheat), canned, made from hard red winter wheat		
Unseasoned[2]	599	87
Seasoned[3]	460	112
Butter[4]	987	23
Buttermilk, fluid, cultured (made from skim milk)	130	140
Cabbage		
Common varieties (Danish, domestic, and pointed types)		
Raw	20	233
Cooked, boiled until tender, drained, shredded, cooked in small amount of water	14	163

For notes, see end of table.

Food and Description	Sodium (mg)	Potassium (mg)
Red, raw	26	268
Cakes		
Baked from home recipes		
Angle food	283	88
Fruit cake, made with enriched flour, dark	158	496
Gingerbread, made with enriched flour	237	454
Plain cake or cupcake, without icing	300	79
Pound, modified	178	78
Frozen, commercial, devil's food, with chocolate icing	420	119
Candy		
Caramels, plain or chocolate	226	192
Chocolate, sweet	33	269
Chocolate coated, chocolate fudge	228	193
Gum drops, starch jelly pieces	35	5
Hard	32	4
Marshmallows	39	6
Peanut bars	10	448
Carrots		
Raw	47	341
Canned		
Regular pack, solids and liquid	236[1]	120
Special dietary pack (low sodium), solids and liquid	39	120
Cashew nuts	15[5]	464
Cauliflower		
Cooked, boiled, drained	9	206
Frozen, cooked, boiled, drained	10	207
Celery, all, including green and yellow varieties		
Raw	126	341
Cooked, boiled, drained	88	239
Chard, Swiss, cooked, boiled, drained	86	321
Cheeses		
Natural cheeses		
Cheddar (domestic type, commonly called American)	700	82
Cottage (large or small curd)		
Creamed	229	85
Uncreamed	290	72
Cream	250	74
Parmesan	734	149
Swiss (domestic)	710	104
Pasteurized process cheese, American	1136[6]	80
Pasteurized process cheese spread, American	1625[6]	240
Cherries		
Raw, sweet	2	191
Canned		
Sour, red, solids and liquid, water pack	2	130
Sweet, solids and liquid, syrup pack, light	1	128
Frozen, not thawed, sweetened	2	130
Chicken, all classes		
Light meat without skin, cooked, roasted	64	411
Dark meat without skin, cooked, roasted	86	321
Chicken potpie, commercial, frozen, unheated	411	153
Chili con carne, canned, with beans	531	233
Clams, raw		
Soft, meat only	36	235
Hard or round, meat only	205	311
Cocoa and chocolate-flavored beverage powders		
Cocoa powder with nonfat dry milk	525	800
Mix for hot chocolate	382	605

Food and Description	Sodium (mg)	Potassium (mg)
Cocoa, dry powder, high-fat or breakfast		
Plain	6	1522
Processed with alkali	717	651
Coconut meat, fresh	23	256
Cod		
Cooked, broiled	110	407
Dehydrated, lightly salted	8100	160
Coffee, instant, water-soluble solids		
Dry powder	72	3256
Beverage	1	36
Coleslaw, made with French dressing (commercial)	268	205
Collards, cooked, boiled, drained, leaves, including stems, cooked in small amount of water	25	234
Cookies		
Assorted, packaged, commercial	365	67
Butter, thin, rich	418	60
Gingersnaps	571	462
Molasses	386	138
Oatmeal with raisins	162	370
Sandwich type	483	38
Vanilla wafer	252	72
Corn, sweet		
Cooked, boiled, drained, white and yellow, kernels, cut off cob before cooking	Trace	165
Canned		
Regular pack, cream style, white and yellow, solids and liquid	236[1]	(97)
Special dietary pack (low sodium), cream style, white and yellow, solids and liquid	2	(97)
Frozen, kernels cut off cob, cooked, boiled, drained	1	184
Corn grits, degermed, enriched, dry form	1	80
Corn products used mainly as ready-to-eat breakfast cereals		
Corn flakes, added nutrients	1005	120
Corn, puffed, added nutrients	1060	—
Corn, rice, and wheat flakes, mixed, added nutrients	950	—
Cornbread, baked from home recipes, southern style, made with degermed cornmeal, enriched	591	157
Cornmeal, white or yellow, degermed, enriched, dry form	1	120
Cornstarch	Trace	Trace
Cowpeas, including blackeye peas		
Immature seeds, canned, solids and liquid	236[1]	352
Young pods, with seeds, cooked, boiled, drained	3	196
Crab, canned	1000	110
Crackers		
Butter	1092	113
Graham, plain	670	384
Saltines	(1100)	(120)
Sandwich type, peanut-cheese	992	226
Soda	1100	120
Cream, fluid, light, coffee, or table, 20% fat	43	122
Cream substitutes, dried, containing cream, skim milk (calcium reduced), and lactose	575	—
Cucumbers, raw, pared	6	160
Custard, baked	79	146
Doughnuts, cake type	501	90
Duck, domesticated, raw, flesh only	74	285

For notes, see end of table.

Food and Description	Sodium (mg)	Potassium (mg)
Eggs, chicken		
Raw		
Whole, fresh and frozen	122	129
Whites, fresh and frozen	146	139
Yolks, fresh	52	98
Eggplant, cooked, boiled, drained	1	150
Farina		
Enriched		
Regular		
Dry form	2	83
Cooked	144	9
Quick-cooking, cooked	165	10
Instant-cooking, cooked	188	13
Nonenriched, regular, dry form	2	83
Flatfishes (flounders, soles, sand dabs), raw	78	342
Fruit cocktail, canned, solids and liquid, water pack, with or without artificial sweetener	5	168
Garlic, cloves, raw	19	529
Grapefruit		
Raw, pulp, pink, red, white, all varieties	1	135
Canned, juice, sweetened	1	162
Grapes, raw, American type (slip skin), such as Concord, Delaware, Niagara, Catawba, and Scuppernong	3	158
Haddock, cooked, fried	177	348
Halibut, Atlantic and Pacific, cooked, broiled	134	525
Ice cream and frozen custard, regular, approximately 10% fat	63[7]	181
Ice cream cones	232	244
Ice milk	68[7]	195
Jams and preserves	12	88
Kale, cooked, boiled, drained, leaves including stems	43	221
Lamb, retail cuts	70	290
Lettuce, raw crisphead varieties such as Iceberg, New York, and Great Lakes strains	9	175
Liver, beef, cooked, fried	184	380
Lobster, northern, canned or cooked	210	180
Macaroni, unenriched, dry form	2	197
Margarine[8]	987	23
Milk, cow		
Fluid (pasteurized and raw)		
Whole, 3.7% fat	50	144
Skim	52	145
Canned, evaporated (unsweetened)	118	303
Dry, skim (nonfat solids), regular	532	1745
Malted		
Dry powder	440	720
Beverage	91	200
Chocolate drink, fluid, commercial		
Made with skim milk	46	142
Made with whole (3.5% fat) milk	47	146
Molasses, cane		
First extraction or light	15	917
Third extraction or blackstrap	96	2927
Muskmelons, raw, cantaloupes, other netted varieties	12	251
Mustard greens, cooked, boiled, drained	18	220
Nectarines, raw	6	294
New Zealand spinach, cooked, boiled, drained	92	463

Food and Description	Sodium (mg)	Potassium (mg)
Noodles, egg noodles, enriched, cooked	2	44
Oat products used mainly as hot breakfast cereals, oatmeal or rolled oats		
Dry form	2	352
Cooked	218	61
Oat products used mainly as ready-to-eat breakfast cereals, with or without corn, puffed, added nutrients	1267	—
Okra		
Raw	3	249
Cooked, boiled, drained	2	174
Olives, pickled; canned or bottled		
Green	2400	55
Ripe, Ascolano (extra large, mammoth, giant jumbo)	813	34
Ripe, salt-cured, oil-coated, Greek style	3288	—
Onions, mature (dry), raw	10	157
Onions, young green (bunching varieties), raw, bulb and entire top	5	231
Oranges, raw, peeled fruit, all commercial varieties	1	200
Orange juice		
Raw, all commercial varieties	1	200
Canned, unsweetened	1	199
Frozen concentrate, unsweetened, diluted with 3 parts water, by volume	1	186
Oysters		
Raw, meat only, Eastern	73	121
Cooked, fried	206	203
Frozen, solids and liquid	380	210
Parsnips, cooked, boiled, drained	8	379
Peaches		
Raw	1	202
Canned, solids and liquid, water pack, with or without artificial sweetener	2	137
Frozen, sliced, sweetened, not thawed	2	124
Peanuts		
Roasted with skins	5	701
Roasted and salted	418	674
Peanut butters made with small amounts of added fat, salt	607	670
Pears		
Raw, including skin	2	130
Canned, solids and liquid, syrup pack, light	1	85
Peas, green, immature		
Cooked, boiled, drained	1	196
Canned, Alaska (early or June peas)		
Regular pack, solids and liquid	236[1]	96
Special dietary pack (low sodium), solids and liquid	3	96
Frozen, cooked, boiled, drained	115	135
Pecans	Trace	603
Peppers, sweet, garden varieties, immature, green, raw	13	213
Perch, yellow, raw	68	230
Pickles, cucumber, dill	1428	200
Piecrust or plain pastry, made with enriched flour, baked	611	50
Pineapple		
Raw	1	146
Frozen chunks, sweetened, not thawed	2	100
Pizza, with cheese, from home recipe, baked		
With cheese topping	702	130
With sausage topping	729	168

For notes, see end of table.

Food and Description	Sodium (mg)	Potassium (mg)
Plate dinners, frozen, commercial, unheated		
Beef pot roast, whole oven-browned potatoes, peas, corn	259	244
Chicken, fried; mashed potatoes; mixed vegetables (carrots, peas, corn, beans)	344	112
Meat loaf with tomato sauce, mashed potatoes, peas	393	115
Turkey, sliced; mashed potatoes; peas	400	176
Plums		
Raw, Damson	2	299
Canned, solids and liquid, purple (Italian prunes), syrup pack, light	1	145
Popcorn, popped		
Plain	(3)	—
Oil and salt added	1940	—
Pork, fresh, retail cuts, trimmed to retail level, loin	65	390
Pork, cured, canned ham, contents of can	(1100)	(340)
Potatoes		
Cooked, boiled in skin	3[9]	407
Dehydrated mashed, flakes without milk		
Dry form	89	1600
Prepared, water, milk, table fat added	231	286
Pretzels	1680[10]	130
Prunes, dried, "softenized," cooked (fruit and liquid), with added sugar	3	262
Pudding mixes and puddings made from mixes, with starch base		
With milk, cooked	129	136
With milk, without cooking	124	129
Pumpkin, canned	2	240
Raspberries		
Canned, solids and liquid, water pack, with or without artificial sweetener, red	1	114
Frozen, red, sweetened, not thawed	1	100
Rice		
Brown		
Raw	9	214
Cooked	282	70
White (fully milled or polished), enriched, common commercial varieties, all types		
Raw	5	92
Cooked	374	28
Rice products used mainly as ready-to-eat breakfast cereals		
Rice flakes, added nutrients	987	180
Rice, puffed; added nutrients, without salt	2	100
Rice, puffed or open-popped, presweetened, honey and added nutrients	706	—
Roe, cooked, baked or broiled, cod and shad[11]	73	132
Rolls and buns, commercial, ready-to-serve		
Danish pastry	366	112
Hard rolls, enriched	625	97
Plain (pan rolls), enriched	506	95
Sweet rolls	389	124
Rusk	246	161
Rutabagas, cooked, boiled, drained	4	167
Rye, flour, medium	(1)	203
Rye wafers, whole grain	882	600

Food and Description	Sodium (mg)	Potassium (mg)
Salad dressings, commercial[12]		
Blue and Roquefort cheese		
Regular	1094	37
Special dietary (low calorie), low fat (approx. 5 kcal/tsp)	1108	34
French		
Regular	1370	79
Special dietary (low calorie), low fat (approx. 5 kcal/tsp)	787	79
Mayonnaise	597	34
Thousand Island		
Regular	700	113
Special dietary (low calorie, approx. 10 kcal/tsp)	700	113
Salmon, coho (silver)		
Raw	48[13]	421
Canned, solids and liquid	351[14]	339
Salt pork, raw	1212	42
Salt sticks, regular type	1674	92
Sandwich spread (with chopped pickle)		
Regular	626	92
Special dietary (low calorie, approx. 5 kcal/tsp)	626	92
Sardines, Atlantic, canned in oil, drained solids	823	590
Sardines, Pacific, in tomato sauce, solids and liquid	400	320
Sauerkraut, canned, solids and liquid	747[15]	140
Sausage, cold cuts, and luncheon meats		
Bologna, all samples	1300	230
Frankfurters, raw, all samples	1100	220
Luncheon meat, pork, cured ham or shoulder, chopped, spiced or unspiced, canned	1234	222
Pork sausage, links or bulk, cooked	958	269
Scallops, bay and sea, cooked, steamed	265	476
Soups, commercial, canned		
Beef broth, bouillon, and consomme, prepared with equal volume of water	326	54
Chicken noodle, prepared with equal volume of water	408	23
Tomato		
Prepared with equal volume of water	396	94
Prepared with equal volume of milk	422	167
Vegetable beef, prepared with equal volume of water	427	66
Soy sauce	7325	366
Spaghetti, enriched, cooked, tender stage	1	61
Spinach		
Cooked, boiled, drained	50	324
Canned		
Regular pack, drained solids	236[1]	250
Special dietary pack (low sodium), solids and liquid	34	250
Frozen, chopped, cooked, boiled, drained	52	333
Squash, summer, all varieties, cooked, boiled, drained	1	141
Strawberries		
Raw	1	164
Frozen, sweetened, not thawed, sliced	1	112
Sweet potatoes		
Cooked, all, baked in skin	12	300
Canned, liquid pack, solids and liquid, regular pack in syrup	48	(120)
Dehydrated flakes, prepared with water	45	140
Tangerines, raw (Dancy variety)	2	126
Tea, instant (water-soluble solids), carbohydrate added		
Dry powder	—	4530
Beverage	—	25

For notes, see end of table.

Food and Description	Sodium (mg)	Potassium (mg)
Tomatoes, ripe		
Raw	3	244
Canned, solids and liquid, regular pack	130	217
Tomato catsup, bottled	1042[16]	363
Regular pack	200	227
Special dietary pack (low sodium)	3	227
Tomato puree, canned		
Regular pack	399	426
Special dietary pack (low sodium)	6	426
Tuna, canned		
In oil, solids and liquid	800	301
In water, solids and liquid	41[17]	279[17]
Turkey, all classes		
Light meat, cooked, roasted	82	411
Dark meat, cooked, roasted	99	398
Turkey potpie, commercial, frozen, unheated	369	114
Turnips, cooked, boiled, drained	34	188
Turnip greens, leaves, including stems		
Canned, solids and liquid	236[1]	243
Frozen, cooked, boiled, drained	17	149
Veal, retail cuts, untrimmed	80	500
Waffles, frozen, made with enriched flour	644	158
Walnuts		
Black	3	460
Persian or English	2	450
Watermelon, raw	1	100
Wheat flours		
Whole (from hard wheats)	3	370
Patent		
All-purpose or family flour, enriched	2	95
Self-rising flour, enriched (anhydrous monocalcium phosphate used as a baking acid)[18]	1079	—[19]
Yogurt, made from whole milk	47	132

[1]Estimated average based on addition of salt in the amount of 0.6% of the finished product.

[2]Processed, partially debranned, whole-kernel wheat with salt added.

[3]Processed, partially debranned, whole-kernel wheat with chicken fat, chicken stock base, dehydrated onion flakes, salt, monosodium glutamate, and herbs.

[4]Values apply to salted butter. Unsalted butter contains less than 10 mg of either sodium or potassium per 100 g. Value for vitamin A is the year-round average.

[5]Applies to unsalted nuts. For salted nuts, value is approximately 200 mg per 100 g.

[6]Values for phosphorus and sodium are based on use of 1.5% anhydrous disodium phosphate as the emulsifying agent. If emulsifying agent does not contain either phosphorus (P) or sodium (Na), the content of these two nutrients in milligrams per 100 g is as follows:

	P	Na
American process cheese	444	650
Swiss process cheese	540	681
American cheese food	427	—
American cheese spread	548	1139

[7]Value for product without added salt.

[8]Values apply to salted margarine. Unsalted margarine contains less than 10 mg/100 g of either sodium or potassium. Vitamin A value based on the minimum required to meet federal specifications for margarine with vitamin A added, 15,000 IUA/lb.

[9]Applies to product without added salt. If salt is added, an estimated average value for sodium is 236 mg/100 g.

[10]Sodium content is variable. For example, very thin pretzel sticks contain about twice the average amount listed.

[11]Prepared with butter or margarine, lemon juice or vinegar.

[12]Values apply to products containing salt. For those without salt, sodium content is low, ranging from less than 10 to 50 mg/100 g; the amount usually is indicated on the label.

Continued.

Footnotes to table, pp. A-41 to A-49, cont'd.

[13]Sample dipped in brine contained 215 mg sodium/100 g.

[14]For product canned without added salt, value is approximately the same as for raw salmon.

[15]Values for sauerkraut and sauerkraut juice are based on salt content of 1.9% and 2.0%, respectively, in the finished products. The amounts in some samples may vary significantly from this estimate.

[16]Applies to regular pack. For special dietary pack (low sodium), values range from 5-35 mg/100 g.

[17]One sample with salt added contained 875 mg of sodium/100 g and 275 mg of potassium.

[18]The acid ingredient most commonly used in self-rising flour. When sodium acid pyrophosphate in combination with either anhydrous monocalcium phosphate or calcium carbonate is used, the value for calcium is approximately 120 mg/100 g; for phosphorus, 540 mg; for sodium, 1360 mg.

[19]90 mg of potassium/100 g contributed by flour. Small quantities of additional potassium may be provided by other ingredients.

E

Sodium Levels in Mineral Waters

Sodium Levels	Beverage (8 fl oz)
Low (less than 5 mg)	Black Mountain spring water
	Bel-Air mineral water
	Perrier
	Poland Springs sparkling water
	Sheffield's O_2 sparkling spring water
Moderate-low (30-60 mg)	Calistoga mineral water
	Canada Dry club soda
	Napa Valley springs mineral water
	Schweppes club soda
Moderate-high (100-110 mg)	Calso water
High (more than 400 mg)	Lady Lee club soda

Adapted from Sodium in mineral waters—8 fluid ounce servings, American Heart Association, Alameda County Chapter, Oakland, Calif., Feb. 1981.

F

Sodium Levels in Popular Soft Drinks

Regular	Sugar-Free
Less than 20 mg/12 fl oz	
Aspen, Bubble-Up, Canada Dry ginger ale, Canada Dry tonic water, Orange Crush, Pepsi, Schweppes ginger ale, Schweppes tonic water, Shasta cola, Squirt	
20-40 mg/12 fl oz	
Canada Dry collins mix, Coca-Cola, Dr. Pepper, Fanta (orange, grape, root beer), Mountain Dew, Mr. Pibb, Seven-Up, Shasta (all flavors except cola, strawberry, lemon-lime), Sunkist, Teem	Sugar-free Dr. Pepper, Diet Shasta grape, Diet Squirt
40-60 mg/12 fl oz	
Fanta ginger ale, Schweppes bitter lemon, Shasta (lemon-lime, strawberry), Sprite	Fresca, Sugar-free Mr. Pibb, Pepsi Light, Diet Seven-Up, Diet Shasta (all flavors except grape), Tab, Tab-Strawberry
60-80 mg/12 fl oz	
	Diet-Rite Cola, Diet Pepsi, Sugar-free Sprite, Tab (black cherry, ginger ale, grape, lemon-lime, orange, root beer)
80-100 mg/12 fl oz	
	Sugar-free Bubble-Up, Diet Mug Root Beer, Diet Sunkist

Adapted from Sodium in soft drinks—12 fl oz servings, American Heart Association, Alameda County Chapter, Oakland, Calif., Feb. 1981.

G

Nutritional Analyses of Fast Foods

	Wt (g)	Energy (kcal)	PRO (g)	CHO (g)	Fat (g)	Chol (mg)	A (IU)	B₁ (mg)	B₂ (mg)	Nia. (mg)	B₆ (mg)	B₁₂ (µg)	C (mg)	D (IU)
Arby's														
Roast Beef	140	350	22	32	15	45	X	0.30	0.34	5	—	—	X	—
Beef and Cheese	168	450	27	36	22	55	X	0.38	0.43	6	—	—	X	—
Super Roast Beef	263	620	30	61	28	85	X	0.53	0.43	7	—	—	X	—
Junior Roast Beef	74	220	12	21	9	35	X	0.15	0.17	3	—	—	X	—
Ham & Cheese	154	380	23	33	17	60	X	0.75	0.34	5	—	—	X	—
Turkey Deluxe	236	510	28	46	24	70	X	0.45	0.34	8	—	—	X	—
Club Sandwich	252	560	30	43	30	100	X	0.68	0.43	7	—	—	X	—

From Consumer Affairs, Arby's, Inc, Atlanta, Ga. Nutritional analysis by Technological Resources, Camden, N.J.

	Wt (g)	Energy (kcal)	PRO (g)	CHO (g)	Fat (g)	Chol (mg)	A (IU)	B₁ (mg)	B₂ (mg)	Nia. (mg)	B₆ (mg)	B₁₂ (µg)	C (mg)	D (IU)
Burger Chef														
Hamburger	91	244	11	29	9	27	114	0.17	0.16	2.7	0.16	0.26	1.2	—
Cheeseburger	104	290	14	29	13	39	267	0.18	0.21	2.8	0.17	0.36	1.2	—
Double Cheeseburger	145	420	24	30	22	77	431	0.20	0.32	4.4	0.31	0.73	1.2	—
Fish Filet	179	547	21	46	31	43	400	0.23	0.22	2.7	0.04	0.10	1.0	—
Super Shef Sandwich	252	563	29	44	30	105	754	0.31	0.40	6.0	0.45	0.87	9.3	—
Big Shef Sandwich	186	569	23	38	36	81	279	0.26	0.31	4.7	0.31	0.63	1.0	—
TOP Shef Sandwich	138	661	41	36	38	134	273	0.35	0.47	8.1	0.56	1.16	0	—
Funmeal Feast	—	545	15	55	30	27	123	0.25	0.21	4.6	0.16	0.26	12.8	—
Rancher Platter*	316	640	32	33	42	106	1750*	0.29	0.38	8.6	0.61	1.01	23.5	—
Mariner Platter*	373	734	29	78	34	35	2069*	0.34	0.23	5.2	0.09	0.56	23.5	—
French Fries, small	68	250	2	20	19	0	0	0.07	0.04	1.7	—	0	11.5	—
French Fries, large	85	351	3	28	26	0	0	0.10	0.06	2.4	—	0	16.2	—
Vanilla Shake (12 oz)	336	380	13	60	10	40	387	0.10	0.66	0.5	0.1	1.77	0	—
Chocolate Shake (12 oz)	336	403	10	72	9	36	292	0.16	0.76	0.4	0.1	1.07	0	—
Hot Chocolate	—	198	8	23	8	30	288	0.93	0.39	0.3	0.1	0.79	2.1	—

From Burger Chef Systems, Inc, Indianapolis, Ind. Nutritional analysis from *Handbook No. 8*. Washington; U.S. Dept of Agriculture.
*Includes salad.

	Wt (g)	Energy (kcal)	PRO (g)	CHO (g)	Fat (g)	Chol (mg)	A (IU)	B₁ (mg)	B₂ (mg)	Nia. (mg)	B₆ (mg)	B₁₂ (µg)	C (mg)	D (IU)
Burger King*														
Hamburger	110	290	15 (25%*)	29	13	—	tr	10%	10%	10%	—	—	tr	—
Cheeseburger	124	350	18 (30%)	30	17	—	tr	8%	10%	10%	—	—	tr	—
Double Cheeseburger	179	530	30 (50%)	32	31	—	tr	10%	10%	20%	—	—	tr	—
Whopper	261	630	26 (40%)	50	36	—	tr	4%	15%	20%	—	—	tr	—
Whopper w/Ch	289	740	32 (50%)	52	45	—	tr	8%	20%	15%	—	—	tr	—
Double Beef Whopper	337	850	44 (70%)	52	52	—	tr	6%	25%	30%	—	—	tr	—
Double Beef Whopper w/Ch	365	950	50 (80%)	54	60	—	tr	6%	25%	30%	—	—	tr	—
Whopper Jr.	144	370	15 (25%)	31	20	—	tr	15%	10%	15%	—	—	tr	—
Whopper Jr. w/Ch	158	420	18 (30%)	32	25	—	tr	15%	10%	15%	—	—	tr	—
Bacon Double Cheeseburger	202	600	35 (50%)	36	35	—	8%	20%	25%	35%	—	—	2%	—
Whaler	—	540	24 (35%)	57	24	—	tr	15%	10%	10%	—	—	tr	—
Whaler w/Ch	—	590	26 (40%)	58	28	—	4%	15%	15%	10%	—	—	tr	—
Chicken Sandwich	—	690	26 (40%)	26	42	—	4%	20%	15%	50%	—	—	2%	—
Veal Parmagiana	—	600	28 (45%)	65	25	—	20%	25%	30%	35%	—	—	10%	—
Regular Fries	68	210	3 (4%)	25	11	—	tr	4%	tr	4%	—	—	4%	—
Regular Onion Rings	76	270	3 (4%)	29	16	—	tr	4%	tr	tr	—	—	tr	—
Apple Pie	85	240	2 (4%)	32	12	—	tr	tr	2%	tr	—	—	tr	—
Chocolate Shake	282	340	8 (10%)	57	10	—	tr	8%	15%	tr	—	—	tr	—
Vanilla Shake	282	340	8 (10%)	52	11	—	tr	10%	20%	tr	—	—	tr	—

From Burger King Corp., Miami, Fla. Nutritional analysis by Raltech Scientific Services, Inc. (formerly WARF), Madison, Wis., and Campbell Labs, Camden, N.J.
*NOTE: Analyses for vitamins and minerals shown with percent signs indicate percent U.S. RDA.

From Young, E.A.: Update: nutritional analysis of fast foods, Public Health Currents, 1981, Reprinted with permission of Ross Laboratories, Columbus, Ohio 43216.
See Burger King section for that restaurant's source for nutritional analysis.
Dashes indicate no data available; X, less than 2% U.S. RDA; *tr*, trace.
NOTE: Older Pizza Hut data are invalid because of reformulation of the products.

			Minerals						Crude
Ca (mg)	Cu (mg)	Fe (mg)	K (mg)	Mg (mg)	P (mg)	Na (mg)	Zn (mg)	Moisture (g)	Fiber (g)
80	—	3.6	—	—	—	880	—	—	—
200	—	4.5	—	—	—	1220	—	—	—
100	—	5.4	—	—	—	1420	—	—	—
40	—	1.8	—	—	—	530	—	—	—
200	—	2.7	—	—	—	1350	—	—	—
80	—	2.7	—	—	—	1220	—	—	—
200	—	3.6	—	—	—	1610	—	—	—
45	0.08	2.0	208	9	106	—	1.6	41	0.2
132	0.08	2.2	218	9	202	—	1.9	46	0.2
223	0.10	3.2	360	15	355	—	3.6	67	0.2
145	0.04	2.2	271	19	302	—	1.2	72	0.4
205	0.21	4.5	578	25	377	—	4.5	143	0.5
152	0.05	3.6	382	14	280	—	3.4	80	0.3
194	0.13	5.4	612	26	445	—	5.9	91	0.1
61	0.24	2.8	688	26	183	—	1.6	70	0.8
66	0.38	5.3	1237	53	326	—	5.6	209	1.3
63	0.32	3.3	996	49	397	—	1.2	195	1.8
9	0.16	0.7	473	16	62	—	<0.1	29	0.6
13	0.23	0.9	661	22	86	—	<0.1	40	0.9
497	—	0.3	622	40	392	—	1.3	—	—
449	—	1.1	762	54	429	—	1.6	—	—
271	0.09	0.7	436	50	245	—	1.1	—	—
tr	6%	15%	240	6%	10%	525	10%	—	—
4%	6%	15%	230	6%	15%	730	15%	—	—
8%	6%	15%	360	10%	30%	990	30%	—	—
4%	6%	15%	520	10%	25%	990	15%	—	—
15%	6%	15%	590	10%	35%	1435	20%	—	—
2%	6%	25%	760	10%	40%	1080	40%	—	—
15%	6%	20%	730	15%	50%	1535	45%	—	—
tr	2%	10%	280	6%	10%	560	15%	—	—
8%	2%	10%	270	8%	20%	785	15%	—	—
25%	—	25%	540	—	45%	985	—	—	—
8%	—	15%	150	—	25%	745	—	—	—
20%	—	15%	160	—	35%	885	—	—	—
6%	—	10%	340	—	20%	775	—	—	—
30%	—	25%	340	—	35%	1130	—	—	—
tr	tr	2%	380	6%	tr	230	tr	—	—
8%	2%	2%	140	2%	6%	450	tr	—	—
tr	tr	2%	50	tr	tr	335	tr	—	—
25%	4%	tr	340	10%	25%	280	6%	—	—
30%	tr	tr	210	4%	10%	320	4%	—	—

Continued.

	Wt (g)	Energy (kcal)	PRO (g)	CHO (g)	Fat (g)	Chol (mg)	Vitamins A (IU)	B₁ (mg)	B₂ (mg)	Nia. (mg)	B₆ (mg)	B₁₂ (μg)	C (mg)	D (IU)
Church's Fried Chicken														
White Chicken Portion	100	327	21	10	23	—	160	0.10	0.18	7.2	—	—	0.7	—
Dark Chicken Portion	100	305	22	7	21	—	140	0.10	0.27	5.3	—	—	1.0	—
From Church's Fried Chicken, San Antonio, Tex. Nutritional analysis by Medallion Laboratories, Minneapolis, Minn.														
Dairy Queen														
Frozen Dessert	113	180	5	27	6	20	100	0.09	0.17	X	—	0.6	X	—
DQ Cone, small	71	110	3	18	3	10	100	0.03	0.14	X	—	0.4	X	X
DQ Cone, regular	142	230	6	35	7	20	300	0.09	0.26	X	—	0.6	X	X
DQ Cone, large	213	340	10	52	10	30	400	0.15	0.43	X	—	1.2	X	8
DQ Dip Cone, small	78	150	3	20	7	10	100	0.03	0.17	X	—	0.4	X	X
DQ Dip Cone, regular	156	300	7	40	13	20	300	0.09	0.34	X	—	0.6	X	X
DQ Dip Cone, large	234	450	10	58	20	30	400	0.12	0.51	X	—	0.9	X	8
DQ Sundae, small	106	170	4	30	4	15	100	0.03	0.17	X	—	0.5	X	X
DQ Sundae, regular	177	290	6	51	7	20	300	0.06	0.26	X	—	0.6	X	X
DQ Sundae, large	248	400	9	71	9	30	400	0.09	0.43	0.4	—	1.2	X	8
DQ Malt, small	241	340	10	51	11	30	400	0.06	0.34	0.4	—	1.2	2.4	60
DQ Malt, regular	418	600	15	89	20	50	750	0.12	0.60	0.8	—	1.8	3.6	100
DQ Malt, large	588	840	22	125	28	70	750	0.15	0.85	1.2	—	2.4	6	140
DQ Float	397	330	6	59	8	20	100	0.12	0.17	X	—	0.6	X	X
DQ Banana Split	383	540	10	91	15	30	750	0.60	0.60	0.8	—	0.9	18	X
DQ Parfait	284	460	10	81	11	30	400	0.12	0.43	0.4	—	1.2	X	8
DQ Freeze	397	520	11	89	13	35	200	0.15	0.34	X	—	1.2	X	X
Mr. Misty Freeze	411	500	10	87	12	35	200	0.15	0.34	X	—	0.12	X	X
Mr. Misty Float	404	440	6	85	8	20	100	0.12	0.17	X	—	0.6	X	X
"Dilly" Bar	85	240	4	22	15	10	100	0.06	0.17	X	—	0.5	X	X
DQ Sandwich	60	140	3	24	4	10	100	0.03	0.14	0.4	—	0.2	X	X
Mr. Misty Kiss	89	70	0	17	0	0	X	X	X	X	—	X	X	X
Brazier Cheese Dog	113	330	15	24	19	—	—	—	0.18	3.3	0.07	1.22	—	23
Brazier Chili Dog	128	330	13	25	20	—	—	0.15	0.23	3.9	0.17	1.29	11.0	20
Brazier Dog	99	273	11	23	15	—	—	0.12	0.15	2.6	0.08	1.05	11.0	23
Fish Sandwich	170	400	20	41	17	—	tr	0.15	0.26	3.0	0.16	1.20	tr	40
Fish Sandwich w/Ch	177	440	24	39	21	—	100	0.15	0.26	3.0	0.16	1.50	tr	40
Super Brazier Dog	182	518	20	41	30	—	tr	0.42	0.44	7.0	0.17	2.09	14.0	44
Super Brazier Dog w/Ch	203	593	26	43	36	—	—	0.43	0.48	8.1	0.18	2.34	14.0	44
Super Brazier Chili Dog	210	555	23	42	33	—	—	0.42	0.48	8.8	0.27	2.67	18.0	32
Brazier Fries, small	71	200	2	25	10	—	tr	0.06	tr	0.8	0.16	—	3.6	16
Brazier Fries, large	113	320	3	40	16	—	tr	0.09	0.03	1.2	0.30	—	4.8	24
Brazier Onion Rings	85	300	6	33	17	—	tr	0.09	tr	0.4	0.08	—	2.4	8
From International Dairy Queen, Inc., Minneapolis, Minn. Nutritional analysis by Raltech Scientific Services, Inc. (formerly WARF), Madison, Wis. (Nutritional analysis														
Jack-in-the-Box														
Hamburger	97	263	13	29	11	26	49	0.27	0.18	5.6	0.11	0.73	1.1	20
Cheeseburger	109	310	16	28	15	32	338	0.27	0.21	5.4	0.12	0.87	<1.1	20
Jumbo Jack Hamburger	246	551	28	45	29	80	246	0.47	0.34	11.6	0.30	2.68	3.7	42
Jumbo Jack Hamburger w/Ch	272	628	32	45	35	110	734	0.52	0.38	11.3	0.31	3.05	4.9	41
Regular Taco	83	189	8	15	11	22	356	0.07	0.08	1.8	0.14	0.5	<0.9	6
Super Taco	146	285	12	20	17	37	599	0.10	0.12	2.8	0.22	0.77	1.6	9
Moby Jack Sandwich	141	455	17	38	26	56	240	0.30	0.21	4.5	0.12	1.1	1.4	24
Breakfast Jack Sandwich	121	301	18	28	13	182	442	0.41	0.47	5.1	0.14	1.1	3.4	51
French Fries	80	270	3	31	15	13	—	0.12	0.02	1.9	0.22	0.17	3.7	<1
Onion Rings	85	351	5	32	23	24	—	0.24	0.12	3.1	0.07	0.26	<1.2	<1
Apple Turnover	119	411	4	45	24	17	—	0.23	0.12	2.5	0.03	0.17	<1.2	1
Vanilla Shake*	317	317	10	57	6	26	—	0.16	0.38	0.5	0.20	1.36	<3.2	41
Strawberry Shake*	328	323	11	55	7	26	—	0.16	0.46	0.6	0.15	1.25	<3.3	43
Chocolate Shake*	322	325	11	55	7	26	—	0.16	0.64	0.6	0.19	1.55	<3.2	45
Vanilla Shake	314	342	10	54	9	36	440	0.16	0.47	0.5	0.18	1.1	3.5	44
Strawberry Shake	328	380	11	63	10	33	426	0.16	0.62	0.5	0.18	0.92	<3.3	30
Chocolate Shake	317	365	11	59	10	35	380	0.16	0.60	0.6	0.18	0.98	<3.2	38

	Minerals							Moisture (g)	Crude Fiber (g)
Ca (mg)	Cu (mg)	Fe (mg)	K (mg)	Mg (mg)	P (mg)	Na (mg)	Zn (mg)		
94	—	1.00	186	—	—	498	—	45	0.10
15	—	1.3	206	—	—	475	—	48	0.20
150	—	X	—	—	100	—	—	—	—
100	—	X	—	—	60	—	—	—	—
200	—	X	—	—	150	—	—	—	—
300	—	X	—	—	200	—	—	—	—
100	—	X	—	—	80	—	—	—	—
200	—	0.4	—	—	150	—	—	—	—
300	—	0.4	—	—	200	—	—	—	—
100	—	0.7	—	—	100	—	—	—	—
200	—	1.1	—	—	150	—	—	—	—
300	—	1.8	—	—	250	—	—	—	—
300	—	1.8	—	—	200	—	—	—	—
500	—	3.6	—	—	400	—	—	—	—
600	—	5.4	—	—	600	—	—	—	—
200	—	X	—	—	200	—	—	—	—
350	—	1.8	—	—	250	—	—	—	—
300	—	1.8	—	—	250	—	—	—	—
300	—	X	—	—	250	—	—	—	—
300	—	X	—	—	200	—	—	—	—
200	—	X	—	—	200	—	—	—	—
100	—	0.4	—	—	100	—	—	—	—
60	—	0.4	—	—	60	—	—	—	—
X	—	X	—	—	X	—	—	—	—
168	0.08	1.6	—	24	182	—	1.9	—	—
86	0.13	2.0	—	38	139	939	1.8	—	—
75	0.79	1.5	—	21	104	868	1.4	—	—
60	0.08	1.1	—	24	200	—	0.3	—	—
150	0.08	0.4	—	24	250	—	0.3	—	—
158	0.18	4.3	—	37	195	1552	2.8	—	—
297	0.18	4.4	—	42	312	1986	3.5	—	—
158	0.21	4.0	—	48	231	1640	2.8	—	—
tr	0.04	0.4	—	16	100	—	tr	—	—
tr	0.08	0.4	—	24	150	—	0.3	—	—
20	0.08	0.4	—	16	60	—	0.3	—	—

not applicable in the state of Texas.)

82	0.10	2.3	165	20	115	566	1.8	43	0.2
172	0.10	2.6	177	22	194	877	2.3	47	0.2
134	0.22	4.5	492	44	261	1134	4.2	139	0.7
273	0.24	4.6	499	49	411	1666	4.8	153	0.8
116	0.11	1.2	264	36	150	460	1.3	47	0.6
196	0.18	1.9	415	53	235	968	2.1	92	1.0
167	0.08	1.7	246	30	263	837	1.1	57	0.1
177	0.11	2.5	190	24	310	1037	1.8	59	0.1
19	0.10	0.7	423	27	88	128	0.3	29	0.6
26	0.07	1.4	109	16	69	318	0.4	24	0.3
11	0.06	1.4	69	10	33	352	0.2	45	0.2
349	0.06	0.2	599	38	312	229	1.0	243	0.3
371	0.10	0.6	613	40	328	241	1.1	253	0.3
348	0.13	0.7	676	53	328	270	1.1	247	0.3
349	0.06	0.4	536	48	318	263	1.0	238	0.3
351	0.07	0.3	556	47	316	268	1.0	242	0.3
350	0.16	1.2	633	57	332	294	1.2	235	0.3

	Wt (g)	Energy (kcal)	PRO (g)	CHO (g)	Fat (g)	Chol (mg)	Vitamins							
							A (IU)	B_1 (mg)	B_2 (mg)	Nia. (mg)	B_6 (mg)	B_{12} (μg)	C (mg)	D (IU)
Ham & Cheese Omelette	174	425	21	32	23	355	766	0.45	0.70	3.0	0.18	1.44	<1.7	64
Double Cheese Omelette	166	423	19	30	25	370	797	0.33	0.68	2.5	0.14	1.33	1.7	61
Ranchero Style Omelette	196	414	20	33	23	343	853	0.33	0.74	2.6	0.18	1.51	<2.0	78
French Toast	180	537	15	54	29	115	522	0.56	0.30	4.4	0.47	1.62	9.2	22
Pancakes	232	626	16	79	27	87	488	0.63	0.44	4.6	0.19	0.56	<26.2	23
Scrambled Eggs	267	719	26	55	44	259	694	0.69	0.56	5.2	0.34	1.31	<12.8	80

*Special formula for shakes sold in California, Arizona, Texas and Washington. From Jack-in-the-Box, Foodmaker, Inc. San Diego, Calif. Nutritional analysis by Raltech

Kentucky Fried Chicken

Original Recipe Dinner

	Wt (g)	Energy (kcal)	PRO (g)	CHO (g)	Fat (g)	Chol (mg)	A (IU)	B_1 (mg)	B_2 (mg)	Nia. (mg)	B_6 (mg)	B_{12} (μg)	C (mg)	D (IU)
Wing & Rib	322	603	30	48	32	133	25.5	0.22	0.19	10.0	—	—	36.6	—
Wing & Thigh	341	661	33	48	38	172	25.5	0.24	0.27	8.4	—	—	36.6	—
Drum & Thigh	346	643	35	46	35	180	25.5	0.25	0.32	8.5	—	—	36.6	—
Extra Crispy Dinner*														
Wing & Rib	349	755	33	60	43	132	25.5	0.31	0.29	10.4	—	—	36.6	—
Wing & Thigh	371	812	36	58	48	176	25.5	0.31	0.35	10.3	—	—	36.6	—
Drum & Thigh	376	765	38	55	44	183	25.5	0.32	0.38	10.4	—	—	36.6	—
Mashed Potatoes	85	64	2	12	1	0	<18	<0.01	0.02	0.8	—	—	4.9	—
Gravy	14	23	0	1	2	0	<3	0.00	0.01	0.1	—	—	<0.2	—
Cole Slaw	91	122	1	13	8	7	—	—	—	—	—	—	—	
Rolls	21	61	2	11	1	1	<5	0.10	0.04	1.0	—	—	0.3	—
Corn (5.5-in ear)	135	169	5	31	3	X	162	0.12	0.07	1.2	—	—	2.6	—

*Includes two pieces of chicken, mashed potato and gravy, cole slaw, and roll. From Kentucky Fried Chicken, Inc. Louisville, Ky. Nutritional analysis by Raltech Scientific

Long John Silver's

	Wt (g)	Energy (kcal)	PRO (g)	CHO (g)	Fat (g)	Chol (mg)	A (IU)	B_1 (mg)	B_2 (mg)	Nia. (mg)	B_6 (mg)	B_{12} (μg)	C (mg)	D (IU)
Fish w/Batter (2 pc)	136	366	22	21	22	—	—	—	—	—	—	—	—	—
Fish w/Batter (3 pc)	207	549	32	32	32	—	—	—	—	—	—	—	—	—
Treasure Chest	143	506	30	32	33	—	—	—	—	—	—	—	—	—
Chicken Planks (4 pc)	166	457	27	35	23	—	—	—	—	—	—	—	—	—
Peg Legs w/Batter (5 pc)	125	350	22	26	28	—	—	—	—	—	—	—	—	—
Ocean Scallops (6 pc)	120	283	11	30	13	—	—	—	—	—	—	—	—	—
Shrimp w/Batter (6 pc)	88	268	8	30	13	—	—	—	—	—	—	—	—	—
Breaded Oysters (6 pc)	156	441	13	53	19	—	—	—	—	—	—	—	—	—
Breaded Clams	142	617	18	61	34	—	—	—	—	—	—	—	—	—
Fish Sandwich	193	337	22	49	31	—	—	—	—	—	—	—	—	—
French Fryes	85	288	4	33	16	—	—	—	—	—	—	—	—	—
Cole Slaw	113	138	1	16	8	—	—	—	—	—	—	—	—	—
Corn on the Cob (1 ear)	150	176	5	29	4	—	—	—	—	—	—	—	—	—
Hushpuppies (3)	45	153	3	20	7	—	—	—	—	—	—	—	—	—
Clam Chowder (8 oz)	170	107	5	15	3	—	—	—	—	—	—	—	—	—

From Long John Silver's Food Shoppes, Lexington, Ky. Nutritional analysis by L.V. Packett, PhD., The Department of Nutrition and Food Science, University of Kentucky.

McDonald's

	Wt (g)	Energy (kcal)	PRO (g)	CHO (g)	Fat (g)	Chol (mg)	A (IU)	B_1 (mg)	B_2 (mg)	Nia. (mg)	B_6 (mg)	B_{12} (μg)	C (mg)	D (IU)
Egg McMuffin	138	327	19	31	.15	229	97	0.47	0.44	3.8	0.21	0.75	<1.4	46
English Muffin, Buttered	63	186	5	30	5	13	164	0.28	0.49	2.6	0.04	0.02	0.8	14
Hotcakes w/Butter & Syrup	214	500	8	94	10	47	257	0.26	0.36	2.3	0.12	0.19	4.7	5
Sausage (Pork)	53	206	9	tr	19	43	<32	0.27	0.11	2.1	0.18	0.53	0.5	31
Scrambled Eggs	98	180	13	3	13	349	652	0.08	0.47	0.2	0.19	0.93	1.2	65
Hashbrown Potatoes	55	125	2	14	7	7	<14	0.06	<0.01	0.8	0.13	0.01	4.1	<1
Big Mac	204	563	26	41	33	86	530	0.39	0.37	6.5	0.27	1.8	2.2	33
Cheeseburger	115	307	15	30	14	37	345	0.25	0.23	3.8	0.12	0.91	1.6	13
Hamburger	102	255	12	30	10	25	82	0.25	0.18	4.0	0.12	0.81	1.7	12
Quarter Pounder	166	424	24	33	22	67	133	0.32	0.28	6.5	0.27	1.88	<1.7	23
Quarter Pounder w/Ch	194	524	30	32	31	96	660	0.31	0.37	7.4	0.23	2.15	2.7	25
Filet-O-Fish	139	432	14	37	25	47	42	0.26	0.20	2.6	0.10	0.82	<1.4	25
Regular Fries	68	220	3	26	12	9	<17	0.12	0.02	2.3	0.22	<0.03	12.5	<1
Apple Pie	85	253	2	29	14	12	<34	0.02	0.02	0.2	0.02	<0.04	<0.8	2
Cherry Pie	88	260	2	32	14	13	114	0.03	0.02	0.4	0.02	<0.02	<0.8	<2
McDonaldland Cookies	67	308	4	49	11	10	<27	0.23	0.23	2.9	0.03	0.03	0.9	10
Chocolate Shake	291	383	10	66	9	30	349	0.12	0.44	0.5	0.13	1.16	<2.9	44
Strawberry Shake	290	362	9	62	9	32	377	0.12	0.44	0.4	0.14	1.16	4.1	32
Vanilla Shake	291	352	9	60	8	31	349	0.12	0.70	0.3	0.12	1.19	3.2	26

		Minerals							Crude
Ca (mg)	Cu (mg)	Fe (mg)	K (mg)	Mg (mg)	P (mg)	Na (mg)	Zn (mg)	Moisture (g)	Fiber (g)
260	0.14	4.0	237	29	397	975	2.3	94	0.2
276	0.13	3.6	208	26	370	899	2.1	88	0.2
278	0.14	3.8	260	29	372	1098	2.0	117	0.4
119	0.11	3.0	194	27	256	1130	1.8	78	0.9
105	0.12	2.8	237	36	633	1670	1.9	104	0.7
257	0.24	5.0	635	55	483	1110	3.0	137	1.3

Scientific Services, Inc. (formerly WARF), Madison, Wis.

—	—	—	—	—	—	—	—	—	—
—	—	—	—	—	—	—	—	—	—
—	—	—	—	—	—	—	—	—	—
—	—	—	—	—	—	—	—	—	—
—	—	—	—	—	—	—	—	—	—
—	—	—	—	—	—	—	—	—	—
—	—	—	—	—	—	—	—	—	—
—	—	—	—	—	—	—	—	—	—
—	—	—	—	—	—	—	—	—	—
—	—	—	—	—	—	—	—	—	—
—	—	—	—	—	—	—	—	—	—

Services, Inc. (formerly WARF). Madison, Wis.

—	—	—	—	—	—	—	—	—	—
—	—	—	—	—	—	—	—	—	—
—	—	—	—	—	—	—	—	—	—
—	—	—	—	—	—	—	—	—	—
—	—	—	—	—	—	—	—	—	—
—	—	—	—	—	—	—	—	—	—
—	—	—	—	—	—	—	—	—	—
—	—	—	—	—	—	—	—	—	—
—	—	—	—	—	—	—	—	—	—
—	—	—	—	—	—	—	—	—	—
—	—	—	—	—	—	—	—	—	—
—	—	—	—	—	—	—	—	—	—
—	—	—	—	—	—	—	—	—	—
—	—	—	—	—	—	—	—	—	—
—	—	—	—	—	—	—	—	—	—
—	—	—	—	—	—	—	—	—	—
—	—	—	—	—	—	—	—	—	—

226	0.12	2.9	168	26	322	885	1.9	70.7	0.1
117	0.69	1.5	71	13	74	318	0.5	21.7	0.1
103	0.11	2.2	187	28	501	1070	0.7	97.8	0.2
16	0.05	0.8	127	9	95	615	1.5	22.9	0.1
61	0.06	2.5	135	13	264	205	1.7	68.1	<0.1
5	0.04	0.4	247	13	67	325	0.2	30.9	0.3
157	0.18	4.0	237	38	314	1010	4.7	100.4	0.6
132	0.11	2.4	156	23	205	767	2.6	108.4	0.2
51	0.10	2.3	142	19	126	520	2.1	48.0	0.3
63	0.17	4.1	322	37	249	735	5.1	83.7	0.7
219	0.18	4.3	341	41	382	1236	5.7	96.0	0.8
93	0.10	1.7	150	27	229	781	0.9	59.5	0.1
9	0.03	0.6	564	27	101	109	0.3	25.4	0.5
14	0.05	0.6	39	6	27	398	0.2	38.3	0.3
12	0.06	0.6	35	7	27	427	0.2	38.9	0.1
12	0.07	1.5	52	11	74	358	0.3	2.2	0.1
320	0.19	0.8	580	49	335	300	1.4	203.0	0.3
322	0.07	0.2	423	31	313	207	1.2	207.9	<0.3
329	0.09	0.2	422	31	314	201	1.2	211.3	<0.3

	Wt (g)	Energy (kcal)	PRO (g)	CHO (g)	Fat (g)	Chol (mg)	Vitamins							
							A (IU)	B$_1$ (mg)	B$_2$ (mg)	Nia. (mg)	B$_6$ (mg)	B$_{12}$ (μg)	C (mg)	D (IU)
Hot Fudge Sundae	164	310	7	46	11	18	230	0.07	0.31	1.1	0.13	0.7	2.5	16
Caramel Sundae	165	328	7	53	10	26	279	0.07	0.31	1.0	0.05	0.6	3.6	14
Strawberry Sundae	164	289	7	46	9	20	230	0.07	0.30	1.0	0.05	0.6	2.8	16

From McDonald's Corporation, Oak Brook, Ill. Nutritional analysis by Raltech Scientific Services, Inc. (formerly WARF), Madison, Wis.

Taco Bell

	Wt (g)	Energy (kcal)	PRO (g)	CHO (g)	Fat (g)	Chol (mg)	A (IU)	B$_1$ (mg)	B$_2$ (mg)	Nia. (mg)	B$_6$ (mg)	B$_{12}$ (μg)	C (mg)	D (IU)
Bean Burrito	166	343	11	48	12	—	1657	0.37	0.22	2.2	—	—	15.2	—
Beef Burrito	184	466	30	37	21	—	1675	0.30	0.39	7.0	—	—	15.2	—
Beefy Tostada	184	291	19	21	15	—	3450	0.16	0.27	3.3	—	—	12.7	—
Bellbeefer	123	221	15	23	7	—	2961	0.15	0.20	3.7	—	—	10.0	—
Bellbeefer w/Ch	137	278	19	23	12	—	3146	0.16	0.27	3.7	—	—	10.0	—
Burrito Supreme	225	457	21	43	22	—	3462	0.33	0.35	4.7	—	—	16.0	—
Combination Burrito	175	404	21	43	16	—	1666	0.34	0.31	4.6	—	—	15.2	—
Enchirito	207	454	25	42	21	—	1178	0.31	0.37	4.7	—	—	9.5	—
Pintos'N Cheese	158	168	11	21	5	—	3123	0.26	0.16	0.9	—	—	9.3	—
Taco	83	186	15	14	8	—	120	0.09	0.16	2.9	—	—	0.2	—
Tostada	138	179	9	25	6	—	3152	0.18	0.15	0.8	—	—	9.7	—

From (menu item portions) San Antonio, Tex.: Taco Bell Co., July 1976; Adams C.F.: Nutritive value of American foods in common units, in *Handbook No. 456.* H.N., eds.: Food values of portions commonly used, ed. 12, Philadelphia, 1975, J.B. Lippincott Co.; Valley Baptist Medical Center. Food Service Department: Descriptions

Wendy's

	Wt (g)	Energy (kcal)	PRO (g)	CHO (g)	Fat (g)	Chol (mg)	A (IU)	B$_1$ (mg)	B$_2$ (mg)	Nia. (mg)	B$_6$ (mg)	B$_{12}$ (μg)	C (mg)	D (IU)
Single Hamburger	200	470	26	34	26	70	94	0.24	0.36	5.8	—	—	0.6	—
Double Hamburger	285	670	44	34	40	125	128	0.43	0.54	10.6	—	—	1.5	—
Triple Hamburger	360	850	65	33	51	205	220	0.47	0.68	14.7	—	—	2.0	—
Single w/Ch	240	580	33	34	34	90	221	0.38	0.43	6.3	—	—	0.7	—
Double w/Ch	325	800	50	41	48	155	439	0.49	0.75	11.4	—	—	2.3	—
Triple w/Ch	400	1040	72	35	68	225	472	0.80	0.84	15.1	—	—	3.4	—
Chili	250	230	19	21	8	25	1188	0.22	0.25	3.4	—	—	2.9	—
French Fries	120	330	5	41	16	5	40	0.14	0.07	3.0	—	—	6.4	—
Frosty	250	390	9	54	16	45	355	0.20	0.60	X	O	X	0.7	—

From Wendy's International, Inc. Dublin, Ohio. Nutritional analysis by Medallion Laboratories, Minneapolis, Minn.

	Wt (g)	Energy (kcal)	PRO (g)	CHO (g)	Fat (g)	Chol (mg)	Vitamins							
							A (IU)	B$_1$ (mg)	B$_2$ (mg)	Nia. (mg)	B$_6$ (mg)	B$_{12}$ (μg)	C (mg)	D (IU)
Beverages														
Coffee*	180	2	tr	tr	tr	—	0	0	tr	0.5	—	—	0	—
Tea*	180	2	tr	—	tr	—	0	0	0.04	0.1	—	—	1	—
Orange Juice	183	82	1	20	tr	—	366	0.17	0.02	0.6	—	—	82.4	—
Chocolate Milk	250	213	9	28	9	—	330	0.08	0.40	0.3	—	—	3.0	—
Skim Milk	245	88	9	13	tr	—	10	0.09	0.44	0.2	—	—	2.0	—
Whole Milk	244	159	9	12	9	27	342	0.07	0.41	0.2	—	—	2.4	100
Coca-Cola	246	96	0	24	0	—	—	—	—	—	—	—	—	—
Fanta Ginger Ale	244	84	0	21	0	—	—	—	—	—	—	—	—	—
Fanta Grape	247	114	0	29	0	—	—	—	—	—	—	—	—	—
Fanta Orange	248	117	0	30	0	—	—	—	—	—	—	—	—	—
Fanta Root Beer	246	103	0	27	0	—	—	—	—	—	—	—	—	—
Mr. Pibb	245	95	0	25	0	—	—	—	—	—	—	—	—	—
Mr. Pibb w/o Sugar	236	1	0	tr	0	—	—	—	—	—	—	—	—	—
Sprite	245	95	0	24	0	—	—	—	—	—	—	—	—	—
Sprite w/o Sugar	236	3	0	0	0	—	—	—	—	—	—	—	—	—
Tab	236	tr	0	tr	0	—	—	—	—	—	—	—	—	—
Fresca	236	2	0	0	0	—	—	—	—	—	—	—	—	—

From Adams, C.F.: Nutritive value of American foods in common units, in *Handbook No. 456.* Washington: U.S.D.A. Agricultural Research *American Hospital Formulary Service,* Washington, D.C., American Society of Hospital Pharmacists, Section 28:20, March 1978.
*6 oz serving; all other data are for 8 oz serving.
†Caffeine content depends on strength of beverage.
‡Value when bottling water with average sodium content (12 mg/8 oz) is used.

| Minerals | | | | | | | | | Crude |
Ca (mg)	Cu (mg)	Fe (mg)	K (mg)	Mg (mg)	P (mg)	Na (mg)	Zn (mg)	Moisture (g)	Fiber (g)
215	0.13	0.6	410	35	236	175	1.0	97.9	0.2
200	0.09	0.2	338	30	230	195	0.9	93.2	<0.2
174	0.11	0.4	290	28	80	96	0.8	101.0	0.2
98	—	2.8	235	—	173	272	—	—	—
83	—	4.6	320	—	288	327	—	—	—
208	—	3.4	277	—	265	138	—	—	—
40	—	2.6	183	—	140	231	—	—	—
147	—	2.7	195	—	208	330	—	—	—
121	—	3.8	350	—	245	367	—	—	—
91	—	3.7	278	—	230	300	—	—	—
259	—	3.8	491	—	338	1175	—	—	—
150	—	2.3	307	—	210	102	—	—	—
120	—	2.5	143	—	175	79	—	—	—
191	—	2.3	172	—	186	101	—	—	—

Washington USDA. Agricultural Research Service. November 1975; Church, E.F., and Church, of Mexican-American Foods. Fort Atkinson, Wis., NASCO.

Ca (mg)	Cu (mg)	Fe (mg)	K (mg)	Mg (mg)	P (mg)	Na (mg)	Zn (mg)	Moisture (g)	Crude Fiber (g)
84	—	5.3	—	—	239	774	4.8	110.6	0.8
138	—	8.2	—	—	364	980	8.4	162.1	1.1
104	—	10.7	—	—	525	1217	13.5	204.6	1.4
228	—	5.4	—	—	315	1085	5.5	133.4	1.0
177	—	10.2	—	—	489	1414	10.1	179.2	1.3
371	—	10.9	—	—	712	1848	14.3	216.4	1.6
83	—	4.4	—	—	168	1065	3.7	195.9	2.3
16	—	1.2	—	—	196	112	0.5	54.9	1.2
270	—	0.9	—	—	278	247	1.0	169.8	0.0

| Minerals | | | | | | | | | |
Ca (mg)	Cu (mg)	Fe (mg)	K (mg)	Mg (mg)	P (mg)	Na (mg)	Zn (mg)	Caffeine (mg)	Sacchar. (mg)
4	—	0.2	65	—	7	2	—	100†	0
5	—	0.2	—	—	4	—	—	40†	0
17	—	0.2	340	18	29	2	—	0	0
278	—	0.5	365	—	235	118	—	—	0
296	—	0.1	355	—	233	127	—	—	0
188	—	tr	351	32	227	122	—	—	0
—	—	—	—	—	40	20‡	—	28	0
—	—	—	—	—	0	30‡	—	0	0
—	—	—	—	—	0	21‡	—	0	0
—	—	—	—	—	0	21‡	—	0	0
—	—	—	—	—	29	23‡	—	27	0
—	—	—	—	—	28	37‡	—	38	76
—	—	—	—	—	0	42‡	—	0	0
—	—	—	—	—	0	42‡	—	0	57
—	—	—	—	—	30	30‡	—	30	74
—	—	—	—	—	0	38	—	0	54

Service, November 1975; The Coca-Cola Company, Atlanta, Ga., Jan. 1977;

H

Food Guide: Exchange Lists for Meal Planning

The *exchange system of dietary control,* developed by professional organizations such as the American Dietetic Association, is based on a simple grouping of common foods according to generally equivalent nutritional values. This system may be used for any situation requiring caloric and food value control.

The foods are divided into six basic groups (some with subgroups), called the "exchange groups" (pp. 402-403). Each food item within a group or subgroup contains approximately the same food value as any other food item in that group, allowing for exchange within groups, thus providing for variety in food choices as well as food value control. Hence the term *food exchanges* is used to refer to food choices or servings. The total number of exchanges per day depends on individual nutritional needs, based on normal nutritional standards. Although there is some variation in the composition of foods within the exchange groups, for simplicity the following values for carbohydrate, protein, fat, and calories are used.

Food	Approximate Measure	Carbohydrate (g)	Protein (g)	Fat (g)	Calories
Milk	1 cup				
A (skimmed)		12	8	trace	90
B (low fat)		12	8	5	120
C (whole)		12	8	8	150
Vegetable	½ cup	5	2	—	25
Fruit	Varies	15	—	—	60
Starch/Bread	1 slice	15	3	trace	80
Meat	28 g (1 oz)				
A (lean)		—	7	3	55
B (medium fat)		—	7	5	75
C (high fat)		—	7	8	100
Fat	1 tsp	—	—	5	45

List 1: Milk exchanges (Cream portion of whole milk equals two fat exchanges. Hence 1 cup whole milk equals 1 cup skim milk plus two fat exchanges.)

Group A (nonfat)	
Skim or nonfat milk	1 cup
Buttermilk	1 cup
Canned, evaporated skim milk	½ cup
Powdered, nonfat dry milk (before adding liquid)	⅓ cup
Yogurt made from skim milk (plain, unflavored)	1 cup
Group B (low fat)	
Low-fat milk (2% butterfat)	1 cup
Yogurt made from low-fat milk (plain, unflavored)	1 cup

Food	Approximate Measure	Carbohydrate (g)	Protein (g)	Fat (g)	Calories
Group C (full fat)					
Whole milk	1 cup				
Canned, evaporated whole milk	½ cup				
Powdered, whole dry milk (before adding liquid)	⅓ cup				
Yogurt made from whole milk (plain, unflavored)	1 cup				

List 2: Vegetable exchanges (As served plain, without fat, seasoning, or dressing. Any fat used is taken from the fat exchange allowance.)
(One exchange equals ½ cup)

Artichoke	Green pepper, chili pepper	Pimientos
Asparagus	Greens	Rhubarb
Bok choy, gai choy	Beet	Rutabagas
Bamboo shoots	Chard	Sauerkraut
Bean sprouts	Collards	String beans: green, yellow, wax
Beets	Dandelion	Summer squash
Broccoli	Kale	Tomato juice
Brussels sprouts	Mustard	Tomatoes
Cabbage	Spinach	Turnips
Carrots	Turnip	Vegetable juice, mixed
Cauliflower	Mushrooms	Zucchini
Celery	Okra	
Cucumber	Onions	
Eggplant		

Vegetables for use as desired: chicory, Chinese cabbage, endive, escarole, lettuce, parsley, radishes, and watercress. For starchy vegetables, see List 4.

List 3: Fruit exchanges (Unsweetened: fresh, frozen, canned, cooked. One exchange is the portion indicated by the fruit.)

Berries		*Other fruits*	
Blackberries	½ cup	Apple	1 small
Blueberries	½ cup	Apple cider	⅓ cup
Raspberries	½ cup	Apple juice	⅓ cup
Strawberries	¾ cup	Applesauce	½ cup
Citrus fruits		Apricots	2 medium
Grapefruit	½ small	Banana	½ small
Grapefruit juice	½ cup	Cherries	10 large, 17 small
Orange	1 small	Fig	1 large
Orange juice	½ cup	Fruit cocktail	½ cup
Tangerine	1 medium	Grape juice	¼ cup
Melons		Grapes	10 medium
Cantaloupe	¼ medium	Kiwi fruit	1 medium
Honeydew	⅛ medium	Mango	½ small
Watermelon	1 cup diced (approx. ½ center slice)	Nectarine	1 small
		Papaya	⅓ medium, ½ small
Dried fruits		Peach	1 medium
Apricots	4 halves	Pear	1 medium
Dates	2 medium	Persimmon	1 medium
Figs	1 medium	Pineapple	½ cup; 1 round center slice
Peaches	2 halves		
Pears	2 halves	Pineapple juice	⅓ cup
Prunes	2 medium	Plums	2 medium
Raisins	2 tbsp	Prune juice	¼ cup
		Prunes, fresh	2 medium

Food	Approximate Measure	Carbohydrate (g)	Protein (g)	Fat (g)	Calories

List 4: Bread exchanges (Equivalent portions indicated by each item.)

Bread

Food	Approximate Measure
Bagel	½
Bread (loaf, average size slice)	1 slice
French	
Italian	
Pumpernickel	
Raisin	
Rye	
White	
Whole wheat	
Bread crumbs, dried	3 tbsp
English muffin	½
Hamburger bun	½
Roll, frankfurter	1
Roll, plain	1 small
Tortilla (6 inches diameter)	1

Cereal

Food	Approximate Measure
Bulgur, cooked	½ cup
Cereal, cooked	½
Cereal, dry (ready-to-eat, unsweetened)	
Bran flakes	½ cup
Grape nuts	¼ cup
Other (flake, puff)	¾ cup
Cornmeal, dry	2 tbsp
Flour	2½ tbsp
Grits, cooked	½ cup
Pasta, cooked (spaghetti, noodles, macaroni)	½ cup
Popcorn (popped, no fat)	1½ cup
Rice, cooked	½ cup
Wheat germ, plain	3 tbsp

Crackers

Food	Approximate Measure
Arrowroot	3
Graham, 2½-in square	2
Matzoth, 4 × 6 in	1
Oyster crackers	20
Pretzels, 3⅛ × ⅛ in	25
Round butter type crackers	6
Rye wafers, 2 × 3½ in	3
Saltines	5
Soda crackers, 2½-in square	3

Dried beans, peas, lentils

Food	Approximate Measure
Beans, peas, lentils (dried and cooked)	⅓ cup
Baked beans, no pork	¼ cup

Starchy vegetables

Food	Calories
Corn	⅓ cup
Corn on the cob (6-in ear)	½ ear
Lima beans	½ cup
Parsnips	½ cup
Peas, green	½ cup
Potato, white	1 small
Potato, white mashed	½ cup
Pumpkin	1 cup
Sweet potato	½ small; ⅓ cup
Winter squash (acorn, butternut, banana)	½ cup
Yam	½ small; ⅓ cup

Prepared foods

Food	Calories
Angel food cake (1½-in cube or small slice)	1 slice
Biscuit, 2-in diameter (omit 1 fat exchange)	1
Chips, potato or corn (omit 2 fat exchanges)	15
Corn muffin, 2-in diameter (omit 1 fat exchange)	1
Cornbread, 2 × 2 × 1¼ in (omit 1 fat exchange)	1 square
Crepe, 6-in diameter (omit 1 fat exchange)	1
Ice milk, ½ cup scoop (omit 1 fat exchange)	1 scoop
Muffin, plain, 2-in diameter (omit 1 fat exchange)	1
Pancakes, 4-in diameter (omit 1 fat exchange)	1
Potatoes, french fried (length 2-3 in; omit 1 fat exchange)	8 pieces
Sherbet, fruit ice, ½-cup scoop	1 scoop
Waffle, 4-in diameter (omit 1 fat exchange)	1

List 5: Meat exchanges

Food	Approximate Measure	Carbohydrate (g)	Protein (g)	Fat (g)	Calories
Group A (lean)					
I. Lean meats, less tissue fat					
Fish (any fresh or frozen)	28 g (1 oz)				
Canned salmon, tuna, mackerel	¼ cup				
Sardines, drained	3				
Shellfish					
Clams, oysters, scallops	5				
Crab, lobster	¼ cup				
Poultry (no skin)	28 g				
Chicken, turkey, cornish hen, guinea hen, pheasant					
Veal (any lean trimmed cut)	28 g				
II. Lean meats, more tissue fat					
Beef	28 g				
Very lean young beef; chipped beef; lean cuts of chuck, flank steak, tender loin, plate ribs and skirt steak, round (top, bottom), rump, spare ribs, tripe					
Lamb	28 g				
Lean cuts: leg, rib, sirloin, loin (roast, chops), shank, shoulder					
Pork	28 g				
Lean cuts of leg (rump, center shank), ham (smoked center cut)					
III. Cheese	28 g				
Cottage cheese	¼ cup				
Dry curd					
Low fat, partially re-creamed					
Other cheeses	28 g				
Less than 5% butterfat; partially skim milk					
Group B (medium fat)					
Beef	28 g				
Ground (15% fat), corned beef (canned)					
Pork	28 g				
Loin (roast, chops), shoulder arm (picnic), shoulder blade, Boston butt, Canadian bacon, boiled ham					
Cheese	28 g				
Mozzarella, ricotta, Swiss, Jack, farmer's cheese, Neufchâtel					
Parmesan	3 tbsp				
Cottage cheese, re-creamed	¼ cup				
Cholesterol foods					
Egg	1				
Organ meats	28 g				
Liver, kidney, sweetbreads, heart					
Shrimp	5 large				
Other					
Peanut butter (omit 2 fat exchanges)	2 tbsp				
Tofu	98 g (3½ oz)				
Group C (high fat)					
Beef	28 g				
Brisket (fresh or corned), ground (20% or more fat)					
Lamb breast	28 g				
Pork	28 g				
Spare ribs, back ribs, ground pork, sausage, country style ham, deviled ham					
Cheese, cheddar types	28 g				
Cold cuts	1 slice				
Frankfurter	1 small				
Poultry	28 g				
Capon duck, goose					

Food	Approximate Measure	Carbohydrate (g)	Protein (g)	Fat (g)	Calories
List 6: Fat exchanges					
Group A (polyunsaturated plant fats)					
Margarine,* soft (stick or tub)	1 tsp				
Mocha mix (cream substitute)	2 tbsp				
Salad dressings*					
French	1 tbsp				
Italian	1 tbsp				
Mayonnaise	1 tsp				
Seeds (sunflower, sesame, pumpkin)	1 tbsp				
Vegetable oils (safflower, corn, soy, cottonseed, sesame)	1 tsp				
Walnuts	4-5 halves				
Group B (monounsaturated plant fats)					
Avocado	⅛				
Nuts					
Almonds	10 whole				
Peanuts	20 whole				
Pecans	2 whole				
Olives	5 small				
Vegetable oils (olive, peanut)	1 tsp				
Group C (saturated animal fats)					
Butter	1 tsp				
Cheese spreads	1 tbsp				
Cream					
Half & Half (10% cream)	2 tbsp				
Light (20% cream)	2 tbsp				
Heavy (40% cream)	1 tbsp				
Sour (light)	2 tbsp				
Cream cheese	1 tbsp				
Pork fat					
Bacon crisp	1 strip				
Bacon fat	1 tsp				
Lard	1 tsp				
Salt pork	¾-in cube				

Miscellaneous foods allowed as desired (negligible carbohydrate, protein, fat)

Artificial sweeteners, as permitted
Bouillon, broth, clear fat free
Catsup, mustard, horseradish, meat sauce
Coffee, tea
Cranberries, cranberry juice (unsweetened)
Garlic

Gelatin, plain or D-Zerta
Herbs and spices
Lemon, lime
Pickles, dill and sour
Salt and pepper
Vinegar

*Made with safflower, corn, soy, cottonseed oil.

I

Calculation Aids and Conversion Tables

More than 185 years ago a group of French scientists set up the metric system of weights and measures. Today, with refinements over years of use, it is called the "Systeme International" (SI). In 1975 our American Congress passed the Metric Conversion Act, which provides for conversion of our customary British/American system to the simpler metric system used by the rest of the world. We are now in the midst of this conversion, as evidenced by distance signs along highways and labels on many packaged foods in supermarkets. Here are a few conversion factors to help you make these transitions in your necessary calculations.

Metric System of Measurement

Like our money system, this is a simple decimal system based on units of 10. It is uniform and used internationally.

Weight units: 1 kilogram (kg) = 1000 grams (gm or g)
1 g = 1000 milligrams (mg)
1 mg = 1000 micrograms (mcg or µg)

Length units: 1 meter (m) = 100 centimeters (cm)
1000 meters = 1 kilometer (km)

Volume units: 1 liter (L) = 1000 millimeters (ml)
1 milliliter = 1 cubic centimeter (cc)

Temperature units: Celsius (C) scale, based on 100 equal units between 0° C (freezing point of water) and 100° C (boiling point of water); this scale is used entirely in all scientific work.

Energy units: Kilocalorie (kcal) = Amount of energy required to raise
1 kg water 1° C
Kilojoule (kJ) = Amount of energy required to move
1 kg mass 1 m by a force of 1 newton
1 kcal = 4.184 kJ

In 1970 the American Institute of Nutrition's Committee on Nomenclature recommended that the term *kilojoule* (kJ) replace the kilocalorie (kcal). This change is gradually coming about.

British/American System of Measurement

Our customary system is a confusion of units with no uniform relationships. It is not a decimal system, but rather a jumbled collection of different units collected in usage and language over time. It is used mainly in America.

Weight units: 1 pound (lb) = 16 ounces (oz)
Length units: 1 foot (ft) = 12 inches (in)
1 yard (yd) = 3 feet (ft)
Volume units: 3 teaspoons (tsp) = 1 tablespoon (tbsp)
16 tbsp = 1 cup
1 cup = 8 fluid ounces (fl oz)
4 cups = 1 quart (qt)
5 cups = 1 imperial quart (qt), Canada

Approximate Metric
Conversions

When You Know	Multiply by	To Find
Weight		
Ounces	28	Grams
Pounds	0.45	Kilograms
Length		
Inches	2.5	Centimeters
Feet	30	Centimeters
Yards	0.9	Meters
Miles	1.6	Kilometers
Volume		
Teaspoons	5	Millimeters
Tablespoons	15	Millimeters
Fluid ounces	30	Millimeters
Cups	0.24	Liters
Pints	0.47	Liters
Quarts	0.95	Liters
Temperature		
Fahrenheit temperature	5/9 (after subtracting 32)	Celsius temperature

British/American System of Measurement, cont'd

Temperature units: Fahrenheit (F) scale, based on 180 equals units between 32° F (freezing point of water) and 212° F (boiling point of water) at standard atmospheric pressure

Conversions between Measurement Systems

Weight: 1 oz = 28.35 g (usually used as 28 or 30 g)
2.2 lb = 1 kg
Length: 1 in = 2.54 cm
1 ft = 30.48 cm
39.37 in = 1 m
Volume: 1.06 qt = 1 L
0.85 imperial qt = 1 L (Canada)

Temperature:		
Boiling point of water	100° C	212° F
Body temperature	37° C	98.6° F
Freezing point of water	0° C	32° F

Interconversion formulas:

$$\text{Fahrenheit temperature (°F)} = \tfrac{9}{5}° \text{C} + 32$$
$$\text{Celsius temperature (°C)} = \tfrac{5}{9} (°\text{F} - 32)$$

Retinol Equivalents

The following definitions and equivalences that are internationally agreed on provide a basis for calculating retinol equivalent conversions.

Definitions International units (IU) and retinol equivalents (RE) are defined as follows:

$$1 \text{ IU} = 0.3 \text{ } \mu\text{g retinol (0.0003 mg)}$$
$$1 \text{ IU} = 0.6 \text{ } \mu\text{g beta-carotene (0.0006 mg)}$$
$$1 \text{ RE} = 6 \text{ } \mu\text{g retinol}$$
$$1 \text{ RE} = 6 \text{ } \mu\text{g beta-carotene}$$
$$1 \text{ RE} = 12 \text{ } \mu\text{g other provitamin A carotenoids}$$
$$1 \text{ RE} = 3.33 \text{ IU retinol}$$
$$1 \text{ RE} = 10 \text{ IU beta-carotene}$$

Conversion formulas On the basis of weight beta-carotene is ½ as active as retinol; on the basis of structure the other provitamin carotenoids are ¼ as active as retinol. In addition, retinol is more completely absorbed in the intestine, whereas the provitamin carotenoids are much less well utilized, with an average absorption of about ⅓. Therefore in overall activity beta-carotene is ⅙ as active as retinol, and the other carotenoids are ¹⁄₁₂ as active. These differences in utilization provide the basis for the 1:6:12 relationship shown in the equivalences given and in the following formulas for calculating retinol equivalents from values of vitamin A, beta-carotene, and other active carotenoids, expressed either as international units or micrograms:

If retinol and beta-carotene are given in micrograms:
Micrograms of retinol + (Micrograms of beta-carotene ÷ 6) = RE
If both are given as IU:
International units of retinol ÷ 3.33) + (International units of beta-carotene ÷ 10) = RE
If beta-carotene and other carotenoids are given in micrograms:
(Micrograms of beta-carotene ÷ 6) + (Micrograms of other carotenoids ÷ 12) = RE

Glossary

Pronunciation Key

ə	banana, collect
ˈə, ˌə	humdrum
ə̄	as in one pronunciation used by *r*-droppers for bird (alternative \əi\)
ə̇	two-value symbol equivalent to the unstressed variants \ə\, \i\, as in habit, duchess (\ˈhabə̇t\ = \ˈhabət, -bit\)
ᵊ	immediately preceding \l\, \n\, \m\, \ŋ\, as in battle, mitten, and in one pronunciation of cap **and** bells \-ᵊam-\, lock **and** key \-ᵊŋ-\; immediately following \l\, \m\, \r\, as in one pronunciation of French table, prisme, titre
əi	as in one pronunciation used by *r*-droppers for bird (alternative \ə̄\)
ər	operation; stressed, as in bird as pronounced by speakers who do not drop *r;* stressed and with centered period after the \r\, as in one pronunciation of burry (alternative \ə̄r\) and in one pronunciation of hurry (alternative \ə·r\); stressed and with centered period between \ə\ and \r\, as in one pronunciation of hurry (alternative \ər·\)
a	mat, map
ā	day, fade, date, aorta
ä	bother, cot; most American speakers have the same vowel in father, cart
ȧ	father as pronounced by speakers who do not rhyme it with bother; farther and cart as pronounced by *r*-droppers
aa	bad, bag, fan as often pronounced in an area having New York City and Washington, D.C., on its perimeter; in an emphatic syllable, as before a pause, often \aaə\
ai	as in some pronunciations of bag, bang, pass
au̇	now, loud, some pronunciations of talcum
b	baby, rib
ch	chin, nature \ˈnāchə(r)\ (actually, this sound is \t\ + \sh\)
d	elder, undone
d·	as in the usual American pronunciation of latter, ladder
e	bet, bed
ˈē, ˌē	beat, nosebleed, evenly, sleepy
ē	as in one pronunciation of evenly, sleepy, envious, igneous (alternative \i\)
ee	(in transcriptions of foreign words only) indicates a vowel with the quality of *e* in *bet* but long, not the sound of *ee* in *sleep: en arrière* \äⁿ nȧryeer\
eu̇	as in one pronunciation of elk, helm
f	fifty, cuff
g	go, big
h	hat, ahead
hw	whale as pronounced by those who do not have the same pronunciation for both *whale* and *wall*
i	tip, one pronunciation of banish (alternative unstressed \ē\), one pronunciation of habit (alternative \ə\; see ə̇)
ī	site, side, buy (actually, this sound is \ä\ + \i\, or \ȧ\ + \i\)
iu̇	as in one pronunciation of milk, film
\	slant line used in pairs to mark the beginning and end of a transcription: \ˈpen\
ˈ	mark preceding a syllable with primary (strongest) stress: \ˈpenmən,ship\
ˌ	mark preceding a syllable with secondary (next-strongest) stress: \ˈpenmən,ship\
ˈˌ	combined marks preceding a syllable whose stress varies between primary and secondary: *backbone* \ˈ=ˈˌ=\
˗	inferior minus sign canceling a stress in the same position in a preceding pronunciation or emphasizing that a following syllable is without stress: *optimism* \ˈäptə,mizəm\, *optimist* \-˗mə̇st\
·	mark of syllable division inserted in a sequence of sounds that can have more than one syllable division: *nitrate* \nī·,trāt\
(), (	indicate that what is symbolized between or after is present in some utterances but not in others: *factory* \ˈfakt(ə)rē\, *bar* \ˈbär, ˈbȧ(r\

The system of indicating pronunciation is used by permission from Webster's Third New International Dictionary ©1981 by Merriam-Webster, Inc., publisher of the Merriam-Webster® Dictionaries.

j	**j**ob, **g**em, ed**g**e, procedure \prə'sējə(r)\ (actually, this sound is \d\ + \zh\)
k	**k**in, coo**k**, a**ch**e
k̲	as in one pronunciation of lo**ch** (alternative \k\), as in German i**ch**-laut
l	**l**i**l**y, poo**l**
m	**m**ur**m**ur, di**m**, ny**m**ph
n	**n**o, ow**n**
ŋ	si**ng** \'siŋ\, si**ng**er \'siŋə(r)\, fi**ng**er \'fiŋgə(r)\, i**nk** \'iŋk\
ō	b**o**ne, sn**ow**, b**eau**; one pronunciation of gl**o**ry
ȯ	s**aw**, **a**ll, s**au**rian; one pronunciation of h**o**rrid
œ	French b**oeu**f, German H**ö**lle
œ̄	French f**eu**, German H**ö**hle
ȯi	c**oi**n, destr**oy**, straw**y**, saw**i**ng
o̅o̅	(in transcriptions of foreign words only) indicates a vowel with the quality of o in *bone* but longer, not the sound of oo in *food: comte* \koo^{n}t\
p	**p**e**pp**er, li**p**
r	**r**a**r**ity, one pronunciation of ta**r**
s	**s**ource, le**ss**
sh	with nothing between, as in **sh**y, mi**ss**ion, ma**ch**ine, spe**ci**al (actually, this is a single sound, not two); with a stress mark between, two sounds as in death'**s-h**ead \'deths,hed\
t	**t**ie, a**tt**ack; one pronunciation of la**tt**er (alternative \d·\)
th	with nothing between, as in **th**in, ei**th**er (actually, this is a single sound, not two); with a stress mark between, two sounds as in knig**ht-h**ood \'nīt,hu̇d\
t̲h̲	**th**en, ei**th**er (actually, this is a single sound, not two)
ü	r**u**le, f**oo**l, y**ou**th, union \'yünyən\, few \'fyü\
u̇	p**u**ll, w**oo**d, curable \'kyu̇rəbəl\
ue	German f**ü**llen, h**ü**bsch
u̅e̅	French r**u**e, German, f**ü**hlen
v	**v**i**v**id, gi**v**e
w	**w**e, a**w**ay
y	**y**ard, cue \'kyü\, union \'yünyən\
ʸ	(in transcriptions of foreign words only) indicates that during the articulation of the sound represented by the preceding character the tip of the tongue has substantially the position it has for the articulation of the first sound of *yard*, as in French *digne*\dēn^y\
yü	**y**outh, **u**nion, c**ue**, few
yu̇	c**u**rable
z	**z**one, rai**s**e
zh	with nothing between, as in vi**s**ion, a**z**ure \'azhə(r)\ (actually, this is a single sound, not two); with a stress mark between, two sounds as in ro**s-eh**ill \'rōz,hil\
|	facilitates the placement of a variant pronunciation: *flightily*\'flīd·|ᵊlē, -īt|, |ᵊli, |ᵻi-\

Absorption \əb'sȯrpshən\ (L. *ab*, away; *sorbere*, to suck in) Process by which digested food materials pass through the epithelial cells of the alimentary canal (mainly of the small intestine) into the blood or lymph.

Acetone \'asə,tōn\ (*acetic*, sour; *ketone*) A by-product of the breakdown of fats for energy. It builds up when the body's glycogen stores are depleted, which happens when carbohydrate is not available for fuel. High urine levels are one sign of poor diabetes control.

Acetylation \ə,se·ᵊ|'āshən\ Key reaction in cell metabolism, introduction of the monovalent acetyl group (—CH_3CO) into an organic compound.

Acetyl-CoA \ə'sēd·ᵊl\ (acetylcoenzyme A) (L. *acetum*, vinegar; Gr. *hyle*, matter; Gr. *en*, in; Gr. *zyme*, leaven) Chief precursor of lipids, an important intermediate in the Kreb's cycle; formed by an acetyl group attaching itself to coenzyme A during the oxidation of amino acids, fatty acids, or pyruvate.

Achlorhydria \|ā,klȯr'hīdrēə\ (Gr. *a*-, without; *chlorohydria*, excess gastric hydrochloric acid) Lack of hydrochloric acid (HCl) secretion in the stomach.

Acid \'asȧd\ (L. *acidus*, sour) Substance that neutralizes base substances by donating H ions. Acids are essentially ionized hydrogen donors—in solution they provide H ions.

Acidosis \,asə'dōsȧs\ Disturbance in acid-base balance in which there is a reduction of the alkali reserve. Acidosis may be caused by an accumulation of acids, as in diabetic acidosis, or by an excess loss of bicarbonate, as in renal disease.

Acinus \'asənəs\ *pl.* acini (L. *acinus*, grape) Groups of secretory cells in glands such as the salivary glands, the pancreas, and the liver. These organized clusters of cells are called acini because their shape resembles that of a bunch of grapes. Their secretions of enzymes and bile feed into the ducts that empty into the gastrointestinal lumen.

Actin \'aktȧn\ Myofibril protein that acts with myosin to cause the contraction and relaxation of muscle.

Active transport \aktiv tranz'pō(ə)rt\ Movement of solutes in solution (for example, products of digestion such as glucose) across a membrane *against* the usual opposing forces. Such movement requires energy, which is supplied by the cell. Sometimes an additional transporting substance is required, such as sodium, for absorbing glucose.

Acute renal failure \ə'kyüt 'rēn³l 'fālyə(r)\ Total shutdown of renal function; requires emergency treatment.

Adenocarcinoma \|ad³n(,)o,kärs³n'ōmə\ Cancer derived from glandular tissue or in which tumor cells form recognizable glandular structures; may be classified according to predominant pattern of cell arrangement.

Adenosine triphosphate (ATP) \ə'denə,sēn (')trī'fä,sfāt\ A compound of adenosine (a nucleotide containing adenine and ribose) that has three phosphoric acid groups. ATP is a high-energy phosphate compound important in energy exchange for cellular activity. The splitting off of the terminal phosphate bond (PO_4) of ATP to produce adenosine diphosphate (ADP) releases bound energy and transfers it to free energy available for body work. The reforming of ATP in cell oxidation again stores energy in high-energy phosphate bonds for use as needed. They may be considered to act as biologic storage batteries that can be charged and discharged according to conditions in the cell.

Adipocytes Fat cells.

Adipose \'adə,pōs\ (L. *adeps*, fat; *adiposus*, fatty) Fat present in cells of adipose—fatty—tissue.

Adrenergic \,adrə¦nərjik\ Activated by or secreting adrenal hormones such as epinephrine or similar acting substances; characteristic of such substances.

Adrenocorticotropic hormone (ACTH) Anterior pituitary hormone; stimulates secretion of glucocorticoids from the adrenal cortex; insulin antagonist.

Adult beriberi \ə'dəlt¦berē'berē\ Typically occurs in young adults in reaction to added physiologic stress such as pregnancy or lactation.

Aerobic \'a(ə)¦rōbik\ (Gr., L., *aer*, air or gas) Requiring oxygen to proceed.

Ageism \'ā(,)jizəm\ Discrimination on the basis of age, usually applying to older persons.

Aldosterone \al'dästə,rōn\ Potent hormone of the cortox of the adrenal glands, which acts on the distal renal tubule to cause reabsorption of sodium in an ion exchange with potassium. The aldosterone mechanism is essentially a sodium-conserving mechanism but indirectly also conserves water since water absorption follows the sodium reabsorption.

Alkalosis \,alkə'lōsəs\ Disturbance in acid-base balance in which there is a reduction of the acid partner in the buffer system or an increase in the base. In either case, the necessary 20:1 ratio between base and acid is upset by an increase in the relative amount of base.

Alpha-lipoprotein \'alfə ,līpə'prō,tēn\ High-density lipoprotein (HDL) that carries cholesterol to the liver to be excreted.

Alpha-tocopherol equivalent (αTE) \¦alfə tə'käfə,ròl ə'kwiv(ə)lənt\ Standard unit of measurement (in mg) for designating vitamin E requirements, since potencies of the other members of the vitamin E group vary; a change from the former measure of international units (IU) for greater precision and clarity.

Alveolus \al'vē'ə-ləs\ *pl.* alveoli (L., *alveus*, hollow) Small, dilated, saclike structures in the lungs; point of oxygen and carbon dioxide gas exchange during respiration.

Alzheimer's disease \'älts,hīmə(r)z də'zēz\ Named for a German neurologist, Alois Alzheimer; a form of senile dementia that may occur in middle as well as in old age.

Ameloblasts \'aməlō,blast\ (Old Fr. *amel*, enamel; Gr. *blastos*, germ) Special epithelial cells surrounding tooth buds in gum tissue that form cup-shaped organs for producing the enamel structure of the developing teeth. Insufficient vitamin A causes faulty production of ameloblasts, and it therefore impairs the soundness of the tooth structure.

Amino acid \ə'mē(,)nō 'asəd\ These compounds form the structural units of protein. Out of a total of 20 or more, 10 are considered dietary essentials, indispensable to life (see *essential amino acid*). The term *amino* represents the presence of the NH_2 group—a base. The various food proteins, when digested, yield their specific constituent amino acids. These amino acids are then available for use by the cells as the cells synthesize specific tissue proteins.

Amphoteric \,amfə¦terik\ (Gr. *amphoteros*, both) Having properties of both an acid and a base and therefore able to function as either. Amino acids have this dual chemical nature because of their structure—they contain both an acid (carboxyl, COOH) and a base (amino, NH_2) group.

Ampulla \am-pu'ə\ (L., "a jug") Flasklike dilation (stretched part) of a tubular structure.

Amylopectin \,amə(,)lō'pektən\ (Gr. *amylon*, starch; *pektos*, congealed) Polysaccharide, the insoluble part of starch, forms a paste with hot water and thickens during cooking.

Amylose \'amᵊ,lōs\ (Gr. *amylon*, starch; *-ose*, sugar) Simple single sugar; a carbohydrate containing a single saccharide (sugar) unit.

Amyotropic lateral sclerosis \'ā·mīə'trōpik 'lad·ərəl sklə'rōsəs\ Muscular weakness and atrophy in the arm and hands caused by damage to motor neurons. Deterioration continues without remission.

Anabolism \ə'nabə,lizəm\ (Gr. *anabole*, a building up) Constructive metabolic processes that build up the body substances; the synthesis in living organisms of more complex substances from simpler ones. Anabolism *uses* energy; available energy generated by catabolic processes is taken up in forming the chemical bonds that unite the components of the increasingly complex molecules as they are developed in the anabolic processes. Anabolism is the opposite of catabolism.

Anachronism \ə'nakrə,nizəm\ (Gr. *anachronismos*, a wrong time reference) Thing placed or occurring out of its proper time; an obsolete or archaic form.

Anaerobic \,anə¦rōbik\ (*an*, negative; Gr. *aer*, air) Not requiring oxygen to function.

Analog \'anᵊl,òg\ (or *analogue*) Gr. *analogos*, due ratio, proportionate) In chemistry, a compound having a similar structure to that of another but differing in a particular component.

Analysis \ənəl'əsis\ (Gr. *ana*, so much of each; *lysis*, dissolve) Study of phenomena—things, events, etc.—by separating them into their component parts.

Anemia \ə'nēmēə\ Blood condition characterized by decrease in number of circulating red blood cells, hemoglobin, or both.

Anergy \'a,nərjē\ (*an*-negative + G. *ergon*, work) Abnormal diminished reaction or sensitivity to specific antigens; often occurs in debilitated malnourished persons. A measure of degree of function of body's immune system.

Angina pectoris \an'jīnə 'pektərəs\ Chest pain, usually radiating down the arm, with a feeling of suffocation; caused most often by lack of oxygen to the heart muscle (myocardium), sometimes precipitated by effort or excitement.

Angiotensin \,anjēōtensin\ (Gr. *angeion, vessel;* L. *tensio,* stretching, pressure) Pressor substance produced in the body by interaction of the enzyme renin, produced by the renal cortex, and a serum globulin fraction, angiotensinogen, produced by the liver. Successive products are formed by the interaction—angiotensin I and II. Angiotensin II is the active pressure substance that increases arterial muscle tone and triggers the production of aldosterone by the adrenal gland. Angiotensin I and II therefore are key products in the cycle of the aldosterone mechanism.

Anion \'a͟ͅnīən\ an ion that carries a negative electric charge.

Anorexia nervosa \͵anō'reksēə (')ner'vōsə\ (Gr. want of appetite; *nervosa*, nervous) Psychologic condition manifested by a refusal to eat to achieve a thin—usually abnormally thin—appearance.

Antagonist \an·'tagə͵ nə̇st\ A substance that counteracts the action of another substance. The antagonist prevents the normal action because its molecular structure is so like that of the first substance that it *almost* fits into the first substance's position in a metabolic process. It gets in the way and prevents the reaction from taking place.

Anthropometry \͵an͵ (t)thrə'pämətrē\ Science of measuring size, weight, and proportions of the human body.

Antibody \'antə͵ bädē\ Animal protein made up of a specific sequence of amino acids that is designed to interact with a specific *antigen* during an allergic response or to prevent infection.

Antidiuretic hormone (ADH) \͵an͵ tə͆ diyə͵ red·ik 'hȯr'mōn\ Secreted by the posterior pituitary gland in response to body stress. It acts on the renal tubules, chiefly the distal tubule, to cause reabsorption of water. The ADH mechanism is the body's primary water-conserving mechanism and is therefore essential to life; see also *vasopressin*.

Antigen \'antə̇jən\ (*antibody* + Gr. *gennan*, to produce) Any substance that stimulates the production of an antibody specifically designed to interact with it. Examples of antibodies include toxins, bacteria, and foreign proteins.

Antinutrient \͵antə̇'n(y)ütrēənt\ (Gr. *anti-*, against) Substance acting to block normal utilization of a nutrient.

Antioxidant \'an(͵)tī͆ äksadənt\ A substance added to a product to delay or prevent its breakdown by oxygen.

Anuria \ə'n(y)u̇rēa\ (*an*, negative + Gr. *ouron*, urine + -ia) Complete lack of urine secretion by the kidneys; also known as *anuresis*.

Apo- \͵apō'\ (Gr. *apo*, from) Prefix implying separation or derivation.

Apoferritin \͵apə'ferət°n\ (Gr. *apo*, away, separation; L. *ferr*, iron) Protein base in intestinal mucosa cells, which will bind with iron (from food) to form ferritin, the storage form of iron.

Apoprotein \͵apō'protein\ Protein part of a compound, as of a lipoprotein. For example, apoprotein C II, an apoprotein of HDL and VLDL that functions to activate the enzyme lipoprotein lipase.

Ariboflavinosis \͵ā͵ rībə͵ flāvə'nōsə̇s\ Group of clinical manifestations of riboflavin deficiency.

Arteriosclerosis \är͵ tirēə(͵)ōskləṙōsə̇s\ (*artery* + Gr. *skleros*, hard) Group of cardiovascular diseases, the major one of which is atherosclerosis: characterized by a thickening of the arterial walls and their loss of elasticity.

Ascites \ə'sīd·ēz\ (Gr. *askites*, from; *askos*, bag) Outflow and accumulation of fluid in the abdominal cavity; also known as *abdominal* or *peritoneal dropsy*.

Asterixis \astərixəs\ (*a*, negative + Gr. *sterixis*, a fixed position) Motor disturbance marked by a temporary lapse of an assumed position; result of a sustained contraction in a group of muscles.

Atheroma \͵athə'rōmə\ Characteristic lesion of atherosclerosis; tumor-type growths on inside lining of blood vessels, composed of lipid material (largely cholesterol) and cellular debris.

Atherosclerosis \͵athə(͵)rōsklȯ'rōsə̇s\ (Gr. *athere*, gruel, *sklerosis*, hardness) Condition in which yellowish plaques (atheromas) are deposited within the medium and large arteries.

Atrophy \'a·trəfē\ (Gr. *atrophia*) Wasting away; reduced size of a cell, tissue, or organ.

Azotemia \͵azə'tēmēə\ (Gr. *a*, without; *zoe*, life) Term meaning nitrogen, referring to an excess of urea and other nitrogenous substances in the blood.

Bacteriuria \(͵)bak͵ tirē'yu̇rēa\ (*bacteria* + Gr. *ouron*, urine + -ia) Presence of bacteria in the urine.

Basal ganglion \'bāsəl͆ gangleon\ *pl.* ganglia (basal = base; Gr. *ganglion*, knot) Group of nerve cells found deep in the cerebral hemispheres of the brain and in the upper brainstem.

Basal metabolic rate (BMR) \'bāsəl med·ə͆ bälik 'rāt\ Rate of internal chemical activity of resting tissue.

Basal metabolism \'bāsəl mə'tabə͵ lizəm\ (Gr. *basis*, base; *metabole*, change) The amount of energy needed by the body for maintenance of life when the person is at digestive, physical, and emotional rest. The amount of oxygen consumed at rest is used as a measure of the basal energy requirements and is expressed as kilocalories per sq. meter of body surface per hour. This basal metabolic rate (BMR) is reported as the percent of variation in the person above or below the normal number of kilocalories required for a person of like height, weight, and sex.

Base \'bās\ Chemical substance that is capable of neutralizing acid by accepting hydrogen ions from the acid. A synonymous term is *alkali*.

Base bicarbonate \͵bās (')bī'kärbə͵ nāt\ "Base" in this term refers to *any* base that might be combined with bicarbonate. In the main buffer system of the human body, this base is sodium bicarbonate.

Beikost \'bīkȯst\ (Ger.) Solid and semisolid baby foods.

Benign \bə'nīn\ Not malignant or recurring.

Beriberi \͵berē'berē\ (Singhalese "I cannot, I cannot") A disease of the peripheral nerves caused by a deficiency of thiamin (vitamin B_1). It is characterized by pain (neuritis) and paralysis of the extremities, cardiovascular changes and edema. Beriberi is common in the Orient, where diets consist largely of milled rice with little protein.

Bile \'bīl\ (L. *bilis*) Greenish yellow to golden brown alkaline fluid secreted by the liver and concentrated in the gallbladder, made of bile salts, cholesterol, phospholipid, bilirubin diglucuronide, and electrolytes. Bile salts are essential in the digestion and absorption of fat in the small intestine.

Bioavailability \bī(͵)ōə'vālə'biləd·ē\ Degree to which the amount of a nutrient ingested actually gets absorbed and is available to the body.

Bioflavonoid \͵bīō'flāvə͵ nȯid\ (L. *flavus*, yellow) Compounds that are widely distributed in nature as pigments in flowers, fruits, tree barks, vegetables, and grains. They have been found to have little nutritional value, and thus are not considered essential nutrients.

Biologic activity \͵bīə͆ läjik ak'tivəd·ē\ Degree of effect in an organism of a specific vitamin; a means of measuring required amount of a vitamin to prevent a deficiency.

Blastocyst \'blastō͵ sist\ (Gr. *blastos*, bud, sprout; *kystis*, bag, bladder) Early developmental stage of the embryo; consists of a single layer of cells surrounding a central area.

Blood urea nitrogen (BUN) \'blod yə'rēə 'nī·trəjən\ Blood test used to identify any disorder in kidney function.

Body composition \ˌbädē ˌkämpə'zishən\ Determined by how much of the body weight is fat, and how much is lean body mass.

Bolus \'bōləs\ (Gr. *bolos*, lump) Rounded mass of food that is ready to be swallowed.

Bone compartment \'bōn kəm'pärtmənt\ Body's total content of skeletal tissue. The bone compartment contains 99% of the body's total metabolic calcium pool.

Bowman's capsule \'bōmənz 'kapsəl\ (after Sir William Bowman, British physician, 1816-1892) Cupped membrane surrounding the glomerulus; site of cell-free filtrate formation.

Bradykinin \ˌbrādəˈkīnən\ (Gr. *bradys*, slow; *kinein*, to move) Kinin (member of a group of endogenous peptides that cause vasodilation, increase blood pressure, and induce contraction of smooth muscle) formed from kallidin II by the action of the enzyme kallikrein. It is a very powerful vasodilator; increases capillary permeability, constricts smooth muscle, and stimulates pain receptors.

Brittle diabetes \'brid·ᵊl ˌdīə'bēd·ēz\ A form of type I diabetes, which is difficult to control and is sensitive to hypoglycemia and acidosis.

Brunner's glands \'br'unə(r)z 'gland\ Mucus-secreting glands in the duodenum that provide mucus to protect the mucosa from irritation and erosion by the strongly acid gastric juices entering from the stomach. Emotional tension and stress inhibit these mucous secretions—a primary factor in duodenal ulcer formation.

Buffer \'bəfə(r)\ Mixture of acidic and alkaline components that, when added to a solution, is able to protect the solution against wide variations in its pH, even when strong acids and bases are added to it. If an acid is added, the alkaline partner reacts with it to counteract its acidic effect. If a base is added, the acid partner reacts with it to counteract its alkalizing effect. A solution to which a buffer has been added is called a buffered solution.

Buffer capacity \'bəfə(r) kə'pasəd·ē\ Substance capable of serving as a buffer to excess acid or base materials entering the body.

Bulimia \byü'limēə\ (Gr. *bous*, ox; *limos*, hunger) Abnormal increase in the sensation of hunger; a clinical gorge-purge syndrome associated with anorexia nervosa.

Cachexia \ka'keksēə\ (Gr. *kakos*, bad; *hexis*, habit; + -ia) A specific profound effect caused by a disturbance in glucose metabolism usually seen in cancer patients (see p. 756); general poor health and malnutrition usually indicated by an emaciated appearance.

Calcitonin \ˌkalsə'tōnən\ Quick-acting hormone secreted by the C cells of the parathyroids in response to hypercalcemia; acts to induce hypocalcemia.

Calcium to phosphorus ratio (Ca:P) \'kalsēəm 'fäsf(a)rəs 'rā,shō\ Inverse ratio affecting the absorption rate of each mineral. The *dietary ratio* of 1:1 is ideal for periods of rapid growth, 1:1.5 for normal adult functions. The normal *serum ratio* for adults is 40 (10 mg/dl calcium × 4 mg/dl calcium phosphorus), and for children is 50 (10 mg/dl × 5 mg/dl phosphorus).

Calculus \'kalkyələs\ *pl.* calculi (L. *pebble*.) Any abnormal accretion within the body of material that forms a "stone." Calculi are usually composed of mineral salts.

Callus \'kaləs\ (L. *kalus*) Unorganized meshwork of newly grown, woven bone developed on pattern of original fibrin clot (formed after fracture) and normally replaced by hard

Calorie \'kal(ə)rē\ (L. *calor*, heat) A measure of heat. The *energy* required to do the work of the body is measured as the amount of *heat* produced by the body's work. The energy value of food is expressed as the number of kilocalories a specified portion of that food will yield when oxidized, either in the body or on being burned. Physicists use several different standard calories in investigative work. The calorie commonly used in metabolic studies and dietetic studies is the large calorie or kilocalorie (kcal), which is the amount of heat required to raise 1 kg of water 1° C.

Calorimetry \ˌkalə'rimə·trē\ (L. *calor* heat; Gr. *metron*, measure) The measurement of heat loss. An instrument for measuring heat output of the body or the energy value of foods is called a calorimeter.

Cancer \'kan(t)sə(r)\ (L. "crab") Cellular tumor whose natural course is fatal. Unlike benign tumor cells, cancer growths are invasive and spread easily.

Candidiasis \ˌkandə'dīəsəs\ Superficial fungus infection (genus *Candida*) of moist parts of the body; infection of oral mucous membranes is *thrush*.

Capillary fluid shift mechanism \'kapə,lerē 'flüəd 'shift 'mekə·nizəm\ Process that controls the movement of water and small molecules in solution (electrolytes, nutrients) between the blood in the capillary and the surrounding interstitial area. Filtration of water and solutes out of the capillary at the arteriole end and reabsorption at the venule end are accomplished by shifts in balance between the intracapillary hydrostatic blood pressure and the colloidal osmotic pressure exerted by the plasma proteins.

Carbonic acid \'kärbənik ásəd\ Acid partner in the carbonic acid–base bicarbonate buffer system in the body.

Carboxypeptidase \(ˌ)kär,bäksē'peptə,dās\ Pancreatic enzyme that acts in protein digestion in the small intestine; it breaks the peptide bond of terminal amino acids having a free carboxyl (COOH) group.

Carcinoma \ˌkärsᵊn'ōmə\ Gr. *karkinos*, crab) Tumor, usually malignant, arising from epithelial tissue.

Cardiac arrhythmia \'kärdē,ak ā'rithmēə\ Irregular heart beat. Often caused by nutritional or hormonal imbalances that affect the heart muscle's ability to contract.

Cardiac output \'kärdē,ak 'aù,pùt\ (Gr. *kardia*, heart) Volume of blood propelled from the heart with each contraction; also called *stroke volume*.

Cardiac rate \'kärdē,ak 'rāt\ Number of heart beats per minute; pulse rate.

Carpodedal spasm \ˌkärpəˌpedᵊl 'spasəm\ (Gr. *karpos*, L. *capus*, wrist; L. *pedalis*, foot) tonic contracture of the hands and feet.

Catabolism \kə'tabə,lizəm\ (Gr. *katabole*, a throwing down) The breaking-down phase of metabolism, the opposite of anabolism. Catabolism includes all the processes in which complex substances are progressively broken down into simpler ones. Catabolism usually involves the release of energy. Together, anabolism and catabolism constitute metabolism, which is the coordinated operation of anabolic and catabolic processes into a dynamic balance of energy and substance.

Catecholamine \\,kad·ə¦kōlə¦mēn\ (*catechol,* aromatic chemical substance; *amine,* organic compound containing nitrogen) Group of compounds having similar effects to those of the sympathetic nervous system; includes dopamine, norepinephrine, and epinephrine.

Cation \\'kad·,īən\ Ion that carries a positive electric charge.

Celiac disease \\'sēlē,ak də'zēz\ Malabsorption syndrome brought on by eating gluten-rich foods (wheat, rye, barley, oats). Characterized by steatorrhea, distention, flatulence, weight loss, and malnutrition resulting from poor absorption associated with damage to the mucosal villi; may be a hereditary condition.

Cellular immunity \\'selyələr ə'myünəd·ē\ Specific, acquired immunity in which the role of the T lymphocytes predominates.

Cerebrovascular accident (CVA) \\sə'rēbrō'vaskyələ(r) 'aksədənt\ Stroke; brain tissue damage caused by reduced blood flow from arterial blockage or breakage; may result in *hemiplegia, hemiparesis,* or *hemianopsia.*

Ceruloplasmin \\sə'rülōplazmən\ Plasma protein containing copper-forming ferroxidase, an enzyme that oxidizes iron in preparation for its absorption.

Cheilosis \\kī'lōsəs\ Swelling and reddening of the lips. Chapped appearance. Fissures at corners of the mouth.

Chelate \\'kē,lāt\ (Gr. *chele,* claw) Chemical compound capable of grasping and incorporating a metallic ion into its molecular structure. By binding the metal, the chelate removes it from a tissue or from the circulating blood.

Chelating agent \\'kē,kātiŋ 'ājənt\ (Gr. *chele,* claw) Substance that combines with a metal, firmly binding it; chemotherapeutic use for metal poisoning.

Chemical bonding \\'kemə̇kəl 'bändiŋ\ Mutual attachment of various chemical elements to form chemical compounds. The chemical bonds that hold the elements of a compound together consist of stored potential energy. When the compound is broken up into parts, free energy is released to do the body's work.

Chemotherapy \\'kēmō'therapē\ Treatment of disease with chemicals that destroy unhealthy tissue.

Chief cells \\'chēf 'sels\ Special cells in the lining of the tubular gastric glands that secrete pepsinogen. Previously formed pepsin and hydrochloric acid in the stomach convert the inactive pepsinogen to the active enzyme pepsin, which begins the breakdown of protein to polypeptides.

Chloride-bicarbonate shift mechanism \\'klōr,id (')bī'kärbə, nāt 'shift 'mekə,nizəm\ Exchange of bicarbonate for chloride. In red blood cells, it provides constant bicarbonate buffering for the rapidly forming carbonic acid from water and carbon dioxide (H_2O + CO_2).

Cholecystitis \\'kōlə,si'stīd·ə̇s\ (Gr. *chole,* bile, gall; *kystis,* bladder) Inflammation of the gallbladder.

Cholecystokinin \\'kōlə,sistə,kīnən\ (Gr. *chole,* bile or gall; *kystis,* bladder, *kinein,* to move) A hormone that is secreted

by the mucosa of the duodenum in response to the presence of fat. The cholecystokinin causes the gallbladder to contract. This contraction propels bile into the duodenum, where it is needed to emulsify the fat. The fat is thus prepared for digestion and absorption.

Cholecystokinin mechanism \\'kōla,sistə'kīnən meka, nizəm\ Hormone secreted by mucosa of upper intestine that stimulates contraction of the gallbladder.

Cholelithiasis \\,kōlələ'thīəsə̇s\ (Gr. *chole,* bile, gall; *lithos,* stone) Formation of gallstones.

Cholera \\'kälərə\ Acute infectious disease characterized by severe diarrhea, acidosis, vomiting, muscle cramps, and prostration; associated with drinking contaminated water.

Cholestasis \\'kōlə'stāsə̇s\ (Gr. *chole,* bile; *stasis,* stoppage) Suppression or stoppage of the bile flow.

Cholesterol \\kə'lestər,ȯl\ A fat-related compound, a sterol ($C_{27}H_{45}OH$). It is a normal constituent of bile and a principal constituent of gallstones. In body metabolism cholesterol is important as a precursor of various steroid hormones such as sex hormones and adrenal corticoids. Cholesterol is synthesized by the liver. It is widely distributed in nature, especially in animal tissue such as glandular meats and egg yolk.

Cholestyramine \\'kə,lestirəmīn\ Drug that prevents cholesterol absorption by binding it in the gut.

Chorion frondosum \\'kōrē,än frän'dōsəm\ Fetal portion of the placenta. About 2 weeks after implantation occurs, villi develop at this site.

Chylomicron \\,kīlə'mī,krän\ (Gr. *chylos,* chyle; *mikros,* small) Particle of fat—lipoproteins—appearing in the lymph and blood after a meal rich in fat. These particles are composed largely of triglycerides with lesser amounts of phospholipids, cholesterol, cholesterol esters, and protein. About 2 to 3 hours after a fat meal, the chylomicrons cause lactescense (milkiness) in the blood plasma; this is termed *alimentary lipemia.*

Chyme \\'kīm\ (Gr. *chymos,* juice) Semifluid food mass in gastrointestinal tract following gastric digestion.

Chymotrypsin \\,kīmə'tripsən\ A protein-splitting (proteolytic) enzyme produced by the pancreas that acts in the intestine. Together with trypsin, it reduces proteins to shorter chain polypeptides and dipeptides.

Cis \\,sis\ (L. on the same side) Having certain atoms or radicals in a chemical structure on the same side.

Cisterna chyli \\sī'stərnə ¦kīlē\ Cistern or receptacle of the chyle is a dilated sac at the origin of the thoracic duct, which is the common truck that receives all the lymphatic vessels. The cisterna chyli lies in the abdomen between the second lumbar vertebra and the aorta. It receives the lymph from the intestinal trunk, the right and left lumbar lymphatic trunks, and two descending lymphatic trunks. The chyle, after passing through the cisterna chyli, is carried upward into the chest through the thoracic duct and empties into the venous blood at the point where the left subclavian vein joins the left internal jugular vein.

Clinical ecology \\'klinə̇kəl ē'käləjē\ Term used to indicate study and treatment of allergy and similar problems by attention to multiple environmental agents.

Coenzyme \(')kō'en,zīm\ (L. *co,* together; Gr. *en,* in; *zyme,* leaven). Enzyme activators required by some enzymes to produce their reactions. Coenzymes are diffusible, heat-stable substances of low molecular weight that combine with inactive proteins called apoenzymes. Each such combination of apoenzyme and coenzyme forms an active compound or a complete enzyme called a holoenzyme. A number of the B vitamins function as coenzymes in the energy-producing pathways in cell metabolism.

Collagen disease \'käləjən dəzēz\ Connective tissue diseases such as rheumatoid arthritis, scleroderma, lupus erythematosus, and others.

Colloid \'kä,lȯid\ (Gr. *kollodes,* glutinous) Glutinous, gluelike; a dispersion of matter throughout a medium.

Colloidal osmotic pressure (COP) \kə'lȯid°l (')äz¦mäd·ik 'preshə(r)\ Pressure produced by the protein molecules in the plasma and in the cell. Because proteins are large molecules, they do not pass through the separating membranes of the capillary cells. Thus they remain in their respective compartments, exerting a constant osmotic pull that protects vital plasma and cell fluid volumes in these compartments.

Compactin \'käm,paktin\ Drug that prevents cholesterol production in the liver by inhibiting enzyme activity.

Compartment \kəm'pärtmənt\ The collective quantity of material in a given type of tissue space in the body. For example, in speaking of body water, the physiologist calls all the water in the body that is outside of cells the extracellular fluid compartment (ECF); all the body water inside of cells is the intracellular fluid compartment (ICF).

Complement \'kämpləmənt\ Enzymatic protein that combines with the antigen-antibody complex, separating them when the antigen is an intact cell.

Complete protein \kəm'plēt 'prō,tēn\ A protein that contains the essential amino acids in quantities sufficient for maintenance of the body and for a normal rate of growth. Such proteins are said to have a high biologic value. Egg, milk, cheese, and meat are complete protein foods.

Concept \'kän,sept\ (L. *cum,* with *capere,* to seize) Combined ideas forming a whole.

Coronary \'kȯrə,nerē\ Referring to the arteries that carry nutrients and oxygen to the heart muscle.

Cortex \'kȯr,teks\ Outer layer; the renal cortex contains the glomeruli and tubules.

Corticosteroid \¦kȯrd·ə,kō,sti(ə),rȯid\ Steroid (hormonal substance) secreted by the adrenal cortex to influence the metabolism of nutrients, electrolytes, and water. Clinically they are given to reduce, among other things, inflammation, as in inflammatory bowel disease such as Crohn's disease or ulcerative colitis.

Corticotropin-releasing factor (CRF) Hypothalamus factor stimulating release of anterior pituitary hormone ACTH.

Costochondral \¦kästə'kändrəl\ (L. *costa,* rib) Regarding a rib and its associated cartilage.

Creatinine \'krē¦atinēn\ End product of the breakdown of body tissue; found in muscles and blood and excreted in urine. High levels indicate abnormally high catabolism of body proteins and possibly inadequate intake of carbohydrate and fat, which have a protein-sparing effect.

Cruciferous vegetables \(')krü¦sif(ə)rəs 'vejtəbəls\ Belonging to the botanical family *Cruciferae* or *Brassicaceae,* whose members have crosslike, four-petaled flowers; broccoli, cabbage, brussels sprouts, and cauliflower.

Crypts of Lieberkühn \'kripts -əv 'lēbə(r),k(y)ün\ (Gr. *Kryptein,* to hide) Tubular glands of the intestine that secrete intestinal juice. These special secretory organs open between the bases of the villi. Their walls are lined with special cells that secrete digestive enzymes, water, and electrolytes.

Cystinuria \,sistə'n(y)ùrēə\ (*cystine* + *uria,* from Gr. *ouron,* urine) Condition caused by a rare hereditary defect, characterized by excessive urinary excretion of cystine (a sulfur-containing amino acid). Cystine crystals often accumulate and form small, smooth, yellow kidney stones (cystine real calculi).

Cystitis \si'stīd·əs\ (Gr. *kystis, kystides,* sac or bladder) Inflammation of the bladder; can be caused by allergy, bacteria, gonorrhea, and other conditions; often characterized by frequent voiding and burning. Untreated, it may lead to stone formation.

Dalton \'dȯlt°n\ (John Dalton, English physicist and chemist, 1766-1844; founder of the atomic theory) Unit of measuring mass, $\frac{1}{12}$ the mass of carbon-12, equal to 1.657×10^{-24}g; also called atomic mass unit.

Deamination \(¦)dē,amə'nāshən\ Removal of amino group (NH_2) from amino acid.

Decarboxylation \(¦)dē(,)kär,bäksə'lāshən\ Key reaction in cell metabolism; the removal of the carboxyl group (—COOH).

Decidua basalis \də'sijəwə 'bāsələs\ (L. *deciduus,* falling off) Maternal portion of the placenta.

Decubitus ulcer \də'kyübəd·əs 'əlsə(r)\ Bed sore.

Dehiscence \də'his°n(t)s\ (L. *dehiscere,* to gape) Splitting open, separation of the layers of a surgical wound.

Dehydration \(,)dē,hī,drāshən\ (L. *de,* away; Gr. *hydor,* water) Excessive water loss from body tissues.

Delirium \də'lirēəm\ (L. + *de lira,* furrow or track, that is, "off the track") Mental disturbance characterized by hallucinations, delusions, physical restlessness and being incoherent; a sign of toxicity.

Delirium tremens \də'lirēəm 'trēmənz\ (L. *de-,* negative connotation; *lira,* furrow or track, that is, "off the track"; *tremere,* to shake) Mental disturbance marked by delirium with trembling and great excitement.

Delusion \də'lüzhən\ (L. *delusio; de,* front + *ludus,* a game) False personal belief that is firmly held, despite strong evidence to the contrary.

Deoxyribonucleic acid (DNA) \(,)dē¦äksē¦rībō¦n(y)üklēik' asəd\ Complex, double-chain protein of high molecular weight, which is the nucleic acid found in the chromosomes of the cell nucleus. It is the chemical basis of heredity and the carrier of genetic information for specific protein synthesis. DNA is composed of four nitrogenous bases (two purines, adenine and guanine, and two pyrimidines, thymine and cytosine), a sugar (deoxyribose), and phosphoric acid. A similar single-chain nucleic acid, ribonucleic acid (RNA), in which the sugar is ribose, also functions with DNA in protein synthesis in the cell.

Diabetes insipidus \,dīə'bēd·'ēz in'sipədəs\ Condition that shares some of the symptoms of diabetes mellitus: large urine output, great thirst and, sometimes, a large appetite. But these are symptoms of a specific injury, not a collection of metabolic disorders. The impaired pituitary gland produces less antidiuretic hormone, a substance that normally helps the kidneys retain water.

Dialysis \dī'aləsəs\ (Gr. *dia*, through + *lysis*, separate) Separating substances in solution by taking advantage of the different rates at which they pass through a semipermeable membrane.

Diastolic \¦dīə¦stälik\ (Gr. *diastole*, expansion) Referring to the heart's period of dilation; the "relaxation" phase of the heartbeat.

Diffusion \də'fyüzhən\ (L. *diffundere*, to spread or to pour forth) Processes by which particles in solution spread throughout the solution and across separating membranes from the place of highest solute concentration to all surrounding spaces of lesser solute concentration.

Digestion \də'jes(h)chən\ (L. *dis*, apart + *genere*, to carry; *digerere*, to separate, arrange, dissolve, digest) Process by which food is broken down chemically in the gastrointestinal tract through the action of secretions containing specific enzymes. Digestion separates complex food structures into their simpler parts, which are the chemicals needed by the body to sustain life.

1,25-Dihydroxycholecalciferol \1.25 ¦dī,hī¦dräksē,kōlə, kal'sifə,ròl\ The physiologically active hormone form of "vitamin" D.

Disability \¦disə'biləd·ē\ Mental or physical impairment that prevents the individual from performing one or more gainful activities; no longer considered synonymous with *handicap*, which implies serious disadvantage or hopelessness.

Disaccharide \(')dī'sakə,rīd\ Class of compound sugars composed of two molceules of monosaccharide. The three common members are sucrose (table sugar), lactose (milk sugar), and maltose (grain sugar).

Disulfiram \dī'səlfə,ram\ White to off-white crystalline powder antioxidant; inhibits oxidation of the acetaldehyde metabolized from alcohol. It is used in treatment of alcoholism, producing extremely uncomfortable symptoms when alcohol is ingested following oral administration of the drug.

Diuresis \,dīyə'rēsəs\ (Gr. *diourein*, to urinate) Increased urination.

Diuretic \¦dīyə¦red·ik\ (Gr. *diouretikos*, promoting urine) Increasing urine excretion; an agent that promotes urine excretion.

Diverticulitis \,dīvə(r),tikyə'līd·əs\ Inflammation of "pockets" of tissue (diverticuli) in the lining of the mucous membrane in the colon.

"Dumping" syndrome \'dəmpiŋ 'sin,drōm\ Number of physical problems (nausea, vomiting, sweating, palpitations, syncope, diarrhea, and so on) that develop when stomach contents are emptied at an abnormally fast rate; occurs when part of the stomach or intestinal tract is removed.

Dynamic \(')dī¦namik\ Pertaining to change. A dynamic process is one that is constantly changing.

Dysgeusia \dəsgüsiə\ (Gr. *dys*, disordered, abnormal; *geusis*, taste) Altered sense of taste.

Dysphagia \dəsfāzh(ē)ə\ (Gr. *dys*, bad, painful, difficult; *phagein*, to eat) Difficulty swallowing.

Dyspnea \'dis(p)nēə\ (Gr. *dyspnoia*, difficulty of breathing) Labored, difficult breathing.

Ecchymosis \,ekə'mōsəs\ *pl.* ecchymoses (Gr. *ekchymosis*) Bruiselike hemorrhagic spot in the skin or mucous membranes.

Eclampsia \e'klampsēə\ (Gr. *eklampein*, to shine forth) Advanced pregnancy-induced hypertension (PIH) manifested by convulsions.

Ecology \ē'käləjē\ (Gr. *oikos*, house) Relations between organisms and their environments.

Ectoderm \'ektə,dərm\ (Gr. *ektos*, article; *derma*, skin) Layer of embryonic tissue from which the nails, skin glands, nervous system, external sensory organs, and mucous membrane of the mouth are formed.

Eczema \÷ig'zēmə, 'eksəmə\ Inflammation of the skin, characterized by redness, itching, crusting, and eventually scaling or pigmentation.

Edema \ə'dēmə\ (Gr. *oidema*, swelling) Large abnormal amounts of fluid filling the intercellular tissue spaces; may be either localized or systemic.

Educate \'ejə,kāt\ (L. *educatus*, from *educere*, to lead forth; from *e*, out + *ducere*, to lead) To develop and cultivate by systematic instruction.

Electrolyte \ə'lektrə,līt\ (Gr. *electron*, amber [which emits electricity if it is rubbed]; *lytos*, soluble) Chemical compound, which in solution dissociates by releasing ions. (An ion is an atomic particle that carries a positive or a negative electric charge.) The process of dissociating into ions is termed *ionization*.

Electroneutrality \ə'lektrə'n(y)ütrələdē\ Condition of a solution of charged particles in which there are equal numbers of positive and negative ions, a balanced neutral state.

Elemental formula \¦elə¦mənt°l 'förmyələ\ Formula whose components cannot be broken down into simpler parts.

Embolus \'embələs\ Circulating blood clot that may lodge in a blood vessel, causing an embolism.

Emulsifier \ə'məlsə,fī(a)r\ An agent that breaks down large fat globules to smaller, uniformly distributed particles. This action is accomplished in the intestine chiefly by the bile acids, which lower surface tension of the fat particles. Emulsification greatly increases the surface area of fat, facilitating contact with fat-digesting enzymes.

Encephalopathy \ən,sefə'läpəthē\ Any degenerative disease of the brain.

Endarteritis \¦end,ärd·ə'rīd·əs\ (end-; Gr. *arteria*, artery; -itis) Inflammation of the inner lining of an artery.

Endoderm \'en(,)dō,dərm\ (Gr. *endo*, inside; *derma*, skin) The layer of embryonic tissue from which the epithelium of the respiratory and digestive tract, as well as bladder and urethra, are formed.

Endogenous \(')en¦däjənəs\ (Gr. *endon*, within; *gennan*, to produce) Developing within an organism.

Endometrium \(')en¦dō'mē·trēəm\ (Gr. *endon*, within; *metra*, uterus) The inner lining of the uterus.

Endorphin \'en'dȯrfən\ (*endo*genous + mor*phine*) Group of polypeptides in the brain that raise the threshold for pain.

Energy \'enə(r)jē\ (Gr. *en,* in or with *ergon* work) The capacity of a system for doing work; available power. Energy is manifest in various forms—motion, position, light, heat, and sound. Energy is interchangeable among these various forms and is constantly being transformed and transferred among them.

Enkephalin \en'kefələn\ Type of endorphin made up of 5 amino acids that raise the threshold of pain and might also serve as a neurotransmitter; it is found in nerve endings in brain tissue, spinal cord, and gastrointestinal tract.

Enteritis \,entə'rīd·əs\ Inflammation of the intestine.

Enterogastrone \,entərō'ga,strōn'\ Hormone produced by glands in the duodenal mucosa that counteracts excessive gastric activity by inhibiting acid and pepsin secretion and gastric motility.

Enterotoxin \,entərō'täksən\ Substance, usually protein aceous, that has toxic effect on the cells of the intestinal lining.

Enzyme \'en,zīm\ (Gr. *en,* in; *zyme,* leaven) Various complex proteins produced by living cells that act independently of these cells. Enzymes are capable of producing certain chemical changes in other substances without themselves being changed in the process. Their action is therefore that of a catalyst. Digestive enzymes of the gastrointestinal secretions act on food substances to break them down into simpler compounds and greatly accelerate the speed of these chemical reactions. An enzyme is usually named according to the substance (substrate) on which it acts, with the common suffix *-ase;* sucrase is the specific enzyme for sucrose and breaks it down to glucose and fructose.

Epidemiology \,epə,dēmē'äləjē\ Branch of medicine dealing with the study of various factors that determine the frequency and distribution of disease in given populations.

Epilepsy \'epə,lepsē\ (Gr. *epilepsia,* a seizing) Transient disturbances of brain function resulting in loss of consciousness and may be accompanied by convulsive seizures.

Epinephrine Compound secreted by the adrenal medulla; potent stimulator of sympathetic or autonomic nervous system; commonly called adrenalin.

Epiphyses \ə'pifəsəs\ Parts of a long bone separated from the main body of the bone by a layer of cartilage.

Ergogenic \,ərgə'jenik\ (Gr. *ergon,* work; *gennan,* to produce) Tendency to increase work output.

Erythema \,erə'thēmə\ (Gr. *erythema,* flush on the skin) Redness of the skin produced by congestion of the capillaries: results from a variety of causes, one of which can be radiant heat, or burns.

Essential amino acid \ə'senchəl ə'mē(,)nō 'asəd\ An amino acid that is indispensable to life and growth and that the body cannot manufacture; it must be supplied in the diet. Eight amino acids are essential: threonine, leucine, isoleucine, valine, lysine, methionine, phenylalanine, and tryptophan.

Essential fatty acid (EFA) \ə'senchəl 'fad·ē 'asəd\ A fatty acid that is (1) necessary for body metabolism or function and (2) cannot be manufactured by the body and must therefore be supplied in the diet. The major essential fatty acid is linoleic acid ($C_{17}H_{31}COOH$). It is found principally in vegetable oils. The other fatty acids usually classified as essential are linolenic acid and arachidonic acid.

Essential hypertension \ə'senchəl 'hīpə(r)tenchən\ High blood pressure of unknown cause.

Ester \'estə(r)\ A compound produced by the reaction between an acid and an alcohol with elimination of a molecule of water. This process is called esterification. For example, a triglyceride is a glycerol ester. Cholesterol esters are formed in the mucosal cells by combination with fatty acids, largely linoleic acid.

Extravasate \ik'stravə,sāt\ (L. *extra,* outside of, beyond, in addition; *vas,* vessel) Escape or discharge from a vessel into the surrounding tissue (for example, blood leakage forming a bruise).

Exudate \'eksə,dāt\ (L. *exsudare,* to sweat out) Material that escapes from blood vessels and is deposited in tissues or tissue surfaces; characterized by a high content of protein, cells, or other cellular solid matter.

Exudative enteropathy \ig'züdəd·iv ,entə'räpəthē\ Any inflammatory intestinal disease accompanied by cellular components (fluid, debris) escaping the blood vessels to be deposited in or near tissue.

Familial hypercholesterolemia \fə'milyəl ,hīpə(r)kə,lestə(,)rō'lēmēə\ Presence of defective LDL receptors, resulting in an increase in LDL-cholesterol levels.

Fatty acid \'fad·ē 'asəd\ The structural components of fats.

Febrile \'febrəl\ (L. *febrilis*) Condition characterized by fever.

Feedback mechanism \'fēd,bak 'mekə,nizəm\ Mechanism that regulates production and secretion by an endocrine gland (A_g) of its hormone (A_h), which stimulates another endocrine gland (T_g; the *target gland*) to produce its hormone (T_h). As sufficient T_h is produced, blood levels of T_h signal A_g to stop secreting A_h.

Ferritin \'ferət°n\ Protein-iron compound in which iron is stored in tissues; the storage form of iron in the body.

Fetal hydrops \'fēd·°l 'hīdräps\ (Gr. *hydor,* water) Extensive edema of the entire fetus associated with severe anemia.

Fetor hepaticus \'fēd·ə(r) hə'padikəs\ Breath odor resembling the smell of fecal material; a characteristic of liver disease.

Fibrinogen \fī'brinəjən\ Fraction of human plasma given via transfusion to increase coagulation of the blood.

Filtration \fil·'trāshən\ (Medieval L. *filtrum,* felt used to strain liquids) Passage of a fluid through a semipermeable membrane (a membrane that permits passage of water and small solutes but not large molecules) as a result of a difference in pressures on the two sides of the membrane. For example, the net filtration pressure in the capillaries is the difference between the outward-pushing hydrostatic force of the blood pressure and the opposing inward-pulling force of the colloidal osmotic pressure exerted by the plasma proteins retained in the capillary.

Fistula \'fis(h)chələ\ (L. *fistula,* pipe) Abnormal passage, usually between two internal organs, or leading from an internal organ to the surface of the body.

Flavin-adenine dinucleotide (FAD) \'flāvən 'ad°n,ēn (')dī'n(y)üklēə,tīd\ A riboflavin enzyme that operates in many reactions affecting amino acids, glucose, and fatty acids.

Flavin mononucleotide (FMN) \'flāvən ¦mänō'n(y)ü-klēə,tīd\ A riboflavin phosphate compound that acts as a coenzyme in the deamination of certain amino acids.

Flavoprotein \¦flā(,)vō'prō,tēn\ The enzymes of which riboflavin is an important constituent (FMN and FAD).

Fluoridation \,flůrə'dāshən\ Process by which fluorine is added to a substance. Proper fluoridation of public water supplies in areas where the fluorine content is naturally low has been demonstrated to control the incidence of dental caries.

Fluorometric \'flůrəmetrik\ Of or related to fluorometry, an analytic technique that measures small amounts of a substance by the characteristic wavelength of light it emits while being exposed to various wavelengths of light.

Flushing reaction \'fləshiŋ rē'akshən\ Short-term reaction resulting in redness of neck and face.

Folic acid \'fōlik 'asəd\ (vitamin B9) The B-vitamin discovered as a factor in the control of pernicious anemia. It functions in metabolism as a coenzyme for transferring single carbon units for attachment in many reactions. In this role, folic acid is a key substance in cell growth and reproduction through aiding in the formation of nucleoproteins and hemoglobin.

Folinic acid \fō'linik 'asəd\ A derivative of folic acid, which has been used in the treatment of megaloblastic anemia. Vitamin C influences this conversion of folic acid in the liver.

Follicular hyperkeratosis \fə'likyələ(r) ¦hīpə(r),kerə'tōsəs\ A vitamin A deficiency condition in which the skin becomes dry and scaly and small pustules or hardened, pigmented, papular eruptions form around the hair follicles.

"Food jag" \'füd 'jag\ Colloquial expression referring to repeated use of single foods over a brief time.

Fuel factor \'fyüel 'faktə(r)\ The kilocalorie value (energy potential) of food nutrients; that is, the number of kilocalories 1 g of the nutrient yields when oxidized. The kilocalorie fuel factor for carbohydrate is 4; for protein, 4; and for fat, 9. These basic figures are used in computing diets and energy values of foods.

Gastrectomy \ga'strek tamē\ (Gr. *gaster*, stomach; *ektome*, excision) Surgical removal of all or part of the stomach.

Gastrin \'gastrən\ Hormone secreted by mucosal cells in the antrum of the stomach that stimulates the parietal cells to produce hydrochloric acid. Gastrin is released in response to entry of stimulants, especially coffee, alcohol, and meat extractives, into the stomach. When the gastric pH reaches 2.0, a feedback mechanism cuts off gastrin secretion and prevents excess acid formation.

Gastritis \ga'strīd·əs\ Inflammation of the stomach.

Gavage \gə'väzh\ (Fr. *gavage*, cramming) Forced tube feeding into stomach; superalimentation.

Generativity \'jenə,rād·¦ivitē\ Active nurturing transmission of culture from one generation to the next.

Geophagia \'jēō'fāj(ē)ə\ (Gr. *ge*, earth; *phagein*, to eat) Eating of clay or earth.

Geriatrics \,jerē'a·triks\ (Gr. *geron*, old man; *iatrike*, medical treatment) Study and treatment of diseases of old age; a branch of medicine concerned with medical problems associated with old age.

Gerontology \,jerən·'täləjē\ (Gr. *geron*, old man; *logos*, study of) Study of the aging process and its phenomena.

Gestation \je'stāshən\ (L. *gestatio*, from *gestare*, to bear) The period of embryonic and fetal development from fertilization to birth; pregnancy.

Glomerulonephritis \glä¦mer(y)ə(,)lōnə'frīd·əs\ Inflammation of the capillary glomeruli in the kidney; may result after a streptococcal infection.

Glomerulosclerosis \glä¦mer(y)ə(,)lōsklə'rōsəs\ (L. *glomerulus*, dim. of *glomus*, ball; *sklerosis*, hardness) Scarring and aging of the renal glomeruli.

Glomerulus \glä'mer(y)ə,lōs\ (L. diminutive form of *glomus*, ball) Convoluted cluster of blood vessels in the cortex of the kidney at the head of the nephron; site of cell-free filtrate formation.

Glossitis \glä'sīd·əs\ (Gr. *glossa*, tongue +-*itis*) Swollen, reddened tongue; riboflavin deficiency symptom.

Glucagon \'glükə,gän\ Hormone produced by the A cells in the islets of Langerhans and secreted when blood sugar levels are low or in response to growth hormone. It stimulates the breakdown of glycogen in the liver and raises blood sugar levels during fasting states to ensure adequate levels for normal nerve and brain function.

Glucocorticoids Group of corticosteroids (adrenocortical hormones) secreted in response to stress; affect carbohydrate metabolism.

Gluconeogenesis \¦glükō¦nēō'jenəsəs\ (Gr. *gleukos*, sweetness; *neos*, new; *genesis*, production, generation) Formation of glucose from noncarbohydrate sources (protein or fat).

Glucose tolerance factor (GTF) \'glü,kōs 'täl(ə)rən(t)s 'faktə(r)\ Chromium compound associated with glucose and lipid metabolism and insulin activity.

Gluten-sensitive enteropathy \'glüt°n 'sen(t)səd·iv ,entə'räpəthē\ Disorder characterized by the inability to absorb gluten, a protein found in wheat, barley, oats, and rye. The presence of gluten is accompanied by damage to the mucosal villi, which in turn interferes with the absorption of other essential nutrients; commonly found in celiac disease and sprue.

Glycemic index \(')glī¦sēmik 'in,deks\ Blood sugar response value of a food in relation to that of glucose. It is an expression of the area under the blood glucose response curve for each food stated as the percentage of the area after taking the same amount of carbohydrate as glucose.

Glyceride \'glisə,rīd\ Group name for fats; any of a group of esters obtained from glycerol by the replacement of one, two, or three hydroxyl (OH) groups with a fatty acid. Monoglycerides contain one fatty acid; diglycerides contain two fatty acids; triglycerides contain three fatty acids. Glycerides are the principal constituent of adipose tissue and are found in animal and vegetable fats and oils.

Glycerol \'glisə,rȯl\ A colorless, odorless, syrupy, sweet liquid; a constituent of fats usually obtained by the hydrolysis of fats. Chemically glycerol is an alcohol; it is esterified with fatty acids to produce fats.

Glycogen \'glīkəjən\ (Gr. *glykys*, sweet; *gennan*, to produce) Polysaccharide, the main storage form of carbohydrate, largely stored in the liver and to a lesser extent in muscle tissue.

Glycogenesis \ˌglīkə'jenəsəs\ Formation of glycogen, the storage form of carbohydrates in animals.

Glycogenolysis \ˌglīkəjə'näləsəs\ (*glycogen* + Gr. *lysis*, dissolution) Specific term for conversion of glycogen into glucose in the liver; chemical process of enzymatic hydrolysis or breakdown by which this conversion is accomplished.

Glycolysis \glīkäləsəs\ (Gr. *glykys*, sweet; *lysis*, dissolution) Catabolism of carbohydrate (glucose and glycogen) by enzymes with release of energy and production of pyruvic acid or lactic acid.

Glycosuria \ˌglī(ˌ)kō's(h)ûrēə\ (Gr. *glykys*, sweet; *ouron*, urine + -*ia*) Abnormally high concentrations of glucose in the urine.

Goblet cell \ˈgäblòt ˈsel\ Special single secretory cells on the mucosal surface that produce mucus. Mucin droplets accumulate in the cell, causing it to swell. The free surface finally ruptures and liberates the mucus. This mucus coats and protects the mucosa.

Goiter \ˈgòid·ə(r)\ (L. *guttur*, throat) Enlargement of the thyroid gland caused by lack of sufficient available iodine to produce the thyroid hormone, thyroxine.

Handicap \ˈhandē̩kap\ Mental or physical defect that may or may not be congenital that prevents the individual from participating in normal life activities; implies disadvantage.

Hemarthrosis \ˌhēmär'thrōsəs\ Hemorrhage into joint cavities, causing local heat, painful swelling, and immobility.

Hematuria \ˌhēmə'tûrēə\ (Gr. *hemato*, blood; *ouron*, urine) Presence of blood in the urine.

Heme \ˈhēm\ Iron-containing, nonprotein portion of the hemoglobin.

Hemodialysis \ˌhēmōdī'aləsəs\ (Gr. *haima*, blood; *dia*, through; *lysis*, separate) Removal of toxic substances from the blood by passing it through a machine that contains a semipermeable membrane and a liquid into which the substances will be diffused; process by which persons with chronic renal failure are kept alive. The machine is often referred to as an "artificial kidney."

Hemoglobin \ˈhēmə̩glōbən\ (Gr. *haima*, blood; L. *globus*, globe) Protein that gives the color to red blood cells. A conjugated protein composed of an iron-containing pigment called heme and a simple protein, globin. Carries oxygen in the blood; combines with oxygen to form oxyhemoglobin.

Hemopoiesis \ˌhēmō̩pòi'ēsəs\ (Gr. *haima*, blood; *poiein*, to form) The formation of blood.

Hemosiderin \ˌhēmō'sidərən\ (Gr. *haima*, blood; *sideros*, iron) Insoluble iron oxide-protein compound in which iron is stored in the liver if the amount of iron in the blood exceeds the storage capacity of ferritin, for example, during rapid destruction of red blood cells (malaria, hemolytic anemia).

Hepatomegaly \ˌhepəd·ō'megəlē\ Enlargement of the liver.

Hexose \ˈhek̩sōs\ Class of simple sugars (monosaccharides) that contain 6 carbon atoms ($C_6H_{12}O_6$). The most common members of glucose (dextrose), frutose (levulose), and galactose.

Hiatus \hī'ād·əs\ Opening or gap.

Hierarchy \ˈhīə̩rärkē\ (Gr. *hieros*, sacred, holy) System of persons or things in a graded order according to held values, functions, or goals.

High-density lipoprotein \hī ˈden(t)səd·ē ˌlīpə'prō̩tēn\ Carries less total lipid and more protein.

Homeostasis \ˌhōmēō'stāsis\ (Gr. *homoios*, unchanging or resembling; *stasis*, standing) State of internal stability of a body or an organism.

Hormone \ˈhòr̩mōn\ (Gr. *hormaein*, to set in motion, spur on) Various internally secreted substances from the endocrine organs, which are conveyed by the blood to another organ or tissue on which they act to stimulate increased functional activity or secretion. The tissue or substance acted on by a specific hormone is called its target organ or substance. For example, insulin, a hormone secreted by special cells of the pancreas (islets of Langerhans), acts to facilitate glucose metabolism.

Humoral immunity \(h)yümərəl ə'myünəd·ē\ Acquired immunity in which the role of antibodies, produced by B lymphocytes and plasma cells, predominates.

Hydatidiform mole \ˌhīdə̩tidəfòrm ˈmōl\ (L. *hydatis*, a drop of water; *moles*, a shapeless mass) An abnormal pregnancy resulting in a cystic mass resembling a bunch of grapes formed by a pathologic ovum in the uterus; a mole pregnancy.

Hydramnios \hī'dramnē̩äs\ (Gr. *hydor*, water; *amnion*, bowl, the membrane containing the fetus) An excess of amniotic fluid.

Hydrochloric acid (HCl) \ˌhī(ˌ)drō'klōrik ˈasəd\ Acid secreted by special gastric mucosal cells; provides necessary acid medium for enzyme action in the stomach.

Hydrogenation \ˌhīdrəjə'nāshən\ The process of adding hydrogen to unsaturated fats to produce a solid, saturated fat. This process is used to produce vegetable shortening from vegetable oils.

Hydrolysis \hī'drāləsəs\ (Gr. *hydor*, water; *lysis*, dissolution) Process by which a chemical compound is split into other compounds by taking up the elements of water. Common examples are the reactions of digestion, in which the nutrients are split into simpler compounds by the digestive enzymes; that is, the conversion of starch to maltose, of fat to fatty acids and glycerol, and so on.

Hydrophilic \ˌhī(ˌ)drə̩filik\ (Gr. *hydor*, water; *philein*, to love) Readily absorbing water; having strong polar groups that readily interact with water; water soluble. Glycerol is hydrophilic.

Hydrophobic \ˌhīdrə̩fōbik\ (Gr. *hydor*, water; *phobein*, to be frightened by) Not readily absorbing water; lacking polar groups and therefore insoluble in water. Fat is hydrophobic.

Hydrostatic pressure \hī(i)drō̩stadik ˈpreshə(r)\ Pressure exerted by a liquid on the surfaces of the walls that contain it. Such pressure is equal in the direction of all containing walls. In body fluid balance hydrostatic pressure usually refers to the blood pressure, which, together with the plasma proteins, maintains fluid circulation and volume in the blood vessels.

Hygroscopic \ˌhīgrə̩skäpik\ (Gr. *hygros*, moist) Taking up and retaining moisture readily.

Hyperemesis gravidarum \ˌhīpə(r)'eməsəs ˌgravə'da(a)rəm\ (Gr. *hyper*, over + Gr. *emesis*, vomiting) Severe vomiting that is potentially fatal.

Hyperglycemia \ˌhīpə(r)glī'sēmēə\ Elevated blood sugar; above normal levels.

Hyperkalemia \ˌhīpə(r)ˌkā'lēmēə\ (Gr. *hyper;* L. *Kalium,* potassium; Gr. *haima,* blood) Excessive amounts of potassium (K) in blood plasma.

Hyperkeratosis \ˌhīpə(r)ˌkerə'tōsəs\ (Gr. *hyper; keras,* horn or horny tissue) Overgrowth of the corneous or horny layer of the skin, consisting of keratin.

Hyperkinesis \ˌhīpə(r)kə'nēsəs\ (Gr. *hyper; kinesis,* motion) Nerve disorder characterized by abnormally high motor activity; may occur in children and interferes with their learning ability; also known as *hyperactivity.*

Hyperlipoproteinemia \ˌhīpə(r)ˌlīpəˌprō,tē'nēmēə\ Elevation of lipoproteins in the blood.

Hypermotility \ˌhīpə(r)mō'tiləd·ē\ Excessive peristaltic activity along the alimentary canal.

Hypernatremia \ˌhīpə(r)nətrēmēə\ (Gr. *hyper;* L. *natruim,* sodium; Gr. *haima,* blood) Abnormally high levels of sodium in the blood.

Hyperoxaluria \ˌhīpə(r)äksəl'yùrēə\ (Gr. *hyper + oxalate + uria*) Excretion of high levels of oxalate in the urine. Oxalates, found in several vegetables (spinach, tomatoes, rhubarb) combine with calcium to form urinary stones.

Hyperparathyroidism \ˌhīpə(r)ˌparə'thīˌroid,izəm\ (Gr. *hyper + parathyroid + ism*) Greater-than-normal levels of activity by the parathyroid glands, which regulate calcium and phosphorus. High calcium levels increase the chances of developing calcium-containing urinary calculi.

Hyperphagia \ˌhīpə(r)'fājēə\ (Gr. *hyper; phagein,* to eat) Eating more than necessary for optimal body function.

Hyperphosphatemia \ˌhīpə(r)fäsfətēmēə\ High serum phosphorus levels.

Hypertonic dehydration \ˌhīpə(r)'tänik (ˌ)dē,hī'drāshən\ Loss of water from the cell as a result of hypertonicity (excess solutes, thus greater osmotic pressure) of the surrounding extracellular fluid.

Hypertriglyceridemia \ˌhīpə(r)ˌtrī¦glisəˌrī'dēmēə\ Elevated blood level of triglycerides.

Hypochloremic alkalosis \ˌhīpōklōrēmik ˌalkəlōsəs\ Excessive loss of gastric secretion (hydrochloric acid).

Hypocupremia \ˌhī(ˌ)pōˌk(y)ü'prēmēə\ Low serum copper level.

Hypogeusia \hī(ˌ)pōgyüzh(ē)\ Impaired taste associated with zinc deficiency.

Hypoglycemia \ˌhī(ˌ)pōglī'sēmēə\ Low blood sugar; below normal levels.

Hypokalemia \ˌhī(ˌ)pōˌkā'lēmēə\ Low potassium levels in the blood.

Hypophagia \ˌhī(ˌ)pō'fājēə\ (Gr. *hypo; phagein,* to eat) Eating less than necessary for optimal health.

Hypophosphatemia \ˌhī(ˌ)pōˌfäsfə'tēmēə\ Low serum phosphorus levels.

Hypoplasia \ˌhī(ˌ)pō'plāzh(ē)ə\ (Gr. *hypo,* under; *plasis,* formation) Incomplete organ; underdevelopment of an organ.

Hyposmia \ˌhī(ˌ)pozmēə\ Impaired smell acuity associated with zinc deficiency.

Hypotonic dehydration \ˌhī(ˌ)pō'tänik (ˌ)dē,hī'drāshən\ Increase of water in the cell (cellular edema) at the expense of extracellular fluid, resulting from hypotonicity (decreased solutes, thus diminished osmotic pressure) of the extracellular fluid surrounding the cell. A dangerous

shrinking of the extracellular fluid (especially blood) volume follows.

Hypovolemia \ˌhī(ˌ)pōˌvä'lēmēə\ (Gr. *hypo;* volume; *haima,* blood) Abnormal reduction in volume of circulatory plasma.

Hypoxia Condition of lack of oxygen in the blood.

Iatrogenic \īˌa·trō¦jenik\ (Gr. *iatros,* physician; *gennan,* to produce) Illness induced by medical treatment.

Idiopathic \ˌidēə¦pathik\ Of unknown cause.

Immunocompetence \ə'myüno'kämpəd·ən(t)s\ Ability to produce antibodies in response to an antigen.

Incomplete protein \ˌinkəm'plēt 'prō,tēn\ Food protein lacking sufficient amount of one or more of the essential amino acids.

Indole \'in,dōl\ Compound produced in the intestines by the decomposition of tryptophan; obtained from indigo and coal tar.

Infantile beriberi \'infən·tīl ¦berē'berē\ Occurs in the first year of life. Symptoms: convulsions, respiratory difficulties, gastrointestinal disorders; terminal symptoms: cyanosis, dyspnea, tachycardia.

Infarct \'in,färkt\ Death of tissue caused by a loss of blood flow to that area, usually caused by a thrombus (clot) clogging the artery feeding the area.

Insulin \'in(t)sələn\ (L. *insula,* island) Hormone formed in the B cells of the pancreas. It is secreted when blood glucose and amino acid levels rise and assists their entry into the cells. It also promotes glycogenesis and conversion of glucose into fat and inhibits lipolysis and gluconeogenesis (protein breakdown). Commercial insulin is manufactured from pigs and cows; new "artificial" human insulin products have recently been made available.

Intermediate-density lipoprotein (IDL) \ˌintə(r)¦mēdēət' den'(t)səd·ē ˌlīpə'prō,tēn\ Approximately 30% cholesterol; carries triglycerides to body cells.

Intermittent claudication \ˌintə(r)¦mit³nt ˌklòdə'kāshən\ Leg pain induced by walking that is relieved by rest.

Intervillous space \ˌintə(r)'viləs 'spās\ (L. *inter-,* between; *villus,* tuft of hair) Spaces situated between villi, small vascular protrusions.

Intima \'intəmə\ (L.) Innermost layer of a blood vessel.

Intramural nerve plexus \ˌin·trə'myùrəl 'nərv 'pleksəs\ (L. *intra,* within; *murus,* wall; *plexus,* a braid) Network of interwoven nerve structures within a particular organ. The action of smooth muscle layers comprising the gastrointestinal wall is controlled by such a network of nerve fibers.

Intrinsic factor \(')in·¦trinzik 'faktə(r)\ (L. *intrinsecus,* on the inside) Substance situated entirely within a part of the body; common term for component of the gastric secretions, a mucoprotein, also called Castle's factor, necessary for the absorption of cyanocobalamin (vitamin B_{12}).

Ion \'īən\ (Gr. *ion,* to wander) Molecular constituent of one or more atoms that is a free-wandering particle in solution. An ion carries a positive or negative electric charge. Ions carrying negative charges are called anions; those carrying positive charges are called cations.

Ionized free calcium (Ca^{++}) \'īənizd frē 'kalsēəm\ Free, diffusible form of calcium in the blood and other body fluids. Makes up a very small amount of the total body calcium

(1%); the remaining 99% of the total body calcium is deposited as calcium salts in bone tissue.

Ischemia \ə'skēmēə\ (Gr. *ischein,* to suppress, and *haima,* blood) Deficiency of blood to a body part resulting from constriction or actual obstruction of a blood vessel.

Isomer \ˈīsōmə(r)\ (Gr. *isos,* equal; *meros,* part) The possession by two or more distinct compounds of the same molecular formula, each molecule possessing an identical number of atoms of each element but in different arrangement.

Isotonic \ˈīsōˈtänik\ (Gr. *isos,* equal; *tonos,* tone, tension) Having the same tension or pressure. Two given solutions are isotonic if they have the same osmotic pressure and therefore balance each other. For example, the law of isotonicity operates between the gastrointestinal fluids and the surrounding extracellular fluid. Shifts of water and electrolytes in and out of the gastrointestinal lumen are controlled to maintain this state of isotonicity.

Isotope \ˈīsōˌtōp\ (Gr. *isos,* equal; *topos,* place) Element that has the same number of protons (atomic number) as another element but a different number of neutrons (atomic mass).

Joule \jül\ A measure of energy; 1 kcal = 4.184 kJ.

Kallikrein \kalə'krēən\ Any member of a group of peptide enzymes of the subgroup serine proteinases, present in blood plasma and various glands, such as the pancreas and salivary gland. Major action is to liberate polypeptides called *kinins* (bradykinin and kallidin).

Keratinization \ˌkerəd·ənəˈzāshən\ (Gr. *keras, kerat,* horn) A process occurring in vitamin A deficiency states in which the epithelial cells either slough off or become dry and flattened, then gradually harden and form rough horny scales. This process may occur in the cornea, the respiratory tract, the gastrointestinal tract, the genitourinary tract, or the skin.

Keratomalacia \ˌkerəd·ōməˈlās(h)ēə\ Softening of the cornea.

Keto acid \ˈkēd·(ˌ)ō 'asəd\ Amino acid residue after deamination. The glycogenic keto-acids are used to form carbohydrates. The ketogenic keto-acids are used to form fats.

Ketoacidosis \ˈkēd·(ˌ)ōasadōsəs\ Abnormally high concentration of ketone bodies (ketones) in body tissues and fluids; a complication of diabetes mellitus and starvation.

Ketone \ˈkēˌtōn\ Intermediate fat metabolite; large class of organic compounds that contain the carbonyl group $C=O$, where the carbon atom is jointed to two other carbon atoms.

Kinetic \kəˈned·ik\ (Gr. *kinesis,* movement) Regarding or producing motion.

Kinin \ˈkīnən\ Any of a group of endogenous peptides that cause vasodilation, increase vascular permeability, reduce blood pressure, and induce contraction of smooth muscle.

Koilonychia \ˌkȯilōˈnikēə\ (Gr. *koilos,* hollow; *onyx,* nail) Spoon-shaped fingernails.

Kwashiorkor \ˈkwäshēˌȯrkər\ (Gold Coast, Africa, "displaced child") Disease syndrome produced by severe protein deficiency.

Kyphosis \kīˈfōsəs\ (Gr. *hyphos,* a hump) Increased, abnormal convexity of the upper part of the spine; hunchback.

Lactated Ringer's solution \ˈlaktātəd 'rˌŋə(r)s səˈlüshən\ Sterile solution of calcium chloride, potassium chloride, sodium chloride, and sodium lactate in water given to replenish fluid and electrolytes; named for Sydney Ringer (1835-1910), an English physiologist.

Lactic acid \ˈlaktik 'asəd\ (L. *lactis,* milk) Produced by anaerobic glycolysis in the muscles during exertion; can be converted to glucose by the liver.

Lactoflavin \ˈlak(ˌ)tōˈflāvən\ The form in which riboflavin occurs in milk.

Lacuna \ləˈk(y)ünə\ A hollow space (pl. lacunae).

Lean body mass (LBM) \ˈlēn 'bädē 'mas\ All component parts of the body, excluding neutral storage lipid; the entire fat-free mass.

Lecithin \ˈlesəthən\ (Gr. *lekithos,* egg yolk) A yellow-brown fatty substance of the group called phospholipids. It occurs in animal and plant tissues and egg yolk. It is composed of units of choline, phosphoric acid, fatty acids, and glycerol. Commercial forms of lecithin, obtained chiefly from soybeans, corn, and egg yolk, are used in candies, foods, cosmetics, and inks. Lecithin plays an important role in the metabolism of fat in the liver. It provides an effective lipotropic factor, choline, which prevents the accumulation of abnormal quantities of fat.

Lecithin-cholesterol acyltransferase (LCAT) \ˈlesəthən kōˈləˈsterˌrȯl asiltranzfərās\ Enzyme that helps HDLs transport cholesterol.

Lecithinase \ˈlesəthənās\ Enzyme acting on lecithin. Suffix *-ase* indicates an enzyme. Word to which it is attached indicates substrate material on which it acts.

Lethargy \ˈlethə(r)jē\ Drowsiness; indifference.

Linoleic acid \ˈlinəˈlēik àsəd\ (L. *linum,* flax; *oleum,* oil) Essential fatty acid, preferred fuel for the heart muscle.

Lipase \ˈlīˌpās\ (Gr. *lipos,* fat; *-ase,* the suffix for enzyme) Any of a class of enzymes that break down fats. A small quantity of gastric lipase (lipase secreted by the gastric mucosa) acts on emulsified fats of cream and egg yolk. The major digestive lipase is pancreatic lipase, which acts on fats in the small intestine. Enteric lipase acts within the mucosal cells, and lipoprotein lipase clears initial transport fats (chylomicrons) from the bloodstream.

Lipid \ˈlipəd\ (Gr. *lipos,* fat) The group name for organic substances of fatty nature. The lipids include fats, oils, waxes, and related compounds.

Lipogenesis \ˌlīpəˈjenəsəs\ (Gr. *lipos,* fat; *genesis,* formation) Conversion of carbohydrates and protein into body fat; occurs when excessive amounts of these nutrients are consumed.

Lipolysis \līˈpäləsəs\ (Gr. *lipos,* fat; *lysis,* dissolution) Breakdown of fat into its component fatty acids and glycerol.

Lipoprotein \ˌlīpəˈprōˌtēn\ Noncovalent complexes of fat with protein. The lipoproteins probably function as major carriers of lipids in the plasma, since most of the plasma fat is associated with them. Such a combination makes possible the transport of fatty substances in a predominantly aqueous medium such as plasma.

Lipoprotein lipase \ˌlipəˈprōˌtēn 'līˌpās\ Enzyme that helps remove triglycerides from chylomicrons.

Low-density lipoprotein (LDL) \ˈlō 'den(t)səd·ē ˌlipəˈprōˌtēn\ Carries at least 66% of the total amount of cholesterol in plasma.

Luminal segmentation \'lümən^əl ˌsegmən·ˌtāshən\ Formation of divisions, or segments, along the alimentary canal. In diverticulitis, this may occur at the site of diverticula and increase the motility of the gastrointestinal tract, promoting diarrhea.

Lymphocyte Special white blood cell from lymphoid tissue that participates in humoral and cell-mediated immunity.

Macrocytic anemia \ˌmakrō¦sid·ik a'nēmēa\ Anemia characterized by red cells that are larger and paler than normal.

Malignant \mə'lignənt\ (L. *malignans*, acting maliciously) Not improving, worsening; resulting in death.

Malnutrition \ˌmaln(y)ü·'trishən\ Faulty nutrition resulting from poor diet, malassimilation, or overeating.

Marasmus \mə'raz_məs\ (Gr. *marasmos*, withering) Lack of nutrition manifested by wasting.

Medulla \mə'dələ\ Innermost portion of the kidney; site of the loop of Henle.

Megaloblastic anemia \ˌmegəlō¦blastik ənēmēə\ (Gr. *mega*, large; *blastos*, embryo) Anemia characterized by formation of large immature red blood cells, deficient carriers of oxygen; caused by deficiency of folic acid and hence faulty synthesis of heme.

Menarche \mə'när(ˌ)kē\ Onset of menstruation.

Mendel, Gregor Johann \'mendəl\ (1822-1884) Austrian monk and naturalist; discovered the natural laws governing direct inheritance by offspring of certain traits or characters from one or the other parent.

Mesoderm \'me¦zə˛dərm\ Embryonic tissue from which connective tissue, bone, cartilage, muscle, blood, blood vessels, kidney, gonads, lymph, and other organs are derived.

Metabolism \mə'tabə˛lizəm\ (Gr. *metaballein*, to turn about, change, alter) The sum of all chemical changes that take place within an organism by which it maintains itself and produces energy for its functioning. Products of these various reactions are called metabolites. Interrelationships of substances in these processes are called metabolic relationships.

Metabolite \mə'tabə˛līt\ (Gr. *metaballein*, to turn about, alter, change) Any substance that forms as a result of the breakdown (catabolism), growth, or maintenance (anabolism) of living tissue.

Metallothionein \'med˛ə¹lōthīōnē˛ēn\ Copper-binding protein; plasma transport carrier.

Micellar bile-fat complex \(')mī¦selə(r) 'bīl 'fat (')käm¦pleks\ (L. *mica*, crumb, grain; *ella*, diminutive suffix) A micelle is a particle formed by an aggregate of molecules, a microscopic unit of protoplasm. In micellar bile-fat complex the particle is formed by the combination of bile salts with fat substances (fatty acids and glycerides) to achieve the absorption of fat across the intestinal mucosa. Bile salt micelles act as detergents to solubilize lipids for digestion and absorption.

Microcytic hypochromic anemia \ˌmīkro¦sid·ik 'hīpō-krōmik ə'nēmēə\ Iron deficiency anemia characterized by small pale red blood cells.

Microvillus \ˌmīkrō'viləs\ (*pl.* microvilli) Minute surface projections that cover the edge of each intestinal villus; they are visible only through the electron microscope. This vast array of microvilli on each villus is called the brush border.

The microvilli add a tremendous surface area for absorption.

Milliequivalent \ˌmilēə'kwiv(ə)lənt\ Unit of measure used for electrolytes in a solution. It is based on the number of ions (cations and anions) in solution, as determined by their concentration in a given volume, not the weights of the various particles. The term refers to the chemical combining power of the solution and is expressed as the number of milliequivalents per liter (mEq/L).

Mitochondrion \ˌmīd·ə'kändrēən\ (Gr. *mitos*, thread; *chondrion*, granule) Cell's "powerhouse," a small, spheric- to rod-shaped organelle located in the cell cytoplasm; principal site of energy generation (ATP synthesis); contains enzymes of Krebs cycle and cell respiration, as well as ribonucleic and deoxyribonucleic acids (RNA and DNA) for synthesis of some proteins.

Monoamine \'mä(ˌ)nōəmēn\ Amine molecule containing one amino group, for example, serotonin, dopamine, norepinephrine.

Monosaccharide \ˌmä(ˌ)nō'sakə˛rīd\ (Gr. *monos*, single; *sakcharon*, sugar) Simple single sugar; a carbohydrate containing a single saccharide (sugar) unit.

Monozygote \ˌmä(ˌ)nō'zī˛gōt\ (Gr. *monos*, single; *zygotos*, yoked together) Single fertilized ovum; may result in identical twins.

Mucus \'myükəs\ Viscid fluid secreted by mucous membranes and glands, consisting mainly of mucin (a glycoprotein), inorganic salts, and water. Mucus serves to lubricate and protect the gastrointestinal mucosa and to help move the food mass along the digestive tract.

Myelin sheath \'mīəlͣn 'shēth\ Protective lipid membrane covering axon shafts of nerve cells; serves as an electrical insulator and impulse transmittor.

Myelinated \ˌmīələ¦nād·əd\ (Gr. *myelos*, marrow) Having a sheath or covering of myelin, a protective lipid membrane, as that insulating axons of nerve cells.

Myocardial infarction (MI) \ˌmīə¦kärdēəl ən'färkshən\ Death of heart tissue resulting from blockage that prevents the flow of blood to or through its coronary arteries.

Myofibril \ˌmīo'fībrəl\ (Gr. *myo*, muscle; L. *fibrilla*, very small fiber) Slender thread of muscle; runs parallel to the muscle fiber's long axis.

Myoglobin \ˌmīə˛glōbən\ Muscle protein (globin) that contains iron (also called myohemoglobin).

Myosin \'mīəsͣn\ (Gr. *myo*, muscle) Myofibril protein that acts in conjunction with actin to cause the contraction and relaxation of muscle.

Necrosis \nə˛krōsͣs\ (Gr. *nekrosis*, deadness) Cell death.

Neoplasm \'nēə˛plazəm\ (Gr. *neo*, new; *plasma*, a formation) Any new or abnormal growth; uncontrolled or progressive growth. Also called a tumor.

Nephron \'ne˛frän\ (Gr. *nephros*, kidney) The nephron includes the renal corpuscle (glomerulus), the proximal convoluted tubule, the loop of Henle, the distal convoluted tubule, and the collecting tubule, which empties the urine into the renal medulla. The urine passes into the papilla and then to the pelvis of the kidney. Urine is formed by filtration of blood in the glomerulus and by the selective reabsorption and secretion of solutes by cells that comprise the walls of the renal tubules. There are approximately 1 million nephrons in each kidney.

Nephropathy \ne͵fräpəthē\ (Gr. *nephros,* kidney; *pathos,* disease) Disease of the nephrons in the kidneys, a complication of diabetes.

Nephrosis \nə'frōsəs\ Inflammation of the nephron.

Neuritis \n(y)ü͵rīd·əs\ Inflammation of nerve tissue, accompanied by pain, paralysis, atrophy, and loss of reflexes.

Neuropathy \n(y)ü'räpəthē\ (Gr. *neuron,* nerve; *pathos* disease) Presence of disease and/or change in function of the peripheral nervous system. Also defined as noninflammatory injury to the peripheral nervous system, a complication of diabetes.

Neurotransmitter \͵n(y)ürōtran(t)'smid·ə(r)\ (Gr. *neuron,* nerve + transmitter) Chemical substances that relay messages through the central nervous system.

Niacin \'nīəsən\ (nicotinic acid) B vitamin; deficiency produces pellagra. Important niacin compounds (NAD and NADP) function as key coenzymes in glucose oxidation. Niacin's relation to pellagra was discovered by Joseph Goldberger. Meat, peanuts, enriched grains, and legumes are major sources of niacin. The essential amino acid, tryptophan, is a precursor of niacin.

Niacin equivalent (NE) \'nīsən ə'kwiv(ə)lənt\ A measure of the total dietary sources of niacin equivalent to 1 mg of niacin. Thus an NE is 1 mg of niacin or 60 mg of tryptophan.

Nicotinamide-adenine dinucleotide (NAD) \͵nikə'tēna͵mīd 'ad°n͵ēn (')dī'n(y)üklē͵o͵tīd\ A niacin compound that functions in tissue oxidation to release controlled energy.

Nicotinamide-adenine dinucleotide phosphate (NADP) \͵nikə'tēna͵mīd 'ad°n͵ēn (')dī'n(y)üklē͵o͵tīd 'fä͵sfāt\ A niacin compound with three high-energy phosphate bonds, which acts as a vital coenzyme in the "respiratory chains" of tissue oxidation within the cell; controlled energy is made available by this reaction.

Night blindness \'nīt͵ blīnnəs\ Inability to see well at night in diminished light; due to faulty operation of eyes' light adjustment mechanism resulting from lack of required vitamin A.

Nitrogen balance \'nītrəjən 'balən(t)s\ The difference between intake and output of nitrogen in the body. If intake is greater, a positive nitrogen balance exists. If output is greater, a negative nitrogen balance exists. For example, during growth when new tissue protein is being formed, nitrogen is retained for protein synthesis, and a state of positive nitrogen balance prevails.

Nonheme \(͵)nänhēm\ Protein portion of hemoglobin that does not contain the heme.

Nonicteric \(͵)nän(')k͵terik\ Hepatic disease without jaundice (icterus).

Norepinephrine One of the catecholamines; a neurohormone, principal neurotransmitter of adrenergic nerves; also secreted by adrenal medulla.

Nulligravida \͵nələ'gravədə\ (L. *nullus,* none; *gravida,* pregnant) Woman who has never been pregnant.

Obesity \ō'bēsəd·ē\ Excessive adipose tissue, more than required for optimal body function.

Occult bleeding \ə'kəlt 'blēdiŋ\ Such a small blood loss that it can be detected only by a microscope or chemical test.

Oliguria \͵älə'g(y)ůrēə\ (Gr. *oligos,* little; *ouron,* urine) Reduced amount of urine in comparison with fluid intake.

Omega (ω) \ō'megə\ The twenty-fourth and final letter of the Greek alphabet; used in numbering system for fatty acids.

Osmolarity \͵äzmə'larəd·ē\ Concentration of osmotically active particles in solution.

Osmole \'äz͵mōl\ Standard unit of osmotic pressure; equal to the gram molecular weight of a substance divided by the number of ions or particles into which the substance is dissociated in solution.

Osmosis \äz'mōsəs\ (Gr. *osmos,* a thrusting) Passage of a solvent such as water through a membrane that separates solutions of different concentrations. The water passes through the membrane from the area of lower concentration of solute to that of higher concentration of solute, which tends to equalize the concentrations of the two solutions. The rate of osmosis depends on (1) the difference in osmotic pressures of the two solutions, (2) the permeability of the membrane, and (3) the electric potential across the membrane.

Osteoblast \'ästēə͵blast\ (Gr. *osteo,* bone; *blastos,* germ) Bone-forming cells.

Osteoclast \'ästēə͵klast\ (Gr. *osteo,* bone; *klan,* to break) Giant, multinuclear cells found in depressions on bone surfaces, which caused resorption of bone tissue and the formation of canals.

Osteodystrophy \͵ästēō'distrəfē\ (Gr. *osteon,* bone; L. *dystrophia,* faulty nutrition) Disease often accompanying renal failure in which calcium is lost from the bones; poor bone formation. Renal osteodystrophy is a result of chronic kidney disease, which may begin in childhood, and can lead to renal dwarfism.

Osteomalacia \͵ästēōmə'lāsh(ē)ə\ Softening of bone caused by impaired mineral uptake; usually resulting from calcium and vitamin D deficiency.

Osteoporosis \͵ästēōpə'rōsəs\ (Gr. *osteon,* bone; *poros,* passage + -osis) Abnormal thinning of bone tissue due to calcium loss.

Oxidation \͵äksə'dāshən\ Process of cell metabolism resulting in release of energy; involves reactions in which hydrogen atoms are removed from a molecule of substance (oxidation) and transferred to the acceptor molecule (reduction).

Palliative care \'palē͵ād·iv 'ke(ə)r\ (L. *palliatus,* cloaked) Care that gives relief but no cure.

Pantothenic acid \͵pantə͵thenik 'asəd\ (Gr. *pantothen,* "from all sides" or "in every corner") A B vitamin found widely distributed in nature and occurring throughout the body tissues. Pantothenic acid is an essential constituent of the coenzyme A, which has extensive metabolic responsibility as an activating agent of a number of compounds in many tissues.

Paralytic ileus \͵parə͵lid·ik 'ilēəs\ (Gr. *eileos,* from *eilein,* to roll up) Obstruction of the intestines, resulting from inhibition of bowel motility.

Parathyroid hormone (PH) \͵parə'thī͵róid 'hór͵mōn\ Hormone of the parathyroid gland, which controls calcium and phosphorus metabolism by stimulating the intestinal mucosa to increase calcium absorption, mobilizing calcium rapidly from bone, and causing renal excretion of phosphate.

Parenchyma \pə'reŋkəmə\ (Gr. "anything poured in bedside") Functional elements of an organ.

Parenteral \pər'entərəl\ Not through the alimentary canal; given by injection through a subcutaneous, intramuscular, intravenous, or other route.

Paresthesia \ˌpares'thēzh(ē)ə\ (Gr. *para,* beyond; *aisthesis,* perception) Abnormal sensations, such as prickling, burning, and "crawling" of skin.

Parietal cell \pə'riəd·ᵊl 'sel\ (L. *paries,* wall) Cell of the gastric glands in the fundus of the stomach that produces hydrochloric acid.

Parity \'parəd·ē\ (L. *parere,* to bring forth) (1) Number of children born alive. (2) System of regulating prices of farm commodities, usually by government price supports, to provide farmers with the same purchasing power they had in a selected base period.

Paroxysmal \ˌparəkˈsizməl\ Recurring in paroxysms.

Pedal edema \'pedᵊl ə'dēmə\ Edema in the feet.

Pellagra \pə'lāgrə\ (L. *pelle,* skin; Gr. *agra,* seizure) A deficiency disease caused by a lack of niacin in the diet and an inadequate amount of protein containing the amino acid, tryptophan, a precursor of niacin. Pellagra is characterized by skin lesions that are aggravated by exposure to sunlight and by gastrointestinal, mucosal, neurologic, and mental symptoms. Four *Ds* often associated with pellagra are dermatitis, diarrhea, dementia, and death.

Pepsin \'pepsən\ The main gastric enzyme specific for proteins. Pepsin begins breaking large protein molecules into shorter chain polypeptides, proteoses, and peptones. Gastric hydrochloric acid is necessary to activate pepsin.

Peptide linkage \'pep,tīd 'liŋkij\ The characteristic joining of amino acids to form proteins. Such a chain of amino acids is termed a peptide. Depending on its size, it may be a dipeptide fragment of protein digestion or a large polypeptide.

Periodontal disease \ˌperēōˈdäntᵊl də'zēz\ Disease, such as inflammation, occurring in tissue surrounding the teeth; facilitates tooth loss.

Peristalsis \'perə'stȯlsəs\ (Gr. *peri-,* around; *stalsis,* contraction) Coordinated action of circular and longitudinal muscles of the intestine that produces wavelike motions and propels the food mass forward.

Pernicious anemia \pə(r)'nishəs ə'nēmēə\ A chronic, macrocytic anemia occurring most commonly in whites after age 40. It is caused by the absence of the intrinsic factor normally present in gastric juice and necessary for the absorption of cobalamin (vitamin B_{12}). Pernicious anemia is controlled by intramuscular injections of cobalamin.

Peroral \pər·'ōrəl\ (L. *per,* through; *oris,* mouth) Performed or administered through the mouth.

Petechiae \pə'tēkēə\ Pinpoint hemorrhages.

pH Symbol used in chemistry to express the degree of acidity or alkalinity (the concentration of H^+) of a solution. It is mathematically based on the negative logarithm expressed as an exponential power (pH = *p*ower of *H*ydrogen ion concentration). Therefore the acidity of a solution varies inversely with the figure expressing it—the smaller the pH number, the greater the degree of acidity. A neutral solution (pure water) has a pH of 7.0. Solutions with a lower pH are acid; those with a higher pH are alkaline. The blood buffer system maintains the blood at a pH of 7.4.

Phagocytes Cells that ingest microorganisms, other cells, or foreign particles; macrophages.

Phlebothrombosis \ˌflebōthräm'bōsəs\ Presence of a clot in a vein.

Phospholipid \ˌfäsfō'lipəd\ Any of a class of fat-related substances that contain phosphorus, fatty acids, and a nitrogenous base. The phospholipids are essential elements in every cell.

Phosphorylation \ˌfäsˌfȯrə'lāshən\ Combining of glucose with a phosphoric acid radical to produce glucose-6-phosphate as a first step in the cellular oxidation of glucose to produce energy. This reaction is catalyzed by the enzyme glucokinase, the specific hexokinase for this purpose.

Photosynthesis \ˌfōd·ō'sin(t)thəsəs\ (Gr. *photos,* light; *synthesis,* putting together) process by which plants containing chlorophyll are able to manufacture carbohydrate by combining carbon dioxide from the air and water from the soil. Sunlight is used as energy, and chlorophyll is a catalyst. The basic chemical reaction is:

$$6CO_2 + 6H_2O \rightarrow C_6H_{12}O_6 + 6O_2$$

Pinocytosis \ˌpinōsīdōsəs\ (Gr. *pinein,* to drink; *kytos,* cell) Absorption of both fluid and large molecules (products of digestion, such as fat substances) by engulfing them directly into the cell cytoplasm.

Placenta \plə'sentə\ (L. a flat cake) Tissue that becomes active during pregnancy, providing a selective exchange of soluble particles in the blood to and from the fetus.

Plaque \'plak\ Patch or flat area forming on tissue; in coronary heart disease, a buildup of fat and other tissue debris in the inside lining of blood vessels.

Plummer-Vinson syndrome \ˌpləmə(r) ˌvin(t)sən 'sin,drōm\ Difficulty in swallowing.

Polycythemia \ˌpälēˌsī'thēmēə\ Condition characterized by an excess of red blood cells with a high concentration of hemoglobin. May be caused by an excess of cobalt (the core of vitamin B_{12}), an essential factor in red blood cell formation.

Polysaccharide \ˌpälē'sakə,rīd\ Class of complex carbohydrates composed of many monosaccharide units. The common members are starch, dextrins, dietary fiber, and glycogen.

Polyunsaturated \ˌpälēˌən'sachə,rātəd\ Carbon chain containing more than one double bond.

Portal \'pōr|d·ᵊl\ An entryway, usually referring to the portal circulation of blood through the liver. Blood is brought into the liver by the portal vein and out by the hepatic vein.

Postprandial \(ˈ)pōst'prandēəl\ Occurring after dinner or after a meal.

Poverty \'pävə(r)d·ē\ Having little or no money, goods, or means of support; scantiness, insufficiency; meagerness. The 1981 federal government definition of the poverty level was an annual income of less than $9287 for a family of four.

Precipitate \prē'sipə,tāt\ (L. *praecipitare,* to cast down) Solid separated out from a solution or suspension.

Precursor \prē'kərsər\ (L. *praecursor*, a forerunner) Something that precedes; in biology, a substance from which another substance is derived.

Preicteric \prēik¦'terik\ Phase of hepatic disease before jaundice (icterus) appears.

Primary deficiency disease \'prīmerē də'fishənsē də'zēz\ Disease that results directly from dietary lack of a specific essential nutrient. For example, scurvy results if the diet is deficient in vitamin C; beriberi results if the diet is deficient in thiamin.

Primigravida \¦prīmə'gravədə\ (L. *prima*, first; *gravida*, pregnant) A woman pregnant for the first time.

Proenzyme \(')prō'en͵zīm\ An inactive precursor converted to the active enzyme by the action of an acid, another enzyme, or other means. Also called zymogen.

Prostaglandin \͵prästə'glandən\ A group of naturally occurring long-chain fatty acids having local hormonelike actions of widely diverse forms.

Protein-bound iodine (PBI) test \'prō͵tēn 'baünd 'īə͵dīn 'test\ Test used to measure thyroid activity by determining the amount of iodine bound to thyroxine and in transit in the plasma.

Protein-energy malnutrition \prō͵tēn 'enə(r)jē (')maln(y)ü·'trishən\ A state of malnutrition caused by a deficiency of both protein and kilocalories as compared with a protein deficiency in the presence of adequate kilocalories.

Proteinuria \͵prō͵tē'n(y)ůrēə\ Presence of abnormally high levels of serum protein in the urine.

Prothrombin \(')prō'thrämbən\ (Gr. *pro*, before; *thrombos*, a clot) A protein (globulin) circulating in the plasma, essential to the clotting of blood. Prothrombin is produced by the liver. The process requires the presence of vitamin K.

P/S ratio \P/S 'rā͵shō\ Ratio of polyunsaturated to saturated fat (fatty acids) in a diet.

Puerperium \͵pyüə(r)'pirēəm\ The period of "confinement" after labor.

Pulmonary edema \'půlmə͵nerē ə'dēmə\ Fluid accumulation in the lungs.

Purpura \'pərpyərə\ (L. "purple") Hemorrhaging into the skin producing the reddish purple discoloration of a bruise.

Pyridoxine (vitamin B₆) \͵pirə'däk͵sēn\ In its active phosphate form (B₆-PO₄), pyridoxine functions as an important coenzyme in many reactions in the metabolism of amino acids and to a lesser extent in the metabolism of glucose and fatty acids. Clinically, pyridoxine deficiency produces a hypochromic, microcytic anemia and disturbances of the central nervous system.

Pyrosis \pī'rōsəs\ (Gr. burning) Heartburn.

Pyruvate \pī'rü͵vāt\ Metabolic end product of glycolysis, which may then be converted to lactate or acetyl CoA.

Radiation \͵rādē'āshən\ (L. *radiatio*) Electromagnetic phenomena that has properties combining both wave and particle functions; spans the entire spectrum from low-frequency radio waves through white light to high-frequency gamma rays.

Radioactive ¹³¹I uptake tests \¦rādē(͵)ō'aktiv 'əptāk 'test\ Tests of thyroid function using a radioactive isotope of iodine, ¹³¹I.

Renin \'rēnən\ This word is often mispronounced 'renən. (It may then be confused with *rennin*, an enzyme from a calf's stomach used to sour milk to make cheese or puddings.) Enzyme formed in the renal cortex. In response to blood pressure changes, it is secreted to act on its specific substrate, angiotensinogen, to form angiotensin I and II.

Rennin \'renən\ Milk-curdling enzyme of the gastric juice found in human infants and in young animals such as calves. Do not confuse with *renin*, an important enzyme produced by the kidney that plays a vital role in producing angiotensin, a potent vasoconstrictor and stimulant for release of the hormone aldosterone from the adjacent adrenal glands.

Retinol-binding protein (RBP) \'retᵊnəl 'bīndiŋ 'prō͵tēn\ The protein carrier for vitamin A.

Retinol equivalent (RE) \'retᵊnəl ə'kwiv(ə)lənt\ Measure of vitamin A activity currently adopted by FAO/WHO and U.S. National Research Council's Food and Nutrition Board recommendations for vitamin A, replacing the term IU (international units). The measure accounts for dietary variances in preformed vitamin A (retinol) and its precursor, carotene. One RE (retinol equivalent) equals 3.33 IU or 1 μg retinol.

Retinopathy \͵retᵊn'äpəthē\ (L. *retina;* Gr. *pathos*, disease) Noninflammatory disease of the retina. In diabetes it is characterized by small hemorrhages from broken arteries, yellow waxy discharge, and retinal detachment.

Riboflavin (vitamin B₂) \͵ribə'flāvən\ A yellow-green pigment that contains ribose. Vitamin B₂ is found in milk as lactoflavin and also in leafy green vegetables and organ meats. Riboflavin forms coenzymes (FMN and FAD) important in the metabolism of amino acids, glucose, and fatty acids.

Salmonellosis \͵salmə͵ne'lōsəs\ Infection caused by *Salmonella* (a genus of microbes), characterized by violent diarrhea, abdominal cramps, painful straining on defecation (tenesmus), and fever.

Saponification \sə͵pänə͵fə'kāshən\ (L. *sapo*, soap; *facere*, to make) Hydrolysis of fats by alkali to produce soaps.

Sarcoma \sär'kōmə\ (Gr. *sarkoma*, fleshy growth) Tumor, usually malignant, arising from connective tissue.

Satiety \sə'tīəd·ē\ (L. *satis*, sufficient + *-ety*, state or condition) A feeling of fullness or satisfaction as after a meal or quenching one's thirst.

Saturate \'sach(ə)rət\ (L. *saturare*, to fill) To cause to unite with the greatest possible amount of another substance through solution, chemical combination, or the like. A saturated fat, for example, is one in which the component fatty acids are filled with hydrogen atoms. A fatty acid is said to be saturated if all available chemical bonds of its carbon chain are filled with hydrogen. If one bond remains unfilled, it is a monounsaturated fatty acid. If two or more bonds remain unfilled, it is a polyunsaturated fatty acid. Fats of animal sources are more saturated. Fats of plant sources are unsaturated.

Scoliosis \͵skōlē'ōsəs\ (Ger. *skoliosis*, curvature) Lateral curvature of the spine.

Scurvy \'skərvē\ A hemorrhagic disease caused by lack of vitamin C. Diffuse tissue bleeding occurs, limbs and joints are painful and swollen, bones thicken due to subperiosteal hemorrhage, ecchymoses (large irregular discolored skin areas due to tissue hemorrhages) form, bones fracture easily, wounds do not heal well, gums are swollen and bleeding, and teeth loosen.

Sebaceous \sə̇bāshəs\ Secreting the fatty lubricating substance sebum.

Seborrheic dermatitis \ˌsebə̇ˈrēik ˌdərmə̇ˈtīd·ə̇s\ Reddened skin covered with small, greasy flakes. Hard sebaceous plugs may project from pores on the nose, cheeks, or forehead.

Secondary deficiency disease \ˈsekən̩ˌderē də̇ˈfishən̩sē də̇ˈzēz\ Disease that results from the inability of the body to use a specific nutrient properly. Such inability may result from either of two general types of failure: (1) failure to absorb the nutrient from the alimentary tract into the blood or (2) failure to metabolize the nutrient normally after it has been absorbed. For example, the malabsorption syndrome is characterized by failure of absorption of fats through the intestinal wall, so that fat is lost in the stool. Phenylketonuria is the inability of the body to metabolize the essential amino acid phenylalanine, so that phenylalanine is lost in the urine.

Secretin \sə̇ˈkrēd·ə̇n\ Hormone produced in the mucous membrane of the duodenum in response to the entrance of the acid contents of the stomach into the duodenum. Secretin in turn stimulates the flow of pancreatic juice, providing needed enzymes and the proper alkalinity for their action.

Sepsis \ˈsepsə̇s\ (Gr. *sepsis*, decay) Presence in the blood or other tissues of pathogenic microorganisms or their toxins; the condition associated with such presence.

Serotonin \ˌsirə̇ˈtōnə̇n\ (L. *sero-*, serum; *tonos*, normal degree of muscle tension) Vasoconstrictor, central neurotransmitter; produced enzymatically from tryptophan.

Solute \ˈsälˌyüt\ Dissolved substance; particles in solution.

Somatostatin \ˌsōmə̇d·ə̇ˈstatˀn\ (Gr. *somatos*, body; *statin*) Hormone produced by the D cells of the islets of Langerhans and the hypothalamus. It inhibits insulin and glucagon production in the pancreas as needed to maintain normal blood glucose levels.

Spinal cord injury \ˈspīnˀl ˈkȯ(ə)rd ˈinj(ə)rē\ Partial or complete severing of the spinal cord caused by trauma. Partial severance results in general muscle weakness and sensory motor loss. Complete severance results in total paralysis of muscles that are controlled by nerves leaving the spinal cord *below* the level of injury, especially in paraplegia or quadriplegia.

Splanchnic \ˈsplaŋknik\ (Gr. *splanchnikos;* L. *splanchnicus*) Pertaining to the large interior organs of the body, especially those located in the abdomen.

Sprue \ˈsprü\ Alternate term for adult celiac disease, a malabsorption syndrome.

Steatorrhea \stēəd·ə̇ˈrēə\ (Gr. *steatos*, fat; *rhoia*, flow) Excessive fat amounts in the feces; often caused by malabsorption syndromes.

Stenosis \stə̇ˈnōsə̇s\ Narrowing or closing of a canal or duct.

Steroid \ˈsti(ə)ˌrȯid\ Any of a large group of fat-related organic compounds, including sterols, bile acids, sex hormones, hormones of the adrenal cortex, and D vitamins.

Stomatitis \ˌstomə̇ˈtīd·ə̇s\ (Gr. *stoma*, mouth; -itis) Inflammation of the oral mucosa.

Stria \ˈstrīə\ (*pl.* striae) (L. furrow, groove) Streaks or lines on stretched skin caused by weakening of the elastic tissue by constant tension.

Stricture \ˈstrikchə(r)\ Constriction, as in the gastrointestinal tract, that causes a partial or complete obstruction.

Struvite stone \ˈstrüˌvīt ˈstōn\ Urinary stone made up of ammonium magnesium phosphate, a very hard crystal.

Substance P \ˈsəbztən(t)s P\ Peptide composed of 11 amino acids; contracts the intestine and dilates blood vessels; may be a neurotransmitter that helps send pain impulses.

Substrate \ˈsəbzˌtrāt\ (L. *sub*, under *stratum*, layer) The specific organic substance on which a particular enzyme acts.

Sucrose polyester (SPE) \ˈsüˌkrōs ˈpälēˌestə(r)\ "Artificial" fat, manufactured by substitution of sucrose for glycerol in the fat molecule, and thus not usable as fat by the body.

Sulfhydryl group \ˌsəlfˈhīdrə̇l ˈgrüp\ The —SH radical that forms high-energy sulfur bonds in chemical compounds. In such compounds sulfur participates in important tissue respiration (oxidation) reactions.

Syncope \ˈsiŋkə̇(ˌ)pē\ Brief loss of consciousness associated with, among other things, reduced levels of extracellular fluid, as occurs during uncontrolled diarrhea.

Syncytium \sə̇nˈsish(ē)əm\ Mass of protoplasm that results when cells merge.

Synergism \ˈsinərˌjizəm\ (Gr. *syn*, with or together; *ergon*, work) The joint action of separate agents in which the total effect of their combined action is greater than the sum of their separate actions.

Synthesis \ˈsin(t)thəsə̇s\ (Gr. *syn-*, with, together; *thesis*, a stated idea or proposition; hence "a putting together") Study of phenomena or development of concepts or substances by putting together the parts to make a whole.

Systolic \sə̇ˈstälik\ (Gr. *systole*, contraction) Referring to the heart's period of contraction.

Tachycardia \ˌtakə̇ˈkärdēə\ Rapid heart rate above normal.

Tetany \ˈtet(ˀ)nē\ Disorder caused by abnormal calcium metabolism. Characterized by severe, intermittent, tonic contractions of the extremities and muscular pain caused by lowered blood calcium levels.

Thiamin (vitamin B₁) \thīˈamən\ A major B vitamin; essential for the normal metabolism of carbohydrates and fats. It acts as a coenzyme (TPP and TDP) in key reactions.

Thiamin pyrophosphate (TPP) \thīˈamən ˌpīrōˈfäˌsfāt\ Activating coenzyme form of thiamin; plays a key role in carbohydrate metabolism.

Thrombosis \thrämˈbōsə̇s\ Development of a blood clot (thrombus) that lodges in a blood vessel and cuts off the blood supply at that point.

Thyroid-stimulating hormone (TSH) \ˈthīˌrȯid ˈstimyəlātiŋ ˈhȯrˌmōn\ Hormone secreted by the anterior pituitary gland that regulates uptake of iodine and synthesis of thyroxine by the thyroid gland.

Thyroxine \thīˈräkˌsēn\ The iodine-containing hormone produced by the thyroid gland.

Tocopherol \tə̇ˈkäfəˌrȯl\ (Gr. *tokos*, childbirth; *pherein*, to bring) Vitamin E; so named because of its association with reproduction in rats.

Total parenteral nutrition (TPN) \'tōd·ᵊl 'pa(a)rənteral n(y)ü·
ˌtrishən\ Feeding of a nutritionally complete solution
through a large central vein (see Chapter 27).

Toxemia \täk'sēmēə\ Formerly used term (current official
term of American College of Obstetricians and Gynecologists is pregnancy-induced hypertension—PIH); a metabolic disturbance that usually manifests itself in the third
trimester with symptoms of hypertension, abnormal
edema, and albuminemia. If uncontrolled, leads to a coma
or convulsions.

Trans \'tran(t)s\ (L., through) Having certain atoms or radicals
in a chemical structure on opposite sides.

Transamination \(ˌ)tran(t)sˌamə'nāshən\ Transfer of the
amino group (NH₂) from an amino acid to a carbon residue
to form another amino acid. The newly formed compound is
classed a nonessential amino acid, since the body can synthesize it and does not depend on the diet to supply it.

Transcobalamin I \ˌtranz'kōbōləˌmēn\ Cobalamin-bind-
ing protein carrier for transport in bloodstream.

Transferrin \tranz'ferən\ An iron-binding protein complex,
a serum beta-globulin; the transport form of iron in the
body.

Transketolation \tranz'kēdolāshən\ Transfer of the first unit
two-carbon group from one sugar to another in glucose
oxidation.

Transmangamin \tranz'maŋgəmən\ Manganese transport
carrier, a compound with a plasma protein beta-
globulin.

Transmural \tranz'myùrəl\ (L. *trans,* across, through; *mur-
alis,* from *murus,* wall) Through the wall of an organ; extending through or affecting the entire thickness of the
wall of an organ or cavity.

Transpyloric \tranz'pīlȯrik\ Passing through the distal opening of the stomach.

Triglyceride \(')trī'glisəˌrīd\ A compound of 3 fatty acids es-
terified to glycerol. A neutral fat, synthesized from carbohydrate, stored in adipose tissue. It releases free fatty acids
into the blood on being hydrolyzed by enzymes.

Trophoblast \'träfəˌblast\ (Gr. *trope,* nutrition; *blastos,* germ)
Ectodermal tissue that attaches the ovum to the wall of the
uterus and supplies nutrients to the embryo.

Trypsin \'tripsən\ A protein-splitting (proteolytic) enzyme secreted by the pancreas that acts in the small intestine to
reduce proteins to shorter chain polypeptides and dipeptides.

Ultrasound \ˌəltrə'saùnd\ Sound waves at a frequency above
that which can be heard by the human ear (20 kilocycles/
second); in controlled doses can be used as a therapeutic
or diagnostic tool, such as to determine skinfold thickness.

Uremia \yə'rēmēə\ (Gr. *ouron,* urine; *haima,* blood) Presence
in the blood of large amounts of by-products of protein
metabolism; caused by impaired nephron function leading
to the inability to excrete urea and other products. This is
a toxic condition characterized by headache, nausea, vomiting, diminished vision, convulsions, or coma.

Vagotomy \vā'gäd·ə_mē\ (L. *vagus,* wandering; Gr. *tome,* a
cutting) Interruption of the impulses carried by the vagus
nerve(s), resulting in prevention of increased flow or acidity of gastric secretions.

Valence \'vālən(t)s\ (L. *valens,* powerful) Power of an element or a radical to combine with or to replace other elements or radicals. Atoms of various elements combine in
definite proportions. The valence number of an element is
the number of atoms of hydrogen with which one atom of
the element can combine.

Varices \'va(a)rəˌsēz\ Enlarged veins.

Vasoactive \ˌvā(ˌ)zōaktiv\ (L. *vas,* vessel) Having an effect on
the diameter of blood vessels.

Vasopressin (ADH) \ˌvāzō'presᵊn\ Hormone secreted by the
anterior pituitary gland in response to body stress, which acts
primarily on the distal renal tubule, causing the reabsorption
of water. The result is diminished urinary output, thus the
term antidiuretic hormone (ADH).

Very low–density lipoprotein (VLDL) \'verē 'lō 'den(t)səd·
ē ˌlipə'prō,tēn\ Name derived from its position in electrophoresis, a method of analyzing lipoprotein fractions in
the blood.

Villikinin \'viləkinən\ Hormone produced by glands in the
upper intestinal mucosa in response to presence of chyme
entering the intestine. Villikinin stimulates alternating
contractions and extensions of the villi. This motion of the
villi constantly agitates the mucosal surface, which stirs
and mixes the chyme and exposes additional nutrient material for absorption.

Villous adenoma \'viləs ˌadᵊn'ōmə\ (L. *villus,* "tuft of hair";
Gr. *adenos,* gland; -oma) Soft, large protrusion on the mucosa of the large intestine.

Villus \'viləs\ (*pl.* villi) (L. *villus,* "tuft of hair") Small protrusions from the surface of a membrane.

Volition \vō 'lishən\ Deliberate action.

Wilson's disease \'wilsənz də'zēz\ Rare hereditary disease in
which large amounts of copper are absorbed by and accumulate in the liver, brain, kidneys, and cornea. Produces
degenerative changes in brain and liver tissue.

Xanthoma \zan'thōmə\ (Gr. *xanthos,* yellow) Fatty, yellowish
colored plaque deposit in the skin.

Xerophthalmia \ˌziˌräf'thalmēə\ (Gr. *xeros,* dry; *ophthalmos,*
eye) A disease of the eye in which the cornea and conjunc-
tiva become dry.

Zwitterion \ˌtsvid·əˌrīən\ The term given to amino acids to
describe the capacity, when ionized in a solution, to behave
as either an acid or a base depending on the need of the
solution in which they are present. This dual nature makes
amino acids good buffer substances.

Zygote \'zīˌgōt\ (Gr. *zygotos,* yoked together) Fertilized ovum;
the single cell before the division process starts.

Index

Median Heights and Weights and Recommended Energy Intake

Category	Age (years) or Condition	Weight (kg)	Weight (lb)	Height (cm)	Height (in)	FEE[a] (kcal/day)	Multiples of REE	Average Energy Allowance (kcal)[b] Per kg	Average Energy Allowance (kcal)[b] Per day[c]
Infants	0.0–0.5	6	13	60	24	320		108	650
	0.5–1.0	9	20	71	28	500		98	850
Children	1–3	13	29	90	35	740		102	1,300
	4–6	20	44	112	44	950		90	1,800
	7–10	28	62	132	52	1,130		70	2,000
Males	11–14	45	99	157	62	1,440	1.70	55	2,500
	15–18	66	145	176	69	1,760	1.67	45	3,000
	19–24	72	160	177	70	1,780	1.67	40	2,900
	25–50	79	174	176	70	1,800	1.60	37	2,900
	51+	77	170	173	68	1,530	1.50	30	2,300
Females	11–14	46	101	157	62	1,310	1.67	47	2,200
	15–18	55	120	163	64	1,370	1.60	40	2,200
	19–24	58	128	164	65	1,350	1.60	38	2,200
	25–50	63	138	163	64	1,380	1.55	36	2,200
	51+	65	143	160	63	1,280	1.50	30	1,900
Pregnant	1st Trimester								+0
	2nd Trimester								+300
	3rd Trimester								+300
Lactating	1st 6 months								+500
	2nd 6 months								+500

[a] Resting energy expenditure (REE); calculation based on FAO equations, then rounded.

[b] In the range of light to moderate activity, the coefficient of variation is ±20%.

[c] Figure is rounded.